The Spinal Cord
Injured Patient

The Spinal Cord Injured Patient

SECOND EDITION

Edited by

Bok Y. Lee, MD, FACS
Professor of Surgery
New York Medical College
Valhalla, New York

Director of Surgical Research
Sound Shore Medical Center
New Rochelle, New York

Adjunct Professor
Rensselaer Polytechnic Institute
Troy, New York

and

Lee E. Ostrander, PhD
Associate Professor
Biomedical Engineering Department
Rensselaer Polytechnic Institute
Troy, New York

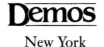

New York

Demos Medical Publishing, Inc., 386 Park Avenue South, New York, New York 10016

Library of Congress Cataloging-in-Publication Data
The spinal cord injured patient / edited by Bok Y. Lee and Lee E. Ostrander. — 2nd ed.
    p. cm.
  Includes bibliographical references and index.
  ISBN 1-888799-51-X (alk. paper)
    1. Spinal cord—Wounds and injuries—Treatment. 2. Spinal cord—Wounds and injuries—Patients—Rehabilitation. I. Lee, Bok Y., 1928– II. Ostrander, Lee E.
RD594.3 .S6656 2001
617.4'82044—cd21

                                                  2001028984

Made in the United States of America

Acknowledgments

We thank Diana M. Schneider, Ph.D., President and Publisher of Demos Medical Publishing, and Joan Wolk, Managing Editor, for their efforts in bringing this book to publication.

Contents

Preface

SPINAL CORD INJURY is a devastating physical, emotional, and socioeconomic event for an individual. It occurs in people of all ages and is one of the most complex and challenging areas of medical-surgical and rehabilitative management. Optimal treatment calls for the integration of a broad array of skills, a team effort, and incorporation of many diverse professional knowledge bases. Because professional participants in the care of spinal cord injured patients can best serve the patient's needs if they appreciate all aspects of treatment and support, this book covers the broad issues involved in providing this care.

This second edition updates and describes refinements in diagnosis and in acute and chronic care as well as advances in medical-surgical management and rehabilitation. All chapters are written by experts who are deeply involved with various aspects of spinal cord injury management.

The scope of this book includes diagnostic methods, evaluation methods, spinal cord injury pathophysiology, medical-surgical management and rehabilitation, and issues of specialized care. Topics include the role of electrical stimulation, the management of neurogenic dysfunction of the bladder, surgical management of the upper limb in tetraplegia, pressure ulcer management, and experimental model and prevention of spinal cord ischemic injury. Of special interest are the discussions of hand reconstruction essential to functional use following spinal cord injury, hemodynamic monitoring that incorporates automated patient profiling, and noninvasive assessment and prevention of deep vein thrombosis and pulmonary embolism using external pneumatic compression. Specialized research aspects that are covered include the effective use of omentum, which may improve the spinal cord blood supply and which is transposed to the spinal cord, and the preservation of nutritional status in improving the prognosis in spinal cord injured patients.

Although no book can cover every aspect of so complex a field, this volume does provide a broad array of advice and suggestions. It is a compendium of otherwise difficult to assemble knowledge replete with time-tested methods as well as new ideas, techniques, and concepts.

B.Y.L.
L.E.O.

The Spinal Cord Injured Patient

1 Immediate Management of the Spinal Cord Injured Patient

THOMAS T. LEE, MD
BARTH A. GREEN, MD, FACS

THE GOAL OF TREATMENT of spinal cord injury (SCI) is to preserve residual neurologic function and aid recovery, stabilize hemodynamic and pulmonary function, and restore spinal alignment and stability. The future of the treatment of SCI patients may involve combination protocol utilizing neurotrophic factors, nerve grafting, and other innovative techniques, but the present treatment protocols merely minimize secondary injury and allow natural recovery of the injured neural tissues. This chapter addresses the many problems unique to the immediate management of a spinal cord injured patient.

ACUTE MANAGEMENT OF SPINAL CORD INJURY

All patients sustaining major blunt trauma must be presumed to have am SCI until proven otherwise. Any motor or sensory signs, pain, incontinence, or external sign of trauma especially should alert the medical personnel of the possibility of spine fracture and SCI. Complaint of focal axial spinal pain should alert the evaluating physician of a possible spinal injury. A cervical collar in combination with a rigid spine backboard should be utilized to immobilize the entire spine and to expedite transport to the emergency department. Continuous movement of an injured spinal cord may cause further neu-

rologic deterioration (1,2). The same guidelines should be implemented in patients with altered mental status, in whom an adequate neurologic assessment is not possible.

The initial emergency department evaluation of SCI should proceed in an orderly fashion. Significant head injuries, as well as systemic trauma, can be associated with spinal cord injuries (3–5). For example, the high velocity required to cause a thoracic fracture frequently leads to thoracic trauma such as rib fractures, pneumothorax, hemothorax, pulmonary contusion, cardiac contusion, and at times, aortic shearing injury. Spinal shock and respiratory muscle failure should be considered in patients with cervical or high thoracic injuries, which can cause a sympathectomy syndrome consisting of hypotension and bradycardia because of unopposed vagal tone. This must be distinguished from a hemorrhagic shock from other etiologies. Fluid support, appropriate hemodynamic monitoring, which includes a pulmonary artery catheter and arterial line, and pressors may be necessary. A baseline full neurologic examination should then be performed. Once the patient is stabilized and the neurologic status is assessed from the hemodynamic and respiratory standpoints, radiographic evaluation for the spine should be performed.

If the patient shows any sign of a SCI, the high-dose methylprednisolone protocol outlined by parts II and III of the National Spinal Cord Injury Study (NASCIS II & III) is recommended (5). The loading dose can be given within 8 hours of the injury; 30 mg/kg of methylprednisolone is given as slow bolus in the first hour, followed by a 5.4 mg/kg/hr hourly infusion for 23 hours. The NASCIS III protocol advocates 48 hours of methylprednisolone if the loading dose of the methylprednisolone is given between 3 and 8 hours after the initial trauma. Appropriate gastritis/ulcer prophylaxis should be given (6). In NASCIS II, the benefit of high-dose steroid was observed in incomplete SCI, but complete motor injury with or without sensory sparing did not show major improvement. This study, however, excluded patients who subsequently underwent decompression and stabilization. The benefit of the steroid must be weighed against the possible complication of infection and gastrointestinal hemorrhage. NASCIS III demonstrated 48 hours of steroid treatment to be associated with higher motor recovery, but the incidence of sepsis and pneumonia was correspondingly higher. In general, no steroid is infused in cases of penetrating missiles through the abdominal cavity, because contamination by bowel bacterial flora is possible.

CERVICAL TRACTION

The authors generally do not place patients under cervical traction until appropriate radiographic studies are obtained in the emergency department (Fig. 1-1). A significant risk of increasing neurologic deficits exists, especially in young patients with distraction-type injury and ligamentous laxity and patients with ankylosing spondylitis (7). Overdistraction and increased spinal deformity are definite considerations in these patients. When there is obvious cervical fracture or dislocation on plain cervical radiographs, traction with a magnetic resonance imaging (MRI)-compatible Gardner Wells tong is applied, and 5 pounds per interspace of total traction is initiated. For example, a C4 fracture would start with 20 pounds of traction, unless gross distraction is seen on radiographs. The same amount of traction is applied

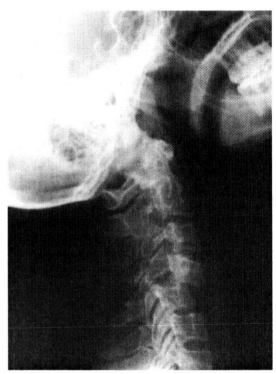

FIGURE 1-1. Cervical spine radiograph of a bilateral locked facet. Note that C7–T1 junction is well-visualized. Surgical intervention was eventually needed to reduce the subluxation, after traction and manual reduction attempts failed.

for patients without clear fracture or malalignment but presenting with a definite cervical level of injury. Posttraction plain radiographs are obtained to ascertain the realignment and to check for overdistraction. The amount of traction can be increased to 10 pounds per vertebral segment. When possible, care also should be taken to avoid traction in patients with ankylosing spondylitis because further fracture and distraction of the vertebral column are likely. These patients may spontaneously reduce the fracture in a cervical collar or under minimal traction and manipulation.

If reduction cannot be achieved, the patient is fiberoptically intubated with minimal neck manipulation. After benzodiazepine and muscle relaxants are administered, manual reduction and realignment under fluoroscopy is attempted. The manual reduction should be performed, taking into consideration the mechanism of injury (i.e., rotation, flexion, etc.). From the authors' experience, the absolute majority of the patients could be reduced by these means, and generally no acute surgical realignment and stabilization are needed. After adequate reduction is achieved, the weight of traction should be reduced to half that used to achieve reduction. To minimize unwanted motion, the patient is maintained in a cervical collar under traction on a Rotorest treatment table.

After cervical fracture reduction and other spine plain films, computed tomography (CT) can be utilized to image areas poorly visualized or suspected injury on the plain film and to identify any other fractures. Up to 2 percent of cervical fractures can be missed on a complete series of cervical spine radiographs, in addition to a 28 percent false-positive rate (8). The utilization of an MRI-compatible traction device alalows an MRI to be performed, if no other contraindication exists.

In the rare instance where manual reduction under general anesthesia and fluoroscopy cannot be achieved, surgical reduction and stabilization should be performed. Most often this is done with a posterior approach to unlock the facet joints, and a concurrent posterior fusion can be performed.

RADIOGRAPHIC EVALUATION

In suspected or known spinal trauma, plain anteroposterior (AP) and lateral radiographs of the cervical, thoracic, and lumbar spines should all be obtained. The cervical spine radiographs should include open-mouth odontoid views, if possible. The cervical–thoracic junction must be visualized, with swimmer's view if necessary. If adequate lateral images through the lower cervical spine cannot be obtained, an axial CT scan with sagittal reconstruction may be obtained to further delineate the regional anatomy.

If a fracture is identified on plain radiographs, or if uncertainty of the anatomy exists, thin-cut CT images through the level of question should be obtained to fully evaluate the bony anatomy. With focal neurological deficit or pain syn-

drome, magnetic resonance imaging (MRI) should be performed. The advantages of MRI are its ability to evaluate soft tissue and neural tissue pathology and its capability of multiplanar imaging. The disadvantages of MRI include relatively long scanning time and poor visualization of bony injury. CT scan with myelogram may be used instead if an MRI is indicated but not obtainable.

Acute dynamic lateral radiographs are generally not very helpful or advisable. Owing to the severe paraspinal muscle spasm associated with a spinal injury, flexion-extension radiographs shortly after an injury may not demonstrate instability. Short-term immobilization and follow-up radiographs, including dynamic lateral radiographs, should be obtained in patients with persistent axial spine pain or new-onset neurologic deficit.

MEDICAL MANAGEMENT OF ACUTE SPINAL CORD INJURED PATIENTS

Multisystem problems are frequently associated with a vertebral fracture or SCI. Some are related to the systemic effect of SCI, and others are related to paralysis and prolonged immobilization.

Cardiovascular Management

Neurogenic shock must be recognized and remedied early in the course after a SCI (9). This usually occurs after a cervical or upper thoracic injury, which interrupts the thoracic sympathetic outflow. The combination of hypotension and bradycardia may cause secondary neurologic injury, as well as pulmonary, renal, and cerebral insults. Such an impact is especially important in patients who sustain multisystem trauma.

A baseline electrocardiogram (EKG) and serum cardiac enzyme profile are taken upon admission for patients over the age of 40 or patients with a cardiac history. A central venous catheter may be inserted for fluid status monitoring, fluid resuscitation, and possible pressor infusion. In a patient with unstable hemodynamic parameters, an arterial line is useful for continuous blood pressure monitoring and blood sample collection. In general, asymptomatic bradycardia is not treated because it tends to recover after the acute injury. Symptomatic bradycardia is treated with intravenous (IV) atropine (0.5–1.0 mg) as necessary. Because of the aforementioned secondary effect of hypotension, a pressor is used to sustain adequate perfusion pressure. Dopamine is generally the drug of choice, unless significant side effects prevent its further usage. (In such cases dobutamine is used.) The dosing starts in the renal dose range (3–5 μg/kg/hr) and is titrated up to the cardiac dose (>10 μg/kg/hr) as necessary.

High-velocity chest injuries leading to thoracic spine fracture may be associated with cardiac contusion and possible tamponade. An echocardiogram can generally diagnose such an occurrence. An echocardiogram can also rule out contractile dysfunction. Specific use of an inotropic agent for cardiac contusion and appropriate hemodynamic monitoring, as mentioned above, should be implemented.

Pulmonary Management

Pulmonary complications are the most common problems faced by an acute SCI patient. The problem is most severe in patients sustaining mid- to upper-cervical SCI because the output to the phrenic nerve (C3–5) is impaired. These patients generally require careful awake fiberoptic intubation to maintain cervical alignment, avoidance of neck hyperextension, and the provision of subsequent ventilatory support. A lateral cervical radiograph should be obtained to reassess cervical alignment after manipulation, including after intubation. Because of the inability of these patients to effectively expand lung volume and clear airway secretions, pulmonary atelectasis and bronchiopulmonary infection ensue. Mucus plugging is another potentially disastrous problem associated with inadequate ventilatory effort and secretion pooling. Acute respiratory failure with inability to ventilate is the usual presentation. Other concurrent pulmonary and thoracic trauma—for example, rib fracture, pulmonary contusion, pneumothorax, hemothorax, and aspiration—further compromise pulmonary function. The use of a halo vest may also diminish pulmonary function.

To aid secretion clearance, patients can be placed on Rotorest beds (Kinetic Concepts, San Antonio, Texas) and put on full rotation. Respiratory treatment with bronchodilator and intermittent positive pressure breathing (IPPB) or increased positive end-expiratory pressure (PEEP) may be necessary to reexpand lung volume. Supplemental oxygen is given to unintubated patients to maintain a pulse oximetry saturation of greater than 95 percent. Even with aggressive efforts, mucus plug formation may continue to be a problem. This requires aggressive suctioning, chest physiotherapy, and possible intubation for bronchoscopic evacuation of the mucus plug.

Thromboembolic Complications

Spinal cord injury patients are frequently immobilized for an extensive period of time. Such prolonged immobilization increases the incidence of deep venous thrombosis (DVT) and hence pulmonary embolism (PE). When lower extremity or pelvic fracture is also present, the risk of a PE is even higher.

Unless an absolute contraindication exists, both the low-dose subcutaneous heparin protocol (5000 U SQ bid) and lower extremity pneumatic compressive devices are used. These tools have been found to reduce the incidence of deep venous thrombosis and pulmonary embolism (10). Even with these preventive methods, DVT and PE occur frequently and should be considered when a patient presents with respiratory difficulty or when a low-grade fever persists despite successful treatment of other sources of fever.

Gastrointestinal/Nutritional Management

In acute SCI, many patients present with at least a partial ileus. A naso- or orogastric tube should be inserted initially to prevent gastric distension and possible perforation. Standard H2-antagonist or carafate is used as gastritis prophylaxis. These agents are employed because of the immediate stress created by the trauma, as well as the possibility of developing peptic ulcer disease while patients are receiving high-dose IV steroid. A spinal cord injured patient requires nutritional support of approximately 150 percent that of the basal caloric requirement, and inadequate nutritional support can lead to catabolic energy process, impaired wound healing, and immune response (11). Oral or enteric feeding is not always possible because of the decrease in GI motility. Early IV hyperalimentation, supplemented with lipid, should be started and switched over to tube feeding or supplemented diet as soon as the patient can tolerate PO intake.

Pancreatitis can occur, especially in cervical and high-thoracic cord injured patients, possibly because of the predominant visceral parasympathetic tone (12). The patient is followed with serial pancreatic enzymes to track recovery, while receiving IV hyperalimentation. Others have advocated enteric feeding through a feeding jejunostomy in these patients. Acalculous cholecystitis can occur, especially after prolonged GI immotility or when a patient has been on chronic central IV hyperalimentation. If this occurs, abdominal ultrasonography can aid the diagnosis. Cholecystectomy in a stable patient, and cholecystostomy in an unstable patient, should be performed. Bowel perforation and ischemic bowel disease should also be suspected under the appropriate clinical setting. It should be noted that not all the cardinal signs of an acute abdomen are present in a spinal cord injured patient.

Genitourinary Management

Many patients with SCI cannot void spontaneously and initially require insertion of a Foley catheter. This serves the dual purpose of bladder drainage and accurate urine output measurement. The existence of the indwelling catheter, even if temporary, may lead to a urinary tract infection. The authors generally remove the catheter when the patient is hemodynamically and neurologically stable. This is followed by a q 4- to 6-hour sterile in-and-out catheterization protocol. This tends to produce a lower incidence of infection rate but is associated with possible urethral injury.

Cutaneous and Musculoskeletal Management

Decubitus ulcers may occur from the time of injury if care is not taken to avoid prolonged pressure points. Subsequent immobilization can be even more hazardous. Both the skin and the underlying soft tissues may be involved. Constant position and pressure of greater than 1 to 2 hours can cause decubitus formation. This is further complicated by the fact that paralyzed patients may not feel the pressure on the dependent portion of their bodies. They are best treated by prevention. In the acute phase of SCI, the patient should be mobilized on a kinetic treatment bed or table to aid even distribution of weight and pressure (13,14). Subsequently, a frequent turning protocol should be instituted. Daily bathing, lotion application, and careful skin inspection should also be carried out. If superficial ulcers are detected early, daily sterile occlusive dressing can be applied to aid healing. Occasionally, chemical or surgical debridement and/or grafting may become necessary with deeper, infected, and poorly vascularized wounds.

CONCLUSION

Numerous secondary neurologic and systemic complications may occur in the face of SCI. The goal of immediate treatment is early spine immobilization and realignment, stabilization of hemodynamic and pulmonary status, prompt radiographic evaluation, and prevention of medical complications. These measures should optimize the chances for neurologic recovery.

REFERENCES

1. Green BA, Eismont FJ. Acute spinal cord injury: a systems approach. *Central Nerv Sys Trauma* 1984; 1(2):173–195.

2. Green BA , Eismont FJ, O'Heir JT. Pre-hospital management of spinal cord injuries. *Paraplegia* 1987; 25:229–238.

3. Eisenburg HM, Cayard C, Papancolaua FF. The effects of three potentially preventable complications on outcome after severe closed head injuy. In Ishar S, Nagai H, and Brock M, eds. *Intracranial Pressure*. 5th ed. Tokyo: Springer-Verlag, 1983.

4. Klauber MR, Toutant SM, Marshall LF. A model for predicting delayed intracranial hypertension following severe head injury. *J Neurosurg* 1984; 61:695–699.

5. Bracken MB, Shepard MJ, Collins WF, et al. A randomized, controlled trial of methyl-prenisolone or naloxone in the treatment of acute spinal-cord injury. Result of the Second National Acute Spinal Cord Injury Study. *N Engl J Med* 1990; 322:1405–1411.

6. Bracken MB, Shepard MJ, Holford TR, et al. Administration of methylprednisolone for 24 or 48 hours or tirilazad mesylate for 48 hours in the treatment of acute spinal cord injury. Results of the Third National Acute Spinal Cord Injury Randomized Controlled Trial. National Acute Spinal Cord Injury Study. *JAMA* 1997; 277(20): 1597–604.

7. Green BA, David C, Falcone S, Razack N, Klose KJ. Spinal cord injuries in adults. In Youmans JR, ed. *Neurological Surgery*. 4th ed. Philadelphia: W.B. Saunders, 1996.

8. Borock EC, Gabram SG, Jacobs LM, et al. A prospective analysis of a two-year experience using computed tomography as an adjunct for cervical spine clearance. *J Trauma* 1991; 31(7): 1001–1005.

9. Gilbert, J. Critical care management of the patient with acute spinal cord injury. *Crit Care Clin* 1987; 3:549–567.

10. Nicolasides AN, Fernandez J, Pollock AV. Intermittent sequential pneumatic compression of the legs in the prevention of venous stasis and postoperaetive deep venous thrombosis. *Surg* 1980; 87(1):69–76.

11. Apelgren KN, Wilmore DW. Nutritional care of the critically ill patient. *Surg Clin North Am* 1983; 63:497–507.

12. Gore R, Mintzer R, Galenoff L. Gastrointestinal complications of spinal cord injury. *Spine* 1981; 6:538–544.

13. Green BA, Green KL, Klose KJ. Kinetic nursing for acute spinal cord injury patients. *Paraplegia* 1980; 18:181–186.

14. Green BA, Green KL, Klose KL. Kinetic therapy for spinal cord injury. *Spine* 1983; 8:722–728.

2 Management of the Multiply Injured Patient

SUBHASH U. KINI, MD
C. GENE CAYTEN, MD, MPH

THIS CHAPTER DESCRIBES the management of patients with multiple injuries and therefore a high probability of spinal cord injuries. In any patient who has suffered multiple injuries, all maneuvers are done with care not to further injure the spinal cord. Such maneuvers include airway control and examination of the back, rectum, and pelvis. The treatment is prioritized as per usual ABCDEs—Airway, Breathing, Circulation, Disability, Exposure, and Environment (1). It should be emphasized that the primary assessment, investigation, and treatment of a patient with severe injuries should be a continuous and integrated process rather than a stepwise progression.

PREHOSPITAL CARE

Management at the scene includes extricating persons who are trapped in a vehicle, immobilizing the cervical spine, placing the patient on a spine board, securing and maintaining an airway, assisting with ventilation, controlling external hemorrhage, and stabilizing long bone fractures. Ischemic tolerance of the central nervous system mandates that oxygenation of the brain be established within 3 to 5 minutes, otherwise there will be irreversible damage. Intravenous (IV) access is advantageous, but it should not retard transport. This is especially so when there has been a delay between the injury and paramedic help reaching patient. It is essential to have good communication between the prehospital personnel and the receiving hospital. This includes alerting the receiving hospital before the arrival of the patient so that the trauma team is ready and waiting in the emergency department at the time the patient arrives. Rapid transportation is important, and if the distance is more than 25 miles, it may be better to use a helicopter.

EMERGENCY DEPARTMENT TRIAGE

Triage is the process by which patients are sorted depending on their injuries and the available resources to deal with those injuries. As the patient is being assessed (primary survey), a member of the team should simultaneously be obtaining history. A careful history and thorough physical examination are of utmost importance in the care of the trauma victim. The history can be obtained from a variety of sources, which include the patient, paramedics, and family members. Obviously, a detailed history taking should not delay providing the appropriate care for an unstable patient. The patient must be completely undressed so that the entire body surface can be examined.

The primary and secondary surveys are done repeatedly; any deterioration is identified and necessary treatment commenced before proceeding to the next step in the evaluation.

Primary Survey

The primary goal of resuscitation is maintenance of oxygenation of tissues. Thus, the airway must be clear, and adequate ventilation must be present. Also, trauma victims are frequently hypovolemic and adequate fluid resuscitation is necessary to maintain an adequate circulating volume.

Airway

The airway must be established as soon as possible; after this has been established, attention is turned to a thorough assessment of every body area and initiation of care necessary to restore homeostasis. The airway can be maintained using any of the following maneuvers: chin lift, jaw thrust, oropharyngeal airway, or nasopharyngeal airway until a definitive airway can be established. A definitive airway implies a cuffed tube in the trachea that can be of three types: orotracheal tube, nasotracheal tube, and surgical airway (cricothyroidotomy or tracheostomy). Patients who need special attention to their airway and who have a higher chance of requiring operative airway management are those with maxillofacial trauma, neck trauma, and laryngeal trauma. Airway obstruction is generally regarded as the most rapidly fatal problem seen in the emergency setting. All forms of airway control require cervical stabilization. Cervical stabilization equipment used to protect the patient's spinal cord should be left in place until cervical spine injury is excluded. Once secretions or foreign bodies are removed, or their presence excluded, the next step is the jaw thrust–chin lift maneuver. If the airway can be opened, a well-fitted mask can be used to ventilate the patient with oxygen for 2 to 3 minutes. If this is not possible, one should immediately intubate the patient. If one fails to be able to intubate, one should proceed to a surgical airway.

Breathing

Airway patency by itself does not ensure adequate ventilation. Every injured patient should have supplemental oxygen, and the adequacy of ventilation should be assessed clinically and confirmed by checking the oxygen saturation by pulse oximetry.

The primary survey should be able to pick up tension pneumothorax, flail chest, open pneumothorax, and massive hemothorax. These must be treated before moving on to the next step in the primary survey. A *tension pneumothorax* occurs whenever a one-way valve from the lung or the chest wall causes air to accumulate in the pleural cavity. This trapped air causes the lung to collapse and decreases the venous return. A tension pneumothorax is a clinical diagnosis; the features are chest pain, respiratory distress, tachycardia, hypotension, unilateral absence of breath sounds, tracheal deviation, and distension of the neck veins.

In a *flail chest*, there are at least two adjacent ribs, each fractured in two or more places. This leads to the formation of an unstable segment that moves paradoxically with the rest of the chest (Fig. 2-1). It is usually associated with significant injury, especially pulmonary contusion. There can be significant hypoxia. In the past, the pathophysiology was thought be due to pendular movement of air, resulting in ineffectual respiration, but now it is thought to be more related to the alteration of the chest wall mechanics and underlying lung contusion. The pain associated with this causes hypoventilation, leading to atelectasis. An *open pneumothorax* is usually easy to diagnose, and the immediate treatment is an occlusive dressing secured with tape to the skin on three sides to prevent the build-up of a tension pneumothorax secondary to the underlying lung injury that is usually present. This can be followed by a tube thoracostomy and by securing the fourth side of the occlusive dressing.

A *massive hemothorax* is diagnosed when there is shock associated with absence of breath sounds and dullness on one side of the chest. Massive hemothorax is managed by volume replacement

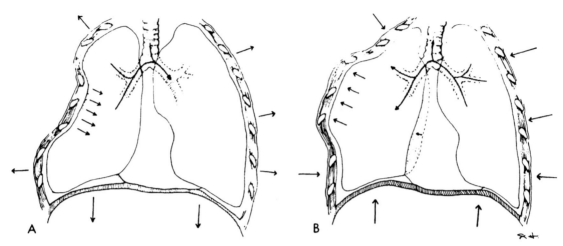

FIGURE 2-1   Paradoxical movement of the unstable "flail" segment of the chest wall. **A.** During inspiration. **B.** During expiration. (From: Symbas PN. Specific presentations of thoracic trauma. In Schwartz GR, ed., *Principles and Practice of Emergency Medicine*. Philadelphia: Lea and Febiger. 1992, p. 1052.)

with crystalloids and packed red blood cells (RBCs) and decompression of the pleural cavity by a tube thoracostomy. If a patient has either an initial drainage of 1500 ml of blood or an output of more than 200 ml/hr for 2 to 4 hours, it is an indication for a thoracotomy.

Circulation

External hemorrhage is identified and controlled in the primary survey. This is achieved in many cases by direct pressure. A tourniquet is indicated only for unmanageable, life-threatening hemorrhage or after traumatic amputation.

Two large-bore IV catheters (preferably size 14) are inserted in each forearm or antecubital fossae. While this being done, blood is drawn for a complete blood count, routine chemistries, and blood gases. A blood sample is also sent to the blood bank for typing and cross-matching, so that blood will be available if needed at short notice later. An IV fluid infusion is begun with a balanced salt solution. IV fluids are given to attempt to rapidly restore an adequate circulating blood volume. If the patient is hypotensive, 2 liters of lactated Ringer's solution are infused within 15 to 30 minutes. If the patient's blood pressure does not rise, consideration should be given to administration of colloid. Figure 2-2 is

an algorithm for patients who are unresponsive to fluid resuscitation.

Colloids and balanced salt solutions have been found to be equally effective in resuscitation. Balanced salt solutions equilibrate rapidly with the interstitial space and thus have a greater volume of distribution than colloids. As a result, two or three times as much balanced salt solution as colloid solution is required for an equivalent intravascular filling. An additional consideration is that colloid solutions cost about 50 times more than balanced salt solutions.

Ongoing blood loss is usually indicated by a failure of blood pressure to return to normal. Management requires immediate hemorrhage control and replacement with IV fluids and blood.

The first indication of hypovolemia is tachycardia followed by a decrease in pulse pressure. The early symptoms and signs of hypovolemic shock are given in Table 2-1.

TABLE 2-1   Signs and Symptoms of Shock

Tachycardia and skin pallor
Thirst
Hypotension
Confusion, aggression, drowsiness, and coma
General weakness
Reduced urine output

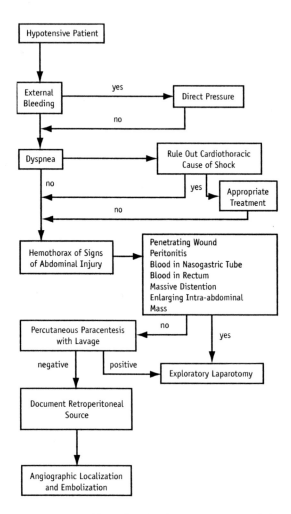

FIGURE 2-2 Algorithm for the management of the hypotensive patient. (From: Cayten CG. Abdominal trauma. In Schwartz GR, ed., *Principles and Practice of Emergency Medicine*. Philadelphia: Lea and Febiger, 1992, p. 1069.)

In most cases, the signs and symptoms can be related to the amount of blood loss, which can be classified in four broad classes (I–IV); this is given in Table 2-2.

In previously healthy young adults, systolic pressure is often preserved despite quite appreciable blood loss (1.5–2.0 liters) due to the effective response to sympathetic stimulation. Conversely, patients with coronary artery disease may become hypotensive because of myocardial insufficiency after only modest blood losses (e.g., 500 ml).

Blood transfused rapidly should be warmed to maximize flow rates and minimize the risk of cardiac arrhythmia and core hypothermia. The transfusion of blood should not be taken lightly because, in addition to the risk of infection, it has associated problems such as immunosuppressive effects (2).

All sources of hypovolemic losses should be ruled out before entertaining the diagnosis of neurogenic shock. An important difference between neurogenic shock and the other types of shock seen in the trauma setting is that neurogenic shock causes *warm shock*. Fluid management also differs in a patient with neurogenic shock. First, the amount of fluid required for resuscitation is much greater. Second, even after adequate fluid administration, if the blood pressure is low, one may have to use vasopressors cautiously. It cannot be emphasized too strongly that vasopressors should be used judiciously and only after an adequate attempt has been made to replace volume in an expanded intravascular space.

Emergency room thoracotomy (ERT) offers the best results when it is directed for potential thoracic injury, especially for potential cardiac tamponade (3). The results of ERT are dismal when performed on patients with abdominal and severe head trauma because survival approaches zero when they do not exhibit signs of life upon arrival in the emergency department (4). Cardiac arrest from blunt trauma has a dismal prognosis, and survival cannot be expected if the patient had no signs of life at the scene after sustaining any type of trauma (5).

Emergency room thoracotomy is technically demanding and should be performed by trained surgeons. The usual incision is a left anterolateral thoracotomy through the fourth interspace. By inspecting and palpating the pericardium, one can rapidly determine if there is cardiac tamponade. If present, a pericardiotomy should be performed anterior to the phrenic nerve. In penetrating wounds of the abdomen with continuing bleeding, the thoracic aorta can be clamped. This is best performed by manual compression. Alternatively, the aorta can be

TABLE 2-2   Classification of Shock

	Class I	Class II	Class III	Class IV
Blood Loss (ml)	Up to 750	750–1500	1500–2000	>2000
Blood Loss (% Blood Volume)	Up to 15%	15%–30%	30%–40%	>40%
Pulse Rate	<100/min	>100/min	>120/min	>140/min
Blood Pressure	Normal	Normal	Decreased	Decreased
Pulse Pressure (mm Hg)	Normal or increased	Decreased	Decreased	Decreased
Respiratory Rate (/min)	14–20	20–30	30–40	>35
Urine Output (ml/hr)	>30	20–30	5–15	Negligible
CNS/Mental Status	Slightly anxious	Mildly anxious	Anxious, confused	Confused, lethargic
Fluid Replacement (3:1 Rule)	Crystalloid	Crystalloid	Crystalloid and blood	Crystalloid and blood

(From: American College of Surgeons Committee on Trauma: Shock. *In Advanced Trauma Life Support® Program for Doctors.* 6th ed. Chicago, American College of Surgeons, 1997, p. 98.)

located by following the ribs. It can then be bluntly dissected out by finger dissection, and a vascular clamp can be applied at a point just above the diaphragm.

Disability (Neurologic Evaluation)

A rapid neurologic examination is performed at the end of the primary survey. The classification of patients depends on the level of consciousness: alert, responsive to commands, responsive only to painful stimuli, and totally unresponsive.

Exposure and Environment Control

Although clothing must be removed to facilitate access, one should ensure that the patient is adequately covered and kept warm and dry. A patient with multiple injuries can easily become hypothermic, and this must be prevented.

Adjuncts to Primary Survey and Resuscitation

All trauma patients need to have EKG monitoring (6). Dysrythmias and ST segment changes may indicate blunt cardiac injury. Pulseless electrical activity may be seen in tension pneumothorax, severe hypovolemia, and cardiac tamponade. Indwelling bladder catheters and nasogastric tubes should be considered as routine for all trauma patients.

Pulse oximetry is an extremely important noninvasive method of assessing the adequacy of ventilation in injured patients. It measures the oxygen saturation of the patient, with the aim of keeping the saturation above 90–95 percent. It is not reliable in poorly perfused extremities, such as in shock and carbon monoxide poisoning.

A urinary catheter is inserted, and hourly measurements of urine volume are started. Transurethral catheterization of the bladder is contraindicated whenever a urethral injury is suspected (this is discussed in detail later). Also, difficulty may be encountered in the placement of a Foley catheter in the presence of a urethral stricture or prostatic hypertrophy.

Patients with fractures of the midface may have a fracture of the cribriform plate. For these patients, an orogastric intubation may be required instead of a nasogastric intubation.

Radiological Studies

The three radiographic evaluations that are considered basic are the chest X-ray, the cervical spine series (AP, lateral, and open mouth), and the AP pelvis. These films can be taken in the resuscitative area. They can be interspersed with clinical examination and resuscitation at appropriate times.

SECONDARY SURVEY

The secondary survey does not begin until the primary survey has been completed and the patient is showing normalization of vital functions. It involves additional patient history, a detailed physical examination, a reassessment of all vital signs, and other investigations. It begins with evaluation of the head and neck; continues with the chest, abdomen, and perineum; and goes on to the extremities. It is completed with a focused but detailed neurologic examination.

The history should include the mechanism of injury, relevant past medical history, current medications, allergies, and the time of the last meal.

During the secondary survey, continuous monitoring of vital signs and urinary output is essential. Pulse oximetry, end-tidal carbon dioxide monitoring, and central venous pressure monitoring should be performed.

Effective analgesia requires IV opioid analgesics. Intramuscular injections should be avoided until definitive diagnoses and/or management plans are established. If opioids are given, it should be recognized that monitoring of pupillary changes might be inaccurate.

Tetanus prophylaxis depends on the previous immunization status. An immunized patient with a contaminated wound requires a booster of tetanus toxoid if more than 5 years have elapsed since his or her last immunization. In addition, tetanus immunoglobulin is required if no immunity exists or the immunization status is not known.

Head and Neck Trauma

Head Injuries. The entire scalp and head should be examined for lacerations, contusions, and evidence of fractures. Scalp lacerations are one of the sites of substantial blood loss leading to hypovolemia. The eyes should be examined for visual acuity, pupillary size, hemorrhages of the conjunctiva and fundi, and any penetrating injury.

Neurotrauma. Head injury is a broad term used to describe traumatic brain injury (TBI) as well as injuries of the skull, mandible, and soft tissues of the head; differentiation is important for the purposes of management and prognostication. A useful classification of TBI is to divide it into focal and nonfocal injuries. Focal lesions include epidural, subdural, and intraparenchymal hematomas.

The Glasgow Coma Scale (GCS) is a simple clinical method for evaluating TBI. Its advantages include reproducibility, consistency, and the fact that it does not take very long to perform. Thus, its greatest use is that it can be repeated at very short intervals. The details of Glasgow Coma Scale are described in Table 2-3.

A computed tomographic (CT) examination of the head without IV contrast is the initial diagnostic procedure of choice for the evaluation of head injury. Neurosurgical intervention usually depends on CT findings, but if a burr hole is to be made before CT, it should be placed on the side of the dilated pupil. An algorithm is described in the initial resuscitation of a patient with severe head injury (Fig. 2-3).

TABLE 2-3   Glasgow Coma Scale

Component	Patient response	Score
Eye opening		
	Spontaneous	4
	To verbal command	3
	To pain	2
	None	1
Best motor response		
	Follows commands	6
	Localizes to painful stimulus	5
	Flexion withdrawal to pain	4
	Abnormal flexion response to pain (decorticate)	3
	Abnormal extension response to pain (decerebrate)	'2
	None	1
Best verbal response		
	Oriented conversation	5
	Disorientation but converses	4
	Inappropriate words	3
	Incomprehensible sounds	2
	None	1
TOTAL		3–15

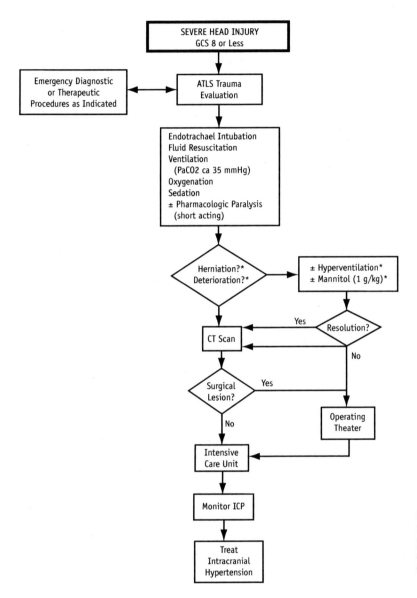

FIGURE 2-3 Initial resuscitation of the severe head injury patient. Guidelines for the management of severe head injury. (Brain Trauma Foundation, 1995, pp. 3–6).

Maxillofacial Injuries. Airway maintenance assumes even greater significance in patients with maxillofacial injuries,. When a patient is unable to maintain the airway or to ventilate adequately, endotracheal intubation is mandatory. The other alternatives are nasotracheal intubation and cricothyroidotomy.

Maxillofacial trauma that is not associated with airway obstruction or major bleeding should be treated only after the patient is stabilized.

Cervical Spine and Neck Injuries. Any patient with multiple injuries is assumed to have a spine injury. This is especially so when there is an altered level of consciousness or a blunt injury above the clavicle. The absence of a neurologic deficit does not exclude cervical spine injury, and such an injury should be presumed until complete cervical spine radiographs interpreted by a skilled radiologist have ruled this out (7). The Guidelines of the Eastern Association for the Surgery of Trauma for ruling out injury to the spinal cord are given in Table 2-4.

TABLE 2-4. Eastern Association for the Surgery of Trauma Guidelines for Ruling Out Spinal Cord Injury.

1. Trauma patients who are alert, awake, have no mental status changes, no neck pain, no distracting pain, and no neurologic deficits may be considered to have a stable cervical spine and need no radiologic studies of their cervical spine.
2. All other trauma patients should have the following three cervical spine x-rays: lateral view revealing the base of the occiput to the upper border of the first thoracic vertebrae, anteroposterior view revealing the spinous processes of the second cervical through the first thoracic vertebra, and an open mouth odontoid view revealing the lateral masses of the first cervical vertebra and entire odontoid process.
   Axial CT scans with sagittal reconstruction should be obtained for any questionable level of injury, or through the lower cervical spine if this area cannot be visualized on plain radiographs. All life-threatening hemodynamic and pulmonary problems should be addressed before a prolonged c-spine evaluation is undertaken. Before removing cervical spine immobilization devices, all radiographs should be read by an experienced emergency medicine physician, neurosurgeon, orthopedic spine surgeon, radiologist, or other physician with expertise in interpreting these studies.
3. If the cervical spine radiographs are normal but the patient complains of significant neck pain, cervical spine radiographs with the patient actively positioning his neck in extreme flexion and extension positions should be obtained.
4. If the patient has a neurologic deficit that may be referable to a cervical spine injury, he should have an immediate surgical subspecialty consultation and MRI scan of the cervical spine.
5. Trauma patients who have an altered level of consciousness due to a traumatic brain injury, or due to other causes which are considered likely to leave the patient unable to complain of neck pain or neurologic deficits for 24 or more hours after their injury, may be considered to have a stable cervical spine if adequate three-view plain x-rays (CT supplementation as necessary) and thin cut axial CT images through C-1 and C-2, are read as normal by an experienced physician.
6. If the patient has abnormalities of the cervical spine discovered on any of the radiographic or MRI images as recommended above, the surgical subspecialty responsible for spine trauma should be consulted.

Source: Pasquale M, Fabian T, and EAST Ad Hoc Committee on Practice Management Guideline Development. Practice management guidelines for trauma from the Eastern Association for Surgery of Trauma. *J Trauma* 1998; 44:941–957.

Traumatic spinal cord injury is discussed in greater details in Chapters 1, 10, and 14.

Injuries that have penetrated the platysma should not be explored in the emergency department.

Ocular and Orbital Trauma. The eyes should be evaluated early in the examination because swelling around the eyes may develop rapidly and prevent a detailed examination. Visual acuity, pupillary size and reaction to light, and penetrating injury to the eye should evaluated.

Cervical Vascular Injury. Active bleeding from a neck wound requires direct pressure to stop the bleeding and an early surgical evaluation.

Chest Injuries

Chest Wall Injury. Although blunt injury to the chest wall is usually minor, it may serve as a clue to intrathoracic injury, especially in children.

Injuries to the Trachea, Bronchi, and Lungs. Patients who have massive subcutaneous or mediastinal emphysema and who have a major air leak from a chest tube are suspected to have a tracheobronchial disruption. Control of the airway and ventilation presents a challenge in these patients. A double-lumen endotracheal tube may be required. Management of pulmonary contusion is the same as that for a flail chest as far as the fluid management and treatment of hypoxia are concerned.

Simple Pneumothorax. Simple pneumothrorax is suspected clinically when there is absence of breath sounds on one side of the chest, and a radiograph usually confirms it. The treatment is a tube thoracostomy through the fourth or fifth intercostal space, just anterior to the midaxillary line. A chest radiograph should be repeated to confirm reexpansion of the lung. General anesthesia, transport via an air ambulance, or positive pressure ventilation should never be administered in a patient with a traumatic pneumothorax before the placement of a chest tube. A simple pneumothorax, which is usually of no hemodynamic consequence, can be converted to a tension pneumothorax, which can be potentially lethal.

Heart Injury. Cardiac tamponade usually occurs from penetrating injuries in the region of the heart (Fig. 2-4). It is less common with blunt injuries to the chest. The classic triad of Beck consists of the presence of distended neck veins, muffled heart sounds, and hypotension. These three features are rarely seen together. Kussmaul's sign, a rise in venous pressure with inspiration during spontaneous respiration, is another feature of cardiac tamponade. Pulseless electrical activity in the absence of severe hypovolemia and tension pneumothorax points to a diagnosis of cardiac tamponade, as does hypotension despite adequate fluid replacement, especially when a mechanism exists for a cardiac tamponade. In such a situation, pericardiocentesis can be performed, purely on clinical grounds.

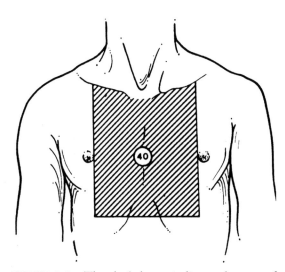

FIGURE 2-4 The shaded area indicates the area of penetrating injury that ultimately was found to produce cardiac arrest. (From: Richardson JR. Thorax. In Ivatury R, Cayten CG, eds. *Textbook of Penetrating Trauma*. Baltimore: William & Wilkins, 1996, p. 274.)

It is both diagnostic and therapeutic. Even aspiration of a small amount of blood, on the order of 15–20 ml, can cause a relief of the pressure. A more definitive procedure is a pericardial window; if this reveals an injury that requires a thoracotomy, an anterolateral thoracotomy should be performed.

Esophageal Injury. The esophagus is most commonly injured in the cervical region, accounting for more than 80 percent of injuries. The diagnosis is sometimes very difficult to make. A bloody aspirate in a nasogastric tube is very nonspecific and can be caused by a traumatic insertion or swallowed blood. Patients with cervical injuries may have one or more of the following features: subcutaneous emphysema, spitting blood, and hoarseness of voice without oral injury. Thoracic injuries can initially be silent, especially in an unconscious patient. The initial chest radiograph may show no findings in up to one-third of patients. However, the typical picture is that of mediastinal emphysema with an accompanying left-sided pleural effusion. If the pleural effusion contains a high level of amylase, it is diagnostic of esophageal injury. These injuries should be diligently looked for and treated urgently. A delay in diagnosis or treatment may progress rapidly to septic shock, and the mortality can increase up to 90 percent. Subdiaphragmatic injuries present like any other hollow viscus perforation.

Aortic Injury. Injuries to the aorta and its branches can produce catastrophic hemorrhage. The most common location of ruptured aorta is just distal to the origin of the subclavian artery and ligamentum arteriosum. This is because of the forward movement of the heart and proximal aorta, whereas the distal aorta is immobile. Immediate survival depends on the formation of an acute false aneurysm. The diagnosis depends on a high index of suspicion. Mediastinal widening on a chest radiograph is the most common finding that alerts the clinician to the possibility of a traumatic aortic rupture. The other features include a tracheal shift to the right, blurring of the aortic outline, opacification of the angle between the aorta and left pulmonary artery, pleural capping, and depression of the left main bronchus. This should be followed by a dedicated study to diagnose or rule out aortic injury. Indications for operative repair of a thoracic great vessel injury are described in Table 2-5.

Abdominal Injuries

One should remember that the abdomen extends from the fourth intercostal space to the groin crease anteriorly, and from the tip of the scapula to the buttock crease posteriorly (Fig. 2-5). The evaluation of acute abdominal trauma, whether from blunt or penetrating injury, can be difficult. Injury to the abdominal viscera following blunt trauma is easily missed, and in the past it was a frequent cause of preventable death. When a patient who is hypotensive is being evaluated, and there is an obvious source of bleeding from a site distant from the abdomen, evaluation of the abdomen can be deferred until the obvious source of hemorrhage is controlled.

Blunt Injury. Motor vehicle collisions are one of the most common causes of blunt injuries. A pattern of blunt abdominal trauma that is specific to seat belts has emerged. This includes avulsion injuries of the mesentery of the small bowel. The symptoms and signs of blunt abdominal trauma can be subtle, and consequently, diagnosis is difficult. Blunt abdominal trauma is usually associated with trauma to other areas, especially the head, chest, and pelvis.

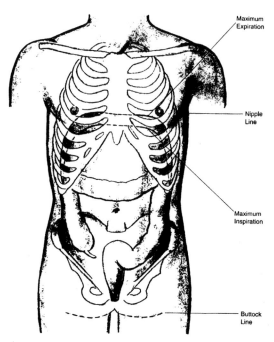

FIGURE 2-5 The extent of the abdomen as applicable to trauma. (From: Cayten CG, Nassoura ZE. Abdomen. In Ivatury R, Cayten CG, eds. *Textbook of Penetrating Trauma.* Baltimore: Williams & Wilkins, 1996, p. 283.)

Penetrating Injury. All patients with penetrating wounds that are in close proximity to the abdomen and are either hypotensive or have signs of peritonitis require an emergency laparotomy. Gunshot wounds are associated with intraabdominal injuries greater than 90 percent of the time, compared with approximately 30 percent of the time for stab wounds. Any gunshot wound that traverses the peritoneum or retroperitoneum also necessitates an emergency laparotomy. However, asymptomatic patients who have stab wounds are evaluated as outlined in Figure 2-6.

Abdominal Vascular Injury. The incidence of vascular injuries is rather high after penetrating injuries to the abdomen. Only one-third of patients present with hypotension after abdominal vascular injuries. The rest remain hemodynamically stable until laparotomy, when the tamponading effect is removed, at which time the patient may become profoundly hypotensive.

TABLE 2-5 Indications for Operative Repair of a Thoracic Great Vessel Injury

Initial Loss of a 1500 ml of blood from the chest tube.
Continuing hemorrhage > 200ml/hr from a tube thoracostomy
Posttraumatic hemopericardium
Pericardial tamponade
Expanding hematoma at the thoracic outlet
Exsanguinating hemorrhage presenting from a supraclavicular penetrating wound
Imaging evidence of acute thoracic great vessel injury

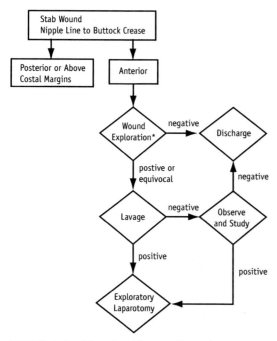

FIGURE 2-6 The algorithm outlines the management of the stable patient with a stab wound of the abdomen who does not have obvious indication for surgery. (From: Cayten CG. Abdominal trauma. In Schwartz GRm ed., *Principles and Practice of Emergency Medicine*. Philadelphia: Lea and Febiger, 1992, p. 1071.)

Spleen Injury. The spleen is the most common organ that requires treatment during laparotomy in patients who have sustained blunt trauma. Blunt injury causing splenic injury is more common than penetrating injury. Diagnostic peritoneal lavage (DPL) is the most sensitive test for detecting splenic injuries, whereas CT scan is the most specific. Experience with ultrasonography is increasing and may soon replace DPL as the diagnostic test of choice when a trained sonographer is available in the emergency department.

Liver Injury. Although the liver is the most commonly injured organ in patients with blunt abdominal trauma with an estimated incidence of 30–40 percent, most of the injuries do not require surgical intervention (8,9). Selective arteriography and transcatheter embolization, CT-guided drainage of perihepatic collections and endoscopic cholangiopancreatography with sphincterotomy can be used to treat the untoward sequelae of hepatic trauma, namely, bleeding and biliary leaks (10).

Small Bowel and Colonic Injuries. Bowel injury is common after penetrating injury (90% after gunshot wounds and 30% in the case of stab wounds) but occurs infrequently after blunt injury. DPL is sensitive in picking up intraperitoneal fluid, whereas CT scan is less sensitive in defining hollow viscus injury.

Rectal Injuries. A rectal examination should be performed before placing a urinary catheter. Anorectal injury is diagnosed during the secondary survey. The details of management are given below.

Genitourinary Tract Injury. Blood at the urethral meatus, a scrotal hematoma, and a high-riding prostate are signs of urethral injury. This subject is discussed at greater length in Chapter 6.

Pelvic Fracture and Perineal Lacerations. Radiographic examination of the pelvis is part of the basic x-ray evaluation of the patient and is usually done after the primary survey. It may pick up many clinically important abnormalities. There are two aspects of pelvic injuries—hemodynamic instability and pelvic stability (11). Hemodynamic stability is more important both initially and prognostically. Patients who are not hemodynamically stable do much worse than those who are stable (mortality of 38% vs. 3%).

Response to initial fluid resuscitation is more important than the class of hemorrhage. One should look for other sources of blood loss in patients who show evidence of ongoing bleeding.

Pneumatic antishock garments (PASG), also known as medical antishock trousers (MAST), were used very liberally in the past for hypotension (12). The suit consists of inflatable sections for each leg and the abdomen and is radiolucent with access for urinary catheterization and digital rectal examination. It has been suggested that when a PASG is applied, it produces an autotransfusion of 0.5–1.0 liters of homologous blood, a reduction in hemorrhage from tissues beneath the suit, and a reduction in the total functioning volume of the vascular compartment. Despite these theoretical advantages, prospective studies have shown either no benefit—even harm—resulting from its use except in the severely hypotensive patient (13). It may have value, however, for temporary immobilization of pelvic fractures.

Ancillary Studies

Diagnostic Peritoneal Lavage. DPL is a rapidly performed invasive procedure in which the peritoneal cavity is reached, usually through a small incision. If gross blood or gastrointestinal (GI) contents are not aspirated, a peritoneal lavage is carried out with 1 liter of warmed Ringer's lactate. If GI contents, gross blood, or urine are not obviously seen, the fluid is sent for microscopy. A positive test, and hence an indication for a laparotomy, are indicated by a RBC count >100,000 RBCs/mm^3, white blood cell (WBC) count >500/mm^3, or a Gram's stain with bacteria.

Indications for the use of DPL include the patient who is comatose from a head injury, a patient who is severely intoxicated or paralyzed, a physical examination that is equivocal in a patient who is hypovolemic, and when a prolonged loss of contact with the patient is anticipated.

The only absolute contraindication for a DPL is an absolute indication for a laparotomy, such as a patient going to the operating room for management of fractures or head injuries. DPL has a sensitivity of 98 percent for intraperitoneal bleeding, but its role is decreasing with the increasing use of ultrasonography in unstable patients.

Role of Ultrasonography. Ultrasonography is a rapid (14), noninvasive, and inexpensive test that can be done in the emergency department and repeated as often as necessary (15). However, it requires a trained sonographer and is less inaccurate in the obese, if there is subcutaneous air, and in the presence of multiple abdominal operations. The *focused assessment for the sonographic examination of the trauma patient* (FAST) is a rapid diagnostic test that sequentially surveys for hemopericardium and then surveys the right upper quadrant, left upper quadrant, and pelvis for hemoperitoneum in patients with potential truncal injuries (16). It has replaced DPL in some centers (17).

Computed Tomography. CT is used in the place of DPL in a stable patient. Oral and IV contrast should be used. The use of rectal contrast also should be considered to rule out retroperitoneal colorectal injuries.

Role of Laparoscopy. Laparoscopy and thoracoscopy are being used increasingly to evaluate stable patients with possible thoracoabdominal injury; unstable patients must have open surgery immediately. There also has been a modest rise in therapeutic procedures. Although most centers perform laparoscopies in the operating room under general anesthesia, a few centers are using microinstruments and performing laparoscopies in the emergency department. Both laparoscopy and thoracoscopy obviate the need for formal laparotomy and thoracotomy up to 40% (18) , especially in patients with stab injuries. Laparoscopy is very sensitive for diagnosing a hemoperitoneum, but it is less sensitive for diagnosing a bowel injury (19). Moreover, it does not reliably rule out retroperitoneal injury. Thoracoscopy gives a better view than laparoscopy for the diagnosis of diaphragmatic injury (DI). Those patients who have DI diagnosed on laparoscopy should have a thoracoscopy, and vice versa. The complication that causes the most anxiety to the surgeon is missed injury.; conducting a formal laparotomy whenever the surgeon has any doubts about the existence of this possibility can minimize this. In addition to all the complications of laparoscopy, there is a higher risk of developing a tension pneumothorax secondary to DI when it is performed for trauma.

Extremity Trauma

Severe limb injuries should not distract the resuscitation team from the priorities of establishing an airway, optimizing ventilation, and restoring circulatory volume because limb injuries are rarely immediately life-threatening, except those that cause exsanguination. A compressive bandage or hand pressure over a sterile pad can reduce blood loss from wounds. Femoral and pelvic fractures can result in significant loss of blood; in the case of pelvic fractures, this can be from 1 to 4 liters of blood.

Open fractures constitute an emergency, whereas a closed fracture requires stabilization. The limb should be splinted when moving a patient.

Of prime importance to limb survival is competence of the vasculature distal to any injury. In the hemodynamically stable patient, examination of the distal pulses is crucial in assessing the peripheral circulation. A diminished or absent pulse strongly suggests a vascular injury and must be explained and managed promptly. Pallor or a blue-gray skin color should arouse suspicion of inadequate tissue perfusion. A sensitive indicator is the capillary return—the normal prompt pink flush of the nailbed seen after transient compression. This response will be slowed or blue if the circulation is inadequate. Perfusion of the distal limb must be checked after any manipulation.

Coagulopathy

Coagulation problems occur in patients with massive blood loss because of dilution with blood substitutes and the fact that coagulation factors deteriorate rapidly in stored blood. Compounding this is the fact that many patients are hypothermic, and this interferes with the enzymes involved in the clotting mechanism. The coagulation process should be monitored, and deficiencies should be treated appropriately with fresh frozen plasma, platelets, or clotting factors rather than on an arbitrary basis.

DEFINITIVE TREATMENT

Head and Neck Trauma

Neurotrauma. Approximately one-third of patients with cervical spine and/or spinal cord

injuries have moderate or severe head injuries (20). Epidural hematomas classically manifest with a lucid interval between the initial concussion and later neurologic deterioration. A biconvex lesion can be seen on CT scan. Unless decompressed, epidural hematomas are fatal, but prognosis usually is excellent if they are decompressed early. Subdural hematomas appear as concave lesions on a CT scan. The prognosis depends on the underlying brain injury. Mass effect is uncommon in subarachnoid hemorrhage. The two complications of this condition are vasospasm, which can be severe enough to cause cerebral hypoxia, and the formation of posttraumatic hydrocephalus secondary to accumulation of blood in the ventricular system.

Cerebral perfusion pressure (CPP) is the difference of the mean arterial pressure (MAP) and intracranial pressure (ICP). Some investigators believe that CPP is a more reliable indicator of cerebral perfusion than ICP. More important, the goal is to maintain a CPP of more than 60–70 mmHg while keeping the ICP to less than 20–25 mm Hg (21). In patients who require ICP monitoring, a ventriculostomy catheter connected to an external strain gauge transducer or catheter tip pressure transducer device is the most accurate and reliable method of monitoring ICP and enables therapeutic CSF drainage (22). In addition to measurement of MAP, the central venous pressure (CVP) and urine output can be monitored to provide an indicator of the volume status because an adequate intravascular volume is essential to prevent low CPP. It previously was believed that raising the head of the bed was beneficial in TBI because it reduced the ICP. However since pathophysiology is better understood now, it has been found that CPP is the same or lower when the head of the bed is elevated because MAP also falls.

The recent reduction in the use of prophylactic corticosteroids and antiseizure medication has signaled a change in the management of diffuse head injuries. In addition, hyperventilation is limited to control transient periods of raised ICP.

Mannitol decreases ICP by drawing fluid out of the brain parenchyma into the intravascular space. Two studies have shown that the outcome has been improved in patients who were administered for raised intracranial tension (23,24). Although the CVP initially rises, it subsequently falls as it acts as an osmotic diuretic.

The mainstay of the treatment of cerebrospinal fluid (CSF) leakage usually is elevation of the head of the bed to 60 degrees. This is not possible in patients with SCI. The use of prophylactic antibiotics is controversial because it may only result in the selection of antibiotic-resistant microbes.

Penetrating injuries to the brain can have catastrophic results. Mortality is > 80 percent in patients who have a GCS score of 3 to 4. Penetrating brain injury is often accompanied by disseminated intravascular coagulation (DIC). Operative goals are dural closure and debridement of necrotic tissue.

Diabetes insipidus is one of the complications of TBI. Treatment includes maintenance of intravascular status and correction of electrolyte abnormalities. Administration of vasopressin (DDAVP) depends on the level of serum sodium; it should not be based solely on urine output. On the other hand, excess antidiuretic hormone (ADH) can cause syndrome of inappropriate antidiuretic hormone secretion (SIADH). Treatment consists of withholding free water. Rarely is hypertonic saline required, and when given, it should be administered cautiously (correction of serum sodium < 0.5 mEq/l/hr) to prevent central pontine myelinolysis.

Maxillofacial Wounds. Facial wounds should be closed once the patient is hemodynamically and neurologically stable. Irrigation with plenty of sterile saline, preferably with a pulsatile jet, is especially beneficial in the management of contaminated facial wounds and will minimize tattooing if it is done early.

Plain radiographs of the face with special views are useful in the management of facial wounds. CT scan—especially three-dimensional CT—provides the most accurate imaging.

Ocular and Orbital Trauma. Funduscopic examination after dilation of the pupils usually gives the best results, but it makes subsequent examination of the pupil difficult, and it is important to highlight this in the patient's chart. The most useful investigations in the evaluation of ocular trauma are plain radiograph to rule out foreign bodies, CT scan with thin cuts, and ultrasonography.

Cervical Vascular Injury. Blunt arterial trauma is not very common and is difficult to diagnose because of its delayed presentation. CT scanning is a good test for detecting blunt cervical arterial injury (25).

In the past, the neck was divided into three zones for further diagnostic procedures in patients with penetrating injuries to the neck. This is no longer appropriate in centers in which arteriography is readily available because the location of the skin wound is not a reliable indicator of the location of underlying vascular injury. Furthermore, the practice of surgical examination of all patients with penetrating injuries in the middle of the neck is outdated.

An anterior sternocleidomastoid incision should be used because it gives a good exposure. When possible, proximal and distal control should be obtained before the injured area is explored. Small injuries should be repaired primarily. Complex injuries should be repaired in stable patients with no serious associated injuries. The injured artery should be ligated in patients who are unstable or have serious associated injuries. If there is a defect in the artery, the repair depends on the length of the defect; a less than 2-cm defect can be repaired primarily with a circumferential end-to-end anastomosis. If the defect is greater than 2 cm or an anastomosis cannot be performed without tension, a vein patch or vein graft should be used. Synthetic graft material should be used only if autogenous vein is not available.

Vertebral artery injuries usually are not amenable to repair and should be ligated. The distal vertebral artery injury is approached as follows: The proximal artery is ligated and a Fogarty catheter passed distal to the injury through an arteriotomy. The balloon is then inflated. If the bleeding does not stop, direct exposure of the distal vertebral artery is required, although the bleeding does stop in most cases. In these patients, the balloon is left inflated for 48 to 72 hours and then deflated. The balloon can be removed at the bedside if there is no further bleeding.

Injuries to the veins in the neck usually can be managed by ligation. The only exception is a bilateral internal jugular vein injury. In such a case, efforts should be made to repair the vein on at least one side.

Chest Trauma

Chest Wall Injury. Both penetrating and blunt injuries can cause chest wall injuries. Seat belt injury is a common cause of breast hematoma in women. Treatment is symptomatic.

Rib fractures are the most common chest wall injuries. If anteroposterior compression followed by lateral compression does not cause pain in an alert patient, it can almost conclusively rule out significant rib fractures. Pain leads to splinting, and this leads to atelectasis and pneumonia. Chest wall strapping, a form of treatment that has now been abandoned, only increases this splinting. Thus, pain relief is important and can be best achieved with intercostal blocks and epidural analgesia. Chest physiotherapy is started after pain has been relieved.

If a chest tube is inserted, it is recommended that prophylactic antibiotic usage, such as a first-generation cephalosporin, last for no longer than 24 hours (26).

Epidural analgesia dramatically improves ventilation in a flail chest. A combination of an opioid and a long-acting local anesthetic agent such as bupivacaine usually is used. Chest physiotherapy commences after pain has been relieved. If, despite all measures, there is continuing hypoxia (PO_2 less than 60 mmHg), the patient may need to be intubated and ventilatory support instituted. Administration of crystalloids should be carefully monitored because the injured lung is sensitive to both underresuscitation and fluid overload.

There are two kinds of sternal fractures. The isolated sternal fracture is seen in restrained motor vehicle occupants and is associated with a low incidence of cardiovascular and pulmonary complications, especially if there are no EKG changes and the chest radiograph is normal. Sternal fractures should be internally fixed only when they are unstable.

Injuries to the Trachea, Bronchi, and Lungs. The diagnosis of tracheobronchial disruption is confirmed by bronchoscopy. Repair is done by thoracotomy. The approach most often is from the right side. The approach is from the left side only if bronchoscopy confirms a left main-stem bronchus injury. Repair of the trachea usually is done with a patch either from the pleura or an intercostal muscle pedicle.

Blunt Cardiac Injury (BCI). *Blunt cardiac injury* is a term used for a condition formerly called *myocardial contusion.* Clinically, there are few reliable signs and symptoms that are specific for BCI. The diagnosis is entertained by maintaining a high index of suspicion in patients with an appropriate mechanism of injury or in those who manifest an inappropriate or abnormally poor cardiovascular response to their injury. Many patients have evidence of external chest trauma, such as fractures or the imprint of a steering wheel. Chest pain, usually due to associated injuries, is common, and patients occasionally describe anginal-type pain that is unrelieved by nitrates. Because there is no gold standard for the diagnosis of BCI, there is confusion with respect to making a diagnosis and difficulty interpreting the literature. The diagnosis of BCI will be directly proportional to the aggressiveness with which it is sought. Key issues involve identifying patients at risk for adverse events from BCI and then appropriately monitoring and treating them. Conversely, patients not at risk could potentially be discharged from the hospital with appropriate follow-up.

All patients in whom BCI is suspected should have an EKG on admission. If the admission EKG is abnormal (arrhythmia, ST changes, ischemia, heart block, unexplained ST), the patient should be admitted for continuous EKG monitoring for 24 to 48 hours. On the other hand, if the admission EKG is normal, the risk of having a clinically significant BCI is negligible, and the pursuit of diagnosis should be terminated. An echocardiogram is not useful as a screening modality, although it is useful in hemodynamically unstable patients. If an optimal transthoracic echocardiogram cannot be performed, the patient should have a transesophageal echocardiogram (TEE) (27).

Patients may be discharged if they are hemodynamically stable, younger than 55 years of age with no history of cardiac disease, require no surgery or neurologic observation, and have a normal admission ECG (27).

Most studies have shown that cardiac enzyme analysis does not aid in the management of patients with BCI.

Esophageal Injury. Definitive diagnostic studies include contrast radiography and endoscopy. A water-soluble contrast, such as Gastrografin, can miss 15–50 percent of esophageal injuries, so these negative studies should be followed by a thin barium study. Rigid esophagoscopy is contraindicated in a patient suspected of having cervical spine trauma. A flexible endoscopy can be performed (28), carefully monitoring for the development of a tension pneumothorax.

Most injuries can be managed by primary repair and reinforcement or flap closure if surgery is performed within 24 hours. Small injuries in the cervical esophagus can be closed transversely, whereas injuries longer than 2–3 cm can be closed longitudinally. The repair should be reinforced with tissue and drained.

Simple thoracic injuries should be closed primarily. A flap of pericardium should be used to buttress this. In the case of traumatic injuries in which the pleura is not chronically inflamed, it is usually too thin to be used as a flap.

Abdominal injuries are best dealt with by reinforcement of the stomach using either a Nissen's fundoplication or a Thal patch.

Esophageal injuries are dealt with differently when diagnosis is delayed for more than 24 hours or when the patient is unstable because these injuries are associated with a significant degree of inflammation and sepsis. This may prevent the surgeon from primarily closing the defect. Instead, a complex exclusion-diversion procedure br required. Cervical wounds require open drainage and debridement. The mediastinum should also be drained if the inflammation has spread to the upper mediastinum. The two ends of the esophagus may require exteriorization. Thoracic injuries require a thoracotomy with extensive pleural debridement and wide drainage with two chest tubes.

Aortic Injury. The chest radiograph is a good screening tool for determining the need for further investigation in blunt aortic injury. The most significant chest film findings include (but are not limited to) widened mediastinum, obscured aortic knob, deviation of the left mainstem bronchus or nasogastric tube, and opacification of the aortopulmonary window (29). The diagnostic modalities that are used to confirm aortic injury are spiral CT scan, aortography, and TEE. All have similar accuracy, and the deciding factor is the relative speed at which a particular modality can be performed in a particular hospital. For example, if it requires time for the gastroenterologist to come in and to set up the TEE, one of the two other tests should be used for diagnosis.

If an aortic injury is confirmed, the treatment is by surgery and should take priority over all but immediately life-threatening hemorrhage. During preparation for the operating room, the patient's blood pressure is kept below 100 mmHg by avoiding aggressive volume expansion and infusion of afterload-reducing agents, such as nitroprusside, if necessary. Aortic repair is by direct suture of the laceration or graft replacement of the injured area.

Abdominal Trauma

A single preoperative dose of prophylactic antibiotics with broad-spectrum aerobic and anaerobic coverage is usually given for patients who have sustained penetrating abdominal wounds. Furthermore, no further antibiotics are administered in the absence of a hollow viscus injury, whereas antibiotics are continued for 24 hours in the presence of injury to any hollow viscus.

Abdominal Vascular Injury. Control of hemorrhage is temporarily achieved by packing all four quadrants while resuscitation continues. Aortic compression at the level of the diaphragm is applied temporarily. A right-sided mobilization maneuver, along with kocherization of the duodenum, is used when the inferior vena cava (IVC) or right renal pedicle must be exposed. A left-sided medial mobilization maneuver exposes the abdominal aorta from the aortic hiatus of the diaphragm to the aortic bifurcation. Repair of the injured vessel is carried out in the usual manner. Salvage of autologous blood may be appropriate.

Diaphragmatic Injury. Diaphragmatic injury occurs in approximately 15 percent of patients with stab wounds and 46 percent of patients with gunshot wounds that involve the lower thorax and upper abdomen. The signs are subtle, and the classic physical findings of scaphoid abdomen, absent breath sounds, and audible bowels in the affected hemithorax are rarely encountered (30). The chest radiograph is normal in up to 50 percent of patients with diaphragmatic injury; in the remainder of the cases only a pneumothorax or a hemothorax is detected. DPL is relatively insensitive, with a false-negative rate of 12–40 percent. Even laparoscopy can fail to detect up to 15 percent of injuries, particularly posterior defects.

Acute diaphragmatic injuries should be managed by laparotomy because of the associated intraabdominal injuries. Most injuries are small and the repair usually is simple. Right-sided posterolateral injuries can be approached with a thoracotomy. Right-sided penetrating diaphragmatic injuries in stable patients are managed expectantly by some clinicians because they are often of little clinical significance.

Spleen Injury. In recent years, splenic injury has been being managed increasingly with splenic conservation (31). Conservative management is less successful in patients who are over 55 years of age, who have bled substantially, and who have multiple injuries. The grades of splenic injury are described in Table 2-6.

Small capsular tears usually stop bleeding promptly. For higher grades of splenic injuries, the surgeon must decide at laparotomy whether to perform a splenectomy or a splenorrhaphy. Surgeons are less likely to perform splenectomy for children because of the higher risk for overwhelming postsplenectomy infection (OPSI). Immunization is indicated for patients who have a splenectomy. A 23-valent pneumococcal vaccine is used, and evidence is accumulating for the use of *H. influenza* and *N. meningitidis* vaccines in asplenic patients. Asplenia may also be associated with an increase in thromboembolism.

Liver Injury. The grading scale for liver injuries is given in Table 2-7.

TABLE 2-6 Splenic Injury Scale (1994 Revision)

Grade	Injury	Description
I	Hematoma	Subcapsular, <10% surface area
	Laceration	Capsular tear, <1 cm parenchymal depth
II	Hematoma	Subcapsular, 1050% surface area Intraparenchymal, <5 cm in diameter
	Laceration	13 cm parenchymal depth but does not involve a trabecular vessel
III	Hematoma	Subcapsular, >50% surface area or expanding. Ruptured subcapsular or parenchymal hematoma
	Laceration	>5 cm parenchymal depth or involving trabecular vessels
IV	Laceration	Involving segmental or hilar vessels producing major devascularization (>25% of spleen)
V	Laceration	Shattered spleen
	Vascular	Hilar vessel injury with devascularized spleen

(From Hulka F and Mullins RJ, in Trunkey DD and Lewis FR, eds. *Current Therapy of Trauma.* St. Louis: Mosby, 1999)

TABLE 2-7 Grades of Liver Injury

Grade	Injury	Description
I	Hematoma	Subcapsular, nonexpanding <10% of surface area
	Laceration	Capsular tear, nonbleeding, < 1 cm deep
II	Hematoma	Subcapsular, nonexpanding 10–50%; Intraparenchymal, nonexpanding <2 cm diameter
	Laceration	<3 cm deep; <10 cm long
III	Hematoma	Subcapsular >50% or expanding Ruptured subcapsular with active bleeding Intraparenchymal >2 cm diameter
	Laceration	>3 cm parenchymal depth
IV	Hematoma	Ruptured central hematoma
	Laceration	Parenchymal destruction 25–75 % of hepatic lobe
V	Laceration	Parenchymal destruction >75% of hepatic lobe
	Vascular	Juxta venous injuries (retrohepatic vena cava/major hepatic veins)
VI	Vascular	Hepatic avulsion

(Modified from Moore EE et al. Organ Injury Scaling: Spleen, Liver and Kidney. *J Trauma* 1989; 29:1665.)

There is extensive literature on the safety of nonoperative management of selected patients with liver injuries. Ideal candidates for nonoperative management are hemodynamically stable patients with minimal peritoneal fluid and no evidence of other abdominal injury. Grades I, II, and often III do not require intensive treatment. Topical hemostatic agents, omentum, or occasionally direct suture ligation of bleeding vessels are used to control hemorrhage. However, there are insufficient data to suggest nonoperative management as a Level I recommendation for the initial management of blunt injuries to the liver and/or spleen in the hemodynamically stable patient (32).

Liver resection or damage control (liver packing, which is discussed subsequently) is indicated for more severe injuries (33). Injuries to the hepatic vein and retrohepatic IVC injury may necessitate damage control or a technique to achieve a bloodless field. The three most common approaches to obtain a bloodless field are Heaney's maneuver (clamping of the suprahepatic and infrahepatic IVC), venovenous bypass, and intraluminal atriocaval shunting. In all three techniques, inflow occlusion is provided by a Pringle maneuver.

Pancreatic and Duodenal Injuries. Routine DPL is negative in >50 percent of patients because the pancreas and duodenum are retroperitoneal organs and most patients have no associated intraperitoneal injuries. The retroperitoneal location makes clinical evaluation of these structures very difficult, and even a CT scan yields nonspecific findings. Thus, these injuries are often missed, and indeed many patients are sent home after being "cleared" by the trauma team.

Although an elevated serum amylase level is nonspecific, rising levels of amylase in conjunction with increasing peritoneal signs are significant. Abdominal radiographs may show scoliosis and blurring of the psoas shadow in duodenal injury. Small injuries of the pancreas are best treated with hemostasis and closed suction drainage. More severe injuries require reconstruction.

Simple injuries of the duodenum can be closed primarily. When this is not possible, a serosal patch repair with a Roux-en-Y loop of jejunum may be used to maintain the normal luminal diameter of the duodenum.

More severe duodenal injuries may require a pancreaticoduodenectomy (34).

When the operation is performed more than 24 hours after injury, mortality is significantly increased. Such patients require a duodenal diverticularization to provide internal decompression.

Small Bowel and Colonic Injuries. Isolated small bowel and mesenteric injuries are uncommon in blunt injury to the abdomen. They are more common in penetrating injury. In blunt injury, the mechanism of injury should raise the suspicion of this possibility. Findings on abdominal CT that may suggest isolated small bowel and mesenteric injury are free fluid, thickened bowel, and extraluminal air (35). Primary repair of small bowel injuries is safe even when the operation is delayed, as long as basic surgical principles are followed, viz., anastomosing well-vascularized segments of bowel. Hence, serial examinations aid in the diagnosis of small bowel injury. Only in damage control laparotomy are bowel ends left stapled and the anastomosis is carried out at relaparotomy.

The management of colonic injuries has changed dramatically over the last 15 to 20 years (27). There is abundant literature on the safety of managing simple injuries with primary repair (36–38), even when the operation is delayed up to 12 hours. The trend toward primary repair of nondestructive colon injuries is related to the lower morbidity rates and lower costs associated with avoidance of colostomy. When stable patients who have no significant associated injuries or underlying disease and are being operated on without undue delay have destructive penetrating colon wounds, the standard of care continues to be resection and anastomosis. Patients with serious associated injuries or significant underlying disease fare better with resection and colostomy. Colostomies performed following colon and rectal trauma can be closed within 2 weeks if a contrast enema is performed to confirm distal colon healing, provided the patient is stable and does not have unresolved wound sepsis.

Damage Control.   Damage control is a relatively new method of managing patients who have had major trauma: intraabdominal injury with associated hypothermia, acidosis, and coagulopathy. A staged, repeated laparotomy is the optimal strategy under such circumstances. At the first laparotomy, any bleeding from the liver is packed and bowel resection is carried out without anastomosis for any bowel disruption [a gastrointesinal anastomosis (GIA) stapler is used to expedite the resection]. The abdomen is left open or a synthetic mesh is sutured to the fascia to facilitate subsequent relaparotomy. The patient is then returned to the operating room

24 to 48 hours after being adequately resuscitated. A time interval greater than this may increase the incidence of sepsis (39). At relaparotomy, the divided bowel is anastomosed and a liver resection is carried out if there is continuing blood loss upon removing the packs.

Abdominal Compartment Syndrome (ACS).   ACS has been recognized with increasing frequency over the past years. Initially, by compressing the splanchnic venous system, there is an increase in venous return, but this is soon followed by compression of the splanchnic vessels, which leads to an increase in peripheral vascular resistance and thus a decrease in venous return. Abdominal hypertension also increases the intrathoracic pressure, which causes a decreased venous return, increased physiologic dead space, and intrapulmonary shunting. An elevated IAP also causes a progressive decrease in renal perfusion and urine output. Similarly, it also decreases the blood supply to the anterior abdominal wall. This has been postulated as a cause of slower wound healing.

The most frequently used method of measuring IAP is by connecting a needle, placed in the sampling port of a clamped indwelling urinary catheter, to a transducer after instilling 50 ml of saline in an emptied bladder. A value greater than 30–35 mm is diagnostic of severe abdomen compartment syndrome. This test is accurate and reliable.

ACS is both prevented and treated by temporary partial closure of the abdomen.

Rectal Injuries.   Intraperitoneal injuries of the rectum are managed in the same way as colonic injuries (40). Management of an incomplete extraperitoneal injury includes IV antibiotics and close observation. If doubt exists whether the injury is full or partial thickness, it should be treated as full thickness. If the injury is a full-thickness extraperitoneal injury, the principles of treatment are fecal diversion, rectal washout, and presacral drainage. After a laparotomy and copious (8–10 liters) saline irrigation of the peritoneal cavity, a loop of sigmoid is brought out through the left lower quadrant. The loop of sigmoid is then opened along its most distal aspect and a Foley catheter is inserted to allow for distal colorectal washout. A rigid proctoscope is inserted transanally to assist this process. After clearing the rectum, the distal loop of the sigmoid is stapled and placed in a subcutaneous pocket adjacent to the stoma site. A skin incision is made anterior to the coccyx. This permits access to the presacral space; a closed suction drain is placed in this space. Closure of the colostomy is done after 4 to 6 weeks in the usual fashion.

Gynecologic Injury

Vulva and Vagina Injuries. Trauma to the vulva can result in a large hematoma. If the hematoma continues to expand or is larger than 5 cm in diameter, surgical evacuation is usually required. All necrotic or foreign matter removed should be removed from a penetrating wound of the vulva and vagina, and surgical repair is accomplished with absorbable sutures to restore normal anatomic relationships as needed.

Upper Reproductive Tract. Gunshot wounds and lacerations to the uterus usually can be repaired by placement of interrupted absorbable sutures. When adnexal structures are injured, at least one ovary should be preserved whenever possible for endogenous hormonal function and assisted reproductive technologies, such as in vitro fertilization.

Extremity Trauma

Evidence of nerve injury may be difficult to obtain in the unconscious or multiply injured patient. There is a higher incidence of neurologic damage with dislocations than with fractures. The more proximal innervation of the muscle bellies must be appreciated when testing distal motor function,. Division of a peripheral nerve must be assumed to have occurred if there is altered sensation in the distribution of that nerve and a wound overlying its course. Neurologic function should be documented to allow later comparison. Thorough evaluation of extremity injuries should include anteroposterior and lateral radiographs of the injured area and the joints above and below.

Miscellaneous Injuries

Trauma in Pregnancy. Early recognition of pregnancy by palpation and human chorionic gonadotopin (HCG) testing is important to be able to address the special problems of the pregnant woman. IV fluids should be given liberally in the prehospital setting because the relative hypervolemia in a pregnant patient usually masks signs and symptoms of shock. Additionally, the patient should be transported on a backboard tilted to the left. This improves venous return to the heart by relieving pressure on the IVC. Essential diagnostic radiographs should not be avoided in the pregnant patient.

Trauma in the Elderly. The aging process decreases the physiologic reserve and reduces the ability to respond to stress in the same manner as a younger person. Similarly, overresuscitation is very easily achieved. Thus, early invasive monitoring is frequently a valuable adjunct to management. Elderly patients, even those with relatively minor injuries, have higher than expected mortality due to comorbidity (41). An increased incidence of pneumonia and pulmonary embolism is also a factor.

Trauma in Children. Children with multisystem injuries can deteriorate rapidly. As the ratio of the surface area to weight of a child is much higher than in an adult, body heat is lost much more easily, and hypothermia can develop quickly.

AIRWAY. The placement of an oral airway should be done directly, without inserting it backwards and then rotating it 180 degrees. Because the smallest area of the child's airway is the cricoid ring, which forms a natural seal with the endotracheal tube, cuffed endotracheal tubes are rarely needed. Cricothyroidotomy is rarely needed for a small child but should be performed by a surgeon when it is necessary.

BREATHING. The child's skeleton is more pliable, so children often can sustain significant intrathoracic injuries without evidence of trauma to the thoracic cage. Hypoventilation is the most common cause of cardiac arrest in children.

CIRCULATION. The increased physiologic reserve means that even though significant blood loss may occur, most of the hemodynamic parameters that are being measured may be normal. In fact >25 percent of the circulating blood volume must be lost before even minimal signs of shock are seen. Another difference is that the child may have bradycardia rather than tachycardia. One can observe the response of the child to a bolus of 20 ml/kg of crystalloid; this may be repeated twice. When the third bolus is being given, consideration must be given to transfuse packed RBCs. IV access in a small hypovolemic child can be challenging. This problem can be overcome by intraosseous access or a venous cutdown on the saphenous vein at the ankle.

Injuries Due to Burns and Cold. Burns may occur either as an isolated problem or in combination with another significant injury. Inhalation injury and carbon monoxide poisoning often complicate burn injury. The so-called "classic" feature of cherry red mucous membranes is a rarely seen and totally unreliable clinical sign. Arterial blood gas tensions, analysis of carboxyhemoglobin concentrations, and, if the patient is able to comply, peak expiratory flow rates should be repeated. Deep circumferential burns over the limbs, neck, and chest can produce a tourniquet-like effect because the damaged skin is unable to expand as tissue edema develops. If this occurs, escharotomies (longitudinal incisions of the skin) are required to permit adequate circulation. If escharotomy of the chest is required, vertical incisions along anterior and posterior axillary lines should be made. If sufficient chest expansion does not occur, further incisions in the midline and midclavicular lines as well as transverse incisions may be required. For rapid assessment of the percentage of the body surface area involved, the rule of nine is useful. Areas of simple erythema are not included in the esti-mate. The size of small burns can be judged roughly by considering the palmar surface of the patient's hand as about 1 percent of the total body surface area. The volume of crystalloids, such as lactated Ringer's, required for IV replacement for the first 4 hours after injury should be judged roughly as the percentage of body surface area of the burn multiplied by the body weight (in kg). The same volume calculated as above should be infused over the next 4 hours and double that volume should be infused over the next 16 hours (42).

CONCLUSION

Patients with SCI usually have multiple injuries. Adequate management of such patients presents a unique challenge and requires a team approach with an aggressive emphasis on the ATLS ABCDEs. The team must be organized properly and must work in a well-equipped resuscitation room. In the case of severe neurologic damage, this team approach must be continued for an extended period to provide for the rehabilitation of the patient.

REFERENCES

1. American College of Surgeons Committee on Trauma. Initial assessment and management. In *Advanced Trauma Life Support® Program for Doctors*, 6th ed. Chicago: American College of Surgeons, 1997, pp. 21–46.
2. Agarwal N, Murphy JG, Cayten CG, Stahl WM. Blood transfusion increases the risk of injection after trauma. *Arch Surg* 1993; 128:171–177.
3. Ivatury RR, et al. "Directed" emergency room thoracotomy: a prognostic prerequisite for survival. *J Trauma* 1991; 31:1076.
4. Millham FH, Grindlinger GA. Survival determinants in patients undergoing emergency room thoracotomy for penetrating chest injury. *J Trauma* 1993; 34:332.
5. Boyd M, Vaneck VW, Bourget CC. Emergency room thoracotomy: when is it indicated? J Trauma 1992; 33:714.
6. Pasquale MD, Nagy K, Clarke J. *Practice Management Guidelines for Screening of Blunt Cardiac Injury*. Eastern Association for the Surgery of Trauma. Practice Management Guidelines Workgroup. 1999.

7. Davis JW, Phreaner DL, Hoyt DB, Mackersie RC. The etiology of missed cervical spine injuries. *J Trauma* 1993; 34(3):342–346.

8. Croce MA, et al. Nonoperative management of blunt hepatic trauma is the treatment of choice for hemodynamically stable patients: results of a prospective trial. *Ann Surg* 1995; 221:744–753.

9. Pachter HL, et al. Status of nonoperative management of blunt hepatic injuries in 1995: a multicenter experience with 404 patients. *J Trauma* 1996; 40:31–38.

10. Carillo EH, Spain DA, Wohltmann CD, et al. Interventional techniques are useful adjuncts in nonoperative management of hepatic injuries. *J Trauma* 1999; 46:619–624.

11. Gruen GS, Leit ME, Gruen RJ, Peitzman AB. The acute management of hemodynamically unstable multiple trauma patients with pelvic ring fractures. *J Trauma* 1994; 36(5):706–711.

12. Cayten CG, Berendt BM, Byrne DW, Murphy JG, Moy FH. A study of pneumatic antishock garments in severely hypotensive trauma patients. *J Trauma* 1993; 34(5):728–730.

13. Cayten CG, Berendt BM, Moy FH, Murphy JG, Byrne DW. A study of pneumatic anti-shock garment in severely hypotensive trauma patients. *J Trauma* 1993; 34:728–734.

14. Rozycki GS, Feliciano DV, Ochsner MG, et al. The role of ultrasound in patients with possible penetrating cardiac wounds: a prospective multicenter study. *J Trauma* 1999; 46:543–552.

15. Hilty W, Snoey ER. Trauma ultrasonography. In Simon BC, Snoey ER, eds., *Ultrasound in Emergency and Ambulatory Medicine*. St. Louis: Mosby, 1997.

16. Rozycki GS, Ochsner MG, Feliciano DV, et al. Early detection of hemoperitoneum by ultrasound examination of the right upper quadrant: a multicenter study. *J Trauma* 1998; 45(5):878–883.

17. McKenney M, Lentz K, Nunez D, et al. Can ultrasound replace diagnostic peritoneal lavage in the assessment of blunt trauma? *J Trauma* 1994; 37(3):439–441.

18. Ortega AE, Tang E, Froes ET, et al. Laparoscopic evaluation of penetrating thoracoabdominal injuries. *Surg Endosc* 1996; 10: 19–22.

19. Ivatury RR, Simon RJ, Stahl WM. A critical evaluation of laparoscopy in penetrating abdominal trauma. *J Trauma* 1993; 34(6):822–827.

20. Iida H, Tachibana S, Kitahara et al. Association of head trauma with cervical spine injury, spinal cord injury, or both. *J Trauma* 1999; 46:450–452.

21. Juul N, Morris GF, Marshall SB, Marshall LF. Intracranial hypertension and cerebral perfusion pressure: influence on neurological deterioration and outcome in severe head injury. The Executive Committee of the International Selfotel. *J Neurosurg* 2000; 92(1):1–6.

22. Bullock R, Chesnut RM, Clifton G, et al. Guidelines for the management of severe head injury. Brain Trauma Foundation. *Eur J Emerg Med* 1996; 3(2):109–127.

23. Schwartz M, Tator C, Towed D, et al. The University of Toronto Head Injury Treatment Study: a prospective, randomized comparison of pentobarbital and mannitol. *Can J Neurol Sci* 1984; 11:434–440.

24. Smith HP, Kelly D Jr, McWhorter JM, et al. Comparison of mannitol regimens in patients with severe head injury undergoing intracranial monitoring. *J Neurosurg* 1986; 65:820–824.

25. Rogers FB, Baker EF, Osler TM, et al. Computed arteriographic angiography as a screening modality for blunt cervical arterial injuries: preliminary results. *J Trauma* 1999; 46:380–385.

26. Luchette FA, Barie P, Oswanski M, Spain DA. Parameters for prophylactic antibiotics in tube thoracostomy for traumatic hemopneumothorax. Eastern Association for the Surgery of Trauma. Practice Management Guidelines Workgroup. 1999.

27. Pasquale M, Fabian T, EAST Ad Hoc Committee on Practice Management Guideline Development. Practice management guidelines for trauma from the Eastern Association for Surgery of Trauma. *J Trauma* 1998; 44:941–957.

28. Flowers JL, Graham SM, Ugarte MA, et al. Flexible endoscopy for the diagnosis of esophageal trauma. *J Trauma* 1996; 40(2):261–265.

29. Nagy K, Fabian T, Rodman G, et al. Guidelines for the diagnosis and management of blunt aortic injury. Eastern Association for the Surgery of Trauma. Practice Management Guidelines Workgroup. 1999.

30. Guth AA, Pachter HL, Kim U. Pitfalls in the diagnosis of blunt diaphragmatic injury. *Am J Surg* 1995; 170(1):5–9.

31. Ivatury RR, Simon RJ, Guignard J, et al. The spleen at risk after penetrating trauma. *J Trauma* 1993; 35(3):409–414.

32. Alonso M, Brathwaite C, Garcia V, et al. Patient management guidelines for the non-operative management of blunt injury to the liver and spleen. EAST Practice Parameter Workgroup for Solid Organ Injury Management. 1999.

33. Cue JI. Packing and planned reexploration for hepatic and retroperitoneal hemorrhage: critical refinements of a useful technique. *J Trauma* 1990; 30:1007–1011.

34. Feliciano DV, et al. Management of combined pancreatoduodenal injuries. *Ann Surg* 1987; 205:673–680.
35. Frick EJ, Pasquale MD, Cipolle MD. Small-bowel and mesentery injuries in blunt trauma. *J Trauma* 1999; 46:920–926.
36. Gonzalez RP, Merlotti GJ, Holevar MR. Colostomy in penetrating colon injury: is it necessary? *J Trauma* 1996; 41(2):271–275.
37. Sasaki LS, Allaben RD, Golwala R, Mittal VK. Primary repair of colon injuries: a prospective randomized study. *J Trauma* 1995; 39(5):895–901.
38. Murray JA, Demetriades D, Colson M, et al. Colonic resection in trauma: colostomy versus anastomosis. *J Trauma* 1999; 46(2):250–254.
39. Ivatury RR, Nallathambi M, Gunduz Y, et al. Liver packing for uncontrolled hemorrhage: a reappraisal. *J Trauma* 1986; 26(8):744–753.
40. McGrath V, Fabian TC, Croce MA, Minard G, Pritchard FE. Rectal trauma: management based on anatomic distinctions. *Am Surg* 1998; 64(12): 1136–1141.
41. Cayten CG, Stahl WM, Agarwal N, Murphy JG. Analyses of preventable deaths by mechanism of injury among 13,500 trauma admissions. *Ann Surg* 1991; 214:510–521.
42. Warden GD, Heimbach DM. Burns. In Schwartz SI, ed., *Principles of Surgery*. New York: McGraw Hill, 1999.

3 Hemodynamic Monitoring in Spinal Cord Injured Patients

JOHN A. SAVINO, MD

THE ACUTE MANAGEMENT of spinal cord injury begins at the scene of the accident, the moment that such an insult is suggested. The goals of treatment remain consistent throughout the patient's course and include maximizing neurologic recovery, restoring normal alignment, correcting deformity, promoting spinal stability and fusion, minimizing pain, facilitating early mobilization and rehabilitation, minimizing hospitalization and cost, and preventing secondary complications of disability.

PREHOSPITAL COURSE

The development of rapid emergency transport systems with trained technicians emphasizing prehospital spinal immobilization and trauma resuscitation ranks among the greatest advances in the care of spinal cord injured patients over the past several decades. Management of these patients begins by maintaining a high index of suspicion for such insults. Frequently, concomitant injuries—such as altered mental status caused by head trauma or intoxication, peripheral nerve injuries, or extremity fractures—limit the ability to detect neurologic compromise, and injury to the spinal cord must be inferred from the mechanism alone. Victims of high-speed motor vehicle accidents, ejection, or falls greater than 15 feet are at high risk for spinal cord injury; however, severe cord injury can result from unimpressive minor trauma as well.

Due to early immobilization and extrication techniques, the percentage of spinal cord injured patients presenting to tertiary care facilities with complete transection had decreased from 65 percent in the late 1960s to about 39 to 46 percent in the late 1990s. In spite of these efforts, however, it is estimated that up to 10 to 25 percent of patients will suffer additional injury to the spinal cord during the prehospital and early acute care phases of treatment from manipulation of the inadequately stabilized spine.

Additional prehospital care focuses on adequate ventilatory and circulatory support and attention to associated injury. Only 40 percent of patients with spinal cord injury will have isolated cord damage; the remaining 60 percent will have significant trauma to the head, chest, abdomen, or other regions of the body. The presence or absence of neurologic deficit are poor predictors of the existence of associated injuries. Patients with high-level cervical cord injuries may frequently mask the manifestations of intraabdominal injury. Prehospital resuscitative measures may include administration of supplemental oxygen or plasma expanders, positioning the head lower than the rest of the body to avoid shock, and insertion of a nasogastric tube to prevent emesis.

EMERGENCY CARE OF SHOCK STATES

Emergency management attends to adequate airway establishment, ventilation and oxygenation, and circulatory support before neurologic evaluation and resuscitation. Support of ventilation and oxygenation must be provided in patients who lack the capacity for adequate gas exchange, whether from cervical cord injury with paralysis of muscles or respiration, associated chest trauma, or other causes. Hypoxia exacerbates the pathophysiologic cascade of spinal cord injury and must be prevented by supplemental oxygen, mechanical ventilation, or both.

Maintenance of systemic blood pressure and spinal cord perfusion is also crucial to minimize secondary ischemic insults, especially in the face of impaired autoregulation of spinal cord blood flow. Circulatory depression following cord injury may be of several types, including neurogenic shock (the hemodynamic consequence of "spinal shock"). This condition may result from selective denervation of the sympathetic chain in the cervical and high thoracic (Tl–T5) region with consequent loss of vascular tone and unopposed vagal activity leading to brachycardia, or from skeletal muscle paralysis and venous pooling below the level of injury. It is characterized by systemic hypotension and inappropriately low heart rate from unopposed parasympathetic function and warm, hyperemic skin. The treatment of choice is inotropic support with dobutamine, pressors such as dopamine that increase vascular tone, and moderate volume infusion.

In contrast, hypovolemic shock resulting from concomitant hemorrhage is manifest by tachycardia and cool, clammy skin from peripheral vasoconstriction. Its management consists of controlling ongoing blood loss, blood transfusion, and aggressive fluid replacement with crystalloid or colloid. The aim of treating post-spinal cord injury hypotension is to restore arterial pressure to normotensive levels. Hypertension should be avoided because of the theoretic risk of enhancing intramedullary hemorrhage and edema.

With respect to trauma in general, it has been reported that up to 50 percent of deaths occur from exsanguination or central nervous system complications within the initial hour after injury. Another 30 percent are caused by major organ injury during the next 2 hours. Of those who do survive initial resuscitation and operative and critical care management, the remaining mortalities are related to infections and multiple organ failure. These patients frequently develop either compensated or decompensated septic shock. Shock, as mentioned, represents the failure of the circulatory system to maintain adequate delivery of oxygen and other nutrients to tissues, thus causing cellular and other organ dysfunction. The ultimate goals of hemodynamic therapy in shock are to restore effective tissue perfusion and normalize cellular metabolism. Septic shock is the prototypical form of distributive shock and differs from other forms of shock, which result from a decrease in cardiac output. In septic patients, tissue hypoperfusion results not only from decreased perfusion pressure attributable to hypotension but also from abnormal shunting of a normal increased cardiac output.

Bedside clinical assessment provides a good indication of global perfusion. In general, hypotension in sepsis refers to a mean arterial pressure below 60 mmHg, although the chronic level of pressure must be considered. Hypotension is usually accompanied by tachycardia. Indications of decreased perfusion include oliguria, clouded sensorium, delayed capillary refill, and cool skin. Some caution is necessary in interpreting these signs in septic patients, however, because organ dysfunction can occur in the absence of global hypoperfusion.

END POINTS OF RESUSCITATION AND THE USE OF PULMONARY ARTERY CATHETERS

Our current ability to recognize early shock "inadequate blood flow to meet the demands of the tissue"—is limited. Traditional parameters such as blood pressure, heart rate, and urine output are not helpful because early guides of shock and areas of ischemia in various organs may go unrecognized until cellular damage has already occurred. Although it is easy to recognize patients in trouble when hypotension occurs, it is difficult to identify patients in occult shock, who may need invasive monitoring. A common error is to wait for patients to demonstrate hemodynamic instability before inserting a pulmonary artery catheter (PAC) and administrating treatment. Patients with a cardiac or pulmonary history who have sufficient multiple injuries, including spinal cord damage, to warrant aggressive fluid resuscitation should be considered for PAC monitoring. Even younger patients with signs of chest trauma may not be able to augment an appropriate cardiac output response due to myocardial contusion when they most need it early in the post-injury phase. Other candidates for invasive monitoring may include patients who are unresponsive to several liters of fluid treatment and sustain abnormal blood pressure, urine output, and lactic acidosis.

Older patients who sustain trauma may demonstrate deceptively normal vital signs, despite a low cardiac index, low mixed venous oxygen saturation (SVO_2), and a high mortality rate. Even healthy older subjects are unable to respond to exercise with the same degree of stroke volume as younger subjects, thus making them susceptible to decompensation during times of stress. As the incidence of myocardial problems increases with age, critically ill surgical patients 50 years of age and older are less capable of increasing cardiac output in response to increasing metabolic demands.

Biochemical parameters such as lactic acidosis may provide another clue to tissue ischemia, provided the pitfalls are understood. Lack of oxygen utilization and anaerobic metabolism after injury results in posttraumatic acidosis secondary to increased lactate in the blood. Lactate, a by-product of anaerobic metabolism, is reflective, as it increases, of a progressive increment of oxygen debt. In a prospective resuscitation study involving trauma patients, all patients who normalized lactate at 24 hours survived, whereas those who required 24 to 48 hours to clear lactate had a mortality rate of 25 percent, and those who required more than 48 hours had a mortality rate of 86 percent. Increased lactate levels are caused by pathologic overproduction, impaired clearance by the liver, or a combination of both problems. Examining markers of both conditions is frequently helpful. A low SVO_2 (<50 percent) in the face of an increasing lactate value indicates continued shock and impaired oxygen utilization. Persistently, increased lactate levels in patients with increased hepatic transaminases or impaired hepatic function, however, could be caused by inadequate clearance by the liver. Rapid determination of lactate levels at the bedside coupled with invasive monitoring of hemodynamics and oxygen transport status enables the clinician caring for injured patients, particularly with associated spinal cord injury, to comprehensively assess the adequacy of circulation and interventions directed toward ameliorating the effects of posttraumatic shock

Another parameter easily available that reflects posttraumatic acidosis is the base deficit. This variable is calculated from directly measured values of arterial pH and PCO_2 from an arterial blood gas sample and provides the clinician with a nonspecific marker of lactate, and therefore anaerobic metabolism and oxygen debt. Persistently increased values of base deficit throughout the resuscitation period have been correlated with impaired oxygen utilization and may provide insight into the adequacy of ongoing resuscitation and therapy.

Intestinal ischemia and reperfusion play important roles in the development of post-injury multiple organ failure. Gut perfusion can be indirectly assessed using tonometric techniques to measure the gastric intramucosal pH (pHi). This technique involves instilling saline into a semipermeable balloon at the end of a modified nasogastric tube, followed, after a period of equilibration, by removing the saline and measuring the PCO_2 of the saline sample. Mucosal ischemia leads to the production of increased CO_2 within the stomach lumen, which is detected as an increased PCO_2 in the saline sample. This gastric mucosal PCO_2 is then used, along with simultaneously measured arterial bicarbonate, in a modified version of the Henderson–Hasselbach equation to calculate the pHi.

Trauma patients with a pHi of <7.32 and otherwise adequate central hemodynamic and oxygen transport 24 hours after intensive care unit admission have a higher rate of multiple organ failure and death than a comparable group of patients with both central and intestinal perfusion. Attempts have been made to improve global perfusion status by optimizing cardiac index and systemic acid–base status with the hope of improving intestinal hypoperfusion. Unfortunately, there has been no improvement in morbidity and mortality. The ideal patients to study would be those with adequate systemic perfusion with selective gut hypoperfusion. Recent technical innovations have led to the development of the semicontinuous gas tonometer, which samples mucosal CO_2 intermittently at short intervals rather than depending on normal sampling of a saline sample in a tonometer balloon. Gut hypoperfusion using this technique is detected by an elevated mucosal arterial CO_2 gap, rather than by calculating the pHi. A recent study described a gap of 18 torr and pHi of 7.25 as appropriate threshold values for identifying trauma patients at risk for multiple organ failure and death.

HEMODYNAMIC GOALS

The key concepts in resuscitation are 1) to deliver enough oxygen to meet the demands of the tissues while the cells are still able to respond by utilizing oxygen; 2) early (<12 to 24 hour) reversal of shock, if already present, and repayment of oxygen debt; and 3) prevention of inflammatory mediator response to ischemia.

Normal values of primary and derived hemodynamic variables are listed in Table 3-1 and 3-2. Studies have utilized combinations of augmented hemodynamic goals as end points of therapy, specifically: A) cardiac index of $\geq$ 4.6 to 6.0 L/min/m²; B) oxygen consumption VO_2 of $\geq$170 ml/min/m² with DO_2 of $\geq$ 600 ml/min/m², or C) all three variables. All the environmental and patient factors (temperature, nursing maneuvers, mechanical ventilation, paralyzing agent, vasopressors, and endocrine state) that affect VO_2 must remain constant for the VO_2 change to imply a favorable response in oxygen utilization.

Some authors have advocated augmenting oxygen delivery (DO_2) until the VO_2 demonstrates no change or a "plateau" (i.e, oxygen debt has been satisfied). A compromise to the concept that mathematical coupling between DO_2 and VO_2 values caused by shared variables would be to use the DO_2 $\geq$ 600 ml/min/m² goal for patients 75 years of age and younger. A DO_2 value of 450 to 500 ml/min/m² may be considered "high" in a sedentary octogenarian, while a 30-year-old previously active male in respiratory failure may need a DO2 of $\geq$700 ml/min/m².

A simple way to look at the balance between DO_2 and VO_2 is the oxygen extraction ration (O_2ER). A normal O_2ER (VO/DO_2) is approximately 0.25 in a nonexercising patient. Critically ill patients can be stratified to their O_2ER and

TABLE 3-1   Parameters of Cardiovascular Performance

Parameter	Abbreviation	Normal Range
Central Venous Pressure	CVP	1–6 mmHg
Pulmonary Capillary Wedge Pressure	PCWP	6–12 mmHg
Cardiac Index	CI	2.4–4.0 L/min/m²
Stroke Volume Index	SVI	40–70 ml/Beat/m²
Left Ventricular Stroke Work Index	LVSWI	40–60 g.m/m²
Right Ventricular Stroke Work Index	RVSWI	4–8 g.m/m²
Ejection Fraction	RVEF	46–50%
End-Diastolic Volume	RVEDV	80–150 ml/m²
Systemic Vascular Resistance Index	SVRI	1600–2400 dynes.sec.m²/cm⁵
Pulmonary Vascular Resistance Index	PVRI	200–400 dynes.sec.m²/cm⁵

TABLE 3-2   Oxygen Transport Parameters

Parameter	Symbol	Normal Range
Mixed Venous Oxygen Saturation	SvO_2	70–75%
Oxygen Delivery	DO_2	520–570 ml/min.m^2
Oxygen Uptake	VO_2	110–160 ml/min.m^2
Oxygen Extraction Ratio	O_2ER	20–30%

their oxygen demands. Patients with an O_2ER of ≤ 0.20 increase their VO_2, while patients with O_2ER of ≥ 0.20 increase their cardiac output. Because spontaneous increase in cardiac output is not a luxury available to all myocardium, maintaining a higher DO_2 in relationship to VO_2 may place the patient at a physiologic disadvantage, with the ability to consume more oxygen when the metabolic demand increases. Patients with a lower oxygen extraction ratio have increased survival.

Achieving an adequate blood pressure in the first 24 hours after severe injury is the minimum standard of care, along with a urine output > 30 to 50 ml/hr, SVO_2 of > 65 percent, and DO_2 of ≥ 600 ml/min/m^2 in patients 75 years of age and younger, or a DO_2 of 450 to 550 ml/min/m^2 in patients 75 years of age and older (to achieve an O_2ER of ≤ 0.20).

Three parameters are important when assessing oxygen delivery: arterial saturation, hemoglobin, and cardiac index. (Refer to Table 3-3.)

TABLE 3-3   Calculation of Derived Cardiovascular and Oxygen Transport Parameters

CVP	= RAP	= RVEDP	
PCWP	= LAP	= LVEDP	
CI	= CO ÷ BSA		
SVI	= CI ÷ HR		
RVEF	= SV ÷ RVEDV		
RVEDV	= SV ÷ RVEF		
LVSWI	= (MAP − PCWP) × SVI (×0.0136)		
RVSWI	= (PAP − CVP) × SVI (×0.0136)		
SVRI	= (MAP − RAP) × 80 ÷ CI		
PVRI	= (PAP − PCWP) × 80CI		
DO2	= CI × 13.4 × Hb × SaO_2		
VO2	= CI × 13.4 × Hb × (SaO_2 − SvO_2)		
O2ER	= VO2 ÷ DO2 (×100)		

Optimizing Arterial Saturation

Respiratory failure frequently presents with an inappropriately normal PCO_2 despite metabolic acidosis because the patient is unable to compensate by hyperventilating to a lower PCO_2. Respiratory insufficiency may also be present or impending despite normal blood gases when the patients require use of their accessory cervical and thoracic muscles.

Ventilatory dependent patients need to be maintained with an optimal level of oxygenation and ventilation with the ultimate goal to decrease the work of breathing. Ideally, the arterial hemoglobin saturation should be maintained above 90% on a fractional inspired oxygen level between 50 and 60 percent. These goals must be attained by utilizing the lowest mean airway pressure, because when these pressures increase the mean intrathoracic pressure increases concomitantly with deleterious effects on the cardiopulmonary system.

As stated, there must be a low threshold for insertion of pulmonary artery catheters in patients with spinal cord injury, especially if concomitant chest injuries are present or the patient is elderly with associated cardiac or pulmonary disease. Frequently, there are nonpulmonary causes by hypoxia (decreased SaO_2) including low hemoglobin or cardiac output and increased oxygen consumption in a patient with significant right-to-left shunting of blood without oxygenation (pulmonary shunt >20 percent). Inevitably, these patients have a decreased SVO_2, which leads to a decreased arterial saturation of hemoglobin. Inappropriate increase and ventilatory support with positive and expiratory pressure (PEEP), particularly when the decrease in arterial saturation of hemoglobin (SaO_2) is caused by a decrease in cardiac output, is ominous because the increase in end expiratory pressure can further compromise the cardiac output, SvO_2, and subsequently, SaO_2. Therefore, all changes in the pulmonary system must be done in conjunction with evaluation of the hemoglobin, cardiac output, oxygen consumption, and venous and arterial saturation of hemoglobin.

Optimizing Hemoglobin

If there is a drop in the hemoglobin, the cardiac output must increase to maintain an optimal oxygen transport. Cardiac output is derived from the stroke volume times the pulse rate. The stroke volume is derived from preload, afterload, and cardiac contractility (Fig. 3-1). For every gram of hemoglobin lost in the trauma patient, the cardiac output needs to increase 9 percent to maintain the same oxygen transport level. Obviously, in patients with poor myocardial reserve, the cardiac output cannot be increased adequately.

The myocardial tissue is at maximum oxygen extraction under normal conditions. Coronary blood flow increases when there is a drop in hemoglobin by vasodilation of the coronary arteries or an increase in the cardiac output to maintain adequate oxygen delivery to the myocardium. One must recall that the coronary perfusion pressure equals the arterial diastolic pressure minus the central venous pressure. Consequently, if the trauma patient with spinal cord injury has a decreased diastolic pressure, especially if coronary artery disease is present, the above stated response is compromised with inevitable myocardial ischemia.

Patients with cardiac risks suffer fewer myocardial complications or have a lower mortality if hemoglobin is maintained greater than 12 g/dl in trauma victims over the age of 60. Patients unable to produce a cardiac output response in the acute phase of trauma and anemia, when a higher cardiac output is essential to meet the increased metabolic demands, may need more than the traditional accepted hemoglobin value of 10 g/dl. Specifically, in spinal cord injured patients who are hypotensive and unable to increase the pulse rate due to the sympatheticolytic effect of cervical cord injury, the level of hemoglobin becomes even more significant. Blood transfusion should be administered on an individual basis, depending on the myocardial function, SvO_2, O_2ER, timing of disease, patient's age, cardiopulmonary reserve, and expected future blood loss. Administering liberal amounts of blood to older, critically ill surgical patients up to a level of 13.5 g/dl in the first 24 hours of resuscitation did not result in short-term complications, but it did lead to an improved survival rate by augmenting oxygen delivery.

Optimizing Cardiac Output

As mentioned, the cardiac output is dependent on preload, afterload, contractility of the myocardium, and pulse rate. The preload at the bedside is measured by the use of the standard pulmonary artery catheter with measurement of the pulmonary capillary wedge pressure. With the use of a volumetric pulmonary artery catheter, the right ventricular end—diastolic volume—is reflective of the preload. The PCWP can be deceptive, particularly in patients with noncompliant ventricles. Compliance of the ventricles may be affected by inherent myocardial problems (contusion, ischemia, infarction) or extramyocardial causes (intrathoracic or intraabdominal pressures, pericardial pressure).

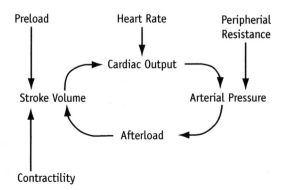

FIGURE 3-1 Determinants of stroke volume, cardiac output, and arterial pressure.

Therefore, a high PCWP and increased volume administration may be necessary if the above circumstances exist. Catecholamines may also induce pulmonary venous constriction, which may result in a higher wedge pressure that is not reflective of left atrial pressures, with a paradoxical increase in the PCWP with volume administration.

Despite the inherent technical and interpretation problems in obtaining PCWP values, the pressure values serve as a guide in avoiding hydrostatic pulmonary edema. Pulmonary and systemic edema are related to three principle factors: 1) increased hydrostatic pressures; 2) decreased colloid osmotic pressure; and 3) increased microvascular permeability. The acceptable pulmonary capillary wedge pressure is dependent on the clinical situation in the spinal cord injured patient. However, blood pressure, heart rate, urine output, Starling's curve for cardiac output (Fig. 3-2), chemistry evaluation or organ functions, metabolic derangements, SVO_2, DO_2, and O_2ER are all assessed concomitantly in the hemodynamically unstable patient.

Controversy frequently exists in spinal trauma patients who are resuscitated with associated brain and lung injuries. Most clinicians abide by the dictum to keep the brain and the lung as dry as possible. However, blood volume deficits may contribute to the development of adult respiratory distress syndrome (nonhydrostatic pulmonary edema) by stimulating mediator release from tissue ischemia. Late volume resuscitation of patients may cause reperfusion injury leading to fulminant respiratory failure and multiple oxygen dysfunction syndrome, which frequently is erroneously blamed on excessive fluid resuscitation. High-risk surgical patients have a higher survival rate if adequate fluid resuscitation maintains organ perfusion.

Afterload reduction is clearly not an option in the hypotensive trauma patient, and more important, in the spinal cord injured patient. However, if there is a lower cord injury without hypotension, hypertension may occur, especially in the elderly. The cautious use of vasodilators with fluid infusion may be beneficial to the cardiac output. However, vasodilators are almost never required early in the course of these patients. If they are used in any patient, whether trauma is the inherent problem or another surgical disorder, the important rule is to reassess the preload, because the afterload and cardiac output may change. As PCWP decreases, more fluid may be necessary to place the heart in an optimal position in ventricular performance curves (PCWP vs. LVSW or CI). In critically ill patients, vasodilator management has the benefit of increasing cardiac output without increasing myocardial oxygen consumption if tachycardia is not induced. Arterial desaturation may occur with all vasodilators because of attenuation of the hypoxic vasoconstrictive response and aggravation of the pulmonary shunt. Consequently, arterial oxygen saturation of hemoglobin must be monitored closely in these patients.

The use of inotropic agents to increase myocardial contractility, and subsequently, cardiac output, to reach oxygen delivery values higher than traditionally accepted is fraught with controversy. Theoretically, an increase in myocardial oxygen consumption may occur with associated myocardial ischemia and infarction. Clearly, the benefit of increasing DO_2 is to

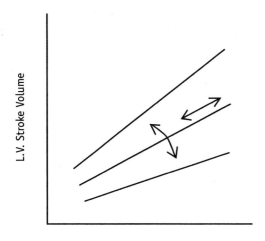

FIGURE 3-2 Starling Principle: relationship between stroke volume and diastolic pressure.

improve oxygen transport to the coronary arteries and the rest of the body to compensate for the increased myocardial work induced by inotropic agents. In spinal cord injured patients, and in trauma patients in general, all efforts should be made early in their resuscitation to optimize DO2 and prevent multiple organ dysfunction by using volume resuscitation and by a judicious use of inotropic and pressor support despite the risks of inducing myocardial ischemia.

In summary, the achievement of an optimal oxygen delivery in trauma patients with associated spinal cord injury is usually met by crystalloid bolus of 250 to 500 ml or more or blood infusion if hemoglobin is less than 10 g/dl to achieve a PCWP of 15 to 18 mmHg. Blood is given more liberally to patients with a history of coronary artery disease or myocardial dysfunction but not above a hemoglobin of 13 to 14 g/dl. Afterload reduction (in patients without complete cord transections) with nitroprusside, enalapril, hydralazine, or calcium channel blockers is instituted with frequent reassessment of preload if systemic vascular resistance is high in a patient with a stable blood pressure. If hemodynamic goals are not obtained, dobutamine is started at 3 to 5 micrograms/Kg/min if blood pressure is adequate or dopamine at the same dose if hypotensive, titrated to as high as 20 micrograms/Kg/min. If tachycardia >120 beats/minute or 10 percent above baseline is a problem with these agents, phosphodiesterase inhibitors are used. The next line of vasopressors is norepinephrine and epinephrine, starting at 1 microgram/min and titrated to the appropriate level to attain an adequate hemodynamic profile. Norepinephrine has less deleterious effects on gastric mucosal pH (pHi) than epinephrine. By adding dobutamine to epinephrine, gastric mucosal flow may be improved. Tailoring of vasopressors and other vasoactive agents should be closely monitored systemically with pulmonary artery catheters and, if tonometers are used, at the level of the stomach with monitoring of pHi or intramucosal PCO_2.

When the acute problem is resolved, patients who require DO_2 augmentation during the first 48 hours after injury may be able to subsequently meet metabolic demands by generating an adequate cardiac output without vasoactive support. Ventilatory and hemodynamic support should be progressively withdrawn, with reassessment of parameters after each step in the withdrawal process. Frequently, these patients may develop a septic crisis or a systemic inflammatory response later in the course requiring further use of invasive hemodynamic monitoring.

RECOMMENDED READING

1. Fessler RG, Masson RL. Management of thoracic fractures. In Menezes AH, Sonntag VKH, eds., *Principles of Spinal Surgery*. New York: McGraw-Hill, 1996. pp. 899–918.
2. Welberger J. Acute spinal injury. In Menezes AH, Sonntag VKH eds., *Principles of Spinal Surgery*. New York: McGraw-Hill 1996. pp. 753–768.
3. Tator CH, Duncan EG, Edmonds VE. Changes in epidemiology of acute spinal cord injury from 1947–1981. *Surg Neurol* 1993; 40:207–215.
4. Bachulus BL, Long WB, Hynes GD, Johnson MC. Clinical indications for cervical spine radiographs in the traumatized patient. *Am J Surg* 1987; 153:472–478.
5. Stover SL, Fine PR. The epidemiology and economics of spinal cord injury. *Paraplegia* 1988; 25:225–228.
6. Podolsky S, Baraff LJ, Simon RR. Efficacy of cervical spine immobilization methods. *J Trauma* 1997; 23:461–465.
7. Chapman JR, Anderson PA. Thoracolumbar spine fractures with neurologic deficit. *Orthop Clin North Am* 1994; 25:595–612.
8. Reiss SJ, Raque GH, Shields DB, Garretson HD. Cervical spine fractures with associated trauma. *Neurosurgery* 1986; 18:327–330.
9. Rhee KJ. Oral intubation in the multiple injured patient: the risk of exacerbating spinal cord damage. *Am Emerg Med* 1990; 19:511–514.
10. Talucci RC, Shaikeh KA, Schwab CW. Rapid sequence induction with oral endotracheal intubation in the multiply injured patient. *Am Surg* 1998; 54:185–187.
11. Dolan EJ, Tator CH. The effect of blood transfusion, dopamine, and gammahydroxybutyrate on posttraumatic ischemia of the spinal cord. *J Neurosurg* 1982; 56:350–358.
12. Shoemaker WC, Montgomery ES, Kaplan E. Physiologic patterns in surviving and nonsurviving shock patients. *Arch Surg* 1973; 106:630–636.

13. Gattinoni L, Brazzil, Pelosi P. A trial of goal oriented hemodynamic therapy in critically ill patients. *N Engl J Med* 1995; 333:1025–1032.

14. Shoemaker WC, Kram HB, Appel PL. Prospective trial of supranormal values as goals of resuscitation in severe trauma. *Arch Surg* 1992; 127:1175–1181.

15. Hayes MA, Timmons AC, Yau EHS. Elevation of systemic oxygen delivery in the treatment of critically ill patients. *N Engl J Med* 1994; 330: 1117–1122.

16. Scalea TM, Simon HM, Duncan AD. Geriatric blunt multiple trauma: Improved survival with early invasive monitoring. *J Trauma* 1990; 30: 129–136.

17. Siegel JH, Fabian M, Smith JA. Use of recombiant hemoglobin solution in reversing lethal hemorrhagic hypovolemic oxygen debt shock. *J Trauma* 1997; 42:199–212.

18. Abramson D, Scalea TM, Hitchcock R. Lactate clearance and survival following injury. *J Trauma* 1993; 35:584–588.

19. Davis JW, Shockford SR, Holbrook TL. Base deficit as a sensitive indicator of compensated shock and tissue oxygen utilization. *Surg Gynecol Obstet* 1991; 173:473–476.

20. Davis JW, Parks SN, Kaups KL. Admission base deficit predicts transfusion requirements and risk of complications. *J Trauma* 1996; 41:769–774.

21. Davis JW, Kaups KL. Base deficit in the elderly: a marker of severe injury and death. *J Trauma* 1998; 45:873–877.

22. Chang MC, Cheatham MC, Nelson LD. Gastric tonometry supplements information provided by the systemic indicators of oxygen transport. *J Trauma* 1994; 37:488–494.

23. Guitierrez G, Palizas, Doglio G. Gastric tonometry adds a therapeutic index of tissue oxygenation in critically ill patients. *Lancet* 1992; 339: 195–199.

24. Guzman JA, Kruse JA. Development and validation of a technique for continuous monitoring of gastric intramucosal pH. Am J Respir Crit Care Med 1996; 153:694–700.

25. Del Guercio LRM, Savino JA. Physiologic monitoring of the surgical patient. In Schwartz SI ed., *Principles of Surgery*, 5th ed. New York: McGraw Hill, 1989. pp.499–509.

26. Savino JA, Del Guercio LRM. Preoperative assessment of high-risk surgical patients. *Surg Clin North Am* 1985; 65:763–774.

27. Mehta VK, Savino JA. Cardiac support. In Ivatury RA, Cayten CG, ed. *The Textbook of Penetrating of Trauma*. Baltimore: Williams and Wilkins, 1996. pp.909–926.

28. Bishop MH, Shoemaker WC, Appel, PL, et al. Relationships between supranormal circulatory values, time delays, and outcome in severe traumatized patients. *Crit Care Med* 1993; 21:56–63.

29. Weissman C, Kemper M. The oxygen uptake-Oxygen delivery relationship during ICU interventions. *Chest* 1991; 99:430–435.

30. Chiolero R, Flatt JP, Revelly JP, et al. Effects of catecholamines on oxygen consumption and oxygen delivery in critically ill patients. *Chest* 1991; 100:1676–1684.

31. Yu M, Levy MM, Smith P, et al. Effect of maximizing oxygen delivery on morbidity and mortality rates in critically ill patients. A prospective, randomized, controlled study. *Crit Care Med* 1993; 21:830–838.

32. Weissman C, Kemper M, Harding J. Response of critically ill patients to increased oxygen demand: Hemodynamic subsets. *Crit Care Med* 1994; 22:1809–1816.

33. Tuchschmidt J, Fried J, Swinney R, et al. Early hemodynamic correlations of survival in patients with septic shock. *Crit Care Med* 1989; 17:719–723.

34. Baxter BT, Minion DJ, McCanoe CL, et al. Rational approach to postoperative transfusion in high-risk patients. *Am J Surg* 1993; 166:720–724.

35. Hebert PC, Wells G, Tweeddale M, et al. Does transfusion practice affect mortality in critically patients? *Am J Respir Crit Care Med* 1997; 155: 1618–1623.

36. Yu M, Takiguchi SA, Takanishi D, et al. Elevation of clinical usefulness of thermodilution volumetric catheters. *Crit Care Med* 1995; 23: 681–686.

37. Tuchschmidt J, Mecher C, Wagers P, Jung R. Elevated pulmonary capillary wedge pressure in a patient with hypovolemia. *J Clin Monit* 1987; 3:67–69.

38. Wood G. Effect of antihypertensive agents on the arterial partial pressure of oxygen and venous admixture after cardiac surgery. *Crit Care Med* 1997; 25:1807–1812.

39. Levy B, Bollaert, P, Lucchelli J, et al. Dobutamine improves the adequacy of gastric mucosal perfusion in epinepherine-treated septic shock. *Crit Care Med* 1997; 25:1649–1625.

4 Neurologic Evaluation and Neurologic Sequelae of the Spinal Cord Injured Patient

THOMAS T. LEE, MD
JACK STERN, MD, PhD

EGYPTIAN PHYSICIANS FIRST RECOGNIZED spinal cord injury syndromes in the seventeenth century B.C. (1). Even in the recent past, the treatment of spinal cord injuries has been approached with a sense of futility and hopelessness. This is an injury that causes a tremendous life-long physiologic, emotional, social, and economic alterations. This fatalistic attitude was changed in large part through the pioneering work of individuals such as Guttman and Borrs (2,3), who identified the need for an organized and systematic approach to this devastating injury. Other significant contributions have been the United States Veterans' Administration and its continued support and establishment of federally designated spinal cord injury centers. Recent spinal cord injuries sustained by some celebrities have also raised public awareness and funding for spinal cord injury research and treatment.

The primary goals in the management of the spinal cord injured patient include the early identification of the degree of neurologic impairment and prevention from further neurologic deterioration. Whenever spinal cord injury is suspected, the goal is to prevent further development of a worsening neurologic condition.

This can be accomplished by adequate immobilization. To more fully evaluate the degree of spinal cord injury, both in its intial stages and possible evolution, it is imperative that the examiner understand the anatomy of the spinal canal and the classifications of spinal cord injury syndromes (4).

NEUROLOGIC EVALUATION

Neurologic characterization of a spinal cord injury requires definition of the level and extent of injury. Motor levels are most objectively determined using specific tests for each nerve root of the brachial and lumbosacral plexuses. Thoracic motor levels are less exactly localized but can be approximated by careful evaluation of intercostal and abdominal muscles. Sensory levels tend to be less precise but must be assessed and carefully documented. Sensory levels are most accurately determined by beginning in the area of sensory deficit and proceeding into areas of normal sensation. The dermatomal pattern must be followed to obtain an accurate appraisal of the sensory level. There is an interface between the C4 and T3/4 dermatomes between the clavicles and the nipples because the dermatomes of the brachial plexus (C5 to T1) extend onto the upper limb. Confusion can be avoided if the upper extremity is placed in the "anatomic" position (palm up) and if sensation is sequentially tested on the clavicle (C4), lateral aspect of the arm (C5), forearm and thumb (C6), middle finger (C7), little finger (C8), medial aspect of the forearm just below the elbow (T1), medial aspect of the arm (T2), and axilla (T3). The nipples approximate the T4 sensory level and the umbilicus T10. The groin crease corresponds to L1, knee to L3, the medial aspect of the dorsum of the foot to L5, and the lateral aspect to S1. Sensory testing of the sacral dermatomes is of critical importance in determining whether an injury is complete. Lifting the leg allows testing of the posterior aspect of the calf and thigh (S2). The perineum and perianal areas are innervated by S4 and S5. Anorectal sensation can be evaluated as part of the digital rectal examination.

The baseline motor, sensory, and reflex examination is especially important because the medical and surgical management of patients with a spinal cord injury depends on the completeness of the spinal cord injury and whether neurologic deterioration occurs. Early determination of the direction of the clinical course is crucial, because there is evidence to suggest that the trauma to the spinal cord initiates a secondary injury cascade, which could lead to further deterioration. It is possible that some of these steps can be prevented or even reversed by medical or surgical treatment. However, the window of opportunity for such therapeutic intervention may be rather small. Therefore, detailed documentation of the neurologic examination is imperative.

Neurologic Grading Scales

Various systems for grading spinal cord injuries have been developed, including the Frankel classification (5), motor index score (6), Sunnybrook cord injury scale (7), and the spinal cord injury severity scale (8). All these systems are used to assess the initial neurologic status and to follow

the neurologic status after the treatment is initiated. These tools have been utilized to follow to neurologic outcome of various treatment protocols for spinal cord injuries (SCIs).

The *Frankel classification* is simple and widely used. The grading system assesses the extent of motor and sensory injuries but does not take into account the significance of bowel or bladder function. Grade A denotes a complete injury, and grade E denotes normal function. Grade B denotes complete motor paralysis but some sensory preservation. Grades C–D represent partial motor presevation below the level of injury. Grades C and D imply non-useful and useful motor strengths, respectively. Other pitfalls of the system include the lack of distinction between a patient with paraplegia and a patient with quadriplegia. This is a qualitative and quantitative assessment of the injury, and improvement within categories C or D cannot be well documented.

The *motor index score* was originally defined by Lucas and Ducker (6) and subsequently modified by the American Spinal Injury Association (ASIA) into a 100-point system. Muscle strength of the brachial and lumbosacral plexi are assessed with the traditional 0–5 motor strength scale. Nerve root motor function of C5–T1 and L2–S1 is assessed bilaterally (10 total nerve roots on each side). The muscle strength of the biceps, wrist extensors, triceps, finger flexors, small finger abductors, hip flexors, quadriceps, ankle dorsiflexors, long toe extensors, and plantar flexors is also assessed bilaterally. The preservation of S4–S5 function is now considered an "incomplete" injury. A scoring system for sensation has been added, with 0, 1, and 2 denoting absent, partial, and normal sensations.

CLASSIFICATION OF SPINAL CORD LESIONS (9)

Complete Lesions

Complete lesions result in immediate abolition of segmental reflex responses caudal to the lesion and demonstrate the unequivocal absence of motor and sensory function distal to the injury in the absence of spinal shock.

Complete Cervical Injury.   It is convenient to consider segmental lesions at different cervical levels starting from below, including T1, because of hand involvement. The relationship between the cord segments and vertebral levels must be noted, especially the observation that the spinal cord levels are higher than the vertebral levels. Complete transection of a T1 segment results in a partial loss of power of interossei, lumbricals, and abductor pollicus, plus complete paralysis of the abductor pollicis brevis and all voluntary motion below, except for the diaphragm. Sensation is absent over the medial forearm and in all areas below it, excluding the C3/C4 innervation below the clavicle. Horner's syndrome is present. Complete transection at C8 level results in clinical findings that include the aforementioned signs plus paralysis of the lumbricals and interossei with a clawed hand (*main en griffe*). Although partial weakness of the finger flexors and other hand muscles persists, there is usually good recovery of flexion and extension at the wrist. The sensory loss extends to the hand to include the fourth and fifth fingers. Additionally, injury at the C7 demonstrates marked weakness of the finger and wrist flexors and the triceps muscle. The extensor carpi radialis longus receives innervation from C6; accordingly, extension of the wrist is present and usually predominates in wrist movement with deviation to the radial side. The position of the hand with extended wrist and flexed fingers is often known as a *preacher's hand*, or *main du predicateur*. This retained function is important for later rehabilitation. Horner's syndrome may occur at this or higher levels but is usually not as well defined as the C8, T1, and T2 lesions, presumably because of the involvement of the ciliospinal center of Budge and Waller with lower lesions.

The shift from a C7 to a C6 lesion involves changes that are particularly marked. Triceps and extensor carpi radialis groups are now weaker and may function insignificantly. Biceps, brachialis, and brachioradialis muscle power is abnormal but

is unopposed at the elbow, to produce a fairly constant flexed posture. The deltoid muscle is weakened but remains functional. The arm may be gently abducted if the patient lies in the supine position, because the abductors of the shoulder are preferentially weakened. The clavicular head of the pectoralis major muscle receives innervation from C5, and hence, function may be demonstrable. This is not true for the sternal head because its innervation comes slowly from the lower segment. The bicep reflexes are absent or diminished; the sensory level extends to include the thumb, lateral aspect of the forearm, and arm. Complete transection of the C5 level results in added paralysis of the biceps, brachialis, brachioradialis, and deltoid muscles. Elevation of the shoulder is preserved with some external rotation. The arm is otherwise flail and areflexic. Diaphragmatic breathing is reduced initially but recovers and stabilizes with time. Anesthesia is almost complete over the arm, save for a strip extending down over the shoulder and the anterior aspect of the upper arm.

Complete transection in the upper cervical segments above C5 leads to respiratory failure because of the loss of phrenic innervation (C3–5). Current emphasis on early resuscitation, adequate artificial ventilation, and aggressive pulmonary care result in the survival of significant numbers of quadriplegics with high-level transection. In time, some phrenic nerve function may return and may, with auxillary respiratory muscle function, provide adequate spontaneous respiration. Phrenic nerve stimulators may also be used in selected patients. Acute and complete spinal cord lesions above the C3 segment are almost invariably fatal unless immediate respiratory support is provided. An incomplete lesion in this region may involve the lower cranial nerves nuclei and pyramidal decussation, sensory and motor tracts and nuclei, respiratory and autonomic centers and tracts, and upper cervical nerve roots. Lesions in the upper cervical spinal cord occasionally produce a peculiar pattern of sensory deficit over the face. This is described as the *Dejerine (onion peel) pattern* of sensory loss. This sensory pattern results from the involvement of the descending tract of the trigeminal nerve, which extends down as far as the C4 segment of the spinal cord. The most caudal portion of this tract carries impulses from the outermost part of the face, whereas the central areas are represented at higher levels. Pain and temperature sensation become altered in a centripetal manner from the outermost part of the face as the lesion in the trigeminal tract extends upward, hence an onion peel pattern of sensory loss.

Serious respiratory disturbances (10,11), often follow high cervical cord lesions. Irritation of the phrenic nerve may lead to hiccups, dyspnea, and coughing. Destruction of this nerve results in paralysis of the diaphragm. Bradycardia is less common; it is attributed to interruption of the fibers ascending to the cardiovascular center in the medulla oblongata. Occlusion of the vertebral arteries or thrombosis of the anterior spinal artery may cause a high cervical cord infarction, resulting in quadriplegia, impairment of various sensory modalities, bladder and bowel dysfunction, and respiratory and vasomotor disturbances.

Complete Thoracolumbar Injuries. It is important to differentiate between a cord injury and injury to the nerve roots. Roots just proximal to the cord injury will often be contused and, initially, may malfunction but recover over several months. Also, because the spinal cord terminates between the first and second lumbar vertebrae, fractures and dislocations distal to this level result in causa equina rather than cord or conus injury. The prognosis for recovery for a conus injury is frequently poorer than for cauda equina or pure cord injury.

Syndromes of Incomplete Spinal Cord Injury

Awareness of a common constellation of neurologic signs following incomplete spinal cord injury alerts the examiner through the identification of the following specific syndromes (12,13).

Central Cord Syndrome. This syndrome is commonly seen with hyperextension injuries of the cervical spine. It is particularly noted in football players with spearing injury or in the elderly. It is sometimes without radiographic evidence of vertebral injury. However, it can also occur with flexion injuries. Central cord syndromes are also associated with syringomyelia and intramedullary spinal cord tumors. The cardinal feature of central cord syndrome is the presence of disproportionate weakness of the arms when compared to the legs. Paralysis in the upper extremity is usually profound, particularly in the hands and fingers. Lower extremity functions are more preserved than upper extremity functions. The diagnosis of central cord syndrome carries a relatively good prognosis. Many patients are eventually able to ambulate, at least with some mechanical support. Some regain bowel and bladder continence. Prognosis for gaining useful function of the hand is usually much less favorable. As with the other incomplete lesions of the spinal cord, a "pure" syndrome is infrequently encountered.

Anterior Cord Syndrome. This syndrome is usually seen with flexion injuries and may be associated with acute traumatic herniation of an intervertebral disc. The syndrome involves injury to the anterior part of the spinal cord that is supplied by the anterior spinal artery. Only the posterior gray horn and both posterior columns are spared. Thus, below the level of the injury, variable degrees of paralysis coincide with diminution of pain and temperature sensation, but not with light touch, joint position sense, or vibratory sensation. Pure anterior horn cell syndrome is characterized by lower motor neuron signs of flaccid weakness, atrophy, and areflexia.

Lateral Cord Syndrome (Syndrome of Brown–Sequard). The Brown–Sequard or hemisection syndrome was originally seen with sharp hemisection of the cord in war injuries. It is seen with unilateral lesions of the cord and presents with ipsilateral motor neuron weakness, posterior column sensory loss, and vasomotor and pseudomotor changes, plus contralateral loss of pain and temperature sensations. These findings are present at a level of one or more segments distal to a lesion. Ipsilateral lower motor neuron weakness and analgesia or hypalgesia are found over a narrow band at the site of injury. In practice, the classic Brown–Sequard syndrome is rarely seen. In contrast, the type of sensory loss produced by peripheral nerve transection, in which all modalities of somatic sensation are lost together, demonstrate anesthesia in the involved area.

Posterior Column Syndrome. This rare syndrome is associated with hyperextension injuries. In its purest form, only posterior column sensation (proprioception, vibration, and crude touch) is lost. In general, prognosis for recovery relatively good.

Root Syndromes. Above the cauda equina, one, or perhaps two, nerve roots are frequently compressed as a result of vertebral subluxation or even acute disc herniation. Cervical unilaterally perched facets are known to present with neck and radicular pain alone. At times, the patient may complain of tingling or numbness. Objective sensory changes referable to a single nerve root are unusual due to an overlap of adjacent dermatomes. However, isolated weakness at the involved root is often demonstrable. Traumatic lesions of the cauda equina due to thoracolumbar or lumbar spinal injuries usually involve multiple roots with highly variable, often asymmetric patterns of motor and sensory loss. Some or all deep tendon reflexes are usually absent. Involvement of midsacral roots may denervate the bladder even if the motor and sensory function of lumbar roots is found to be intact. It is important to test sacral root function as well because injuries of the lumbosacral spine usually involve nerve roots rather than the spinal cord itself; the occurrence of isolated sacral root involvement producing saddle hypalgesia is just as possible as sacral root sparing. Because spinal roots and nerves are part of the peripheral nervous system, regeneration can occur (12) provided that anatomic continuity of the root or nerve is preserved. Thus, spontaneous motor and sensory recovery is often seen, sometimes even after prolonged intervals. Whenever a nerve root remains compressed, the chances of recovery are usually enhanced by closed or open (operative) decompression.

SEQUELAE OF SPINAL CORD INJURY

Spinal Shock

The term *spinal shock* was introduced by Hall, who described the neurogenic form, with its characteristic early areflexia and flaccidity (13). In humans, this period extends to a few weeks after injury. During the interval, marked hypertonia is present, and virtually all reflex action is absent, with the exception of the anal reflex. The presence of spinal shock indicates that, in the primate and especially in the human cord, function is highly dependent on influence from above and that the capacity for independent action is much less than in lower animals.

Spasticity

Spasticity appears after the period of spinal shock. The latter may be defined as exaggerated activity of the extensor posture mechanism with the interruption of descending inhibitory fibers of the corticobulboreticular, the caudatospinal, cerebelloreticular, and the reticulospinal pathways (14). Hypertonicity is found, together with hyperreflexia and clonus. The latter is, in effect, an expression of repeated stretch reflexes that travel through simple monosynaptic pathways.

Reflex activity other than that found with deep tendon responses appears and precedes the appearance of spasticity. This is of two types: one involves the sacral parasympathetics with reappearance and strengthening of the anal and bulbocavernous reflexes; the other is the primitive withdrawal response, which is quite variable but consists primarily of knee flexion and hip flexion. These movements are often combined with the Babinski's response (extension of the great toe and fanning of the toes). The extension movement is actually a primitive flexion withdrawal; dorsiflexion may be a better term (15). Another manifestation of the withdrawal response is the fact that the afferent discharges from the plantar responses can be elicited from wide areas on the leg and thigh. Its presence points to a wide extension of activity through much of the cord. The stimulus is usually excessive and associated with an infected full bladder or a large pressure sore or sepsis. Fortunately, modern care of the paraplegic or quadriplegic is such that these problems can largely be eliminated, and consequently, the mass reflex is uncommonly seen now. Paraplegia-in-flexion was a frequent finding in the past. Its presence was thought to point to a complete lesion, as opposed to an incomplete one with paraplegia extension. Paraplegia-in-flexion has decreased in incidence because of better nursing care and external orthosis.

The flexor spasm constitutes the third phenomenon in this group. These spasms are frequently violent. They may be initiated by stimulation of intact skin or by stimulation from a pressure sore. These are less common than in the past but have not disappeared. Other indications of the mass reflex, such as reflex sweating, may be seen in isolation. There is a complete loss of all sensory modalities with complete lesions. This is often associated with a zone of hyperpathia at the level of the injury. These patients are later aware of what would normally be appreciated as visceral pain. Sensations may be transmitted by way of the phrenic nerves, which contain sensory fibers although they are primarily motor. These enter the cord at C3, C4, and C5 levels, and hence, are at least partially above most cervical lesions. Impulses may also travel along the autonomic nervous system. A third mechanism associated with autonomic hyperreflexia is a reflex vasoconstriction in the paralyzed area that occurs in response to visceral overdistention, which usually involves the bladder. A hypertensive crisis ensues, and the patient notes severe headache, flushing of the face, stuffiness in the nose, and a pounding heartbeat. Patients are sometimes aware of unpleasant phantom sensations in the acute phase; these often involve localized areas such as the genitals. They may be severe intially but tend to disappear during rehabilitation.

Autonomic Changes

Changes in vasomotor control are very important in considering autonomic changes (16).

Spinal shock has already been discussed. The second type of shock is vascular. This occurs in the acute period and is due to a sudden loss of sympathetic control. Experimental studies place the vasomotor pathways in the ventrolateral white matter. Blood pressures isolated may remain low for a brief period of 1 to 2 days. This hypotension is different from that found with the usual traumatic shock in that it is accompanied by a slow rather than fast pulse.

The second phase is postural hypotension. This persists for many weeks after the injury and can be detected by placing the patient on a tilt table. The presence of postural hypotension reflects the slow return of vasomotor tone. Careful monitoring of blood pressure is required during tilting in this phase. Because the pressure may fall precipitously, it may pass the lower level of autoregulation of blood flow for the brain as well as for the spinal cord above the lesion.

Bladder involvement is also prominent in the state of spinal shock (17,18). There is an absence of active or reflex contraction of the detrusor muscle; therefore, the bladder distends beyond the passive obstruction at the neck. If this is unchecked, urinary retention occurs with overdistention and, eventually, overflowing continence. The period of bladder shock usually parallels the period of spinal shock—1 to 6 weeks. Reflex detrusor contractions then appear under ideal circumstances. Age and quality of bladder care are important factors. These contractions may be noted prior to the reappearance of deep tendon reflexes. The mechanism is that of simple reflex action without afferent and efferent arcs through S1, S3, and S4, paralleling the monosynaptic reflex for skeletal muscle. The end result is a full automatic bladder, which is now common.

Sexual malfunction (19,20) is another prominent manifestation of interruption of the control of the autonomic nervous system. In the male, priapism or passive engorgement is common in the acute phase. Reflex erections return later at about the same time as reflex detrusor action. Ejaculations are usually not possible with complete cervical cord transections. These require more complicated, integrated reflex actions through the lumbar sympathetic system. Gastric sensations are absent with complete lesions, but alternative sites for similar feelings may develop above the level of transection. Ovulation may be suppressed in the female for 1 or 2 months but is unaffected thereafter. Pregnancy and normal delivery are possible.

Gastrointestinal function is also seriously impaired. Ileus and fecal retention are routine in the acute phase. Ulcerations in the upper gastrointestinal tract are uncommon but are clinically well known. These may result from unbalanced actions of the vagus nerve. Bowel function returns after the period of initial spinal shock and proceeds until the establishment of the autonomic rectum with reflex defecation. This parallels reflex bladder and reflex erection activities.

The loss of sweating is another feature of autonomic involvement. Complete cervical transection leads to anhydrosis throughout the body, secondary to interruption of the sympathetic outflow. Pilomotor function is similarly affected. Thermoregulation can become a significant problem.

Posttraumatic Cystic Myelopathy (PPCM) and Posttraumatic Myelomalacic Myelopathy (PPMM)

In 1 to 3 percent of patients with spinal cord injury, tethered spinal cord and myelomalacia occurs (21). Spinal cord cysts (syringomyelia) can occur with similar frequency (22). The local hemorrhagic environment, edematous spinal cord, change in cerebrospinal fluid dynamics, and extrinsic compression predispose the patient to scar formation and secondary injury. Spinal cord cysts can form with or without spinal cord tethering (Fig. 4-1). These two entities have been reported to occur from weeks to years after the initial trauma. Continued traction and distension of the injured spinal cord could lead to neurologic (motor, sensory, sphincter functions) deterioration, axial/radicular pain patterns, and autonomic dysfunction. These two entities should be considered in the differential diagnosis of delayed neurologic deterioration in spinal cord injured patients.

The advent in magnetic resonance imaging MRI and cine-MRI techniques have made the diagnosis easier and more feasible. Surgical lysis

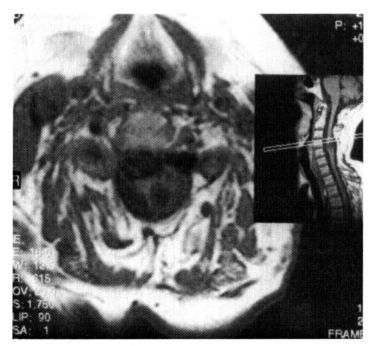

FIGURE 4-1 Axial T1-weighted RI image of a postero-laterally tethered spinal cord with intramedullary cyst formation. Note that cyst can occur with or without cord tethering.

of adhesion (untethering) and duroplasty have been demonstrated to provide some symptomatic relief for patients with PPMM (21). The role of untethering with or without cyst shunting in the PPCM patients is more controversial (22).

REFERENCES

1. Elsberg, CA. The Edwin Smith Surgical Papyrus and diagnosis and treatment of injuries to the skull and spine 5000 years ago. *Ann Med Hist* 1931; 3:271.
2. Guttman L. *Spinal Cord Injuries: Comprehensive Management and Research*. London: Blackwell Scientific Publications, 1973.
3. Borrs E, Comarr AE. *Neurological Urology*. Baltimore: University Park Press, 1971.
4. Albin MS. Acute spinal cord injury. *Crit Care Clin* 1985; 1:267.
5. Frankel HL, Hancock DO, Hysolop G, et al. The value of postural reduction in the initial treatment of closed injuries of the spine with paraplegia and tetraplegia. *Paraplegia* 1969;31:179.
6. Lucas JT, Ducker TB. Motor classification of spinal cord injuries with mobility, morbidity, and recovery indices. *Am Surg* 1979; 45:151.
7. Tator CH, Rowed DW, Schwartz ML. Sunnybrook cord injury scales for assessing neurological injuries and neurological recovery. In Tator CH, ed., *Early Management of Acute Spinal Cord Injury*. New York: Raven Press, 1982.
8. Bracken MB. Characterization of the severity of acute spinal cord injury: implication for management. *Paraplegia* 1978; 15(4):319.
9. Schneider RC, Crosby EC, Russo RH, Gosh HH. Traumatic spinal cord syndromes and their management. *Clin Neurosurg* 1973; 20:424.
10. Bellamy R, Pitts FW, Stauffer ES. Respiratory complications in traumatic quadriplegia: analysis of 20 years' experience. *J Neurosurg* 1973; 39:596.
11. Frost ER. The physiopathology of respiration in neurosurgical patients. *J Neurosurg* 1979; 50:669.
12. McQueen JD, Khan MI. Evaluation of patients with cervical spine lesions. In: The Cervical Spine. Philadelphia: JB Lippincott, 1983.
13. Hall M. *Four Memories of the Nervous System.* London, 1840.
14. Lindsley DF, Schriner LH, Magoun WH. Electromyographic study of spasticity. *J Neurophysiol* 1949; 12:197.
15. Landau WM, Clare MW. The plantar reflex in man with special references to some conditions where the extensor response is unexpectedly absent. *Brain* 1959; 82:321.
16. Kurnick NB. Autonomic hyperreflexia and its control in patients with spinal cord lesions. *Ann Intern Med* 1956; 44:678.
17. O'Flynn JD. Neurogenic bladder in spinal cord injury. *Urol Clin North Am* 1974; 1:155.
18. Thomas DG, Smallwood R, Graham D. Urodynamic observations following spinal trauma. *J Urol* 1975; 47:161.
19. Comarr AE. Sexual function among patients with spinal cord injury. *Urol Int* 1970; 25:134.
20. Weiss HD. Physiology of penile erection. *Ann Intern Med* 1972; 76:793.
21. Lee TT, Arias JM, Andrus HJL, Quencer RM, Falcone SF, Green BA. Progressive posttraumatic myelomalacic myelopathy (PPMM): treatment with untethering and expansile duroplasty. *J Neurosurg* 1997; 86:624.
22. Lee TT, Gromelski EB, Alameda G, Green BA. Surgical treatment outcome of progressive posttraumatic cystic myelopathy (PPCM). In press, *J Neurosurg* 2000.

5

Urologic Evaluation and Management of the Spinal Cord Injured Patient

GEORGE F. OWENS, MD, FACS

THE INCIDENCE OF traumatic spinal cord injury is approximately three per 100,000 population. Motor vehicle accidents and falls account for a majority of the cases. Recreational (especially diving) accidents and gunshot and stab wounds also account for a significant number of spinal cord injuries. A majority of those injured are between 15 and 34 years of age. Associated injuries are the rule in patients sustaining spinal cord injury. Consequently, immediate management of these patients should be approached in a team fashion.

Because of the high incidence of genitourinary tract injury in association with multiple trauma, a complete evaluation of the GU tract is warranted at the time of presentation, regardless of the presence or absence of hematuria. This should include computerized tomography (CT) of the abdomen and pelvis or an intravenous urogram (IVU). Magnetic resonance imaging (MRI) may also prove helpful. If bladder or urethral injury is suspected, a cystogram and retrograde urethrogram should also be performed. Initially, a catheter is placed in the bladder and left indwelling to monitor urine output. The patient is stabilized and, if required, immediate surgical repair of associated injuries is accomplished without delay.

GOALS OF UROLOGIC CARE

The primary concern of the urologist in caring for the spinal cord injured patient is to maintain renal function. Renal failure ranks as one of the most common late causes of death in male patients. The three primary causes of renal failure are: 1) bladder and sphincter dysfunction resulting in high-pressure voiding and impaired renal tubular drainage; 2) urinary tract infection; and 3) amyloid disease as a result of chronic pressure sores.

A second concern of the urologist is with affording the patient an acceptable means of bladder emptying. After a thorough assessment of the dynamics of micturition in each patient, the mechanism of voiding dysfunction can be defined and appropriate therapy instituted.

A third concern is the sexual rehabilitation of the spinal cord injured patient. In the male, this entails providing him with the means to maintain an erection adequate for sexual activity, and for those patients desiring children, an acceptable method of retrieving or producing viable sperm.

ANATOMY AND PHYSIOLOGY

To formulate a complete urologic care plan and understand and properly interpret the radiologic and urodynamic procedures performed on the spinal cord injured patient, one needs at least a basic understanding of the anatomy and neurophysiology of the GU tract.

Anatomic Considerations

The kidneys lie in the retroperitoneum, protected by the lower ribs and perirenal fatty tissue. They are supplied by renal arteries arising directly from the aorta, just below the superior mesenteric artery. Anterior to the artery lies the renal vein, which drains directly into the inferior vena cava. The renal pedicles are relatively fixed, and therefore renal vascular injury must be considered in severe trauma. The renal pelvis lies posterior to the artery. The ureters are fixed at the ureteropelvic junction and, consequently, are susceptible to avulsion at this point in deceleration injury. The remainder of the ureter courses to the bladder freely in the retroperitoneum. Blood supply is from the aorta and iliac arteries. The ureters course below the internal iliac artery and enter the bladder posteriorly and inferiorly through an oblique intramural tunnel. This tunnel provides the antireflux mechanism during voiding. Each ureter is surrounded by an incomplete collar of detrusor smooth muscle. The bladder wall consists of an outer adventitial layer, a smooth muscle layer, and an inner urothelium. The muscle layer is formed by interlacing large–diameter smooth muscle cells. The trigone of the bladder is composed of a deep detrusor layer and a more superficial muscle layer constituted of small diameter smooth muscle cells. This layer extends down into the posterior urethra, which is attached to the pubis by the puboprostatic ligament. The membranous urethra is that portion surrounded by the urogenital diaphragm. The bulbous urethra lies free within the perineum and scrotum. The remainder of the anterior urethra, the pendulous urethra, courses through the penis.

Neuroanatomic and Physiologic Considerations

The spinal cord ends at the level of the first lumbar vertebra. Below this level lies the conus medullaris and the cauda equina. The respective nerve roots exit from the corresponding intervertebral space. Injury below the first lumbar vertebra (L1) results in so-called *lower motor neuron lesions* and injury above L1 results in *upper motor neuron lesions*. On the basis of evolving knowledge of the innervation of the lower urinary tract, this classification is somewhat antiquated. It is, however, still in common use and is therefore mentioned.

Innervation to the lower urinary tract is via parasympathetic, sympathetic, and somatic nerves. The anterior segments of the pelvic plexus serve as the final common pathway for the autonomic innervation of the bladder and urethral sphincter. Preganglionic parasympathetic nerves arise from the intermediolateral gray columns of the third and fourth sacral segments of the spinal cord (S3 and S4) and run in the pelvic nerve to ganglia lying in or on the bladder wall. Postganglionic fibers then course directly to the detrusor muscle bundles. The neurotransmitter for these nerves is acetylcholine (Ach).

Sympathetic preganglionic nerves arise in the intermediolateral gray matter of the thoracolumbar cord from the 10th thoracic to the second lumbar (T10 to L2) These fibers enter the sympathetic ganglia and the postganglionic fibers and then course to the pelvic plexus and the hypogastric nerve. The neurotransmitter for the postganglionic nerves in this case is norepinephrine. The somatic nerves to the external urethral sphincter are derived from the pudendal nerve. Recent studies suggest that these nerves run with the pelvic nerve. They arise from the anterior horn of S2 to S4. They are classified as alpha motor neurons but do not exhibit the behavior typical of alpha motor neurons arising from S3, S3, and S4. The perineal portion of the pelvic floor is innervated mainly by fibers from S3, S3, and S4, and the upper pelvic floor muscles from S3 and S4.

Neuroanatomy of Sexual Excitation

The parasympathetic innervation to the penis responsible for reflex erection is derived from the pelvic nerves (S2 to S4) via the nervi erigentes. The sympathetic nerves arise from the thoracolumbar segments T11 to L2 and innervate the seminal vesicles, vas deferens, and posterior urethra. These nerves are responsible for psychogenic erections. Somatic innervation derived from sacral segments S2 to S4 via the pudendal nerve supply the bulbocavernosus, ischiocavernosus, striate urethral sphincter, and perineal muscles and is responsible for ejaculation. Seminal emission is derived from sympathetic fibers from the thoracolumbar segments T11 to L2 coursing via the hypogastric nerve.

INITIAL MANAGEMENT

Immediate Care—Paraplegic and Quadriplegic

Of paramount importance in the evaluation of the spinal cord injured patient is a systems approach in the assessment of associated injuries. Once the patient has been stabilized and other injuries requiring immediate attention have been cared for, the patient can be transferred to a neurosurgical intensive care unit. A small bore catheter, No. 12 French or No. 14 French, is left indwelling in the bladder for the first 48 hours. This allows close monitoring of urine output during the immediate post-injury period.

Spinal Shock Phase—Paraplegic and Quadriplegic

Once the patient is hemodynamically stable, the indwelling catheter is removed, and intermittent catheterization is started. Both sterile and clean techniques are employed in different spinal injury centers. An acceptable approach is to employ sterile technique when catheterization is performed by the nursing staff in quadriplegics and initially in the paraplegic. When the paraplegic patient has been instructed in self-catheterization, a method of clean self-catheterization (CSIC) is utilized.

Prolonged initial management with an indwelling urethral catheter is to be discouraged. Calcifications can form around the catheter, resulting in refractory urinary tract infections and bladder stones. In males, the incidence of urethritis and epididymitis is greater with indwelling urethral catheters. Fistulas and stricture formation are also more likely after prolonged urethral catheterization.

Bacteriuria occurs in virtually all patients on intermittent catheterization regardless of which technique, clean or sterile, is used. Culture to identify the species of bacteria as well as urinalysis to assess the degree of pyuria should be performed routinely, that is, once monthly, to determine if medical therapy is indicated. Routine antibiotic prophylaxis has not been demonstrated to decrease the incidence of clinically important urinary tract infections and therefore is not recommended. The bacteriuria is, in general, tolerated without adverse effects in the majority of patients. Certainly, if the patient appears clinically ill without any other obvious source of infection, treatment with an appropriate antibiotic on the basis of previous culture results should be instituted to sterilize the urine.

Prompt initiation of intermittent catheterization during the acute phase facilitates the overall long-term urologic management of all patients with injury to the spinal cord. The achievement of a "balanced bladder" is the ultimate goal in management. A balanced bladder can be defined as a bladder with sufficient capacity to store urine reliably and empty sufficiently without undue high pressure or vesicoureteral reflux, so that residual urine is not more than 30 percent of bladder capacity nor greater than 125 cc.

Catheterization can be started at intervals of 6 hours. A small-caliber (i.e., No. 12F or No. 14F), straight catheter should be used. The interval of catheterization should be adjusted to obtain between 300 and 350 cc of urine with each catheterization. Paraplegic patients can be taught self-catheterization during this phase of treatment. Typically, within 2 to 6 weeks the bladder will begin to function in an upper motor neuron (suprasacral) type of injury.

INTERMEDIATE MANAGEMENT

Work-Up and Evaluation—Urodynamic Studies

During this phase of management, the achievement of a balanced bladder is the goal of therapy. A complete evaluation of the patient should be performed in all cases. It is during this period that urodynamic monitoring of the lower urinary tract should be initiated. Carbon dioxide or water can be used as the medium. Water is usually preferable because its properties make it a more reliable and reproducible medium for assessment of bladder capacity and intravesical pressures. Its use, especially in the initial evaluation, is recommended.

Intravesical pressures are monitored by a small (4F or 5F) tube within the bladder. The bladder is filled via a separate larger catheter. Alternatively, a multiple-lumen catheter can be used. Intra-abdominal pressures are monitored by placing a catheter in the rectum; in the female, the vagina can also be used. The electrical activity of the external urethral sphincter of pelvic floor musculature is recorded by placing wire electrodes or needles percutaneously into the muscle. The proper position can be confirmed by observing action potentials on an oscilloscope or other suitable monitoring device. Patch electrodes can be used but are less specific in reflecting activity of the muscle group in question.

In all patients who are voiding, a simultaneous uroflow and EMG should be performed. The finding of detrusorsphincter dyssynergia is apparent when a decrease is present in flow associated with an increase in muscle activity. Monitoring both intravesicle and intra-abdominal pressures permits calculation of the pressure generated by the bladder (detrusor) by subtracting the abdominal pressure from the total intravesical pressure: ($P_{detrusor} = P_{vesical} - P_{abdominal}$). If available, videourodynamics should be performed. This allows for a visualization of the dynamics of voiding while the pressures are recorded simultaneously. It aids in differentiating internal from external sphincter detrusor dyssynergia, identifying low and high pressure reflux, and in confirming the proper location of the pressure monitors within the urinary tract. The response of the bladder to filling and emptying during voiding can thus be visualized and recorded. Cystoscopy can also be performed at this time.

In general, patients can be classified into two broad categories: those having suprasacral lesions and those with cauda equina or conus lesions, which are associated with bladder areflexia. When a management program is planned, preserving renal function and helping the patient to achieve an acceptable lifestyle are the two major considerations. Lesions may be complete or incomplete, and the degree of dyssynergia varies accordingly. In all cases, the treatment should be tailored to the individual rather than fitting the individual into a preconceived treatment protocol.

Quadriplegics with Suprasacral Lesions

In the majority of cases, quadraplegic patients with suprasacral lesions develop spontaneous voiding after a period of spinal shock. Detrusor contractions can be initiated by supropubic tapping or some other stimulus. Dyssynergia is present to varying degrees. Urodynamic studies help identify filling and voiding vesicular pressures and allow measurement of residual urine. If bladder pressure is not significantly elevated (less than 60 to 70 cm H_2O) and the amount of residual urine acceptable (less than 75 cc and uninfected), spontaneous or stimulated voiding is an acceptable method of management.

External urine collection devices, now available for men and women, can be used to protect against incontinence. There are a variety of types of condom catheters on the market. In most cases, one can be found that is acceptable and reliably remains in place. Women can wear any of the high-absorbency pads now marketed by several companies.

When dyssynergia causes significant obstruction, high voiding pressures are generated that accelerate the development of renal failure. In those patients with external sphincter–detrusor dyssynergia, the external sphincter can sometimes be successfully ablated with pharmacologic therapy. Alpha sympatholytics such as phentolamine, phenoxybenzamine, and prazosin have been used successfully in the past. Current treatment employs selective alpha-1 blockers such as terazosin or doxazosin or the newer alpha-1a blocker, tamsulosin. Skeletal muscle relaxants (dantrolene and baclofen) have also been employed successfully. Transurethral external sphincterotomy to ablate the sphincter can also be performed and is without the side effects of long-term medication. Occasionally, transurethral resection of the prostate and bladder neck is required to resect the internal urethral aphincter. In older patients with prostate hyperplasia, transurethral resection may be necessary to relieve the obstructive prostate.

If hyperreflexia results in too-frequent detrusor contractions, anticholinergics such as propantheline or smooth muscle relaxants such as oxybutynin, tolterodine, or hyoscyamine (which also have an anticholinergic type of activity), or musculotropics such as flavoxate can be used to control the bladder. Spontaneous voiding is still an option. In selected patients with some use of their upper extremities or with patients able to have 24-hour care, the bladder can be paralyzed with anticholinergics and intermittently catheterized. Alternatively, a suprapubic cystostomy in the male or an indwelling bladder catheter in the female can be used to collect urine. However, because of the long-term complication of indwelling catheters (urinary tract infection, calculi, contracted bladder, hematuria, catheter blockage) these should be considered a second-line therapeutic choice. The use of transurethral catheters in the male is especially discouraged because of the additional complications of urethritis, epididymitis, urethral stricture, and urethrocutaneous fistulous formation.

Quadriplegics with Areflexic Bladders

In certain patients with multiple levels of injury, the quadriplegic patient will not have any detrusor activity. Oral cholinomimetic therapy with bethanechol has not been demonstrated to be effective in any well-controlled studies. These patients generally require catheter drainage. Currently, clinical trials of sacral nerve stimulation are being conducted. Initial results are promising, and bladder stimulation will probably become a clinically feasible choice in the near future.

Paraplegics with Suprasacral Lesions

In these patients as in others, the achievement of a balanced bladder is the goal of therapy. Patients with an acceptably low vesical voiding pressure can be allowed to void into an external collection device. As mentioned, these are now available for men and women. For those patients with a high vesicular voiding pressure, those few men unable to wear a condom catheter (or similar device), and those women unable to remain satisfactorily dry with a collection device or pad, an alternative management protocol must be devised.

For those patients with hyperreflexia and high intravesicular pressure, the first line of therapy should be medication to paralyze the bladder and intermittent catheterization to empty it. Occasionally, the patient may be able to void with abdominal straining without causing harmful high pressure voiding (> 60 to $70 \ H_2O$). The Crede maneuver should be avoided because it is associated with high voiding pressures. The use of anticholinergics or smooth muscle relaxants or antispasmotics will, in most cases, successfully control the hyperreflexic bladder. Oxybutynin (Ditropan) is the author's drug of choice. The dose must be titrated to obtain the desired response. Typically, a patient is started on 5 mg b.i.d., and the dose is increased as needed up to 5 mg t.i.d. or q.i.d. Complete bladder paralysis is the end point of therapy, to maintain a low pressure system. The patients catheterize themselves, utilizing a clean technique starting with 6-hour intervals and adjusting the time between catheterizations to obtain approximately 350 to 400 cc with each catheterization. Men can apply a condom catheter in between catheterizations and women can wear an appliance or incontinence pad to protect against breakthrough bladder contractions.

Those patients with hyperreflexic bladder who are unresponsive to anticholinergic medication and who exhibit detrusor–sphincter dyssynergia pose a difficult management problem with respect to obtaining a balanced bladder. Medical ablation of the sphincter can be attempted with alpha blockers and/or antispasmodics, however, the success rate is low. Traditionally, male patients have undergone transurethral sphincterotomy, rendering them incontinent, and worn condom catheters to collect the urine. For those patients with the less common detrusor–internal sphincter dyssynergia, a transurethral resection of the bladder neck and prostate can be attempted. The justification for these procedures is that through ablation of the source of obstruction, the patient will be able to void successfully and not experience dangerous high-intravescular pressures. Unfortunately, the success rate of transurethral sphincterotomy is not always high. An alternative treatment is partial cystectomy with bladder augmentation using a segment of detubularized bowel; ileum or colon can be employed. Detubularization is required to obliterate bowel contractions and avoid creation of a high-pressure system.

Paraplegics with Areflexic Bladders

For patients unable to empty the bladder by abdominal straining, the treatment of choice is intermittent catheterization. A regimen of clean intermittent self-catheterization offers significant advantages over the use of indwelling bladder catheters. Urethrocutaneous fistulas, urethritis, bladder calculi, bladder contracture, urinary tract infection, and urosepsis are more common with indwelling catheters. The incidence of hospitalization to treat these complications is also higher with indwelling catheters, increasing the cost of care for these patients.

Patients should be instructed in the method of clean intermittent self-catheterization as well as a program of urinary acidification. Intake should be adjusted to produce a steady urinary output and permit the patients to catheterize themselves on an acceptable schedule.

A certain number of patients will be unable or will refuse to perform self-catheterization. Tapping the suprapubic region or manually stimulating the anal sphincter or pulling on the pubic hair will in some cases induce a detrusor contraction. This can be combined with abdominal straining or the Crede maneuver to empty the bladder.

LONG-TERM MANAGEMENT

Patients should remain in spinal care programs during their rehabilitation and recovery. As time passes, the nature of the bladder dysfunction may change or complications may develop. There is no universally accepted best method of management. In general, especially in males, indwelling urethral catheters should be avoided. Women tolerate catheterization better than men, and acceptable external collection devices are still not widely available. Therefore, catheterization is more often the management option employed in women. The decision to perform any surgical procedure, for example external sphincterotomy, transurethral resection of the prostate, bladder augmentation, or sacral nerve root stimulation, should be postponed until the treating physician is sure that the results of the spinal cord injury are not transient. This usually means waiting several months to a year before performing any definitive surgical procedures.

One must keep in mind the basic tenets of urologic care: to preserve renal function and to aid in providing an acceptable, functional lifestyle. Overall, most patients are managed by condom drainage. Indwelling catheters, mostly in women, and intermittent catheterization are the next most common method of long-term management. Throughout the intermediate phase of management, patients should be observed for spontaneous voiding.

Once the long-term management strategy has been decided, the patient should be evaluated periodically. To date, there are no reliable early predictors of future complications. In long-term management, therefore, problems must be identified as early as possible. Patient awareness and teaching are integral to successful long-term management. They should be instructed to report any changes in their routine or in bladder function. Urinalysis should be monitored on a regular basis. Leukocyte esterase, nitrite, and protein content and pH balance can all be easily monitored at home by dipstick analysis of the urine.

Periodic microscopic examination and culture should also be performed at least every 3 months, and at times, monthly, depending on the clinical situation. Assessment of renal function is also necessary. Serum electrolytes, creatinine, and blood urea nitrogen should be checked at least yearly, if not biannually. Creatinine clearance should be checked annually, because serum creatinine can be misleading as an indicator of renal insufficiency in spinal cord injury patients with muscle atrophy. The intravenous urogram (IVU) has traditionally been used to assess renal function. Its use, however, is not without complications, and other techniques with less potential harmful complications are now available. Evaluation of renal function with radionuclides offers a useful alternative. [131]I of ^{123}I hippuran scans or [99m]TcDTPA or DMSA or MAG3 are simple, effective tests to assess renal function. A plain film of the kidney, ureter, and bladder (KUB) should be performed to check for calculi. When indicated, a renal sonagram, IVU, cystogram, or voiding cystourethrogram can be ordered to further delineate any abnormal finding. A nuclear scan and KUB should be done yearly. Urodynamics are not done routinely. Instead, they are performed if any changes are noted on the routine studies and urodynamic information is necessary to determine proper therapy. Whatever procedures are used and whatever schedule is employed, it is important to continue follow-up because complications can occur many years postinjury. With more patients surviving longer, continued screening is essential.

SEXUAL REHABILITATION

Erection and ejaculation are both parasympathetic and sympathetic nervous responses. Parasympathetic nerves from S2 to S4 innervate the corpora cavernosa, and sympathetic nerves from the thoracolumbar erection center (T11 to L2) contribute to erections. Emission and ejaculation occur through stimulation of the sympathetic nerves from T12 to L2 and pudendal nerves originating from the somatic sacral roots (S2 to S4). Sexual function depends on the level and completeness of the injury. Suprasacral lesions tend to result in reflex erections but not psychologically induced erections. Conus or cauda equina lesions generally are associated with no erections at all. Emission and ejaculation depend on the intactness of the sympathetic outflow from T11 to L2 and the somatic nerves from S2 to S4, the hypogastric and pudendal nerves, respectively.

Approximately 67 percent of spinal cord injury patients have erections, while only about 10 percent will ejaculate. In most patients, it will take up to 6 months for recovery of sexual function. For those patients with satisfactory erections but retrograde ejaculation who desire children, the semen can be obtained from the bladder. The urine is sterilized and alkalinized and the bladder emptied. After ejaculation, the bladder is catheterized and irrigated with a buffered medium such as Ham's F-10, and the semen is collected and washed for insemination. For those patients unable to have erections or those who have a lack of seminal emission, transrectal electroejaculation and glandular vibratory stimulation can be utilized to induce erections and ejaculation. Intrathecal neostigmine injection is no longer used to stimulate erections. Patients with lesions above T6 are at risk of autonomic dysreflexia as a result of the stimulation. Therefore close monitoring of vital signs is especially important in these patients. In patients with retrograde ejaculation desiring children, the semen is collected as described previously. Semen quality is generally impaired, with poor motility being the most common abnormality. There is also a higher percentage of abnormal morphology. This is a developing technology, and one would expect higher success rates as the methods are refined.

Not all patients are candidates for stimulation. Penile prosthesis, either semirigid or inflatable, offers an alternative therapy for these patients. The procedure is relatively simple, and the success rate high and complication rate low.

SPECIAL CONSIDERATIONS

Urinary Tract Infection and Urolithiasis

A general consensus does not exist concerning the use of antimicrobial therapy in the spinal cord injured patient. Most investigators would agree that prophylactic antimicrobials are not necessary in patients who are catheter free. Some authors suggest prophylaxis in patients with indwelling catheters or on intermittent catheterization. However, several excellent large studies have failed to demonstrate an advantage to long-term antimicrobial prophylaxis; therefore, this author does not utilize it. Significant pyuria (>50 leukocytes per high-power field) and symptomatic bacteriuria—bacteriuria associated with fever or significant symptoms—should be treated with an appropriate antibiotic. Empiric therapy can be started on the basis of the results of the most recent routine urine culture and then adjusted on the basis of culture and sensitivities of specimens sent off before therapy was started.

Bladder calculi cause significant irritative signs and are often infected. In general, they should be removed when detected. For calcification around indwelling catheters, a solution of 10 percent hemiacidrin in water can be used to irrigate the bladder. One should take care to monitor the serum magnesium in patients undergoing this therapy because hypermagnesemia is a potential complication. For patients with larger bladder calculi that cannot be irrigated free, transurethral electrohydraulic lithotripsy or laser lithotripsy is usually effective in fragmenting the stone, thus allowing its aspiration to

rid the bladder of the fragments. For very large stones or stones not amenable to lithotripsy, open cystolithotomy is required.

Approximately 8 percent of spinal cord injured patients develop renal calculi. Recurrence rates are high. The incidence of renal calculi is highest in the first year after injury and higher in patients with bladder calculi. The occurrence of struvite stones is greatly increased in the spinal cord injured patient. Up to 98 percent of stones in these patients have some degree of struvite, as opposed to 15 percent of stones in the general population that are struvite in composition. The presence of struvite is associated with deterioration in renal function in up to 50 percent of patients. They are typically infected, usually by urease-producing bacteria, and are associated with chronic urinary tract infection. Because of impaired mobility and calcium resorption, the spinal cord injured patient is also more likely to develop calcium stones.

The presence of any asymptomatic stone does not require intervention. However, urinary obstruction, recurrent infection, and renal impairment are all indications for intervention. For patients able to tolerate the procedure, extracorporeal shock wave lithotripsy (ESWL) offers a nonsurgical approach to elimination of the stone. Alternatively, percutaneous endourologic nephrolithotomy or nephrolithotripsy for renal stones and transureteral endoscopic lithotripsy for removal of ureteral stones are now widely available and are the "surgical" procedures of choice in treatment of urolithiasis. Although the initial treatment of an asymptomatic stone remains conservative, rarely is it justified with the availability of ESWL and endourology to leave a symptomatic stone untreated.

Automatic Dysreflexia (Hyperreflexia)

More than 80 percent of patients with lesions above T6 exhibit signs and symptoms of this disorder. Urinary retention with bladder distention is one of the most common causes of this syndrome. Its occurrence is a medical emergency. Signs and symptoms include hypertension, sweating above the level of the lesion, piloerection, restlessness, anxiety, bradycardia, pounding headache, and flushed face. It is secondary to massive sympathetic outflow. Other urologic causes include catheterization, urinary tract infection, testicular torsion, electroejaculation, distention of the renal pelvis, and urologic procedures. The immediate treatment is removal of the stimulus. In cases of bladder distention, either catheterization to relieve retention or replacement or irrigation of an obstructed indwelling catheter is indicated. The patient should be placed with the head elevated; other potential causes such as fecal impaction should be ruled out. If the patient does not respond to removal of the offending stimulus, pharmacologic therapy is indicated. Rapid decrease in blood pressure can be achieved by continuous intravenous administration of nitroprusside. Alternatively, one can use hydralazine, ganglionic blockers such as pentolinium and trimethaphan, diazoxide, phentolamine, amyl nitrate inhalation, and occasionally spinal anesthesia. Nitroprusside in 100 mg/cc concentration in 5 percent dextrose and water offers the quickest response and the best control. Initial therapy with 1 mg/kg/min is started, and the dose titrated to achieve normal pressure. An arterial line or some other method is required for continuous monitoring of the blood pressure.

Phenoxybenzamine, a nonselective alpha blocker, has been used in treatment of recurrent autonomic dysreflexia. Pentolinium and mecamylamine (ganglionic blockers) have also been suggested, as has guanethidine.

New Treatment Modalities

The artificial urinary sphincter has been successfully placed in patients with spinal cord lesions. In patients with areflexic bladders and incompetent bladder outlets, it has been successfully implanted and used in conjunction with intermittent catheterization. It also has potential as a substitute sphincter for patients requiring sphincterotomy. Initial problems with erosion at the site of cuff placement have been rectified by

design changes. Careful choice of the proper cuff pressure and size is required to prevent complications.

Bladder contraction by selective stimulation of the anterior nerve roots via implantable electrodes is now being performed at several medical centers and offers great promise in the control of bladder function. Inhibition of bladder contractions by nerve stimulation is also in clinical trials, and if successful, will offer another alternative to pharmacologic manipulation. These methods or extradural nerve root stimulation to control detrusor and sphincter activity are perhaps the most exciting advances since the concept of intermittent catheterization was first introduced.

CONCLUSION

As length of survival increases in patients with spinal cord injury, proper urologic management is even more important. As our knowledge of the physiology of micturition extends, we can expect significant advances in treatment methods for the spinal cord injured patient. Further study is needed to identify early predictors of potential complications and bladder functions. These, together with the rapid technologic advances being made, will allow these patients to live longer, more normal lives. In the foreseeable future, we may be able to override the neural dysfunction by externally stimulating selected nerves, thereby reproducing a normal micturition reflex. We have for the most part advanced beyond the need for urinary diversion, and soon patients may be managed catheter-free and without the need for pharmacologic intervention or surgical procedures.

RECOMMENDED READINGS

1. Anderson RU, Hsieh-Ma ST. Association of bacteriuria and pyuria during intermittent catheterization after spinal cord injury. *J Urol* 1983; 130:299.

2. Barrett DM, Goldwasser B. The artifical urinary sphincter; current management philosophy. *AUA Update Serier* 1986; 5:2.

3. Barton CH, Khonsari F, Vaziri ND, et al. Effect of modified transurethral sphincterotomy on autonomic dysreflexia. *J Urol* 1986; 135:83.

4. Bedbrook GM. The development and care of spinal cord paralysis. *Paraplegia* 1987; 25:172.

5. Bennett CJ, Seager SW, Vasher EA, McGuire EJ. Sexual dysfunction and electroejaculation in men with spinal cord injury: review. *J Urol* 1988; 139:453.

6. Berard E, Depassio J, Pangau N, Landi J. Self-catheterization: urinary complications and the social resettlement of spinal cord injured patients. *Paraplegia* 1985; 23:386.

7. Chagnon S, Leroy F, Vallee CH, Blery M. Cinefluoroscopic study of the micturition and cystomanometry in patients with spinal cord injuries: a comparative study in 50 cases. *J Radiologic* 1985; 66:26.

8. Chagnon S, Vallee CH, Laissy JP, Blery M. Comparison of ultrasound and intravenous urography imaging of the urinary tract for investigation of 50 patients with spinal cord injuries. *J Radiologie* 1985; 66:801.

9. Culkin DJ, Wheeler JS, Nemchausky BA, et al. Percutaneous nephrolithotomy in spinal cord injury population. *J Urol* 1986; 136:1181.

10. DeGroat WC. Anatomy and physiology of the lower urinary tract. *Urol Clin of North Am* 1993; 20:3.

11. DeVivo MJ, Fine PR. Predicting renal calculus occurrence in spinal cord injury patients. *Arch Phys Med Rehabil* 1986; 67:722.

12. Dimitrijevic MM, Dimitrijevic MR, Illis LS, et al. Spinal cord stimulation for the control of spasticity in patients with chronic spinal cord injury: II. Neurophysiologic observations. *Cent Nerv Syst Trauma* 1986; 3:129.

13. Dimitrijevic MR, Illis LS, Nakajima K, et al. Spinal cord stimulation for the control of spasticity in patients with chronic spinal cord injury: II. Neurophysiologic observations. *Cent Nerv Syst Trauma* 1986; 3:145.

14. Dimitrijevic MR. Neurophysiology in spinal cord injury. *Paraplegia* 1987; 25:205.

15. Dudognon P, Labrousse C, Lubeau M, et al. Early vesico-ureteral reflux following conus medullaris injury: case report. *Paraplegia* 1986; 24:194.

16. Ergas Z. Spinal cord injury in the United States: a statistical update. *Cent Nerv Syst Trauma* 1985; 2:19.

17. Erickson RP. Autonomic hyperreflexia: pathophysiology and medical management. *Arch Phys Med Rehabil* 1980; 61:431.

18. Falols WF, Stacy WK. A prospective analysis of renal function in patients with spinal cord injuries and persistent bacilluria. *Milit Med* 1986; 151:116.

19. Fellstrom B, Butz M, Danielson BG, Ljunghall S. The effects of methenamine-hippurate upon urinary risk factors for renal stone formation. *Scand J Urol Nephrol* 1985; 19:125.

20. Gardner-Grundy D, Swain A, Russell J. ABC of spinal cord injury. BP, Parsons KF, Soni BM, Krishnan KR. The managemnet of upper urinary tract calculi in spinal cord damaged patients. *Paraplegia* 1985; 23:371.

21. Gardner BP, Parsons KF, Machin DG, et al. The urological management of spinal cord damaged patients: a clinical algorithm. *Paraplegia* 19986; 24:138.

22. Gocking K, Gebhardt K. Indikation und ergebnisse der transurethralen 12-uhr-sphinkterotimie in der therapie der neurogenen blasenentleerungsstorungen bei querschnittslakmung. *Z Urol Nephrol* 1986; 79:207.

23. Gosling JA, Dixon JS, Lendon RG. The autonomic innervation of the human male and female bladder neck and proximal urethra. *J Urol* 1977; 118(2):302FF.

24. Green BA, Eismont FJ. Acute spinal cord injury: a systems approach. *Cent Nerv Syst Trauma* 1984; 1:173.

25. Green BG, Sloan SL. Penile prosthesis in spinal cord injured patients: combined psychosexual counselling and surgical regimen. *Paraplegia* 1986; 24:167.

26. Grundy D, Russell J. ABC of spinal cord injury: urological management. *Br Med J* 1986; 292:249.

27. Grundy D, Swain A, Russell J. ABC of spinal cord injury: early management and complications—I. *Br Med J* 1986; 292:44.

28. Grundy D, Swain A, Russell J. ABC of spinal cord injury: early management and complications—II. *Br Med J* 1986; 292:123.

29. Grundy D, Russell J. ABC of spinal cord injury: Later management and complications—I. *Br Med J* 1986; 292:677.

30. Halstead LS, VerVoort S, Seager SWJ. Rectal probe electrostimulation in the treatment of anejaculatory spinal cord injured men. *Paraplegia* 1987; 25:120.

31. Hoffberg HJ, Cardenas DD. Bladder trabeculation in spinal cord injury. Arch Phys Med Rehabil 1986; 67:750.

32. Hughes JT. Historical review of paraplegia before 1918. *Paraplegia* 1987; 25:168.

33. Kakulas BA. The clinical neuropathology of spinal cord injury: a guide to the future. *Paraplegia* 1987; 25:212.

34. Lockhart JL, Vorstman B, Weinstein D, Politano VA. Sphincterotomy failure in neurogenic bladder disease. *J Urol* 1986; 135:86.

35. Lloyd LK. New trends in urologic management of spinal cord injured patients. *Cent Nerv Syst Trauma* 1986; 3:3.

36. Lloyd LK, Kuhlemier KV, Fine PR, Stover SL. Initial bladder management in spinal cord injury: does it make a difference? *J Urol* 1986; 135:523.

37. McGuire TJ, Kumar VN. Autonomic dysflexia in the spinal cord-injured. *Postgrad Med* 1986; 80:81.

38. Mathe JF, Labat JJ, Lanoiselee JM, Buzelin JM. Detrusor inhibition in suprasacral spinal cord injuries: is it due to sympathetic overactivity? *Paraplegia* 1985; 23:201.

39. Maynard FM, Glass J. Management of the neuropathic bladder by clean intermittent catheterization: 5 year outcome. *Paraplegia* 1987; 25:106.

40. Mohler JL, Barton SD, Blouin RA, et al. Evaluation of creatinine clearance in spinal cord injury patients. *J Urol* 1986; 136:366.

41. Nance PW, Shears AH, Givner ML, Nance DM. Gonadal regulation in men with flaccid paraplegia. *Arch Phys Med Rehabil* 1985; 66:757.

42. Perkash I. Long-term urologic management of the patient with spinal cord injury. *Urol Clin of North Am* 1993; 20:3.

43. Perkash I, Martin DE, Warner H. Reproductive problems of paraplegics and the present status of electroejaculation. *Cent Nerv Syst Trauma* 1986; 3:13.

44. Pietronigro DD, DeCrescito V, Tomasula JJ, et al. Ascorbic acid: a putative biochemical marker of irreversible neurologic functional loss following spinal cord injury. *Cent Nerv Syst Trauma* 1985; 2:85.

45. Raeder JC, Gisvold SE. Perioperative autonomic hyperreflexia in high spinal cord lesions: a case report. *Acta Anaesthesiol Scand* 1986; 30:672.

46. Rao KG, Hackler RH, Woodlief RM, et al. Real-time renal sonography in spinal cord injury patients: prospective comparision with excretory urography. *J Urol* 1986; 135:72.

47. Rossier AB, Fam BA. From intermittent catheterization to catheter freedom via urodynamics: a tribute to Sir Ludwig Guttman. *Paraplegia* 1979; 17:73.

48. Ruuter ML. Cystometrographic patterns in predicting bladder function after spinal cord injury. *Paraplegia* 1985; 23:243.

49. Ruuter ML, Lehtonen TA. Bladder outlet surgery in men with spinal cord injury. *Scand J Urol Nephrol* 1985; 19:241.

50. Stover SL, Lloyd LK, Nepomuceno CS, Gale LL. Intermittent catheterization: follow-up studies. *Paraplegia* 1977–78; 15:38.

51. alalla A, Bloom JW, Nguyen Q. Successful intraspinal extradural sacral nerve stimulation for bladder emptying in a victim of traumatic spinal cord transection. *Neurosurgery* 1986; 19:955.

52. Thomas DG. Spinal cord injury. In Murphy AR, Stephenson TP, Wein AJ, (eds)., *Urodynamics, Principles, Practices and Applications*. New York: Churchill Livingstone, 1984.

53. Viera A, Merritt JL, Erickson RP. Renal function in spinal cord injury: a preliminary report. *Arch Phys Med Rehabil* 1986; 67:257.

54. Warner H, Martin DE, Perkash I, et al. Electrostimulation of erection and ejaculation and collection of semen in spinal cord injured humans. *J Rehabil Res Dev* 1986; 23:21.

55. Wein AJ. Drug treatment of voiding dysfunction. Part I: Evaluation of drugs: treatment of emptying failure. *AUA Update Series* 1988; 7:106.

56. Wein AJ. Drug treatment of voiding dysfunction. Part II: Drug treatment of storage failure. *AUA Update Series* 1988; 7:114.

57. Wu Y, Nanninga JB, Hamilton BB. Inhibition of the external urethral sphincter and sacral reflex by anal stretch in spinal cord injured patients. Arch Phys Med Rehabil 1986; 67:135.

58. Wyndale JJ. Urology in spinal cord injured patients. *Paraplegia* 1987; 25:267.

59. Wyndale JJ. Urethral sphincter dyssynergia in spinal cord injured patients. *Paraplegia* 1987; 25:10.

60. Yalla SV. Spinal cord injury. In Krane RJ and Siroky MB, (eds)., *Clinical Neurology*. Boston: Little, Brown, and Co. 1979.

6 Advantages and Disadvantages of Roentgenograms in the Diagnosis of Odontoid Fractures

ALAIN B. ROSSIER, MD
IL Y. LEE, MD
AY-MING WANG, MD

BECAUSE UNDIAGNOSED fracture-dislocation at the C1 to C2 level may be catastrophic, early correct diagnosis is of the essence. Open-mouth views may be difficult to interpret and misleading. In many instances, only tomograms will allow a correct assessment of the situation.

We report our findings in a patient who was referred to us within 2 hours of injury with a diagnosis of odontoid fracture without neurologic deficit. Subsequent neurologic and roentgenographic work-up negated both of these findings and disclosed other pathologic features of the cervical spine that would not have been discovered if the roentgenograms had been confined to the area suspected of having sustained major trauma. The sequence of events in this particular case seemed of sufficient interest to justify their reporting.

CASE REPORT

While walking in an airport area, a 20-year old man hit the top of his head against the back flap of a plane wing. He fell to the ground and was unconscious for about 5 minutes. The patient was transported in the supine position to a local clinic by emergency paramedics. The sensory and motor neurologic evaluation was reported as normal. However, the roentgenograms of the cervical spine were interpreted as showing posterior displacement of C1 on C2 with questionable fracture of the odontoid. Past history revealed that the patient had sustained a go-cart injury as a child, during which he was knocked into the air and somersaulted, landing on his right side and injuring his right elbow and knee. The patient was unconscious for 5 to 10 minutes and experienced some decrease in the grip strength of the right hand, which eventually fully recovered. Cervical spine roentgenograms were reported as normal.

At the time of admission to our spinal cord injury service 2 hours after injury, the patient did not have any subjective complaints. He was awake and oriented and had tenderness in the

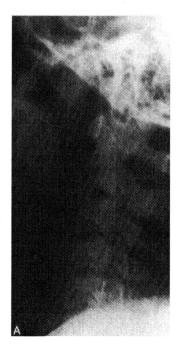
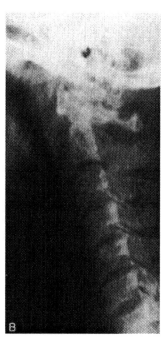

FIGURE 6-1 Initial roentgenograms. **A.** In the referring clinic. Apparent step off C1 to C2 secondary to rotation of the cervical spine below C2. The head is in a nearly true lateral position (superimposition of posterior border of mandibles). **B.** In the Spinal Cord Injury Service. Same misleading step off C1 to C2 secondary to rotation of the head. The cervical spine below C2 is in a nearly true lateral position (superimposition of the articular facets).

upper cervical spine by palpation. Cranial nerves were all normal. Reflexes in the upper and lower extremities were 1+ and 2+, respectively. Horner's syndrome was not present, and there was no sensory deficit. However, the motor examination revealed weakness of hand grip and wrist flexors and extensors bilaterally (3+ out of 5). Paresis was more marked on the right. Supine lateral roentgenograms of the cervical spine that had been done in the referring clinic showed what was diagnosed as posterior displacement of C1 on C2 (Fig. 6-1). The open-mouth view that was carried out in our service was inconclusive. In view of these findings, it was decided to fit the patient with a halo vest. At the time the patient was positioned for its application, another lateral roentgenogram of the cervical spine showed "reduction" of the retrolisthesis C1 on C2 (Fig. 6-2). The halo vest was then fitted. Lateral and anteroposterior tomograms of the suspected area were performed to better define the location of the suspected odontoid fracture (Fig. 6-3). Unexpectedly, they did not show any dens fracture or displacement. In view of the apparent discrepancy in these findings, bone scans with

99^{m}Tc-labeled methylene diphosphonate were carried out 2 and 8 days after injury with the

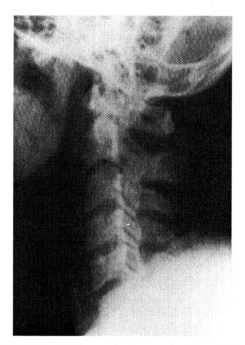

FIGURE 6-2 Radiograph taken at the time the halo vest was fitted. "Correction" of the step off C1 to C2. Head and cervical spine are in a nearly true lateral position.

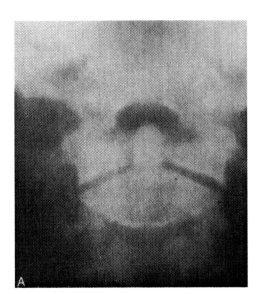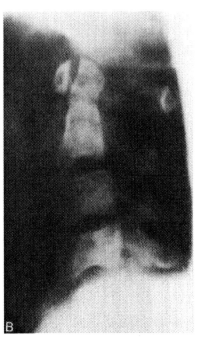

FIGURE 6-3 Tomograms of C1 to C2. **A.** Anteroposteriror view. **B.** Lateral view. Both show no visible fracture or misalignment.

hope that this would aid in making the diagnosis (1,2). No increased uptake of the radiopharmaceutical agent could be observed in the suspected cervical area.

In view of these negative findings, the halo vest was removed. However, it was believed justified to carry out a metrizamide tomomyelogram to exclude any intraspinal pathology that could account for the motor deficit in the hands. No abnormality could be seen at the C1 to C3 levels. Although the cuts in the head neutral and flexion positions did not show any impingement of bone or soft tissue within the spinal canal, the cuts to the right at C6 to C7 in the head extension position were strongly suggestive of spondylotic changes impinging within the spinal canal (Fig. 6-4).

Mid- and left-sided cuts were normal. These findings appeared to correlate well with the motor deficit, which was more pronounced in the right hand and wrist. The patient was fitted with a protective soft collar. At the time of discharge 2 weeks later, the patient had fully recovered and did not show any motor deficit.

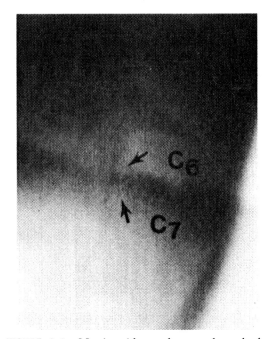

FIGURE 6-4 Metrizamide myelogram through the lumbar route. Tomographic cut to the right: spondylotic changes (arrows) at the posterior border of C6 to C7 vertebral bodies with some impingement within the spinal canal.

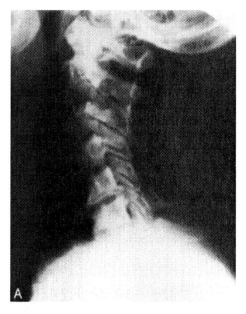

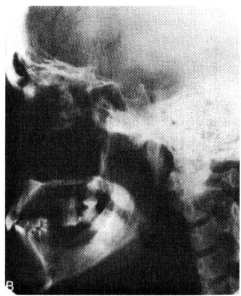

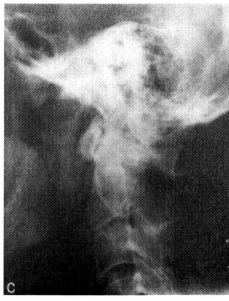

FIGURE 6-5 Normal subject. **A.** Step off C1 to C2 secondary to the rotation of the head. The cervical spine below C2 is in a nearly true lateral position. **B.** Step off C1 to C2 due to the reverse situation: perfect lateral position of the the head but marked rotation of the cervical spine. **C.** True lateral head and neck position: no step off C1 to C2.

DISCUSSION

The sequence of events that took place in the case indicates the fact that roentgenograms may be misleading in the diagnosis of dens fracture dislocation. It appears that the positioning of the patient in an exact lateral projection, not only of the head but also of the cervical spine segments below C2, is of the utmost importance in achieving an accurate diagnosis in traumatic odontoid

pathology. The diagnosis error, based upon the initial radiograms, can be attributed to two factors, the importance of which appear to have been somewhat underestimated in past publications dealing with cervical spine trauma (3–8). In the first instance, one roentgenogram was not taken in a true lateral position of the cervical spine from C2 downward, although the head position was close to a true lateral (superimposition of the posterior border of the mandibles) (see Fig. 6-1A). In the second instance, although the roentgenogram was taken in a nearly true lateral position of the cervical spine from C2 downward, the head position was rotated to a major extent (see Fig. 6-1B). To corroborate this postulate, we have tried to duplicate the mistakes previously described by placing a patient without spine pathology in different positions of the head and neck in relation to each other. The results of these experiments have demonstrated that the aforementioned hypothesis concerning the role of the patient's head and neck positioning was correct (Fig. 6-5).

When the neck is rotated and the head is perfectly lateral, the lateral aspect of the vertebral body of C2 rotates anteriorly and causes a double contour on the film that may be mistakenly interpreted as a fracture. The time relationship between the anterior arch of C1 and the odontoid process of C2 should use a continuous straight line as a landmark.

The posttraumatic transitory neurologic deficit in the patient's hands and wrists, which did not correlate with the suggestive roentgenographic dens pathology, could have been related to the degenerative spondylotic changes at the C6 to C7 levels. The patient's previous history of weakness in the right hand following head and neck injury points to a similar cause-and-effect relationship.

Apart from the interesting misleading roentgenographic findings in the patient, this case also illustrates another important point: investigations should not be limited to the supposedly pathologic area but should cover further possible abnormalities in other locations that could also be involved in the pathologic process, as suggested by a careful neurologic evaluation. Philosophically, it must be acknowledged that our natural tendency as physicians is to focus more on previous abnormal findings than to look for further new pathologic features. In traumatic injuries of the spine, we should not limit our investigations to what first appears to be evident on roentgenograms. It should be remembered that a careful neurologic evaluation takes precedence over radiograms, which should be guided by abnormal neurologic deficits and not vice-versa.

This case seems to represent a good example of how errors may contribute positively to extend our knowledge.

SUMMARY

Missed pathology at the C1 to C2 level following an injury may have tragic consequences. Open-mouth views and lateral roentgenograms may be obscured by technical features that make their interpretation dubious. These difficulties are illustrated in a patient whose posttraumatic condition was diagnosed as odontoid fracture without neurologic deficit. However, further work-up indicated the absence of C1 to C2 pathology but disclosed neurologic deficits related to bone pathology in another region of the cervical spine. Some of the fallacies that are linked to the roentgenographic imaging of the C1 to C2 region are discussed. First, the need is emphasized for radiographic views with both the head and cervical spine in the true lateral position. Second, when one has radiographic evidence of pathology in one part of the spine, one should also study the rest of the spine.

REFERENCES

1. Bell EG, Subnamanian G. The skeleton. In Goncalves Rocha AF, Harbert JC, eds., *Textbook of Nuclear Medicine: Clinical Applications.* Philadelphia: Lea and Febiger, 1979. Pp. 109–128.
2. Matin P. Bone scanning of trauma and benign conditions. In Freeman LM, Weissmann HS, eds., *Nuclear Medicine Annual* 1982. New York: Raven Press, 1982. Pp. 81–118.
3. Braakman R, Penning L. *Injuries of the Cervical Spine.* Amsterdam: Excerpta Medica, 1971.
4. Gerlock AJ, Kirchner SG, Heller RM, Kaye JJ. *Advanced Exercises in Diagnostic Radiology.* Philadelphia: W.B. Saunders, 1978.
5. Harris JH. *The Radiology of Acute Cervical Spine Trauma.* Baltimore: Williams and Wilkins, 1978.
6. Howorth MB, Petrie JG. *Injuries of the Spine.* Baltimore: Williams and Wilkins, 1964.
7. Lob A. *Die Wirbelsäulenverletzungen und ihre Ausheilung* (2nd ed.) Stuttgart: Thieme, 1954.

8. McRae DL. How to look at cervical radiographs. In Tator CH, ed., *Early Management of Acute Spinal Cord Injury*. New York: Raven Press, 1982. Pp. 77–92.

7

Body Composition and Endocrine Profile in Spinal Cord Injured Patients

ALAIN B. ROSSIER, MD
HERVÉ FAVRE, MD
MICHEL B. VALLOTTON, MD

VARIOUS METABOLIC ALTERATIONS have been described in spinal cord injured patients, notably in protein metabolism, electrolyte balance, calcium–phosphorus equilibrium, and hepatic and endocrine functions (1). We have studied the body composition of such patients, using the compartmental analysis as proposed by Moore and coworkers (2). Results have demonstrated a body composition similar to that observed in patients with hyperaldosteronism, so plasma aldosterone, plasma renin activity, and cortisol were measured later in a second group of patients presenting an identical clinical setting.

Global evaluation of these patients showed a persistent increase in plasma aldosterone and plasma renin activity levels with a normal cortisol level that may account for the observed changes in body composition.

MATERIAL AND METHODS

This work is based on the study of 11 paraplegic and six tetraplegic male patients with spinal cord injuries. Patients' ages ranged from 17 to 55 years, with a mean age of 27 years. Each patient

was carefully evaluated to exclude coexisting disturbances of cardiac, hepatic, or renal function. The control group consisted of 24 healthy subjects matched for sex and age.

Serial measurements of total body composition were made at different points in the patients' course—between the 10th and 30th days and during the second, fourth, and 12th months after spinal cord injury. In the control group, body composition was studied on one occasion.

Total body composition was determined by simultaneous tracer dilution method developed in our laboratory and described in detail by Busset, et al.(3). In brief, on the first day of the experiment, ^{42}potassium (K) 150 μCi, ^{24}sodium (Na) 100 μCi, and ^{82}bromide (Br) 30 μCi was injected intravenously between 7 and 8 A.M. Twenty-four-hour urine was collected. On day two, a sample of blood was drawn 24 hours after injection of the isotopes, and urine was again collected. On day three, a second sample of blood was drawn 48 hours after injection and titrated water 1 μCi was injected. Isotopes were counted in each of the urine and blood specimens using a beta counter (B 12 H, 20th Century Electronics, Ltd.) for the potassium and a gamma counter (Auto gamma, Packard 4 10 A) for the ^{24}Na and ^{82}Br. On day three, blood was taken 2 and 3 hours after injection of titrated water. Two-hour urine collection was made after injection of this isotope. Tritium was measured by a beta counter (Tri-Cab, Packard). All these isotopes were purchased from Radiochemical Center Amersham (England). Details concerning the type of column used to separate isotopes and the calculation made are given elsewhere (3). This method permits the simultaneous determination of:

- Total body water (TBW) equivalent to the titrated water space.
- Extracellular water (ECW) equivalent to the diffusion space of ^{82}Br, corrected for both the diffusion of Br into the RBCs and for the true serum H_2O concentration (4).
- Total exchangeable sodium (Na$_e$) equivalent to 70 percent of the total Na obtained by measuring serum isotopic Na dilution in a sample taken 24 hours after injection of ^{24}Na.
- Total exchangeable potassium (K$_e$) equivalent to 90 percent of the total K obtained by measurement of urine isotopic activity 48 hours after injection of ^{42}K.

The error of these determinations, for the simultaneous method, was in our hands of the order of ± 3 percent, and the reproducibility had been shown to be of the order of ± 5 percent (3).

Among the values that may be derived from these direct measurements, we considered the following (2):

- Intracellular water (ICW); the difference between TBW and ECW may be acknowledged as an index of the active cellular mass.
- The Na$_e$/K$_e$ ratio reflects the proportion of the extracellular milieu to the cellular mass.
- The (Na^e+K$_e$)/TBW ratio or the "mean body osmolality;" Edelman et al. (5) have demonstrated the close relationship existing

between TBW and the total body supply of these two exchangeable cations.

In some particular situations, however, this correlation is no longer valid for unknown reasons, as demonstrated by Bartter (6) and confirmed by de Sousa, et al. (7).

Average intracellular potassium concentration (AvICK) is calculated as follows:

AvICK = intracellular potassium (ICK)/ICW (mmol/L), where ICK = K − ECK and ECK = ECW × Kplasma × correction factor (2).

According to Nagant de Deuxchaisnes, et al. (8), a decrease in AvICK may be considered as the hallmark of true potassium depletion, a consequence of a cellular metabolic alteration (anoxia, acidosis, and hypercorticism). The primary metabolic defect must be corrected before potassium depletion may be remedied. This treatment is the opposite of that for potassium deficit from excessive losses, which is easily corrected by the administration of potassium, and pseudodepletion, which corresponds to a reduction in cell mass without change in AvICK and is found in patients suffering from chronic debilitating disease.

Total body fat (TBF) is calculated according to the Pace–Rathbun formula (9) based on the assumption that fat contains no water and lean tissue contains 73.2 percent water. This derivation is subject to significant error (10).

The K$_e$/FFS ratio expresses the part of the lean body mass made up of cellular tissue, where FFS = body weight − (TBW + TBF).

Expression of the Results

Each form of presentation of the results of a compositional study has its drawbacks; the choice of the form of presentation must be made with regard to the ultimate goal of the study. We wished to follow the case developments of our relatively homogeneous group of patients and compare this group with a group of normal subjects. Because we could not a priori discern whether a variation in body weight was due to variations in TBF or TBW or both, we chose to express our results in absolute terms rather than relating them to body weight or TBW.

This form of expression may obscure variations from the normal but will increase the salience of the differences found and facilitate the longitudinal study of the subjects.

Endocrine Study

In view of the results obtained by the study of the body composition in the first group of patients, endocrine studies have been undertaken in a second series of patients to substantiate the mechanism responsible for the alterations found in the body composition of paraplegic and tetraplegic patients. Plasma aldosterone (PA), plasma renin activity (PRA), and cortisol were measured on day one after the injury and one and two months later, in two paraplegic and five tetraplegic male patients. The clinical features and the treatment of these patients, whose ages ranged from 20 to 55 years (mean age 30 years), were similar to those of the patients in the first series.

PRA was estimated according to Poulsen and Jorgensen (11) and Valloton (12); plasma aldosterone and cortisol were measured according to Underwood and Williams (13). Normal values have been previously established by the laboratory for normal subjects ingesting a 150 mmol sodium per day diet in supine position. Blood was drawn at 8 A.M. in supine patients. During the first 3 days, the patients were perfused with an isotonic saline solution containing 20 mmol of potassium per liter at a rate between 1500 and 2500 ml/24 hours. In addition, they received 6 mg of dexamethasone the first day, tapered to 1 mg a day by day six. On this treatment, extracellular fluid volume was maintained constant as judged by the blood pressure. Systolic mean blood pressure $\pm$ SD was 116 + 21 mmHg the first day, and 118 + 14 and 114 + 15 by the end of the first and second months, respectively.

Diastolic blood pressure averaged 68 ± 16 mmHg the first day, and 76 ± 9 and 73 ± 11 by the end of the first and second months, respective-

ly. There were no statistical differences between these values. There were also no significant differences during the three periods of observation in serum sodium, potassium, and total carbon dioxide concentration. Mean serum sodium concentrations averaged 137 ± 2.8 mmol/L on day one, 140 ± 4.0 mmol/L during the first month, and 142 ± 3.3 mmol/L during the second month. The corresponding values for potassium were 4.1 ± 0.23, 4.0 ± 0.21, 4.1 ± 0.31, and for total CO_2, 26.6 ± 1.9, 26 ± 3.32, and 25 ± 2.9, respectively. These values did not differ from those recorded in the patients of the first series.

Statistics

All the values are expressed as mean $\pm$ SD. Statistical comparisons were made with Student's t-test and double variance analysis whenever applicable.

RESULTS

Body Composition

Results and normal values are displayed in Tables 7-1 to 7-3.

Data Comparison Between Patients and Controls. The average weight of our patients is lower than that of control subjects, with an average corpulence index (14) of 12 percent below ideal body weight (Table 7-1). Total body fat is within normal limits.

Average total body weight for the group approaches the lower limits of the normal; the distribution between the intracellular and extracellular compartments is slightly altered as evidenced by a nonsignificant elevation of the Na_e/K_e ratio. Na_e is within normal limits.

K_e is significantly decreased (p < 0.001), with an average absolute value of 2287 mmol. This decrease will be reflected in all the values derived from or dependent on K_e.

The Na_e/K_e ratio is raised (although not significantly) by a reduction of the denominator with a normal numerator. The $(Na_e + K_e)/$

TABLE 7-1 Comparison of Mean Values Observed in
Spinal Cord Injury Patients with Those of Control Subjects

	Normal Controls N=24	Paraplegics or Tetraplegics N = 17		
		Mean ± SD	Difference	Significance
Weight (kg)	67.3 ± 7.4	59.5 ± 7.88	−7.8	NS
TBW (Liter)	40.7 ± 5.66	36.40 ± 4.37	−4.3	NS
ECW (Liter)	16.3 ± 1.70	17.65 ± 1.96	+1.35	NS
Na_e (mEq)	2830 ± 339	2751 ± 351	−79	NS
K_e (mEq)	3096 ± 332	2287 ± 431	−809	P < 0.01
TBF (kg)	9.6 ± 2.4	10.25 ± 5.08	+0.65	NS
ICW (Liter)	21 ± 3	18.53 ± 3.52	−2.47	NS
$Na_e./K_e$	0.85 ± 1.0	1.23 ± 0.26	+ 0.23	NS
AvICK (mEq/L)	150 ± 10	118.06 ± 13.74	−31.94	P < 0.01
$Na_e + K_e$/TBW (mEq/L)	155 ± 5	138.70 ± 11.67	−16.30	p < 0.05
K_e/FFS (mEq/kg)	225 ± 25	174.01 ± 19.31	−50.99	P < 0.01

There is a significant decrease in K_e, AvICK ($Na_e + K_e$) TBW, and K_e/FFS. The other values do not show significant deviation from the normal (NS = not significant).

TBW ratio is reduced significantly (p < 0.05). However, serum sodium concentration remains in the normal range from 135 to 143 mmol/L (average 140 mmol/L) (see Table 7-1). This implies an apparent contradiction—that is, a "low mean body osmolality" in the face of normal serum sodium and potassium values. Such a situation has been reported earlier by Bartter et al. (6) and de Sousa et al. (7) without any definite explanation. In certain circumstances, the Edelman formula may not represent the true mean body osmolality, which could be the consequence of a situation of cationic inactivation.

The K_e/FFS ratio is significantly reduced (p < 0.01). This is logical if the weight loss is at the expense of the lean tissue (with a normal TBF) and, in particular, at the expense of the muscle mass (decrease of K_e proportionally greater than the decrease in fat-free solids (FFS), which includes organs less affected by paraplegia, such as the skeleton). Therefore, the decreased K_e/FFS ratio expresses a relatively greater loss of lean body mass (Table 7-1).

AvICK is significantly reduced (p < 0.01), permitting the classification of this potassium deficiency as potassium depletion.

Finally, in our patients, the serum potassium was found to be within normal limits during the entire course of the study (range 3.8 to 5, average 4.5 mmol/L).

The body of data accumulated from present series of measurements allows the conclusion that as a group, the paraplegics and tetraplegics we treated had potassium depletion, low mean body osmolality, and weight loss at the expense of lean body mass.

Evolution of the Measurements of Parameters in the Paraplegic and Tetraplegic Group

We first tried to differentiate early from late changes. We adopted a period of 1 month after trauma as an arbitrary limit between the early and late stages, because the catabolic posttraumatic phase is estimated to be of about 1 month's duration. Measurements were made from the 10th day to 1 month after trauma for the early period and from 2 months to 12 months after injury for the late period. Table 7-2 summarizes the trend of variations occurring during these two periods.

As can be seen in Table 7-2, compared with those in normal persons, the alterations in body composition of paraplegic and tetraplegic patients exist in varying degrees from the first month after injury and remain unchanged later.

TABLE 7-2 Comparison of Measurements Made During and After One Month Following Spinal Cord Injury in 17 Patients

	During 1st Month	2nd to 12th Months		
	Mean ± SD	Mean ± SD	Difference	Significant
Weight (kg)	59.52 ± 6.02	59.46 ± 8.74	−0.06	NS
TBW (Liter)	37.80 ± 3.97	35.70 ± 4.48	−2.10	NS
ECW (Liter)	17.64 ± 1.89	17.65 ± 2.03	+0.01	NS
Na_e (−Eq)	2643 ± 342	2805 ± 380	+162	NS
K_e (mEq)	2400 ± 380	2231 ± 452	−169	NS
TBF (kg)	9.53 ± 4.23	10.57 ± 5.50	+1.04	NS
ICW (Liter)	20.40 ± 2.75	18.05 ± 3.92	−2.35	NS
Na_e/K_e	1.11 ± 0.13	1.30 ± 0.29	+0.19	$p < 0.05$
AvICK (mEq/Liter)	114.47 ± 16.76	119.86 ± 11.99	+5.39	NS
$Na_e + K_e$/TBW (mEq/Liter)	133.68 ± 14.02	141.21 ± 9.70	+7.35	NS
K_eFFS (mEq/kg)	176.66 ± 22.69	172.84 ± 18.20	−3.82	NS

The *t*-test shows that only the modest elevation of Na_e/K_e reaches significance, as a result of the opposite (and in themselves nonsignificant) variations in both Na_e and K_e.

Within the limits of observation of the selected parameters, with the exception of an increase in the Na_e/K_e ratio, statistical analysis does not reveal any difference between the early and the late periods. Thus, the potassium depletion, the low mean body osmolality ratio, and the weight loss are present from the first month after injury and persist thereafter.

In a second phase of investigation, it was deemed necessary to look at the modifications that might take place under the influence of the patient's resumption of activity. To do so, we compared the measurements carried out before and after wheelchair ambulation, a very important step in the course of rehabilitation, during which the motor activity of the patient increases considerably. Wheelchair ambulation occurs with most of our patients at about 2 to 3 months after injury. Table 7-3 shows the direction and the statistical significance of variations observed

TABLE 7-3 Comparison of Measurements Made Before and After Wheelchair Ambulation in 17 Patients

	Before Wheelchair Ambulation	After Wheelchair Ambulation		
	Mean ± SD	Mean ± SD	Difference	Significant
Weight (kg)	63.13 ± 7.34	55.83 ± 6.82	−7.30	$p < 0.02$
TBW (Liter)	37.18 ± 4.57	35.34 ± 4.01	−1.84	NS
ECW (Liter)	17.93 ± 2.03	17.27 + 1.85	−0.66	NS
Na_e (mEq)	2700 ± 391	2819 ± 343	+199	NS
K_e (mEq)	2300 ± 447	2270 ± 423	−0.30	NS
TBF (kg)	12.02 ± 5.17	8.48 ± 4.49	−3.59	NS
ICW (Liter)	19.40 ± 3.54	18.07 ± 3.91	−1.33	NS
Na_e/K_e	1.20 ± 0.24	1.28 ± 0.28	+0.04	NS
AvICK (mEq/L)	114.82 ± 13.67	122.47 ± 13.02	+7.65	NS
$Na_e + K_e$/TBW (mEq/L)	134.61 ± 12.40	144.25 ± 8.04	+9.64	$p < 0.02$
K_eFFS (mEq/kg)	174.63 ± 19.75	173.40 ± 19.64	−1.23	NS

The *t*-test shows that the only significant variations are a fall in body weight and an elevation of the $(Na_e + K_e)$/TBW ratio.

during the periods under consideration, before and after wheelchair ambulation.

From the foregoing, it would appear that the resumption of physical activity results in a weight loss at the expense of both TBF and TBW and coincides with a partial correction of the mean body osmolality. The potassium depletion persists after wheelchair ambulation, and no argument can be found in favor of an increase in muscle mass.

Endocrine Results

As illustrated in Fig. 7-1, plasma aldosterone and plasma renin activity levels are both above the normal values for people who receive a normal salt diet and remain supine. Elevation of both parameters appears immediately after the injury and persists for months. In contrast, the cortisol values found in the serum of these patients remain normal during the period of observation with the exception of suppressed levels observed on the first day after injury, which could be easily explained by the corticoid treatment these patients received at that time. In these patients,

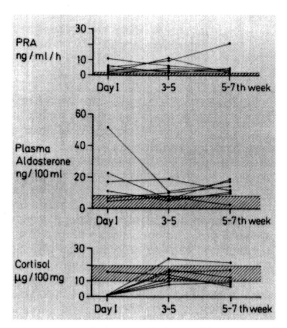

FIGURE 7-1 Above normal plasma aldosterone and plasma renin activity levels for people who receive a normal salt diet and remain supine.

no correlation could be found between PA and PRA.

DISCUSSION

Despite individual variations in patients' courses, three elements were demonstrated to be common to the group: potassium depletion, low mean body osmolality, and loss of weight. The method used shows that the weight loss is a result of combined loss of TBF and TBW, especially at the expense of the intracellular water fraction, which is in agreement with the observations of Cardús et al. (15,16). Because the TBW loss amounts to more than the water contained in adipose tissue, a loss in lean body mass must be present, most probably from the muscle mass.

The persistent fall in total exchangeable potassium is the most important finding in these patients. This fall is probably composed of two elements:

- Loss of muscle mass (pseudodepletion).
- Potassium depletion syndrome, clearly demonstrated in this study by a decreased AvICK. This potassium depletion reveals the existence of a permanent metabolic change in the paraplegic patients.

Decreased AvICK is pronounced in the early course of our patients and persists practically unchanged throughout the period of observation. Such a perturbation is usually secondary to alterations of either metabolic (anoxia and/or acidosis) or endocrine origin (8). The spinal cord injured person is a patient beset by numerous metabolic difficulties that may create and maintain a potassium depletion: there is an initial posttraumatic shock with vasoplegia, hypotension, anemia secondary to capillary stasis, hemolysis and decreased hematopoiesis, disorders of hemostasis, and depression of cellular metabolism reflected in a decreased BMR, resulting from the combined effects of anemia, hypoxia, pain, and increased body temperature loss secondary to vasoplegia (1). Then comes the posttraumatic catabolic phase (2 weeks to 6 months) with a negative nitrogen balance (17,18). From the third day, the urinary potassium losses reach a maximum and a concomitant sodium retention is found (17). In addition, transitory BSP retention (1), disturbances of glucose tolerance (17), occasional feminization syndrome with gynecomastia and testicular atrophy (19), adrenal functional disturbances, and increased urinary aldosterone excretion have been reported (19,20).

Such changes per se are sufficient to explain a true potassium depletion. This potassium depletion is similar to that observed in nonedematous cardiac and cirrhotic patients and differs from that which can be seen in patients with muscular wasting disease, in which AvICK remains normal (8). This fact suggests the presence of some mineralocorticoid hormone disturbance such as secondary hyperaldosteronism or excess of cortisol. The repercussions of hypercorticism on the total body composition are an increase in Na_e/kg and a decrease in K_e. Expressed in absolute terms, we found the Na_e to be normal in our patients. Therefore, in view of the loss of body weight observed, the ratio of Na_e to body weight must be increased, which is in fact the case: the Na_e/kg in our patients averaged 50.4 mmol/kg (normal 43.3 mmol/kg), a value which is close to that found in patients with cirrhosis or cardiac insufficiency without edema (8).

The AvICK remains markedly decreased. Because the $Na_e + K_e/TBW$ ratio becomes partially corrected, a finding that is in agreement with Cardús and McTaggart (16) at this stage for the disease, and the serum sodium concentration remains normal, we must postulate a degree of intracellular substitution of sodium for potassium, as in secondary hyperaldosteronism (8). Increased aldosterone excretion in spinal cord injured patients has already been reported by Claus-Walker et al. (21). Because hyperaldosteronism is the most likely mechanism for the persistent potassium depletion, we have measured plasma aldosterone, plasma renin activity, and cortisol in a second series of patients over a period of 2 months. Compared with results in

normal persons, the results have confirmed that the paraplegics have a high aldosterone level throughout the period of observation (see Fig. 7-1).

Increased aldosterone secretion may be stimulated by different elements, some of which could be relevant to paraplegics. The most classic stimulus is hypovolemia (22). This stimulus could be excluded in our group of patients because their blood pressure remained constant. In addition, hypovolemia implies a low exchangeable sodium and a low Na_e/kg ratio, which is in opposition to our finding of a normal exchangeable sodium and elevated Na_e/kg ratio. Hyperkalemia is another stimulus that is irrelevant to our patients because the serum potassium was found to be within normal limits all during the study (6).

Finally, the most potent stimulus for the aldosterone secretion remains angiotensin II generated by renin. We have found elevated plasma renin activity from the immediate posttraumatic phase throughout the period of observation of 2 months. The initiation of the stimulation of renin secretion, as well as its persistence, could be explained by the vasoplegia accompanying the paraplegic condition. This vasoplegia occurs immediately after the injury and persists for the rest of the paraplegic patient's life. In view of recent in vitro experiments, stimulation of the PGE_2 biosynthesis by the potassium depletion may offer another explanation for the maintenance of elevated PRA and PA in paraplegic patients (23). It should be noted that, although both PRA and PA are elevated, there is no statistical correlation between the two parameters as would normally be expected. However, this situation is not unique and has been described in other pathologic conditions such as uremia (24).

In fact, the most remarkable finding in these patients is the persistence of a high plasma aldosterone level best explained by a permanent vasoplegia. This endocrine abnormality can induce the changes in the body composition; that is, a permanent potassium depletion with a progressive correction of the $Na_e + K_e/TBW$ ratio.

Correction of this ratio depends on the sodium retention resulting from the hyperaldosteronism, which creates a relative increase in the exchangeable sodium despite the continuing potassium depletion. At the end, as it appears from our data, the intracellular volume is reduced and the extracellular volume is slightly increased.

SUMMARY

Various metabolic alterations have been ascribed to spinal cord injured patients; 11 paraplegic and six tetraplegic male patients with spinal cord injuries were studied in regard to body composition as assessed by compartmental analysis. Because body composition was shown to be similar to that observed in hyperaldosteronism, five more tetraplegics and two paraplegics were investigated with regard to plasma aldosterone, renin, and cortisol levels. The most striking finding was the persistence of elevation of both aldosterone and renin activity. This might best be explained by the chronic condition of vasoplegia in these patients. It is suggested that endocrine modifications are responsible for the changes in body composition that is, permanent potassium depletion with progressive correction of the total exchangeable sodium + potassium/total body water ratio. From these longitudinal metabolic studies, it is concluded that potassium depletion, low mean body osmolality, weight loss at the expense of the lean body mass, and elevated plasma aldosterone level and plasma renin activity are some of the metabolic changes that take place in spinal cord injured patients.

REFERENCES

1. O'Connell FB, Gardner WJ. Metabolism in paraplegia. *J Am Med Assoc* 1953; 153:706.
2. Moore FD, Olesen KH, McMurrey JD, et al. *The Body Cell Mass and Its Supporting Environment*, (1st ed)., Philadelphia: W.B. Saunders, 1963. Pp. 535.
3. Busset R, de Sousa RC, Mach RS. Etude de la composition corporelle a l'aide de radio-isotopes chez l'homme normal et au cours de differents etats pathologiques. *Methode Sem Hop Paris* 1967; 43:1312.
4. Lacroix M, Busset R, Mach RS. Utilisation comparative du soufre 35 et du brome 82 pour la determination du volume de l'eau extracellulaire. *Helv Med Acta* 1965; 32:87.
5. Edelman IS, Leibmann J, O'Meara MP, Birkenfeld LW. Interrelations between serum sodium concentration, serum osmolality and total exchangeable sodium, total exchangeable potassium and total body water. *J Clin Invest* 1958; 37:1236.
6. Bartter FC, Barbour BH, Carr AA, Delea CS. On the role of potassium and of the central nervous system in the regulation of aldosterone secretion. In Baulieu EF, Robel P, eds, *Aldosterone: A Symposium.* Oxford: Blackwell Scientific Publications, 1964. Pp. 221–242.
7. de Sousa R, Busset R, Moser C, et al. Correlation entre sodium echangeable, potassium echangeable, eau totale et espace brome (Applications cliniques de la formule d'Edelman). *Helv Med Acta* 1964; 31:623.
8. Nagant de Deuxchaisnes C, Collet RA, Busset R, Mach RS. Exchangeable potassium in wasting, amyotrophy, heart disease and cirrhosis of the liver. *Lancet* 1961; 1:681.
9. Pace N, Rathbun EN. Studies on body composition, III. The body water and chemically combined nitrogen content in relation to fat content. *J Biol Chem* 1945; 158:685.
10. Quoidbach A, Busset R, Dayer AA, Mach RS. Evaluation of body composition in obesity using isotopic dilution techniques. In Vague J, ed., *Physiopathology of Adipose Tissue*, 3rd ed. Amsterdam: Excerpta Medica Foundation, 1969. Pp. 302–317.
11. Poulsen K, Jorgensen J. An easy radioimmunological microassay of renin activity, concentration and substrate in human and animal plasma and tissues based on angiotensin I trapping by antibody. *J Clin Endocrinol Metab* 1974; 39:816.
12. Vallotton MB. Parallel radioimmunoassay of angiotensin I and of angiotensin It for measurement of renin activity and of circulating active hormone in human plasma. In Federlin K, Hales CN, Kracht J, eds., *Immunological Methods in Endocrinology.* Stuttgart: Thierne, 1971. Pp. 94–100.
13. Underwood RH, Williams GH. The simultaneous measurement of aldosterone, cortisol and corticosterone in human peripheral plasma by displacement analysis. *J Lab Clin Med* 1972; 79:848.
14. Monnerot-Dumaine M. L'indice de corpulence

et son calcul chez l'adulte. *Presse Med* 1955; 63:1037.

15. Cardus D, McTaggart WG. Total body water and its distribution in men with spinal cord injury. *Arch Phys Med Rehabil* 1984; 65:509.

16. Cardus D, McTaggart WG. Body sodium and potassium in men with spinal cord injury. *Arch Phys Med Rehabil* 1985; 66:156.

17. Knowlton K, Spence WT, Rioch DMcK, et al. Metabolic changes following transsection of the spinal cord in dogs. *Acta Neurovegetativa* 1957; 15:374.

18. Wyse DM, Pattee CJ. The metabolic alterations of immobilization, injury and paraplegia. Part 1: Protein metabolism. *DVA Treat Serv Bull* 1953; 8:63.

19. Wyse DM, Pattee CJ. The metabolic alterations of immobilization, injury and paraplegia. Part V: Endocrine and physiological alterations. *DVA Treat Serv Bull* 1953; 8:351.

20. McDaniel JW, Sexton AW. Psychoendocrine function in relation to level of spinal cord transection. *Horm Behav* 1971; 2:59.

21. Claus-Walker JL, Carter RE, Lipscomb HS, Vallbona C. Daily rhythms of electrolytes and aldosterone excretion in men with cervical spinal cord section. *J Clin Endocrinol Metab* 1969; 29:300.

22. Laragh JH, Cannon PJ, Ames RP. Aldosterone in man. Its secretion, its interaction with sodium balance and angiotensin activity. In Baulieu EE, Robel P, eds., *Aldosterone: A Symposium*. Oxford: Blackwell Scientific Publications, 1964. Pp. 427–448.

23. Zusman RM, Keiser HR. Regulation of prostaglandin E2 synthesis by angiotensin II, potassium, osmolality, and dexamethasone. *Kidney Int* 1980; 17:277.

24. Louis F, Zwahlen A, Favre H, Vallotton MB. Controle de l'aldosterone plasmatique chez les patients en hemodialyse. *Schweiz Med Wschr* 1980; 110:1882.

8 Renal Insufficiency in Spinal Cord Injured Patients

CYRIL H. BARTON, MD
N.D. VAZIRI, MD

PATIENTS WITH SPINAL CORD INJURY (SCI) are at increased risk for diseases involving the kidneys and urinary tract, which in turn cause substantial morbidity and mortality in this population (1–5). Common urinary tract abnormalities related to SCI that predispose to renal failure include neurogenic bladder dysfunction, vesicoureteral reflux, urinary tract infection, calculous disease, and obstruction (1,2,5,6). Other conditions present in SCI that predispose patients to renal insufficiency include chronic infection complicated by sepsis or secondary amyloidosis, hypertension, and vasomotor instability, as well as exposure to potentially nephrotoxic medications and radiographic contrast agents (1,6–10).

ACUTE RENAL INSUFFICIENCY (ARF)

A variety of factors may cause or predispose SCI patients to acute renal insufficiency (ARF). These include renal ischemia related to intravascular volume depletion, hypotension, and shock; obstructive nephropathy caused by bladder dysfunction or calculous disease; and intrinsic renal injury resulting from trauma, sepsis, and/or nephrotoxin exposure (11–17). Shock may occur early in patients with spinal injury due to *spinal shock*, a condition typically seen with cervical cord lesions, where disruption of descending sympathetic fibers (from the hypothalamus and midbrain) causes a dramatic reduction in sympathetic tone. Shock (occurring in the acute setting of SCI) may also result from blood loss, "third spacing" of fluid, and/or sepsis. In addition, concomitant rhabdomyolysis or exposure to nephrotoxic agents (e.g., aminoglycosides, amphotericin, and intravenous radiographic contrast material) may cause or contribute to ARF in this setting. In the clinical assessment, it is useful to consider that ARF can result from essentially three pathophysiologic conditions: 1) prerenal azotemia, 2) postrenal azotemia or obstructive nephropathy, and 3) intrinsic renal failure.

Prerenal Azotemia

Prerenal azotemia is a common form of acute renal insufficiency that occurs in a variety of conditions characterized by renal hypoperfusion (resulting from either a fall in perfusion pressure or from an intense rise in renal vascular resistance [Table 8-1]). In turn, renal hypoperfusion causes a reduction in glomerular filtration rate, which is accompanied by an increase in tubular reabsorption of filtrate. This results in the retention of nitrogenous waste products (azotemia) and a reduction in urine output (oliguria). It should be noted, however, that urine output

TABLE 8-1 Causes of Prerenal Azotemia

A. Reduction of intravascular volume
  1. Abnormal gastrointestinal losses: diarrhea, emesis, fistulas, drainage
  2. Hemorrhage
  3. Excessive diuresis: diuretics, partial- or post-obstruction, chronic tubulointerstitial nephropathies, potassium depletion, lithium administration, osmotic diuresis, central or nephrogenic diabetes insipidus, hypercalcemia
  4. Sequestration in third space: ileus, burns, peritonitis, pancreatitis, traumatized tissue
B. Cardiovascular disorders: cardiac failure, pericardial tamponade, massive pulmonary embolism, renal arterial occlusion
C. Decreased peripheral vascular resistance: gramnegative sepsis, vasodilatory drugs, etc.
D. Renal vasoconstriction: prostaglandin inhibitors, cyclosporin A, severe liver disease, surgery, and anesthesia

might be inappropriately high in patients with tubular dysfunction (commonly present in SCI, as well as in other conditions listed in Table 8-1). Therefore, the absence of oliguria should not necessarily be construed as evidence against the diagnosis of prerenal azotemia. Other characteristic features of prerenal azotemia include both a low urinary sodium concentration (less than 20 mEq/L) and fractional excretion of sodium (less than 1 percent) caused by enhanced tubular reabsorption of this cation. Fractional excretion of sodium (FENa) is calculated from simultaneous measurements of Na and creatinine concentrations in serum and spot urine samples using the following formula:

$$FENa = UNa/SNa \div U\ Creat/S\ Creat \times 100$$

where UNa and SNa represent urinary and serum sodium concentrations and U Creat and S Creat represent urinary and serum creatinine concentrations, respectively. Once again, a low urinary sodium concentration and FENa may not be attained in patients with sodium-losing states (e.g., diuretic administration, tubulointerstitial nephropathies, or mineralocorticoid deficiency) despite renal hypoperfusion. This is often

the case in patients with long-standing spinal cord injury suffering from neuropathic bladder dysfunction, chronic pyelonephritis, and urolithiasis. Prerenal azotemia is further characterized by a disproportional rise in blood urea nitrogen (BUN) compared to creatinine, where the ratio of BUN/Cr typically exceeds 20. However, this ratio also may be increased in patients with long-standing SCI because of a low serum creatinine related to reduced muscle mass.

Careful attention to the history and physical findings remains an essential part of the assessment in patients presenting with ARF. The presence of thirst, dry mouth, lightheadedness, reduced skin turgor, and orthostatic symptoms suggest intravascular volume depletion. In some critically ill patients, measurement of central venous or pulmonary wedge pressure may be necessary in the diagnosis and management of prerenal failure. Prompt recognition and correction of prerenal azotemia is important because renal hypoperfusion predisposes to ischemic parenchymal injury and acute tubular necrosis. Additionally, hypoperfusion markedly increases the risk of renal damage associated with nephrotoxic antibiotics, radiocontrast material, septicemia, and rhabdomyolysis.

Treatment

Prerenal azotemia is rapidly reversible with restoration of normal renal perfusion, which is usually accomplished by the rapid infusion of isotonic saline. In hypotensive patients, boluses of 250 to 500 ml (0.9 percent saline) should be administered under careful observation, with frequent monitoring of blood pressure, pulse, cardiopulmonary status, and urine output. In the absence of congestive heart failure, saline fluid challenges can be repeated until blood pressure and hemodynamic status has stabilized. Most patients with hypovolemic shock tolerate a rapid infusion of 2 liters of isotonic saline at a rate of 6 ml/min/kg. If a favorable response occurs, infusion of isotonic saline should be continued until common endpoints of volume resuscitation are accomplished which include:

- Central venous pressure of 15mmHg
- Pulmonary wedge pressure of 10 to 12 mmHg
- Cardiac index > 3L/min/m^2
- Oxygen uptake (VO$_2$) > 100 ml/min/m^2
- Blood lactate < 4 mmol/L
- Base deficit −3 to + 3 mmol/L

Of note, it may be both difficult and dangerous to place a central venous pressure line in a patient who is extremely volume-depleted and hypotensive. In such cases, it is more prudent to begin volume resuscitation via any suitable intravenous route followed by frequent clinical assessment of hemodynamic parameters (e.g., blood pressure, pulse rate, and jugular venous pulse), mental status, and urine output.

If a favorable hemodynamic response to isotonic saline infusion does not occur, then colloid fluids and/or blood products (in the case of hemorrhagic shock) may be added to the resuscitation regimen. Administration of vasopressors (e.g., dopamine, phenylephrine, epinephrine, and/or norepinephrine) is indicated in patients who are refractory to volume resuscitation. In most cases, hypotension will respond to fluid-volume resuscitation; however, because SCI patients are more susceptible to pulmonary edema, massive volume infusion generally should be avoided . Therefore, in cases where shock (particularly spinal shock) is refractory to 2 to 3 liters of volume replacement, vasopressor therapy should be initiated.

During the acute-care period (following spinal injury) an indwelling bladder catheter should be placed to facilitate urine drainage because most patients (those with cord lesion above S2) initially develop flacid bladders subject to overdistention. Hypovolemia should be prevented or promptly treated, as there is evidence that, in addition to its well-established adverse affects, ischemia may also play an important role in aggravating spinal cord injury (19,20). Hypoxia, hyperpyrexia, and anemia should also be treated (O2 saturation and hematocrit should be maintained above 95 and 30 percent, respectively). A hematocrit in the range of 30 to 34 percent probably provides the best balance of oxygen-carrying capacity and reduced viscosity. Associated electrolyte and acid–base disturbances should be treated with the priority for correcting multiple concomitant abnormalities as follows: first, volume and perfusion deficits; second, pH; third, potassium, calcium, and magnesium abnormalities; and fourth, sodium and chloride abnormalities. It should be noted that restoration of tissue perfusion often results in improvement in electrolyte and acid–base disturbances.

Postrenal Azotemia

Partial or complete urinary tract obstruction should always be ruled out in the evaluation of ARF, especially in patients with underlying acute or chronic SCI. The various causes of urinary tract obstruction are listed in Table 8-2. SCI patients are particularly prone to urinary tract obstruction, with the most important predisposing factor being neuropathic bladder dysfunction (21,22). Essentially, three types of neuropathic bladder dysfunction occur as a result of spinal

---

TABLE 8-2 Causes of Urinary Tract Obstruction

A. Intrarenal obstruction: uric acid, drugs (e.g., sulfa, acyclovir, and methotrexate), myeloma casts
B. Extrarenal
  1. Intraluminal: Calculi, purulent debris, sloughed papillae, fungal ball, blood clot, tumors and polyps, strictures, trauma, ureteroceles, anterior and posterior urethral valves
  2. Extraluminal
    a. Reproductive system abnormalities: malignant and benign tumors, cysts, pregnancy, endometriosis, ureteral ligation during gynecologic surgery, ovarian and pelvic infections and abscesses
    b. Retroperitoneal: retroperitoneal fibrosis (primary, secondary) tumors, hematoma, urinoma, infection, and surgical disruption
    c. Gastrointestional pathology: malignancies, chronic inflammatory bowel diseases, pancreatic pseudocyst, appendiceal abscess
    d. Vascular abnormalities: aneurysms, aberrant vessels, retrocaval ureters

cord injury: 1) a hyperreflexic or spastic bladder, 2) an areflexic or flacid bladder, and 3) mixed profiles of bladder dysfunction. For the first several weeks following spinal cord injury, the bladder is usually flaccid and subject to hyperdistention, which is caused by the temporary loss of all reflex activity below the level of injury. In patients with upper motor neuron lesions (above S2), after several weeks of flaccidity the bladder becomes a low volume, hyperreflexic spastic organ that is very inefficient in emptying, because of detrusor dyssynergia and sphincter spasm. In contrast, a permanent state of bladder flaccidity and areflexia occurs following injury to the reflex-voiding center (S2–S4), which constitutes a lower motor neuron lesion. As a consequence of incomplete spinal cord injury or with injury involving the conus–cauda equina junctions, mixed bladder lesions may occur. For example, such combinations as flaccid bladder/spastic internal sphincter, spastic bladder/lax external sphincter, or a "sensory" bladder with no control over voiding have been described (22).

Less common causes of obstructive nephropathy occurring during the acute phase of SCI include the traumatic disruption of the ureters, bladder, or urethra, or with obstruction related to retroperitoneal bleeding. In both the acute and chronic phases of spinal cord injury, obstruction of an indwelling bladder catheter should always be ruled out as a possible cause of renal insufficiency. In chronic SCI, the high prevalence of acute and chronic pyelonephritis predisposes patients to papillary necrosis and ureteral obstruction caused by sloughed tissue and purulent debris (15). Another potential cause of obstruction is urolithiasis, which is also quite prevalent in chronic SCI patients (16,17,23). Factors predisposing to urinary tract stone disease (in SCI) include hypercalciuria, hyperuricosuria, and hyperoxaluria (16,24–27). In addition, urinary tract infection (with urease-producing bacteria) results in the formation of urine that is highly alkaline (pH > 7.5) and supersaturated with NH_4^+, PO_4^{3-}, CO_3^{2-}, which in turn predisposes to struvite stone formation. Infection stones or struvite stones are

very difficult to manage and are often complicated by pyonephrosis, sepsis, and renal failure. Other factors thought to predispose ·SCI patients to urinary tract calculous disease include an abnormal urine flow rate and reduced urinary excretion of citrate, pyrophosphate, and orthophosphate, which are major inhibitors of stone formation (16,27–29).

For obstruction to cause significant azotemia, both kidneys must be affected (assuming both kidneys have normal function). Therefore, a single lesion at the level of the urethra or bladder neck can cause azotemia, whereas above the level of the bladder, the obstructing lesions must be bilateral to cause azotemia. Complete obstruction of both kidneys is manifested by anuria, whereas forms of incomplete obstruction may present with polyuria or with fluctuating urinary volumes. It should be noted that due to the associated sensory deficits, acute bladder distention is usually asymptomatic in SCI patients; patients with urinary tract obstruction however, may exhibit hypertension. Moreover, acute bladder distention may lead to autonomic dysreflexia in patients with spinal cord injury above T7, which typically presents with a constellation of signs and symptoms including severe hypertension, flushing, diaphoresis, pounding headache, and cardiac dysrhythmias. In addition, subarachnoid bleeding, convulsions, coma, and even death may complicate this syndrome (30–33).

The clinical and laboratory features of obstructive nephropathy often reflect underlying abnormalities in renal tubular function (34–38). Consequently, the urine sodium concentration and fractional excretion of sodium (FENa) are generally increased (> 20 mEq/L and > 1 percent, respectively). However, early in acute obstruction, the FENa may be quite low (< 1 percent of the filtered load), indicative of normal tubular function that usually remains intact during the initial phase of obstructive nephropathy. Consequently, acute obstruction may transiently mimic prerenal azotemia from a biochemical standpoint. Partial obstruction may also cause a form of hyperkalemic distal renal tubular acidosis, which appears to result from several tubular abnormalities, including a defect in distal sodium reabsorption. This in turn reduces the ability of the distal tubule and collecting duct to generate sufficient luminal electronegativity necessary for normal tubular potassium and hydrogen ion secretion. Acid secretion may be further impaired by diminished collecting duct hydrogen-ATPase activity, while the problem of hyperkalemia may be compounded by increased collecting duct potassium reabsorption related to enhanced activity of H-K-ATPase (an enzyme that promotes potassium reabsorption as well as hydrogen ion secretion). Another common consequence of obstructive uropathy is a vasopressin-resistant urinary concentration defect. This abnormality is primarily responsible for the polyuria associated with partial obstruction as well as postobstruction diuresis.

Diagnosis and Management

Bladder dysfunction, as well as some degree of urinary obstruction, is present in virtually all SCI patients. During the acute phase, placement of an indwelling catheter is usually required to facilitate urinary drainage and to closely monitor urine output. The use of either intermittent bladder catheterization or percutaneous fine-bore suprapubic cystostomy is recommended in the subacute setting (usually 1 to 2 weeks post-injury), because the use of these techniques is shown to reduce the risk of urinary tract infection (39–41). Obstruction should be ruled out in all azotemic patients. A suprapubic mass is generally apparent in patients with bladder distention, and the placement of a bladder catheter may be useful in the diagnosis and initial management of obstruction (at or below the level of the bladder), while patients with an indwelling catheter in place should have the catheter tested for patency.

Renal ultrasonography is the preferred diagnostic imaging procedure, as it is reliable, safe, and readily available (42–45). However, on rare occasions it may be necessary to employ other diagnostic modalities such as intravenous pyelography, retrograde or antegrade pyelography,

computed tomography (CT), or magnetic resonance imaging (MRI). Once the diagnosis of obstruction is established, measures should be taken to restore urine flow as soon as possible to minimize the occurrence of irreversible parenchymal damage. In addition, vigorous antibiotic therapy should be instituted if urinary tract infection is also present. Supportive measures including hemodialysis or peritoneal dialysis should be employed (as indicated) to control severe azotemia, fluid, electrolyte, and acid–base disturbances.

A brisk diuresis usually follows the relief of obstruction, which is often caused by a combination of factors, including volume expansion, increased osmotic load, defective tubular transport of salt and water, and vasopressin resistance. In the majority of cases, postobstructive diuresis is self-limited (generally lasting several days) and appropriate for the state of volume expansion and degree of azotemia. However, a severe persistent diuresis may occur as the result of tubular dysfunction with impaired reabsorption of sodium and water. These patients are at risk for volume and electrolyte depletion, including hypokalemia and hypomagnesemia. Intravenous volume replacement can generally be accomplished with matching volumes of half normal saline (0.45 percent sodium chloride), to which appropriate quantities of KCl, $NaHCO_3$, and, if necessary, $MgSO_4$ are added. The volume and composition of replacement fluid can be determined from measurements of urine output and serum and urine electrolyte concentrations (e.g., Na, K, Cl, and Mg). Should hyponatremia develop, replacement fluid should be changed to normal saline alternating with half normal saline, whereas, if hypernatremia occurs replacement fluid should be changed to quarter normal saline alternating with half normal saline. With massive diuresis, measurement of electrolytes should be performed approximately every 6 hours. Blood pressure, weight, pulse rate, and cardiopulmonary status should also be frequently assessed. In addition, serum calcium, phosphorous, and bicarbonate should be monitored, because hypophosphatemia and/or metabolic acidosis can complicate postobstructive diuresis.

At times it is difficult to differentiate persistent postobstructive diuresis from that driven by volume expansion (related to fluid administration). In such cases it is appropriate to lower the rate of fluid administration while closely monitoring pulse rate, blood pressure, urine output, body weight, BUN, creatinine, and (if available) central venous pressure or pulmonary artery wedge pressure. The continuation of polyuria in the presence of hypotension, tachycardia, and/or a fall in central pressure (CVP or PAWP) is indicative of persistent postobstructive diuresis and appropriate volume replacement should be continued in such instances. In contrast, a reduction in urine output with hemodynamic stability (following a reduction in the rate of fluid administration) suggests iatrogenic polyuria. In this situation, further parenteral fluid replacement may be reduced or discontinued.

Acute Intrinsic Renal Failure

Unlike prenal and postrenal azotemia, acute intrinsic renal failure is associated with renal parenchymal injury and consequently, is not immediately reversible upon withdrawal of the offending factor. However, complete or partial recovery may occur following correction or with resolution of the underlying pathophysiologic process causing injury. Acute intrinsic renal failure with acute tubular necrosis (ATN) is usually caused by ischemic and/or nephrotoxic injury, whereas acute interstitial nephritis (AIN) is thought to be caused by an idiosyncratic or hypersensitivity reaction. A classification of the major causes of acute intrinsic renal failure is provided in Table 8-3.

Typically, a combination of toxic and ischemic insults is operative in the genesis of acute intrinsic renal failure in any given patient. A common example of this would be a septic patient receiving aminoglycosides. Acute renal failure caused by ischemia and/or nephrotoxin exposure is usually associated with histologically demonstrable tubu-

TABLE 8-3 Classification of Acute Intrinsic Renal Failure

A. Ischemic acute tubular necrosis (ATN)
　1. Severe volume depletion: hemorrhage, dehydration, cardiovascular collapse
　2. Surgical complications
　4. Trauma, rhabdomylosis
　4. Septic shock
　5. Severe pancreatitis
B. Nephrotoxic insults
　1. Nephrotoxic antibiotics: aminoglycosides, cephaloridine, amphotericin B, colistin, vancomycin
　2. Iodinated radiographic contrast media
　3. Anesthetic agents: methoxyfluorane, enflurane
　4. Ethylene glycol poisoning (antifreeze)
　5. Cyclosporin administration
　6. Heavy metal poisoning, organic solvents
　7. Anticancer agents: methyl-CCNU, mithramycin, Adriamycin, cis-platinum
C. Acute interstitial nephritis
　1. Drug-induced
　2. Infections
　3. Autoimmunity
　4. Idiopathic

lar epithelial cell necrosis; hence, the term ATN. However, other terms, including acute vasomotor nephropathy (AVN) and lower nephron nephrosis, have been used interchangeably with ATN.

Ischemic Acute Tubular Necrosis (ATN)

As noted, mild to moderate renal hypoperfusion usually causes prerenal azotemia, a condition without any associated renal parenchymal damage that is immediately reversible upon restoration of adequate renal perfusion. With more severe or prolonged renal hypoperfusion "incipient ATN" can occur, where the ability to conserve water is lost. This condition is characterized by nonoliguric renal failure (urine output > 500 ml/day) and a low urine osmolality (< 500 mOsm/kg). Although incipient ATN is not immediately reversible, renal function usually improves within 2 to 3 days following restoration of renal perfusion. A further reduction in renal blood flow may result in established ATN, which is characterized by a severe reduction in GFR with associated oliguria (urine output < 500 ml/day) and marked tubular dysfunction with an inability to conserve sodium (FENa > 3 percent). With established ATN, recovery of renal function generally requires a longer period of time and is often incomplete. The GFR rarely returns to normal (or back to its baseline level of function) and tubular function likewise remains to some extent compromised with the overall prognosis (for functional recovery) being mainly dependent on the severity and duration of the ischemic or toxic insult. Finally, extreme states of renal hypoperfusion can result in partial or complete irreversible cortical necrosis. This latter condition generally occurs in association with profound shock, overwhelming sepsis, and disseminated intravascular coagulation.

Thus, depending on severity, renal ischemia can cause a spectrum of disorders ranging from rapidly reversible prerenal failure to irreversible cortical necrosis. A number of mechanisms have been implicated in the genesis of acute renal failure associated with ischemic and toxic insults (46–52). These include: 1) tubular obstruction by swollen epithelial cells, necrotic epithelial debris, or myoglobin casts in rhabdomyolysis; 2) back-leak of the filtrate through damaged tubular epithelium, thereby negating glomerular filtration; 3) persistent afferent arteriolar constriction and/or efferent arteriolar dilatation leading to a fall in glomerular capillary pressure and net filtration forces (hence the term *acute vasomotor nephropathy*); and 4) a reduction in glomerular capillary wall permeability. Several of these mechanisms are generally operative in most cases of ATN. The histopathologic changes, however, are usually mild and include patchy tubular cell necrosis along with areas of regeneration, proximal tubule brush border loss, dilatation of Bowman's space, the presence of tubular casts, interstitial edema, and inflammation. In general, these changes poorly correlate with both the incidence and severity of ATN; consequently renal biopsy is rarely used in the diagnosis or prognosis of this disorder.

A variety of factors predispose SCI patients to ATN (11,22,53–56). First of all, there is an increased risk for ischemia during the initial posttraumatic period (caused by spinal shock, shock resulting from hemorrhage, and/or shock as a consequence of " third spacing" of fluid into traumatized tissue). Second, there is an increased risk for sepsis and septic shock in SCI patients, with the major sources for infection and sepsis being the lungs, urinary tract, surgical wounds, decubitus ulcers, and osteomyelitis. Third, SCI patients are frequently exposed to various endogenous and exogenous nephrotoxins. An example of the former would be myoglobin, released from muscle as a result of traumatic or ischemic muscle injury, while examples of the latter would include exposure to nephrotoxic antibiotics and intravenous radiographic contrast material.

Laboratory tests (useful in the diagnosis of ATN) are generally those, indicative of tubular dysfunction, that specifically underscore the kidneys' inability to appropriately reabsorb sodium and water and concentrate the urine. Therefore (with established oliguric ATN), urine osmolality is less the 350 mOsm/kg H_2O, urine sodium concentration is increased (> 20 mEq/L), and the fractional excretion of sodium is greater than 1 percent (FENa > 1 percent). However, patients with incipient or mild forms of ATN are typically nonoliguric and may or may not demonstrate abnormalities in sodium reabsorption. Consequently, measurement of urine osmolality and FENa (in nonoliguric ATN) is of dubious diagnostic value.

The urinalysis in ATN characteristically reveals a so called "dirty sediment," that is muddy brown, consisting of tubular epithelial cells and tubular cell casts, as well as a variety of granular casts and other tubular debris. However, in some patients the urine sediment is relatively inactive. The presence of mild proteinuria and microhematuria is also consistent with a diagnosis of ATN. In contrast, heavy proteinuria, hematuria, and red blood cell casts are indicative of glomerulonephritis, while the presence of pyuria with eosinophiluria is presumptively diagnostic for acute interstitial nephritis. Urine that is red, reddish brown, or dark brown suggests the presence of blood, hemoglobin, or myoglobin. However, because all three test positive for blood (by orthotolidine impregnated test strips) further differentiation requires microscopic examination of the urine (which will identify red blood cells); the absence of proportional hematuria provides strong presumptive evidence for either myoglobinuria or hemoglobinuria (more specific laboratory testing is required to differentiate between hemoglobin and myoglobin).

The diagnosis of ATN, therefore, is usually made on the basis of clinical and laboratory evidence and requires the exclusion of other causes of ARF such as prerenal azotemia, postrenal failure, acute interstitial nephritis, renal vascular disorders, and rapidly progressive glomerulonephritis. Close attention should also be given to the sequence of events leading to renal failure (i.e. the clinical setting); therefore, ARF occurring in association with sepsis, shock (related to sepsis or other causes), nephrotoxin exposure, severe trauma, and/or surgery is most likely due to ATN.

Drug-Induced Renal Failure

Despite their relatively small size, the kidneys receive a large portion (approximately 20 percent) of cardiac output. In addition, the kidneys are capable of generating very high intratubular concentrations of potentially toxic substances. Consequently, the kidneys are highly susceptible to injury from various drugs and toxins. The major mechanisms by which pharmaceutical agents cause acute renal failure are listed in Table 8-4. These include: 1) a reduction in glomerular capillary perfusion pressure, causing prerenal failure; 2) tubular injury resulting in acute tubular necrosis (ATN); 3) acute interstitial nephritis; 4) hypersensitivity vasculitis; and 5) tubular obstruction.

Examples of drug-related prerenal failure include volume depletion (caused by the excessive use of diuretics or cathartics) or hypotension (resulting from over-administration of antihy-

TABLE 8-4 Major Mechanisms of Drug-Induced Acute Renal Failure

A. Reduction in glomerular capillary pressure
   1. Preglomerular vasoconstriction (examples include NSAIDs and cyclosporin A)
   2. Postglomerular vasodilatation (examples include ACE-Is and ARBs),
   3. Intravascular volume depletion (examples include diuretics)
B. Renal tubular cell injury and ATN (examples include aminoglycosides and amphotericin)
C. Acute interstitial nephritis (examples include diuretics, NSAIDs, antibiotics, and various miscellaneous drugs)*
D. Hypersensitivity vasculitis (examples include sulfonamides, thiazides, and allopurinol)
E. Intrarenal tubular obstruction (examples include poorly soluble sulfonamides, methotrexate, and acyclovir)

* See Table 8-5.

pertensive agents). In addition, drugs that modulate renal autoregulation such as nonsteroidal anti-inflammatory drugs (NSAIDs), angiotensin converting enzyme inhibitors (ACE-Is), and angiotensin II receptor blockers (ARBs) can predispose patients to prerenal failure (57–64). NSAIDs can reduce glomerular perfusion by causing afferent arteriolar vasoconstriction. This occurs as a result of NSAID inhibition of renal vasodilatory prostaglandin synthesis (i.e., PGI_2 and PGE_2). ACE-Is and ARBs lower glomerular capillary pressure by causing efferent arteriolar dilatation, which is an action resulting from the inhibition of angiotensin II-mediated efferent arteriolar constriction (64–67).

It should be noted that in volume-repleted subjects with normal renal function, the effect of NSAIDs and ARBs on renal perfusion and glomerular filtration is negligible. However, there are a number of conditions that predispose patients to drug-induced vasomotor acute renal failure. These include volume-depleted states (resulting from extracellular fluid losses) and conditions where "effective arterial blood volume" and renal perfusion are reduced (e.g., congestive heart failure, cirrhosis, nephrotic syndrome, sepsis, and traumatic or postoperative settings associated with third spacing of fluid). In volume-depleted states, maintenance of glomerular perfusion is dependent on appropriate renal autoregulatory responses (i.e. afferent arteriolar dilatation and efferent arteriolar constriction). As afferent arteriolar dilatation is mainly a function of vasodilating prostaglandins, the inhibition of prostaglandin synthesis (by NSAIDs) can cause marked reductions in renal perfusion (resulting in ARF) in patients with underlying volume depletion. Furthermore, in the setting of chronic renal failure (CRF), prostaglandins appear to play an important role in the preservation of renal hemodynamics (68). Consequently, even euvolemic CRF patients may be at increased risk for NSAID-induced, vasomotor-related ARF. Furthermore, the concomitant use of NSAIDs with other drugs or agents capable of causing renal vasoconstriction, such as cyclosporin A or intravenous radiocontrast agents, substantially increases the risk for ARF (69,70). The administration of ACE-Is and ARBs may cause acute renal failure in conditions where glomerular capillary pressure and filtration are dependent on angiotensin II-mediated efferent arteriolar vasoconstriction, which again include volume-depleted states, severe congestive heart failure, and cirrhosis (60,62,71,72). In addition, bilateral renal artery stenosis and/or diffuse small vessel disease (nephroangiosclerosis) have been shown to predispose patients (treated with ACE-Is) to ARF (64,73,74).

Nephrotoxic agents can also cause direct injury to renal tubular cells by a variety of mechanisms that include the disruption of plasma membrane integrity, inhibition of enzymatic activity, disruption of mitochondrial function, and/or lysosomal injury. Nephrotoxin exposure can also impair the function of the endoplasmic reticulum, as well as the cell nucleus, resulting in abnormal protein as well as nucleoprotein synthesis. Moreover, the release of toxic substances from damaged tubular cells (e.g., hydrolytic lysosomal enzymes) and increased free radical generation, related to mitochondrial dysfunction and derangements in oxidative metabolism can

compound and accelerate tissue damage. In addition, the presence of underlying renal hypoperfusion and resulting ischemia greatly increases both the incidence and severity of nephrotoxic renal injury.

Drugs Causing Acute Tubular Necrosis

Due to the rapid proliferation and introduction of new pharmacologic agents, the number of drugs capable of causing acute tubular necrosis continues to grow. Currently, these include the nephrotoxic antibiotics, iodinated radiographic contrast media, heavy metals, and certain antineoplastic agents, as well as a growing number of other drugs and chemicals (Table 8-5). The drugs or agents associated with ATN that are most relevant to spinal cord injured patients (aminoglycosides, amphotericin, and radiographic contrast agents) are discussed herein.

Aminoglycoside-induced Acute Tubular Necrosis. Aminoglycoside antibiotics are widely used in the treatment of serious infections caused by gram-negative organisms, particularly *Pseudomonas.* Unfortunately, mild to moderate renal insufficiency occurs with the parenteral use of these

---

TABLE 8-5   Causes of Interstitial Nephritis

A. Drugs (partial list)
  1. Antimicrobial agents: penicillin, synthetic penicillin analogs, cephalosporins, tetracyclines, sulfanamides, rifampin, trimethoprim-sulfa preparations
  2. Nonsteroidal anti-inflammatory drugs: zomepirac, tolmetin, fenoprofen, indomethacin, naproxen, phenylbutazone, diflunisal, mefenamic acid
  3. Miscellaneous: phenindione, warfarin, thiazides, furosemide, allopurinol, azathioprine, phenytoin, cimetidine
B. Infections: diphtheria, leptospirosis, staphylococcal, streptococcal, brucellosis, Legionnaires' disease, toxoplasmosis, mononucleosis, CMV, syphilis, falciparum malaria, etc.
C. Immunologic disorders: systemic lupus erythematosus, Goodpasture's syndrome
D. Idiopathic

---

drugs in about 10 percent of treated patients (75–78). However, the incidence of severe renal failure (requiring dialytic therapy) is considerably less. Factors affecting risk for aminoglycoside nephrotoxicity include (76,79,80):

1. The daily drug dosage, dosing interval, and duration of treatment (i.e. the risk for nephrotoxicity directly correlates with the quantity of drug administered, the frequency of dosing, and duration of treatment). Sequential courses of aminoglycoside therapy (within days or weeks of each other) also increase the risk for nephrotoxicity.
2. The specific aminoglycoside agent used (i.e. based on clinical trial data, the rank order for nephrotoxicity appears to be gentamicin > tobramycin > amikacin > netilmicin) (79–83).
3. Concurrent drug therapy (i.e. the risk for nephrotoxicity is increased when aminoglycosides are administered in conjunction with amphotericin B, vancomycin, cephalothin, clindamycin, cisplatin, furosemide, and intravenous radiocontrast agents).
4. The presence of a coexisting volume, electrolyte, or acid–base disturbance (e.g., volume depletion, hypokalemia, hypomagnesemia, and/or metabolic acidosis have been shown to potentiate aminoglycoside nephrotoxicity).
5. Additional factors that potentiate risk for aminoglycoside toxicity are advanced age, female gender, obesity, preexisting liver disease, and preexisting renal insufficiency.

In SCI patients, because of reductions in muscle mass, serum creatinine values are often substantially lower than expected for the given level of renal function. Therefore, formulas (e.g., the Cockroft and Gault formula) that employ the serum creatinine concentration to estimate renal function require appropriate modification in SCI patients (84,85). (This concept is discussed in more detail under the heading Clinical and Laboratory Features).

Following the administration of aminoglycosides, demonstrable increases in serum creatinine concentration with corresponding reductions in glomerular filtration rate generally do not occur until after 7 to 10 days of therapy, unless drug dosage is excessive or risk factors are present. It is important to emphasize that patients with aminoglycoside-induced ATN are usually nonoliguric, with daily urine output ranging between 500 and 2000 ml. Consequently, the presence of "a normal urine output" should not be regarded as evidence of normal renal function. Instead, daily measurement of BUN and serum creatinine should be used to monitor renal function. Patients should also be monitored for manifestations of aminoglycoside tubular toxicity, including renal potassium and magnesium wasting, which can result in moderate to severe hypokalemia and hypomagnesemia (76,79,86). The earliest laboratory abnormality related to aminoglycoside-induced renal injury is abnormal enzymuria (consisting of lysosomal, brush border, and cytosolic enzymes), which is usually detectable within 1 to 2 days of treatment. However, this finding (indicative of proximal tubular injury) has not been shown to correlate with more serious forms of nephrotoxicity such as ARF. Other manifestations of proximal tubular injury, associated with aminoglycosides, include tubular proteinuria (evidenced by increased urinary excretion of beta$_2$-microglobulin), along with aminoaciduria and glucosuria, while distal tubular dysfunction is evidenced by an inability to normally concentrate urine. This later abnormality generally occurs early in the course of treatment and may persist following discontinuation of therapy (76,79).

Measures that reduce the risk for aminoglycoside nephrotoxicity include:

1. Limiting the use of aminoglycosides to specific indications (i.e. serious gram-negative infections such as *Psuedomonas aeruginosa*) and at the first reasonable opportunity, change to a less nephrotoxic regimen. Other antibiotics shown to be effective in the treatment of serious gram-negative infections include third generation cephalosporins, aztreonam, and imipenem.

2. When forced to use an aminoglycoside, select the appropriate agent with the least nephrotoxicity.

3. Because clinical efficacy is directly related to high peak serum levels, while toxicity is shown to correlate with high trough levels, we do not recommend dosing more frequently than once a day. Recent studies (in patients with normal renal function) show that single daily injections of gentamicin (4–5 mg/kg/day), netilmicin (5 mg/kg/day), and amikacin (15 mg/kg/day) have resulted in a 30 to 50 percent reduction in the cortical concentration of each respective drug when compared with the administration of the same daily dose by continuous infusion (87,88). For most aminoglycosides, regimens using single (once a day) injections have been associated with a lower incidence of nephrotoxicity when compared with regimens where the same daily dose was administered by continuous infusion (89–91). Moreover, a recent randomized study has shown that once-daily dosing of gentamicin (4 mg/kg in patients with normal renal function) was less nephrotoxic and more efficacious than three daily doses of 1.33 mg/kg (92). Once-daily aminoglycoside regimens are also more cost effective than divided dose regimens. In theory, the same loading dose can be administered regardless of renal function; however, with respect to aminoglycosides, smaller loading doses are generally recommended. For example typical loading doses for some of the commonly used aminoglycosides are: gentamicin (1.7 mg/kg); tobramicin (1.7 mg/kg); amikacin (7.5 mg/kg); and netilmicin (2 mg/kg), while maintenance dosing (which can range from every 8 to 24 hours) should be determined by trough levels. Monitoring serum peak and trough levels should begin within 48 hours after starting therapy. Peak aminoglycoside levels, which measure adequacy of dosing, should be obtained 30 minutes after the completion of IV-infusion or 60 minutes following IM injection. Trough levels, which gauge drug accumulation and potential toxicity, should be measured at the end of the dosing interval just prior to the next dose. Recommended trough levels for the commonly used aminoglycosides are: gentamicin (1 to 2 mg/L); tobramicin (1 to 2 mg/L); amikacin (5 to 10 ml/L); and netilmicin (0.5 to 2 mg/L).

4. It is important to correct any preexisting or developing electrolyte abnormalities (e.g., hypokalemia and hypomagnesemia) and maintain an adequate state of volume repletion.

5. If, possible, avoid exposure to other nephrotoxic agents.

6. Because nephrotoxicity is also a function of accumulative dose, attempts should be made to limit the duration of therapy with substitution of less nephrotoxic drugs as soon as it is clinically appropriate. Although acute renal failure associated with aminoglycosides is typically nonoliguric and reversible (following dose reduction or discontinuation), the serum creatinine will often continue to increase for several days (up to a week) before reaching a plateau and returning to baseline values.

Amphotericin Nephrotoxicity. Amphotericin (a polyene antibiotic that is frequently used in the treatment of systemic fungal infections) is also commonly associated with nephrotoxicity (76,79,93–96). Both the antifungal and nephrotoxic actions of amphotericin are related to its interaction with lipid components of cell membranes; where cholesterol–amphotericin complexes formed in cell membranes serve as aqueous channels that allow easy passage of small molecules and ions such as water, potassium, hydrogen ion, and various other solutes. The resulting nephrotoxicity, which can manifest itself in the form of tubular dysfunction or as ARF, is a function of the daily dosage of amphotericin; the accumulative amount administered, as well as the modality of administration. Examples of amphotericin-induced tubular dysfunction include metabolic acidosis (secondary to distal renal tubular acidosis), hypokalemia and hypomagnesemia (resulting from renal potassium and magnesium wasting), and the loss of urinary concentrating ability (secondary to nephrogenic diabetes insipidus) (97–100). Examination of the urinary sediment typically reveals the presence of micro-hematuria, pyuria and cylindruria. Amphotericin-induced ARF is generally dependent on the dosage and duration of therapy, being uncommon when the cumulative dosage is less than 600 mg, whereas up to 80 percent of patients exhibit nephrotoxicity when the cumulative dosage is between 2 and 3 grams (79,93,94,101,102). However, in some patients, ARF occurs early in the course of therapy as a consequence of severe intrarenal vasoconstriction that is usually reversible with either dose reduction or discontinuation of amphotericin. With prolonged treatment, renal insufficiency appears to be a consequence of both vascular dysfunction as well as tubular injury, and recovery is often delayed for weeks or even months. Progressive chronic renal failure, however, is unusual but may occur as a consequence of prolonged therapy or with multiple courses of therapy.

Additional risk factors for amphotericin nephrotoxicity include volume depletion, underlying renal insufficiency, and concomitant exposure to other potential nephrotoxins (e.g., diuretics, aminoglycosides, cisplatin, cyclosporine, radiocontrast agents, and deoxycholate). Ironically, deoxycholate is the standard vehicle in which amphotericin is suspended; consequently, the administration of amphotericin in liposomes or with other lipid vehicles, has been shown to reduce nephrotoxicity without compromising efficacy (103–105). Additional measures shown to diminish risk for amphotericin nephrotoxicity include the maintenance of an adequate state of volume repletion along with the avoidance of diuretic use and the avoidance of the concomitant administration of either intravenous radiocontrast material or nephrotoxic drugs such as aminoglycosides. Because of the high potential risk for nephrotoxicity, all patients receiving amphotericin should undergo frequent monitoring of serum creatinine and serum electrolytes, including sodium, chloride, potassium, bicarbonate, and magnesium.

ACUTE INTERSTITIAL NEPHRITIS (AIN) AND HYPERSENSITIVITY VASCULITIS

It is estimated that AIN causes approximately 10 percent of ARF (106,107). This condition has been described in association with a variety of drugs and infectious diseases (106,108–110). AIN may also develop as a manifestation of a systemic disease such as systemic lupus erythematosus, Sjögren's syndrome, cryoglobulinemia, or Goodpasture's syndrome (111,112). However, in approximately 10 to 20 percent of cases, no discernible cause can be identified, and the AIN is labeled idiopathic (113,114). The causes of AIN are summarized in Table 8-5.

Because SCI patients are frequently exposed to medications (especially antibiotics, diuretics, and NSAIDs) drug-induced AIN should be considered in the differential diagnosis of ARF, particularly when accompanied by pyuria, proteinuria, and/or allergic manifestations. The drugs most commonly associated with AIN are the beta-lactam antibiotics (penicillins and cephalosporins), sulfonamide derivatives, rifampin, diuretics, and NSAIDs (especially those derived from propionic acid such as fenoprofen, ibuprofen, and naproxen) (76,106,108,110). Allergic manifestations (e.g., fever, rash, arthralgias, eosinophilia, and/or eosinophiluria) frequently accompany the type of AIN associated with antibiotics and diuretics. In contrast, NSAID-associated AIN is rarely accompanied by allergic manifestations. However, heavy proteinuria, which is rarely seen with other types of AIN, is a common manifestation of NSAID-associated AIN (76,106,115). Furthermore, the duration of drug exposure is typically much longer with NSAID-associated AIN (0.5 to 18 months) when compared with other types of drug-induced AIN, where duration of drug exposure averages about 15 days (range 1 to 37 days). Although the pathogenesis of AIN remains incompletely understood, most types are thought to involve abnormalities in cell mediated immunity; however, humoral mechanisms may also be important in the genesis of certain forms of this disease.

Typical pathologic features of AIN include the presence of interstitial edema along with cellular infiltrates comprised of mononuclear cells, plasma cells, eosinophils, and neutrophils. In addition, patchy tubular changes are usually apparent, including epithelial cell degeneration, necrosis, and tubular atrophy (106,116). Less commonly reported findings include tubular cell invasion by the inflammatory cells or the presence of interstitial granulomatous lesions (112,117). However, the pathologic features of NSAID-associated AIN are remarkable for tubulointerstitial changes as well as glomerular changes. A focal or diffuse interstitial infiltrate that is predominantly lymphocytic is usually apparent along with vacuolization and degenerative changes involving both the proximal and distal tubules, while the glomeruli characteristically demonstrate epithelial food-process effacement (106,116).

The diagnosis of AIN should be suspected in patients who have ARF associated with pyuria, hematuria, or proteinuria with or without allergic manifestations (e.g., fever, rash, arthralgias, eosinophilia, and/or eosinophiluria)—with the presence of allergic manifestations being characteristic of AIN caused by agents other than NSAIDs. There is also occasional overlap between drug-induced AIN and ATN, as well as between AIN and hypersensitivity vasculitis. For example, in some cases of drug-induced AIN, infiltrating inflammatory cells have been shown to inflict tubular injury, apparently triggering superimposed ATN (117). In addition, a number of drugs, including sulfonamides, thiazides, and allopurinol, have been shown to cause AIN with an associated multiple-organ small-vessel vasculitis involving the skin, liver, heart, and lungs (75,76,118).

Although a definitive diagnosis of AIN generally requires a kidney biopsy, the presence of eosinophiluria in a patient with ARF provides strong presumptive evidence for this diagnosis. In either case, the underlying inciting agent or condition must be identified and removed or effectively treated (i.e. the offending drug discontinued or the infection treated). Following such measures, improvement in renal function should occur, but this may be delayed for several weeks. In patients with drug-induced AIN, where renal function has not improved within 3 weeks (following discontinuation of the offending drug), a 7- to 14-day course of prednisone therapy (1 mg/kg/d) may be beneficial in restoring renal function. Steroid therapy, however, is not recommended in the management of infection-related AIN.

CRYSTALLURIA, TUBULAR OBSTRUCTION, AND ARF

A final mechanism to be discussed with regard to ARF involves renal tubular obstruction related to crystalluria. This occurs when high concentrations of a relatively insoluble substance (e.g., uric acid, calcium oxalate, and certain drugs or their metabolites) precipitate out, causing intrarenal microtubular obstruction (119,121). Drugs and chemicals reported to cause crystalluria-induced ARF include: 1) high doses of certain sulfonamides (e.g., sulfadiazine and sulfamethoxazole) (122,123); 2) high doses of methotrexate ; 3) acyclovir (when given in large doses intravenously) ; 4) uricosuric agents (e.g., probenecid and radiographic contrast agents) when administered in the presence of hyperuricemia; and 5) massive doses of vitamin C as well as ethylene glycol can cause oxalate crystalluria (126,127). It should also be noted that conditions associated with tissue destruction or increased cell turnover (e.g., rhabdomyolysis or tumor lysis syndrome) can cause severe hyperuricemia with ensuing crystalluria and ARF (120).

Acute Tubular Necrosis Associated with Radiographic Contrast Agents

ARF is now a well-recognized complication of intravascularly administered radiographic contrast agents (128–131). The majority of the contrast agents currently available for intravascular administration consist of various salts of the tri-iodinated benzoic acid. As a result of their low PK values, these salts maintain their anionic form in the circulation and as such, are exclusively distributed within the extracellular fluid compartment.

Consequently, they are excreted by the kidney and carry a substantial osmolar load (which is thought to be involved in the genesis of the associated nephrotoxicity). The so-called *nonionic contrast agents* have been made available that contribute substantially lower osmolar loads compared to the older *ionic agents* (132–134). However, it remains unclear whether the newer (nonionic agents) actually reduce the risk of ARF in those patients at high risk for radiographic-contrast nephropathy.

Although the risk for ARF (from radiographic contrast material) is very low in the general population (about 0.1 percent), this risk is substantially increased in patients with underlying renal failure, diabetes mellitus, advanced age, hyperuricemia, multiple myeloma (with associated volume depletion), and in low cardiac output states (129–137). Additional factors shown to increase ARF risk include the use of large amounts of intravenous contrast material, repeated or multiple exposures to radiocontrast, concomitant exposure with other nephrotoxins (e.g., aminoglycosides, amphotericin, and NSAIDs), as well as a previous history for radiocontrast nephrotoxicity (130–138). Preexisting renal disease however, is probably the most important risk factor for radiocontrast nephropathy. Furthermore, the severity of the underlying renal insufficiency generally correlates with the frequency and severity of the superimposed component of ARF.

Diabetes mellitus (with associated diabetic nephropathy) and advanced age (accompanied by diminished nephron mass) have also been reported to increase the risk for radiocontrast nephropathy (135–137). However, additional studies involving diabetic and elderly patients with normal renal function have failed to demonstrate any predisposition to radiocontrast-induced ARF (137–139). These conditions per se (e.g., diabetes and old age), therefore, may not represent independent risk factors for contrast nephropathy. Although volume depletion and low cardiac output states reportedly increase

the risk for radiocontrast-induced ARF, in a similar fashion this risk appears to be only minimally increased in patients with normal renal function, which again emphasizes the importance of renal function with regard to risk. An additional important modulator of risk is the volume status of the patient, where preexisting volume depletion increases the risk for radiocontrast nephropathy irrespective of the underlying condition. For example, in the presence of renal disease, diabetes, or multiple myeloma, the risk for radiocontrast-induced ARF is markedly increased in the presence of volume depletion.

The severity of radiocontrast-induced renal impairment may vary from mild, transient renal insufficiency (with normal urine output) to severe, oliguric ARF requiring dialysis. Most episodes of ARF, however, are reversible and characterized by nonoliguria and a low fractional excretion of sodium. Elevations in serum creatinine and BUN typically occur within 24 hours of radiographic contrast exposure, reaching a peak in several days and returning to baseline within 1 to 2 weeks. In addition, an exceedingly high urine specific gravity (> 1.032), due to the presence of iodinated radiocontrast, is often apparent on urinalysis.

Although the pathogenesis of acute renal failure associated with radiocontrast agents is not completely known, the following mechanisms may be involved: 1) direct tubular epithelial damage as evidenced by vacuolization, degeneration, and necrosis of tubular cells on histologic examination, as well as the appearance of enzymes and other markers of tubular injury, in the urine; 2) intrarenal obstruction by sloughed tubular cells, proteinaceous casts (i.e. Tamm–Horsfall glycoprotein), and uric acid (augmented by the uricosuric effect of radiocontrast agents); and 3) renal vasoconstriction, which generally follows an initial period of vasodilation. Although the vasoconstrictive response is usually transient (lasting a few minutes), it can persist (particularly in the presence of an activated renin–angiotensin system).

Radiographic contrast nephrotoxicity can usually be prevented by observing the following points:

1. Risk factors should be identified and based on a risk-versus-benefit analysis; alternative diagnostic procedures should be considered and used in those patients at increased risk when deemed appropriate (e.g., ultrasonography, MRI, and radionuclide scanning).
2. The co-administration of other potentially nephrotoxic agents should be avoided (i.e. NSAIDs and nephrotoxic antibiotics should be discontinued or avoided, if possible).
3. Dehydrating preparatory measures such as the use of cathartics and overnight fasting should be avoided in high-risk patients.
4. Patients should be maintained in a volume-repleted state prior to, during, and following the administration of radiographic contrast material.
5. Hyperuricemia should be corrected prior to the administration of radiographic contrast material (because these agents are uricosuric and ARF can result from intratubular obstruction due to uric acid sludging).
6. The quantity of contrast material being administered should be kept to a minimum and multiple sequential studies within the same 2- to 3-day period should be avoided in high-risk patients.
7. Other measures reported to reduce the risk for radiocontrast-induced ARF include *a*) Pretreatment with a calcium channel blocker; *b*) the use of nonionic contrast agents and; *c*) the administration of mannitol (132–134,140, 141). Although there is consistent data supporting the prophylactic efficacy of calcium channel blockers in ameliorating radiocontrast-induced nephrotoxicity in high-risk patients, data supporting the beneficial effects of mannitol and non-ionic contrast are less consistent and their use in reducing ARF risk remains controversial.

Acute Tubular Necrosis Associated with Rhabdomyolysis

Rhabdomyolysis and myoglobinuria can occur as a result of the initial trauma responsible for spinal cord injury (22,142,143). In addition, a variety of other conditions (present in SCI) including metabolic disorders, toxic insults, pressure necrosis, seizures, and hyperpyrexia, may cause rhabdomyolysis (142,144–147). Although approximately 33 percent of able-bodied persons with rhabdomyolysis develop ATN , the incidence of ATN in SCI patients with rhabdomyolysis is not known; however, it is expected to be equal to or even greater than that seen in individuals without spinal cord injury.

Patients with rhabdomyolysis characteristically present with reddish-brown or dark brown urine that tests markedly positive for blood (with orthotolidine test strips, which are sensitive to both myoglobin and hemoglobin), but on microscopic examination there are disproportionately few red blood cells present. In addition, the affected muscles typically exhibit pain, tenderness, or swelling. Patients with rhabdomyolysis and ARF are also at risk for pronounced hyperkalemia, hyperuricemia, and hyperphosphatemia as a consequence of an increased flux of potassium, phosphorus, and nucleoproteins from damaged muscle (149). Marked initial hypocalcemia with subsequent hypercalcemia, generally occurring during the recovery phase of ATN has also been reported. The hypocalcemia may be related to the development of hyperphosphatemia, which promotes precipitation of calcium into soft tissues. Other putative mechanisms for hypocalcemia include skeletal resistance to the calcemic action of parathyroid hormone or in some cases, parathyroid gland dysfunction, although remobilization of calcium from damaged muscle appears to be the mechanism responsible for hypercalcemia (150). The proportional increase in serum creatinine is generally greater in ATN associated with rhabdomyolysis because of the release of both creatinine and creatine from the injured muscle.

Serum levels of creatine phosphokinase (CPK), aldolase, aspartate aminotransferase (AST), and lactate dehydrogenase (LDH) rise dramatically in patients with rhabdomyolysis as a result of muscle injury. Therefore, the demonstration of high serum levels of CPK or other intracellular enzymes is essential in the diagnosis of rhabdomyolysis. If positive, the presence of myoglobin in the serum or urine is also diagnostically useful. Although the precise mechanism by which myoglobinuria causes ATN is uncertain, ischemia related to intrarenal vasoconstriction combined with normal or increased oxygen requirements may be involved. In patients with rhabdomyolysis and myoglobinuria, ARF can be prevented by infusion of normal saline to correct any fluid-volume deficit and maintain urine output at 100 to 200 ml/hr along with alkalinization of the urine with sodium bicarbonate administration to maintain urine pH $\geq$7.0 (151,152).

CHRONIC RENAL INSUFFICIENCY

Chronic renal insufficiency is a serious complication of long-standing spinal cord injury that causes substantial morbidity and mortality. In a large necropsy series reported by Tribe and Silver in 1969, renal insufficiency was the primary cause of death in the great majority (75 percent) of cases studied (153). In a subsequent report published in 1977 by Hackler (154), chronic renal failure was found to be the principal cause of death in 45 percent of patients (in a cohort of World War II and Korean War veterans with traumatic spinal cord injury). An additional report by Borges and Hackler (involving a group of Vietnam War veterans with SCI) demonstrated further reduction in the percentage of deaths from renal causes (20 percent), while in 1982 Price reported a renal-related mortality rate of only 14 percent in a long-term follow-up study (involving a large group of civilian SCI patients) . More recent studies have continued to demonstrate this trend; Devivo, et al., through a process of merging survival data (from the National Database, available collaborative studies, and the Social Security Administration) has shown that kidney and urinary tract diseases account for only a small percentage (3.5 percent) of all deaths in SCI patients (3,157). However, diseases of the urinary system were found to be the most frequent secondary contributing cause of death in SCI patients. Much of the progress in the prevention of renal insufficiency and reduction of urinary tract disease-related mortality (in SCI patients) has been achieved by a combination of intensive patient education, prevention and control of infection, prevention of reflux, and most importantly, special attention to the maintenance of urine flow and bladder drainage (2,3,53,157,158).

Pathogenesis

Tubulointerstitial diseases, characterized by progressive renal insufficiency (with associated pyuria but only minimal proteinuria) have been generally described as the predominant type of kidney disease occurring in SCI patients. However, it has been our experience that moderate to heavy proteinuria, indicative of glomerular disease, is frequently present in SCI patients with moderate to advanced renal insufficiency. It would therefore appear that both tubulointerstitial and glomerular injury are involved in the development of chronic renal failure in patients with long-standing spinal cord injury. This concept is consistent with a growing body of evidence indicating that multiple predisposing factors and at least several pathophysiologic processes are likely to be involved in the genesis of chronic renal insufficiency in patients with long-standing SCI. These include chronic pyelonephritis, nephrolithiasis, obstructive nephropathy, reflux nephropathy, amyloidosis, and hypertensive nephrosclerosis (2,4–6,8,10,53, 158,159).

Chronic urinary tract infection with pyelonephritis contributed to renal insufficiency in every one of 43 SCI patients with end stage renal disease reported by our group (160), which is similar to the experience reported by other investigators (153). In SCI patients, bacteria may gain easy access to the bladder via an indwelling catheter or as a complication of intermittent catheterization. Fecal contamination, as well as the dampness associated with absorbent garments, may also increase the frequency and rate of bacterial colonization and subsequent infection. Also, in patients with decubitus ulcers, there is often cross infection between infected pressure sores and the urinary tract (160). Moreover, in SCI patients, urinary tract infections are frequently perpetuated by impaired urinary drainage, the presence of urinary calculi, and/or with the use of indwelling catheters (2,29,53,159,160). Furthermore, the combination of active infection and functional obstruction often leads to vesicoureteral reflux along with a progressive destructive pyelonephritis. In addition to causing tubulointerstitial injury and predisposing to pyelonephritis, reflux nephropathy has been associated with the development of focal glomerulosclerosis (161). This condition generally presents with proteinuria and hypertension and can cause or contribute to progressive renal failure in SCI patients. The mechanism by which vesicoureteral reflux leads to glomerulosclerosis is thought to involve the development of glomerular capillary hypertension with subsequent hyperfiltration injury, related to reflux-mediated progressive nephron loss.

Nephrolithiasis is another frequent finding among patients with long-standing spinal cord injury, particularly in those patients with persistent urinary tract infection; however, a number of factors may be involved in the genesis of this abnormality (16,17,23,162). Although hypercalciuria caused by immobilization is common during the early phase of SCI, it is usually absent or less pronounced during the more chronic phases of the disease (163). In fact, urinary calcium excretion may be reduced in those patients with chronic renal impairment because of an associated impairment in vitamin D metabolism or the development of secondary hyperparathyroidism. In addition, we have noted substantial hyperoxaluria in a group of spinal cord injured patients with varying degrees of renal insufficiency that may be caused by increased intestinal absorption of oxalate occasioned by the associated impairment of bowel motility (26). We have also noted reductions in urinary citrate in SCI patients, and other investigators have confirmed this observation (27,28). Therefore, reduction in the urinary content of citrate, which is a potent inhibitor of

stone formation, may be of significance in the genesis of urolithiasis in this population. However, urinary tract infection (particularly those caused by urease-producing organisms) is probably the most important predisposing factor to urolithiasis. Such infections can facilitate formation of struvite stones by providing an abundance of ammonium while also greatly increasing the urinary pH. Urinary stasis related to functional obstruction, as well as inflammatory debris associated with infection, also facilitate stone formation in SCI patients. Development of urolithiasis may further contribute to renal deterioration by causing obstruction and, more importantly, by complicating the treatment of urinary tract infection. In addition, sequential studies have revealed a significant fall in renal plasma flow in SCI patients with the development of nephrolithiasis (164).

Amyloidosis is another major factor contributing to the development of renal insufficiency in patients with long-standing spinal cord injury. In addition, amyloidosis is the major cause of heavy proteinuria seen in this population. According to the results of autopsy studies reported by Tribe and Silver, 50 percent of the patients studied had evidence for renal amyloidosis (6). In a more recent study involving 43 spinal cord injured patients with end-stage renal disease, we found an even greater prevalence (81 percent) of renal amyloidosis (153). The greater incidence of renal amyloidosis in our patients was thought to be related to their longer survival made possible by the availability of maintenance hemodialysis. Infected pressure sores, osteomyelitis, and urinary tract infections with pyelonephritis (commonly present in SCI patients) appear to be the major predisposing factors in the genesis of secondary amyloidosis.

As a final consideration, hypertensive nephrosclerosis may contribute to the progression of renal failure in SCI patients (particularly in those patients with underlying renal insufficiency) (6,158). This observation is based on clinical experience as well as autopsy data and underscores the importance of maintaining good blood pressure control.

Prevention

Chronic renal insufficiency is an entirely preventable complication of SCI. This is evidenced by the steady decline in mortality from renal causes, which parallels the technical and therapeutic improvements reflected in the data published during the last two decades (154,156). Measures that are effective in the prevention or treatment of urinary obstruction and infection have played and continue to play a most pivotal role in the reduction of renal disease as well as renal-related morbidity and mortality in SCI patients. Good bladder management includes 1) the maintenance of low voiding pressure; 2) the provision of a relatively large capacity low-pressure storage system and; 3) the prevention of infection (53). Ideally, good bladder management will be achievable through reflex voiding. If this is accomplished, however, post-void residual volumes should be less than 100 ml, and bladder pressures (during storage and while voiding) should be below 35 to 40 cm H_2O. In some patients, high voiding pressures may be improved with the use of alpha-adrenergic blocking drugs and/or antispasticity agents, while administration of musculotropic relaxants, tricyclic antidepressants, or anticholinergic agents may improve bladder storage capacity (2,53,165). When reflex voiding is not feasible, the utilization of intermittent bladder catheterization provides a viable option. A clean technique should be used (regarding catheterization), and bladder overdistention must be avoided (through the use of frequent or timely catheterization). Further, the adjunctive use of medication may be effective in increasing bladder capacity and reducing intravesical pressure (2,53). Placement of a chronic indwelling catheter, however, is less desirable due to an increased risk for urinary tract infection, calculous disease, dysreflexia, and bladder cancer (2,53,159). In male patients, external sphincterotomy may be useful in lowering the intra-vesicular pressure and ameliorating vesicoureteral reflux as well as allowing a catheter-free status in patients with detrusor-sphincter dyssynergia

(53,155). It is recommended that annual assessment of the urinary tract be performed to screen for bladder changes, vesicoureteral reflux, and calculous disease. This can usually be accomplished with a cystogram and ultrasonography or with excretory urography (if renal function is normal) (2,53).

Prevention or effective management of urolithiasis is also very important in SCI. Measures that effectively prevent or reduce the frequency and severity of urinary tract infections, as well as treatment designed to minimize obstruction and maintain satisfactory urine flow, are essential in reducing urolithiasis risk (2,29,53,162). Such measures are particularly important in preventing the formation of struvite stones, which are the most common type of calculi seen in SCI patients and the most problematic. In addition, the use of urease inhibitors may prove useful in the management of struvite stones. Patients who form calcium oxalate stones may benefit from a reduction in dietary oxalate, improved bowel care, and pyridoxine supplementation, which decreases endogenous oxalate production. In addition, adequate calcium intake can reduce oxalate absorption by chelation of dietary oxalate within the intestine. Also, patients should be advised against consuming large quantities of vitamin C, which acts as an oxalate precursor, increasing production of endogenous oxalate. Although the use of stone forming inhibitors such as citrate has not to our knowledge been evaluated in SCI, treatment with sodium or potassium citrate may prove useful in those patients who have distal renal tubular acidosis as a risk factor for urolithiasis.

Because secondary amyloidosis is a consequence of chronic infection and suppuration, its prevention is predicated on either the prevention or effective management of infection. SCI patients are at high risk for a number of infections, including urinary tract infections with pyelonephritis, that may be further complicated by abscess formation (renal and perinephric) and sepsis. Decubitus ulcers are also common, with an annual incidence of approximately 23 percent (4,158). Moreover, these lesions often become infected, which may be further complicated by cellulitis and/or osteomyelitis. Respiratory complications, however, are the leading cause of mortality in SCI patients, with atelectasis and pneumonia being particularly problematic in patients who have high cervical lesions (3,4,157). With further progress in the area of infectious disease management both mortality and morbidity rates should continue to improve in SCI patients.

Clinical and Laboratory Features

Progression of renal disease causes not only a reduction in excretory function but also results in renal-related metabolic and endocrine dysfunction. Diminished excretory function is manifested by a reduction in glomerular filtration rate with associated elevations in BUN and serum creatinine levels. As noted, due to reduced muscle mass, the magnitude of serum creatinine elevation in SCI patients may be considerably less than in able-bodied individuals with comparable renal insufficiency. For the same reason, the serum concentration and urinary excretion of creatinine are proportionately lower in quadriplegics when compared with paraplegics having comparable levels of renal function (85). However, it should be noted that creatinine clearance, when calculated from measurements of urinary and plasma creatinine concentration, is not affected by differences in muscle mass or creatinine production and can be reliably used in the assessment of glomerular filtration rate in SCI patients. On the contrary, one should avoid using standard formulas or nomograms to estimate creatinine clearance in SCI patients because these formulas are designed for use in able-bodied individuals who have normal muscle mass. We compared creatinine clearance measurements, obtained from urine and serum collections, with those calculated from the serum creatinine concentration using an equation popularized by Cockroft and Gault: (84,85)

$$Ccr = \frac{(140 - age) \times wt \ (kg)}{72 \times Scr \ (mg \, / \, dl)}$$

for men and

$$Ccr = \frac{(140 - age) \times 0.85 \ wt \ (kg)}{72 \times Scr \ (mg \, / \, dl)}$$

for women, where Ccr represents creatinine clearance (ml/min), wt stands for body weight, and Scr represents serum creatinine concentration (mg/dl). In this study, we found that while the measured and calculated values closely approximated one another (in the able-bodied group) the Cockroft and Gault formula substantially overestimated the true (measured) creatinine clearance in SCI patients. Specifically, the calculated creatinine clearance overestimated the measured value (by 20 percent in paraplegics and 40 percent in quadriplegics), necessitating the use of correction factors (i.e. of 0.8 in quadriplegics and 0.6 in paraplegics) (84,85). In contrast to serum creatinine, the blood urea nitrogen concentration in SCI patients has been shown to be comparable to values obtained from able-bodied persons with similar levels of renal function, dietary protein intake, and metabolic state (165). It should be noted, however, that blood urea nitrogen levels are usually affected to a greater extent than serum creatinine by factors such as dietary protein intake, catabolic rate, and state of hydration. Because moderate to advanced renal insufficiency in SCI is often caused by a combination of glomerular and tubulointerstitial disease, urinary findings may include proteinuria, hematuria, and pyuria. The presence of heavy proteinuria, or the development of nephrotic syndrome (i.e. > 3.5 grams of urinary protein per 24 hours), usually signifies glomerular involvement with secondary amyloidosis or focal glomerulosclerosis. Additional evidence for tubulointerstitial disease may include polyuria, impaired urinary concentrating ability, impaired urinary sodium reabsorption, renal tubular acidosis, and hyporeninemic hypoaldosteronism.

Although the ability to conserve sodium and water is usually impaired in most SCI patients with renal disease, sodium-volume overload may become problematic with the development of hypertension, cardiac failure, and pulmonary edema particularly in patients with moderate to severe renal failure.

The kidneys are the principal organs involved in potassium excretion, and in response to progressive nephron loss, tubular secretion of potassium is increased in the remaining functional nephrons. Increased potassium secretion by colonic mucosa also helps maintain potassium homeostasis. However, in the presence of severe renal insufficiency, these adaptive mechanisms generally fail to prevent hyperkalemia. Severe hyperkalemia can also occur in patients with moderate renal insufficiency when large amounts of potassium enter the extracellular fluid compartment from an exogenous source, such as the ingestion of potassium-rich food or the intravenous administration of fluids containing potassium. In addition, excessive release of potassium from the intracellular compartment due to hemolysis, rhabdomyolysis, tissue necrosis, or hypercatabolic states can cause severe hyperkalemia in patients with impaired renal function. Alternatively, conditions capable of adversely affecting renal tubular transport of potassium—including reduced distal sodium delivery, oliguria, hyperreninemia, hypoaldosteronism, use of potassium-sparing diuretics (e.g., amiloride, triamterene, spironolactone), and prostaglandin synthetase inhibitors (e.g., NSAIDs)—predispose to hyperkalemia, even in patients with mild to moderate renal insufficiency. Likewise, constipation can contribute to hyperkalemia by limiting colonic excretion of potassium. This is of particular significance in SCI patients, who frequently suffer from impaired colonic motility and anal sphincter dysfunction. Hyperkalemia in turn predisposes patients to severe electrophysiologic disorders that can cause life-threatening arrhythmias, cardiac conduction defects, and cardiac arrest, as well as skeletal and smooth muscle weakness or paralysis. Accordingly, hyperkalemia represents one of the most critical complications of renal insufficiency.

Patients with renal insufficiency also have a compromised capacity for magnesium excretion, and as a consequence, they are at risk for hypermagnesemia. This condition can cause skeletal muscle weakness or paralysis, the loss of deep tendon reflexes, and cardiac conduction defects, as well as alterations in mental status. Therefore, the use of magnesium-containing antacids and laxatives generally should be avoided in patients with renal insufficiency.

Endocrinologic Disorders. The metabolic and endocrine functions of the kidneys are multifaceted and include production of specific hormones (e.g., erythropoietin, $1,25(OH)_2D_3$ and prostaglandins) and regulation of the renin–angiotensin–aldosterone system. In addition, the kidneys participate in the metabolism and excretion of various polypeptide and steroid hormones and also serve as target organs for a number of hormones (e.g., aldosterone, parathormone, atrial natriuretic peptide, and antidiuretic hormone). In chronic renal failure, not only are there parallel losses involving both the excretory and endocrine functions of the kidney, in addition, the profound biochemical abnormalities (induced by renal insufficiency) can adversely affect the function of other endocrine glands. Accordingly, severe renal insufficiency is associated with multiple endocrinopathies, the discussion of which is beyond the scope of this chapter. One additional consideration regarding SCI patients with end-stage renal disease is the high incidence of amyloidosis involving various endocrine organs, which may further contribute to endocrine dysfunction in this setting (166)

Hematologic Complications. One of the most constant and disabling consequences of end-stage renal disease is anemia, which is primarily related to erythropoietin deficiency (167). However, impaired iron utilization, a shortened erythrocyte life span, nutritional deficiencies, and blood loss are also involved in the genesis of anemia in chronic renal failure (168). In a study involving the hematopoietic system in end-stage renal disease (ESRD) we found anemia to be of greater severity in SCI patients (treated with hemodialysis) compared to able-bodied hemodialysis patients (169). In addition, we found a high incidence of amyloid deposition in the bone marrow of SCI patients with ESRD, which may also be a contributing factor in the development of anemia in this setting.

Another complication of severe renal insufficiency is platelet dysfunction, which can predispose to bleeding problems. Studies involving coagulation and fibrinolytic pathways conducted by our group, in patients with long-standing spinal cord injury and ESRD have revealed numerous abnormalities in both the intrinsic and extrinsic pathways (170–173). There was also an increased prevalence of antithrombin III deficiency along with decreased protein C anticoagulant activity (in the presence of increased protein C antigen concentration) (173). In addition, significant alterations were noted in the fibrinolytic system, including a marked reduction in tissue plasminogen activator activity (173). Overall the coagulation and fibrinolytic abnormalities observed in this population suggest a predisposition for thrombophilic diathesis.

Disorders of Bone and Mineral Metabolism. The kidneys are the principal producer of $1,25(OH)_2D_3$ (the biologically active metabolite of vitamin D), which is essential in calcium absorption and normal bone metabolism. Advanced renal insufficiency causes $1,25(OH)_2D_3$ deficiency, which in turn can result in a negative calcium balance and osteomalacia. Furthermore, the combination of $1,25(OH)_2D_3$ deficiency, hypocalcemia, and hyperphosphatemia (the latter a consequence of reduced renal phosphate excretion) stimulates parathyroid activity, which often results in secondary hyperparathyroidism. Moreover, complications of secondary hyperparathyroidism, including high-turnover bone disease, metastatic calcifications, and osteitis fibrosa cystica substantially contribute to morbidity and mortality in ESRD (174–176). Recent studies have shown that risk for metastatic soft tissue calcification is significantly increased when the serum calcium phosphate (Ca $\times$ P) product exceeds 60 to 70 mg^2/dL^2 (174,177). Bone disease is further compounded by demineralization (relat-

ed to chronic acidosis and reduced physical activity), which is generally present in SCI patients with advanced renal disease. In addition, aluminum-related bone disease can occur in patients who are receiving aluminum containing compounds (usually in the form of antacids or phosphate binders) (178). Aluminum overload has also been reported in patients inadvertently dialyzed utilizing dialysates prepared from aluminum-contaminated water (179). Aluminum toxicity (which can cause bone disease, dementia, myopathy, and anemia) has been substantially curtailed with the use of better water purification techniques in dialysis and by the diminished use of aluminum-containing phosphate binders. The latter has been accomplished by the substitution of effective nonaluminum containing phosphate binders (e.g., calcium carbonate, calcium acetate, and RenaGel®).

Finally, a peculiar type of amyloidosis has been described in long-term dialysis patients, where there is deposition of amyloid fibrils (containing beta2-microglobulin) in collagen tissue, particularly in the synovia of joints and tendons as well as in subchondral bone (180). The most common clinical manifestations of this disease are carpal tunnel syndrome and a destructive spondyloarthropathy typically involving the shoulders, knees, hips, and axial skeleton. Characteristic radiographic findings include erosions and defects involving the margins of affected bone, particularly at tendon insertion sites, as well as the presence of radiolucent cystic lesions within subchondral bone. The pathophysiology of *dialysis-related amyloidosis* involves tissue accumulation of beta$_2$-microglobulin (a low molecular weight protein expressed by nucleated cells) that is normally filtered and degraded by the kidneys. Even though beta$_2$-microglobulin is removed with dialysis (up to 400 to 600 mg/wk with high flux dialysis), accumulation continues because of the high rate of production (approximately 1500 mg/wk). Consequently, the only known effective treatment for this condition is successful kidney transplantation.

Neurologic Consequences. Both the central nervous system (CNS) and peripheral nervous system (PNS) are affected by uremia. Some of the major CNS manifestations include the reversal of normal sleep patterns, reduction in cognitive function, asterixis, confusion, obtundation, and coma. Uremic peripheral neuropathy can involve both sensory and motor modalities. CNS manifestations readily improve with the institution of adequate dialysis therapy. However, once significant uremic neuropathy develops, the response (if any) to dialysis therapy is slow and often incomplete. For this reason, dialytic therapy should be initiated prior to the development of clinically significant peripheral neuropathy. Because the superimposed neurologic manifestations of uremia can compound and greatly magnify disability in SCI patients, the early institution of renal replacement therapy should be considered in this setting.

Cardiovascular and Pulmonary Complications. Severe renal insufficiency predisposes patients to fluid overload, congestive heart failure, pulmonary edema, and hypertension (181). However, a combination of dietary fluid and sodium restriction, dialysis, and the use of antihypertensive agents can effectively control these problems. Pericarditis is generally a late manifestation of untreated uremia, which can be complicated by cardiac tamponade (181,182). The presence of uremic pericarditis signifies the need for the prompt institution of dialytic therapy. Patients already receiving "adequate dialysis," however, may occasionally develop *dialysis-associated pericarditis* that does not appear to be uremic-related. However, an assessment of dialysis adequacy is indicated in all dialysis patients presenting with pericarditis because a deficient dialysis regimen could predispose to this condition. Patients should also be evaluated for other potential triggering factors or causes of pericarditis, including intercurrent infection, hyperparathyroidism, hyperuricemia, chronic volume overload, and malnutrition. In addition, pericarditis may be a manifestation of an underlying systemic disease (e.g., systemic lupus erythematosus) or related to the use of a drug (e.g., minoxidil). Acute pericarditis should be suspected in patients who present with chest pain and fever; the diagnosis is confirmed by the presence of a pericardial friction rub. Echocardiography is also useful in detecting and monitoring the progress of pericardial effusions. It should be noted, however, that small asymptomatic pericardial effusions (<100ml) are routinely described in dialysis patients and probably have no clinical relevance. Patients with acute pericarditis should be hospitalized and closely monitored for arrhythmias, as well as for signs of impending tamponade (e.g., pulsus paradoxus or unexplained dialysis associated hypotension) (182). The management of dialysis-associated pericarditis includes:

1. Intensifying the dialysis regimen by increasing the frequency of dialysis, usually to five treatments per week for a period of 2 to 4 weeks.
2. Avoidance of anticoagulation (to reduce the risk for tamponade, heparin-free dialysis should be used).
3. Volume depletion should be avoided and patients should not be excessively ultrafiltrated below their targeted dry weight.
4. Adequate pain control using either acetaminophen, codeine, hydrocodone, or in extreme cases, morphine sulfate. It should be noted that neither the use of NSAIDs, systemic steroids, nor intrapericardial steroids have been shown to be particularly beneficial in the management of pericarditis-related pain (182).
5. Cardiac tamponade requires timely surgical attention with drainage, preferably via subxiphoid pericardiostomy. Blind needle pericardiocentesis should only be used as emergency treatment for life-threatening tamponade. Although most patients recover from pericarditis with conservative management, this disease still accounts for 3 to 4 percent of all deaths in dialysis patients, and constrictive pericarditis can occasionally occur as a delayed complication.

In addition to pericarditis, hypertrophy and/or dilatation of the cardiac chambers and ischemic heart disease are more common in patients with advanced renal failure (183,184). Furthermore, in an autopsy study performed at our center involving SCI-ESRD patients, one or more cardiac abnormalities were noted in every patient examined (185). These included fibrinous pericarditis (50 percent), left- and right-ventricular hypertrophy (45 and 20 percent respectively), left- and right-ventricular dilation (40 and 30 percent, respectively), cardiac amyloidosis (25 percent), myocardial fibrosis (45 percent), and coronary arteriosclerosis (45 percent). In addition to pulmonary congestion and edema (thought to be the result of uncontrolled hypervolemia), a number of pulmonary abnormalities were also noted in the majority of patients examined. These included pneumonia, pulmonary interstitial and pleural fibrosis, pulmonary arteriosclerosis, and calcification, as well as the deposition of amyloid and hemosiderin (186).

Infections. Bacterial infections are extremely prevalent in SCI patients with advanced renal failure. In fact, chronic infections involving the urinary tract, pressure wounds, and osteomyelitis are contributing factors in the development and progression of renal disease in this population. In a survey of 43 SCI-ESRD patients, practically all had evidence for chronic active urinary tract infection, while many were noted to have infected pressure ulcers (some with associated osteomyelitis) (160). In addition, vascular access infection, respiratory infection, peritonitis (mainly occurring in those treated with peritoneal dialysis), and sepsis were encountered with considerable frequency. Cross-infection between pressure sores, urinary tract, and blood access or peritoneal access was also frequently observed. Fever and significant leukocytosis were either absent or disproportionately mild, for the severity of the associated infection, and in more than 50 percent of cases, septicemia was the immediate cause of death.

Gastrointestinal Complications and Releated Disease. Gastrointestinal (GI) complications are common in SCI-ESRD patients and may be related to a variety of factors, including spinal cord injury per se, the effects of chronic renal failure, medication side effects, as well as the side effects and complications of renal replacement therapy. With regard to SCI, during the first month post-injury, adynamic ileus and gastric ulcerations are the most frequently reported GI complications, whereas in patients with chronic SCI, fecal impaction is the most frequent GI-related problem (187). Gastroesophageal reflux disease (GERD) is also commonly seen in SCI patients, and this condition may be exacerbated by associated recumbency, immobilization, and irregular mealtime patterns. Furthermore, impaired gastric emptying, reported to be more common in patients with lesions above T-1, may also exacerbate GERD and increase the risk for related complications such as gastritis, esophagitis, and GI-bleeding (188). Additional factors that predispose to GI-bleeding in this setting include stress ulcers, malnutrition, hypovolemic shock, and increased exposure to medications such as NSAIDs, corticosteroids, and anticoagulants (189,190). Another common problem in SCI patients is intestinal obstruction that may occur during the initial post-injury period due to adynamic ileus or pseudoobstruction related to trauma, surgery, anesthesia, or severe medical illness (e.g., pneumonia or sepsis). Because of the loss of autonomic nervous system stimulation and central control of the act of defecation, constipation with fecal impaction may be problematic in patients with chronic SCI. Moreover, the superimposition of renal failure can adversely affect the frequency, severity, and nature of gastrointestinal complications in SCI patients. For example, some of the most common symptoms of uremia per se are gastrointestinal (e.g., anorexia, nausea, and vomiting) while stomatitis, gastritis, duodenitis, and colitis with associated gastrointestinal bleeding are frequent complications of uncontrolled uremia. Characteristically, uremic-related gastrointestinal manifestations should rapidly improve following the institution of dialysis. Therefore, the persistence of any symptoms or manifestations of gastrointestinal disease in a patient receiving adequate dialysis therapy should prompt further evaluation to identify some other cause for the persisting symptomatology.

A second concern involves the apparent increased risk for gastrointestinal disease in "nonuremic" ESRD patients on maintenance dialysis, where a higher prevalence of gastritis, GERD, duodenitis, hiatal hernia, pancreatitis, and gallbladder disease is reported (191–194). Furthermore, gastrointestinal disease related to beta2-microglobulin amyloid infiltration has been reported in long-term chronic dialysis patients, while our group has reported a high incidence of gastrointestinal pathology related to secondary amyloidosis with involvement of both the liver and alimentary tract (195). Also reported (in dialysis patients) is an increased incidence of gastrointestinal angiodysplasia, a condition that can cause life-threatening, difficult to manage, recurrent episodes of gastrointestinal bleeding (196,197). Other conditions that increase GI-bleeding risk in ESRD include esophagitis, gastritis duodenitis, and colitis, as well as the occurrence of single discrete ulcerations usually located in the cecum or ascending colon (192,198, 199). In addition, the use of medications such as aspirin, NSAIDs, prednisone, and oral iron has been associated with upper gastrointestinal bleeding in dialysis patients. Furthermore, underlying platelet dysfunction (commonly present in uncontrolled uremia) can reoccur as a consequence of inadequate dialysis and should, therefore, be ruled out as a cause or contributing factor regarding bleeding in ESRD patients. If present, qualitative platelet dysfunction (as evidenced by a prolonged Ivy bleeding time) should improve or resolve with restoration of adequate dialysis therapy. Furthermore, when indicated, a more rapid improvement in bleeding time (within 1 to 2 hours) can be accomplished with Desmopressin (DDAVP) administration (0.3 mg/kg IV or SC); however, this effect is short in duration (lasting only 6 to 8 hours) and repeat dosing may be ineffective (200). The intravenous administration of estrogen (0.6 mg/kg/day for 5 days) may also be effective in reducing abnormal bleeding times, with an onset in action occurring after approximately 6 hours and duration of effect lasting up to 30 days (201). A final consideration, applicable to any bleeding problem occurring in a dialysis patient, concerns the use of heparin. That is, in patients who are either actively bleeding or are at increased risk for bleeding, hemodialysis should be performed using a heparin-free or regional citrate protocol.

Of additional concern in able-bodied hemodialysis patients, is the disproportionately high incidence of acute abdominal disease presenting with acute abdominal pain with peritoneal signs reported to be caused by diseases such as acute pancreatitis, diverticulitis, spontaneous colonic perforation, bowel infarction, and strangulated abdominal wall hernia (194,202–204). Because the presence of spinal cord injury is also associated with increased risk for acute abdominal disease, it would be logical to assume that SCI-ESRD patients have at least a similar—if not greater—risk for life-threatening acute abdominal disease as able-bodied dialysis patients. Moreover, because visceral sensation is generally impaired in SCI patients, many of the early clues regarding diagnosis (usually obtained from the history and physical examination) are obscured. For example, after bowel perforation, abdominal discomfort may not be apparent until inflammation has reached the upper abdominal peritoneum which receives innervation from high cervical cord segments. Because a timely diagnosis of life-threatening acute abdominal disease is often difficult in SCI patients, even vague or apparently mild symptomatology must be taken seriously.

Other GI-related problems reported to occur with increased frequency in chronic hemodialysis patients include constipation, ascites, and liver disease, and rarely, GI disease related to beta2-microglobulin amyloid infiltration (191,205–208). Constipation (already highly prevalent in SCI patients) may be further aggravated, with development of ESRD as a result of reduced physical activity, the implementation of a "renal diet" and the related fluid restriction, or the use of medications (e.g., calcium-containing phosphate binders, oral iron preparations, and calcium antagonists). To minimize constipation and prevent fecal impaction, patients should be maintained on a good bowel management program that ensures regular and complete evacuation. Meals should be given at regular times, the intake of high-fiber foods encouraged, physical activity should be encouraged, and fluid intake should be as liberal as possible, considering the severity of renal insufficiency and volume of urine output. The use of bulk-forming laxatives and stool softeners (emollient laxatives) are also helpful in establishing and regulating bowel programs, while the intermittent use of a stimulant laxative may be useful in moving stool that has impacted proximal to the rectum.

An idiopathic form of ascites is associated with renal failure and dialysis. However, in patients who develop ascites, underlying causes such as liver disease, abdominal malignancies, heart failure, and constrictive pericarditis should be ruled out, as *hemodialysis-associated ascites* is a diagnosis of exclusion (205). Although the pathogenesis of this condition is not fully understood, it is thought to result from a combination of chronic fluid-volume overload and increased capillary permeability. Support for this comes from the observation that most patients diagnosed with hemodialysis-associated ascites have a history of chronic overhydration with volume expansion and large interdialytic weight gains as a consequence of dietary indiscretion. Because anorexia, progressive malnutrition, and life-threatening cachexia often complicate this condition, aggressive management is warranted. This includes a combination of achieving strict patient compliance regarding dietary salt and fluid restriction and by increasing fluid removal during dialysis. The latter can be facilitated with the use of a high-sodium slightly cooled, bicarbonate-based dialysis solution that helps maintain hemodynamic stability during high volume ultrafiltration. Other techniques effective in increasing fluid removal include: 1) utilizing a regimen of sequential isolated ultrafiltration where several hours of ultrafiltration (without dialysis) are performed, followed by several hours of standard hemodialysis; 2) increasing the frequency and/or duration of hemodialysis, thereby allowing more time for fluid removal; or 3) changing to a different method or modality of dialysis more effective in fluid removal (e.g., slow continuous ultrafiltration with dialysis or peritoneal dialysis).

Liver disease (in dialysis patients) is often due to infection with hepatitis B (HBV) and C (HCV) viruses (206,207). However, because of several factors—including better serologic techniques used in screening blood products, reduced blood transfusion requirements in dialysis patients (related to the routine use of erythropoietin), and the implementation of vaccination programs—the incidence of HBV infection has progressively declined. Consequently, HCV has now emerged as the most common type of viral hepatitis in hemodialysis patients with reported prevalence rates (for anti-HCV positivity in the United States) ranging from 1 to 20 percent (207–209) .

Dialysis patients are also at increased risk for drug-induced toxic hepatitis, which has been reported to occur in association with a variety of different types of drug exposure including allopurinol, methyldopa, fluoxymesterone, diazepam, ampicillin, indomethacin, and iron dextran (210,211). For reasons that remain unclear, ESRD patients not only appear to be more sensitive to drug-induced liver injury, but they also demonstrate an increased tendency for hepatic deposition of metals such as iron and foreign particles such as silicone (211). In patients suspected of having a drug-induced hepatitis, discontinuation of the offending agent is generally followed by improvement in liver function. Iron overload with hemosiderosis can occur in patients who have received large amounts of iron (usually in the form of parenterally administered iron or as a result of multiple blood transfusions). Hepatic siderosis should be suspected in patients exhibiting a combination of elevated transaminases (ALT and AST) and high serum ferritin levels (>1000 μg/L). Treatment involves the discontinuation of any exogenous iron administration along with the mobilization of iron from tissue stores. The latter can be accomplished with the administration of erythropoietin, whereby the resulting increase in red blood cell formation facilitates mobilization of iron from tissue stores. In severe cases, where serum ferritin levels exceed 2000 μg/L, the combination of phlebotomy and erythropoietin administration is shown to be both safe and efficacious in the management of hepatic siderosis (210).

A third consideration concerns gastrointestinal symptomatology related to the dialysis procedure per se. This should be strongly suspected in patients demonstrating a close temporal relationship between the occurrence of symptoms and dialysis, whereas the presence of symptoms at various times (unrelated to dialysis) is more suggestive of underlying gastrointestinal disease. For example, excessive ultrafiltration and intravascular volume depletion often cause nausea and vomiting during hemodialysis, which is also frequently accompanied by hypotension and muscle cramps. Because problems related to excessive ultrafiltration generally stem from the need to remove large volumes of fluid during dialysis, management should be primarily directed at reducing interdialytic weight gains through dietary counseling. Alternatively, the implementation of sequential ultrafiltration (as adjunct therapy to hemodialysis) can be effectively used in the removal of large volumes of fluid with less risk of causing symptomatic hypotension.

Dialysis-associated anorexia, nausea, and vomiting could also be manifestations of the dialysis disequilibrium syndrome (DDS) (212,213). Typically, nausea and vomiting occurring at the end of dialysis, or shortly thereafter, would be suggestive of DDS. This syndrome classically occurs in severely azotemic patients following the initiation of a hemodialysis regimen that is "overly efficient" with regard to the rate and magnitude of solute removal. DDS is characterized by a constellation of signs and symptoms ranging from nausea, vomiting, agitation, and headache in mild cases to stupor, seizures, and coma in severe cases. Although most cases of DDS occur within the first 6 months of hemodialysis therapy, this syndrome can occur virtually anytime in association with a "highly efficient dialysis," especially in patients who have previously been underdialyzed; for example, when a long-duration, high-efficiency hemodialysis treatment is performed as compensation for one or more missed treatments. In addition, DDS is more likely to occur in pedi-

atric and elderly dialysis patients as well as in patients undergoing twice-weekly dialysis as opposed to three-times-a-week dialysis. Although its pathogenesis remains controversial, DDS is thought to result from a rapid increase in brain cell water, causing brain edema. This pathophysiologic shift in water content from the extracellular fluid into the cells is caused by a transient reduction in extracellular fluid osmolality (compared to intracellular osmolality) that is of sufficient magnitude to allow the rapid movement of water into cells along an osmolar gradient. Apparently the combination of an underlying uremic-related increase in brain osmolality, caused by an increase in *idiogenic osmoles* composed of amino acids, organic acids, methyl amines, and polyols, and a dialysis-related rapid reduction in plasma solute content, caused by the removal of urea and other readily dialyzable solutes results in the development of a transient, but substantial, osmolar gradient between the brain and the extracellular fluid compartment. Because the increased brain osmolality is related to an increase in idiogenic osmoles and not to urea per se, the rapid reduction in plasma urea (with high efficiency dialysis) disproportionately lowers plasma and extracellular fluid osmolality despite the fact that urea freely crosses cell membranes and is cleared from both brain and plasma at essentially the same rate. DDS can be avoided by prescribing an initial series of low-efficiency dialysis treatments. With regard to hemodialysis, we recommend:

1. Do not exceed a 30 percent reduction in blood urea nitrogen during the initial two dialysis treatments. This can be accomplished by using a small surface area dialyzer, keeping a low blood flow rate (not to exceed 250ml/min), and limiting the duration of dialysis to 2 hours.

2. The use of dialysate with a sodium concentration approximately equal to the patient's serum sodium concentration and containing at least 200 ml/dL of glucose. Because of its much lower efficiency in clearing small

molecular weight solutes, peritoneal dialysis has not been associated with DDS.

Nutritional Disorders. Many patients with end-stage renal disease have evidence for protein-energy malnutrition as defined by various biochemical and anthropometric parameters (214–216). Moreover, both the prevalence and severity of malnutrition appear to be even greater in SCI patients with chronic renal failure than in their able-bodied counterparts. This was clearly demonstrated in a study involving dialysis patients both with and without spinal cord injury, in which the SCI group exhibited a higher incidence of suboptimal dry body weight along with reduced values (regarding measurements of mid-arm muscle circumference, triceps skin fold thickness, serum albumin concentration, serum transferrin level, and total lymphocyte counts) when compared with the group of able-bodied dialysis patients (217). A variety of factors are thought to be operative in the genesis of protein-energy malnutrition in this population, including chronic infection, amyloidosis, depression, anorexia, and prescribed or self-imposed protein restriction. In addition, factors related to the dialysis procedure per se may adversely affect nutrition. These include the release of proinflammatory cytokines, an increased catabolic effect, and the loss of nutrients (occurring in association with hemodialysis), while substantial losses of protein and other nutrients can occur in association with peritoneal dialysis. In turn, malnutrition has been shown to be an important risk factor for increased morbidity and mortality in ESRD patients (177) Consequently, every effort should be made to maintain a good state of nutrition in SCI patients.

Management

The management of SCI patients with chronic renal disease should begin with the identification and correction of any potentially reversible component of renal insufficiency such as urinary obstruction (functional or mechanical), active infection, renal hypoperfusion, or severe hypertension. In patients with significant residual renal function (glomerular filtration rates greater than 10 ml/min), every effort should be made to delay the progression of renal disease. This can be achieved by maintaining satisfactory urine flow along with effective treatment of urolithiasis and control of infection (e.g., urinary tract, pressure wounds, and osteomyelitis). Additional renal protective measures would include the maintenance of normal blood pressure and the avoidance of nephrotoxin exposure. Furthermore, the administration of an angiotensin-converting enzyme inhibitor or angiotensin-II receptor blocking drug may be beneficial in reducing the rate of progression of renal failure in selected patients (e.g., those with hypertension, proteinuria, and only mild to moderate underlying renal insufficiency). These agents can prevent the development of glomerular capillary hypertension and hyperfiltration, which is a maladaptive process shown to accelerate the progression of nephron loss in patients with underlying renal disease. Mild protein restriction (approximately 0.8 g/kg/day of high biological value protein) has also been shown to reduce glomerular capillary pressure and slow the rate of progression of renal disease (218,219). Although both of the aforementioned treatments effectuate renal protection by the same putative mechanism (i.e. a reduction in glomerular capillary pressure), this appears to be accomplished via different actions on the glomerular microcirculation. In the case of ACE-Is and ARBs, the reduction in glomerular capillary pressure is the result of efferent arteriolar dilatation, caused by inhibition of angiotensin II-mediated vasoconstriction, whereas with protein restriction, glomerular capillary pressure reduction is due to afferent arteriolar vasoconstriction, apparently related to inhibition of vasodilatory prostaglandins (219,220).

As previously noted, SCI patients with renal insufficiency often exhibit an inability to conserve sodium and water. Consequently, they are at increased risk for dehydration and volume depletion; this can result from increased gastrointestinal fluid losses, increased insensible losses, or enhanced renal losses. Conversely, other SCI patients, particularly those with more advanced renal insufficiency, also develop an inability to normally excrete sodium and volume, which accordingly also places them at risk for volume overload and related complications (e.g., hypertension and pulmonary edema). Therefore, close attention should be paid to the fluid-volume and electrolyte status in SCI patients with renal insufficiency, especially in the event of an intervening illness. Moreover, when glomerular filtration falls irreversibly (below 8 to 10 ml/min), renal replacement therapy should be instituted with hemodialysis, peritoneal dialysis, or possibly with renal transplantation. Published data regarding the use of dialysis in SCI patients is still very limited, while information concerning renal transplantation in this setting is practically nonexistent.

Hemodiaylsis. With the development and implementation of dialysis, the mortality associated with acute renal failure has been reduced, and death as a direct consequence of ESRD has been virtually eliminated. Overall, the noted beneficial effects of dialysis reported in able-bodied ESRD patients are likewise seen in SCI-ESRD patients. However, because of the increased prevalence of pneumonia, pulmonary embolism, nonischemic heart disease, septicemia, amyloidosis, and malnutrition, the mortality rate in SCI patients on maintenance dialysis is expectantly higher than that observed in able-bodied patients (221–223).

Like all extracorporeal systems, hemodialysis requires the establishment of an adequate vascular access, while selection of the specific type and anatomic location of the access is generally determined both by the patient's needs as well as practicality. For example, a short-term or temporary access is appropriate for use in the treatment of potentially reversible acute renal failure or for temporary use in an ESRD patient who has a failed permanent access. A variety of single- or double-lumen catheters are currently available for use in either the femoral, subclavian, or jugular vein; however, the internal jugu-

lar vein is the preferred site for catheter placement. This is because subclavian catheters are associated with an increased risk for subclavian vein stenosis, while femoral catheters both restrict lower extremity movement and have a high infection rate when left in place for more than 2 days (224–226). Additional complications shared by all transcutaneous catheters include hemorrhage, thrombosis, and infection. Furthermore, hemothorax and/or pneumothorax can immediately complicate placement of internal jugular and subclavian vein catheters; therefore, a post procedure chest radiograph must be obtained (224,227).

A long-term or permanent blood access should be placed in patients requiring chronic hemodialysis. Currently, the most commonly used permanent vascular accesses are the arteriovenous (AV) fistula and the arteriovenous (AV) graft (224,227). These devices are subcutaneous and may be created or placed in either the upper or lower extremity. The preferred site for an AV fistula is the distal (nondominant) forearm, where the anastomosis is usually created between the radial artery and cephalic vein; however, if this is not feasible, upper arm vessels can be used (e.g., an elbow brachiacephalic anastomosis). If it is not possible to create an AV fistula, an adequate blood access can almost always be established with either an AV graft or a transposed brachial-basilic vein fistula (224). The most widely used AV grafts are composed of synthetic material (polytetrafluoroethylene [PTFE]). The currently recommended sites and types of AV grafts in order of preference are: 1) a forearm curved looped brachial cephalic graft, 2) an upper arm straight graft, 3) a forearm straight radial cephalic graft, and 4) a looped thigh graft (224,227,228). A final option (for vascular access) is the placement of a subcutaneously tunneled, cuffed central venous catheter. The use of this type of catheter should be reserved for patients who are unsuitable for peritoneal dialysis and where either the lack of suitable blood vessels or the presence of complications, such as distal limb ischemia, precludes the use of an AV vascular access.

Important complications of vascular access devices include:(1) infection with or without sepsis; 2) access stenosis or thrombosis; 3) the formation of an aneurism or pseudoaneurysm; 4) access rupture with hemorrhage; and 5) limb ischemia distal to the access (224,227–229). Overall the preferred type of vascular access is the AV fistula, which is proved to be the safest and longest lasting type of permanent access. AV fistulas, however, must be created at least 4 to 6 weeks (preferably 2 to 3 months) before they are suitable for use in hemodialysis. Furthermore, the size and condition of the patient's peripheral blood vessels can limit their application. Although AV PTFE grafts have certain advantages (e.g., the variety of potential placement sites, the ability to bridge distant vessels, and an excellent capacity for high blood flow rates) they are overall less desirable than AV fistulas. This is because of a higher incidence of complications, particularly infection, stenosis, and thrombosis (mainly attributable to the foreign nature of the AV conduit) (224,227,229). The subcutaneously tunneled, cuffed central venous catheter, however, is the type of access most frequently complicated by infection; a recent multicenter study reports the relative risk of bacteremia to be 7.6 compared with AV fistulae (230).

Dialysis centers should have in place a team of trained personnel, including a nephrologist, a vascular surgeon, and an interventional radiologist, as well as nurses and technicians who are responsible for the planning, placement, and maintenance of vascular accesses and who are experienced in managing the related complications. When a patient is initially diagnosed with chronic renal failure, every effort should be made to protect the cephalic veins, especially in the nondominant arm. This vein should not be subjected to venipuncture or the placement of an indwelling catheter; however, veins in the dorsum of the hand may be used for this purpose.

Hemodialysis Treatment in Spinal Cord Injury. Although limited, the clinical experience would indicate that standard dialysis procedures are generally well tolerated in SCI patients (221–223,231,232). However, one potentially problematic area, regarding hemodialysis in SCI patients involves the type of buffer used (the two buffers currently in use being bicarbonate and acetate). Acetate a congener of bicarbonate, is metabolized to bicarbonate primarily by skeletal muscle. Consequently, patients with reduced muscle mass (i.e. SCI patients) are more susceptible to acetate accumulation and toxicity (233). The effects of acetate accumulation include arterial hypoxemia (related to associated hypocapnia and hypoventilation), peripheral vasodilation, decreased myocardial contractility, and metabolic acidosis, as well as associated vasomotor instability, nausea, vomiting, headache, and fatigue. Therefore, in view of the increased potential for acetate accumulation in patients with reduced muscle mass, bicarbonate buffered dialysate should be preferentially used in SCI patients (234).

A second problematic area concerns the relative biocompatibility of the artificial membrane used in hemodialysis. Of the four membrane types currently in use (cellulose, substituted cellulose, cellulose synthetic, and synthetic) the least biocompatible is cellulose (213). Artificial membranes made from unsubstituted cellulose, on contact with blood, can both activate the complement system and stimulate the activation of phagocytic cells. This in turn can result in numerous adverse effects including the activation of pro-inflammatory cytokines, the generation of reactive oxygen species, cell lysis, hypoxemia, and tissue injury (235–237). In contrast, dialyzers utilizing membranes made from substituted cellulose (e.g., cellulose acetate) or synthetics (e.g., polyacrylonitrile, polysulfone, polycarbonate, and polyamine) are associated with considerably less complement activation. In addition, recent studies involving ARF in experimental animals show that both the complement-activating potential of the dialysis membrane to which the animal was exposed and the degree of leukocyte infiltration involving the kidney adversely affected recovery from ARF (238,239). Furthermore, studies in humans with ARF have demonstrated both a reduction in mortality as well as an increased rate in the recovery of renal function, when dialysis was performed using synthetic "biocompatible membranes" compared with dialysis using "nonbiocompatible membranes" (240,241). Therefore, in the management of ARF there are compelling data supporting the preferential use of biocompatiblemembrane dialyzers. There is also data in chronic hemodialysis patients indicating that the use of nonbiocompatiblemembrane dialyzers may have damaging effects such as aggravation of dyslipidemia, an increase in lipid peroxidation, and the generation of reactive oxygen species (235–237). In addition, the use of nonbiocompatible membranes has been shown to cause or aggravate hypoxemia in patients undergoing hemodialysis (213,229). One of the proposed mechanisms for this involves increased leukocyte sequestration in pulmonary capillaries, producing "leukocyte microthrombi" caused by enhanced expression of leukocyte adhesion molecules (apparently resulting from dialysis membrane interaction). However, it should be noted that dialysis-associated hypoxemia appears to be multifactorial, involving mechanisms that include: 1) hypocapnia-induced compensatory alveolar hypoventilation (observed with acetate-buffered dialysate), as a consequence of intradialytic losses of CO_2; 2) compensatory hypoventilation due to alkalemia, as a consequence of bicarbonate-buffered dialysate, where high concentrations of bicarbonate (>35 mEq/L) are used; and 3) histamine-mediated abnormalities involving ventilation and perfusion resulting from complement-induced mast cell degranulation (213,229).

Peritoneal Dialysis. Before the advent of indwelling peritoneal catheters, peritoneal dialysis was used only as a temporary modality in the treatment of acute renal failure. However, during the past two decades peritoneal dialysis has emerged as one of the major therapeutic modalities for the treatment of end-stage renal disease (242). Furthermore, several variations of peritoneal dialysis are now available for use in the management of renal failure. These include intermittent peritoneal dialysis (IPD), continuous cycler-assisted peritoneal dialysis (CCPD), and continuous ambulatory peritoneal dialysis (CAPD). Because IPD is usually performed at night while the patient is asleep (via an automated delivery system), it is often referred to as nocturnal intermittent peritoneal dialysis (NIPD). CCPD is identical to NIPD except that in the former, the patient performs at least one additional long-dwell daytime exchange. With CAPD, usually four intermediate-dwell exchanges (approximately 6 hours per exchange) are performed daily, on a continuous basis.

Although each of these modalities (i.e. CAPD, CCPD, NIPD) are proved to be effective as renal replacement therapy in able-bodied patients, published data regarding the practicality and efficacy of peritoneal dialysis in SCI-ESRD patients is very limited. It has been our experience, however, that long-term IPD is as effective as hemodialysis in SCI patients, with regard to controlling azotemia, volume, and serum electrolytes and acid–base balance (232). Moreover, in this study SCI patients treated with IPD exhibited greater hemodynamic stability compared to those receiving hemodialysis; however, serum albumin levels were substantially lower in IPD treated patients, because of losses from the peritoneal cavity. This recognized complication of peritoneal dialysis might compound the problem of protein-energy malnutrition that is frequently present in SCI-ESRD patients. In our experience, the incidence of peritonitis is not increased in SCI-ESRD patients, compared to able-bodied ESRD patients. However, in patients who develop peritonitis, the infecting organism is often concomitantly present in the urine and/or a decubitus ulcer, indicative of cross-contamination.

With improvements in peritoneal catheter design, method of placement, and maintenance, as well as the implementation of more effective aseptic procedures and improved catheter connection technology, the incidence of peritonitis has markedly decreased in patients treated with peritoneal dialysis (242). It is, therefore, our opinion that CAPD, CCPD, or NIPD can provide a viable alternative form of renal replacement therapy in selected SCI-ESRD patients. However, there are a number of important issues that require careful consideration regarding the use of peritoneal dialysis in SCI-ESRD patients:

1. Because protein loss (associated with peritoneal dialysis) may compound pre-existing protein-calorie malnutrition, the patients' nutritional status should be carefully evaluated and frequently monitored. Furthermore, in our opinion, pre-existing hypoalbuminemia should be considered a relative contraindication to peritoneal dialysis.

2. The observation that bacteria (infecting or colonizing pressure sores and/or the urinary tract) are likely to contaminate the peritoneal cavity via the PD catheter underscores the importance of meticulous observance and use of aseptic measures. In our opinion, the presence of either extensive or infected pressure sores is another relative contraindication to peritoneal dialysis.

3. A further consideration is that respiratory diseases (particularly pneumonia) are currently the leading cause of mortality in patients with SCI. We have also observed a high incidence of acute and chronic pulmonary disorders in SCI patients with advanced renal disease (186). Consequently, there is understandable concern that the instillation of large volumes of fluid into the peritoneal cavity, in SCI-ESRD patients with diminished pulmonary reserve, will further compromise respiratory function and predispose to pulmonary infection. In such circumstances, the use of multiple small-volume exchanges (approximately 1 liter) with shorter dwell times (easily accomplished with a programmable automated cycler) may substantially diminish the risk for pulmonary compromise. However, the use of hemodialysis (with biocompatible dialyzers) may be more appropriate in pulmonary-compromised patients.

4. High concentrations of glucose are required to provide the osmotic force for ultrafiltration in peritoneal dialysis. Consequently, absorption of glucose from the peritoneal cavity can

cause hyperglycemia during the procedure and can also occasionally result in delayed reactive hypoglycemia. This issue is of further concern in view of the reported high incidence of glucose intolerance among spinal cord injured patients (243).

5. Abdominal muscle weakness, impaired intestinal motility, and related constipation, which are often present in SCI patients, can occasionally interfere with peritoneal dialysis (particularly dialysate drainage). In turn, incomplete drainage of dialysate from the peritoneal cavity can cause abdominal distention and bloating and can also result in suboptimal solute and water clearances. Therefore, patients undergoing peritoneal dialysis will require proper bowel care and positional changes.

Dietary Considerations. The primary objectives of dietary regimens in SCI patients receiving long-term dialysis are to provide adequate nutrition while preventing fluid overload, hypertension, hyperkalemia, and hyperphosphatemia. Protein-energy malnutrition is a common complication of CRF, and in turn, a poor nutritional state predisposes ESRD patients to impaired wound healing, increased susceptibility to infection, difficulties with rehabilitation, and increased mortality (177,214–217). The cause of malnutrition in CRF is often multifactorial, involving medical, psychosocial, economic, and possibly, cultural factors.

Anorexia, which is commonly present in patients with CRF, may be due to uremia per se, or related to other factors associated with ESRD (e.g., an intercurrent illness, infection, depression, medications, dialysis, or an altered sensation of taste) (214,215,244). Anorexia, as well as nausea and vomiting, are well known complications of uremia that should resolve with adequate dialysis; however, in certain patients the dialysis procedure itself may cause or contribute to anorexia. With peritoneal dialysis, abdominal distention, related to the instillation of dialysate, can cause sensations of fullness and satiety with resulting anorexia (242,244). This problem can be obviated by draining the peritoneal cavity 30 to 60 minutes prior to meals and by not refilling with fresh dialysate until 30 to 60 minutes after meals. Side effects of hemodialysis such as nausea, vomiting, fatigue, and malaise can also contribute to malnutrition (229,244). These symptoms may be related to excessive ultrafiltration or to dialysis-associated cytokine release. Limiting interdialytic weight gain to approximately 1 liter (by strict adherence to dietary salt and fluid restrictions) obviates the necessity for large-volume or "excessive" ultrafiltration with dialysis. For example, in anuric patients, recommended sodium and water restriction is 2 grams and 1 liter per day, respectively. If the patient is being dialyzed with a poorly biocompatible cellulosic membrane dialyzer, changing to a more biocompatible dialyzer may also improve symptoms such as nausea and anorexia. Some losses of nutrients invariably occur during dialysis, including water-soluble vitamins, amino acids, and intact proteins. With peritoneal dialysis, protein losses average 9 grams/day. Protein losses during hemodialysis are negligible; however, polypeptide and amino acid losses can average 10 to 13 grams per treatment (244).

In the management of malnutrition, it is important to rule out an intercurrent or related illness, (e.g., chronic infection or depression) as a cause or contributing factor. Gastroparesis that is often related to autonomic nervous system dysfunction in SCI patients usually responds to treatment effective in promoting gastric emptying (e.g., metoclopramide or cisapride administered 15 to 30 minutes prior to meals and at bedtime). An altered sense of taste in ESRD patients has been attributed to zinc deficiency, and this condition may improve with oral zinc (20 mg/day). The medications most likely to cause anorexia, nausea, and dyspepsia in dialysis patients are aluminum- or calcium-containing phosphate binders and oral iron preparations. The substitution of Renagel® as a phosphate binder or the use of an intravenous iron dextran preparation in place of oral iron should be effective in minimizing these side effects.

It is also important to recognize that ESRD is associated with numerous hormonal and meta-bolic disturbances, including: 1) insulin resistance; 2) decreased biologic effects of insulin-like growth factors; 3) increased plasma levels of catabolic hormones (e.g., cortisol and glucagon; 4) a high prevalence of secondary hyperparathyroidism; 5) defective erythropoietin production; 6) chronic metabolic acidosis; and 7) abnormal carbohydrate, fat, and protein metabolism. Individually, or in combination, these abnormalities are no doubt responsible for a wide variety of uremic manifestations and in aggregate, they also adversely affect nutritional status by inducing a state of hypercatabolism (215,229,244). Moreover, therapeutic modalities (i.e. dialysis) that ameliorate uremic-induced hormonal and metabolic dysfunction are also shown to improve nutritional status. In addition, effective treatment of anemia (using erythropoietin) or the correction of metabolic acidosis (with bicarbonate), as well as the effective control of hyperparathyroidism, have also been reported to improve nutritional status in ESRD (244–246) Furthermore, there is evidence that the administration of recombinant human growth hormone, as well as the use of intradialytic parenteral nutrition, can increase protein anabolism and improve overall nutritional status in malnourished dialysis patients (247,248).

Dietary recommendations for stable chronic dialysis patients are:

1. Protein intake should be approximately 1.2 g/kg/day, with at least 50 percent being of high biologic value.
2. Because dialysis patients have impaired cell energy metabolism, caloric intake for sedentary, nonobese patients)should be approximately 35 kcal/kg/day, with carbohydrate providing 40 to 50 percent of the total calories. Higher caloric intakes are required in patients who are underweight, those who routinely engage in strenuous activity, or hypercatabolic patients (i.e., related to trauma, surgery or infection).
3. Protein and caloric intake should be based not on the patient's actual body weight, but instead on the average body weight for

healthy subjects of the same age, sex, height, and body frame as that of the patient.

4. Sodium and water restriction (in anuric patients on hemodialysis) should be 1 to 2 g/day (40 to 80mEq/day) and 1 liter/day, respectively. Compliance with sodium restriction is necessary to curb excessive thirst, hypervolemia, and hypertension. In anuric patients receiving peritoneal dialysis, sodium and water intake can usually be liberalized to 3 to 4 g/day (130 to 170mEq/d) and 2 to 2.5 liters/day, respectively.

5. A common and potentially life-threatening problem in ESRD patients is hyperkalemia. Therefore, in most patients, dietary potassium intake should not exceed 2 to 3 g/day (50 to 75 mEq/day). However, in patients with significant residual renal function, only mild potassium restriction may be necessary.

6. Because of renal failure-related vitamin D deficiency, dietary calcium requirements generally exceed the recommended 1 g/day for healthy nonuremic adults. To help achieve positive calcium balance, higher dialysate calcium concentration (3.5 mEq/L) or calcitriol (vitamin D) supplementation may be required in some patients. However, it should be noted that the majority of ESRD patients are already receiving moderate to large quantities of calcium carbonate or calcium acetate (as phosphate-binders) and as a consequence, hypercalcemia can become a problem.

7. In ESRD, dietary phosphate should be restricted to 0.8 g/day to reduce the risk for hyperphosphatemia, which plays a major role in the associated disturbances in calcium and bone metabolism. For example, hyperphosphatemia inhibits the 1-hydroxylation of vitamin D (exacerbating 1,25 dihydroxy vitamin D deficiency) while stimulating parathyroid hormone (PTH) secretion, which can lead to secondary hyperparathyroidism. Furthermore, a reduction in serum ionized calcium, usually resulting from a combination of hyperphosphatemia and vitamin D deficiency, is an additional stimulus for PTH secretion. Hyperphosphatemia is also commonly associated with metastatic soft tissue calcifications (related to high Ca $\times$ P products of > 60 to 70 mg^2/dL^2). Moreover, mortality is shown to be increased when the Ca $\times$ P product exceeded 72 mg^2/dL^2 or when serum phosphate levels were $\geqslant$ 6.6 mg/dL (174). The control of serum phosphate (levels of 6.5 mg/dL or lower but, ideally in the range of 4.5 to 5.5 mg/dL) requires a combination of dietary phosphate restriction (approximately 800 mg/day), adequate dialysis therapy, and the administration of phosphate binders with meals (e.g., calcium acetate, calcium carbonate, and/or Renagel®).

8. Because dialysis patients are at greater risk for developing deficiencies involving water-soluble vitamins and certain minerals as a consequence of reduced intake, diminished absorption, altered metabolism, and losses related to dialysis per se, it is recommended that they routinely receive the following daily vitamin/mineral supplementation: folic acid (1 mg); pyridoxine (20 mg); thiamin (30 mg); and zinc (20 mg), plus the usual daily allowance of other B vitamins (244,249). Although plasma levels of selenium are reported to be low in dialysis patients, the effects or possible benefits of administering this important antioxidant have not been studied in this setting. Likewise, the potentially beneficial effects of vitamin E have not been studied in dialysis patients. However, the administration of vitamin C should be limited to 150 to 200 mg/day because higher doses can cause hyperoxalemia (244). Finally, the administration of vitamin A should be avoided, because serum vitamin A levels are generally already elevated in CRF due to the combination of decreased renal catabolism and increased serum levels of retinal A binding protein.

Medication and Pharmacologic Considerations. In addition to vitamins, trace elements, and phosphate binders (previously discussed), the majority of ESRD patients also require medication for management of anemia and hypertension. The recommended range for target hematocrits of 30 to 36 percent can be achieved with the use of erythropoietin, which is generally administered intravenously (thrice weekly) with hemodialysis or subcutaneously administered (twice weekly) in peritoneal dialysis patients. However, for erythropoietin to be effective, folate, vitamin B12 and iron stores must be replete. Low serum levels of iron and ferritin and/or low transferrin saturation (<20 percent) are indicative of iron deficiency. Iron deficient patients should be evaluated for blood loss, including occult losses from the gastrointestinal tract. However, it should be recognized that hemodialysis patients are at increased risk for iron deficiency anemia due to unavoidable losses of small quantities of blood with dialysis (retained in the extracorporal circulation). In addition to iron deficiency and chronic blood loss, other causes of erythropoietin-resistant anemia include hemolysis, aluminum intoxication, underlying infection or inflammation, secondary hyperparathyroidism, and bone marrow disease. In the treatment of iron deficiency anemia, oral iron preparations (e.g., ferrous sulfite, ferrous fumarate, or ferrous sulfate) may be used in doses providing 100 to 150 mg daily of elemental iron. In patients intolerant or refractory to oral iron, intravenous preparations (e.g., iron dextran, ferric gluconate, or ferric hydroxysaccharate) may be used. Intravenous iron is generally required for correction of anemia in hemodialysis patients who have increased iron losses associated with dialysis, while in uncomplicated peritoneal dialysis, oral iron therapy is usually effective in correcting anemia. Because of the risk for anaphylactic reactions (occurring in < 1 percent of patients) a test dose of 0.5 ml of iron dextran (50 mg/ml) is recommended (250). Delayed milder reactions with fever, myalgia, and lymphadenopathy have also been reported in association with iron dextran administration (250). Regarding therapeutic regimens, we recommend using 100 mg of iron dextran (diluted in 50 ml of normal saline) infused over a 5-minute period at the end of five to 10 successive dialysis sessions. A total dose of 500 to 1000 mg of elemental iron is usually sufficient to correct iron deficiency. Therapeutic

efficacy can be evaluated by the hemoglobin/hematocrit response (usually occurs within 3 to 4 weeks), while the serum iron and ferritin levels, along with the transferrin saturation, are useful in monitoring iron stores. However, a period of at least 1-month is required post iron therapy before these tests accurately reflect the new state of iron stores.

Hypertension in patients with ESRD often has a volume-related component, which may respond to a combination of dietary sodium restriction and fluid removal with dialysis. However, many ESRD patients with hypertension also require antihypertensive medications for blood pressure control. Most antihypertensive agents can be safely and effectively used in the management of hypertension in SCI-ESRD patients. These include calcium channel antagonists, angiotensin converting enzyme inhibitors (ACE-Is), angiotensin II receptor blockers (ARBs), alpha-blockers, beta-blockers, central sympatholytics, and vasodilators. Diuretics, however, are generally ineffective in patients with ESRD, although large doses of loop diuretics (e.g., furosemide) have been used with some success in the management of hypertension and volume overload in selected ESRD patients (i.e. those with a GFR > 5 to 10 ml/min).

SCI patients with advanced renal disease often exhibit a variety of concurrent illnesses and related conditions that necessitate the use of various medications. However, there are also numerous underlying pathophysiologic conditions present in this population that serve to modulate the bioavailability, distribution, and metabolism of pharmacologic agents. For example, drug bioavailability can be affected by alterations in gastrointestinal motility and absorption commonly present in SCI-ESRD patients. Furthermore, increased gastric alkalinization in uremic patients apparently resulting from the action of gastric urease on urea, may reduce the bioavailability of agents dependent on acid hydrolysis for absorption (251). Uremia is also associated with alterations in first-pass hepatic metabolism that can have opposing effects on drug bioavailability (252). For example, an associated inhibition of hepatic biotransformation should function to increase drug bioavailability, whereas an associated reduction in protein binding should decrease drug bioavailability by increasing the availability of unbound drug for hepatic metabolism.

The apparent volume of drug distribution (a mathematical construct useful in estimating the drug dose necessary to achieve therapeutic plasma levels) is also affected in SCI-ESRD patients (252,253). For example, drugs that are water soluble or highly protein bound tend to be restricted to the extracellular fluid compartment and consequently have relatively small volumes of distribution. In contrast, lipid-soluble drugs that can readily enter cells and tissue have comparatively large volumes of distribution. Therefore, conditions associated with impaired or decreased drug-protein binding (e.g., uremia and hypoproteinemia) cause the apparent volume of distribution of protein-bound drugs to increase. The relationship between the apparent volume of distribution of a drug and its degree of binding is demonstrated by the following:

$$Vd = VB + VT \, (FB/FT)$$

where Vd is the apparent volume distribution, VB and VT are the actual volumes of blood and water in tissues, respectively, and FB and FT are the fractions of free drug in blood and tissue, respectively. In addition, the presence of edema or ascites increases the Vd of water soluble and protein bound drugs, whereas muscle wasting (which is highly prevalent in SCI-ESRD) decreases Vd (253,254). Because Vd, after completion of drug absorption, is equal to the fractional absorption of the dose (f $\times$D) divided by the plasma concentration (c) of the drug, Vd can also be calculated using the following:

$$Vd = \frac{f \times D}{c}$$

The most important consideration, however, is that the metabolism and excretion of a wide variety of drugs are profoundly affected by renal insufficiency per se. Although certain drugs are excreted in the urine essentially unaltered, most drugs undergo biotransformation prior to excretion. Hepatic biotransformation, in turn, involves a number of reactions including oxidation, reduction, and hydrolysis, as well as synthetic processes (i.e. conjugation and acetylation) by which the parent drug or agent is transformed into various metabolites. In the presence of renal failure the reaction rates for both hydrolysis and reduction are reduced, whereas the oxidation rate of various drugs is accelerated (253–255). Thus, in addition to its profound influence on drug excretion, renal insufficiency can affect drug metabolism via alterations in hepatic biotransformation.

Of further consideration is that total body clearance or elimination of a drug is determined by the summation clearance of all involved organ systems (i.e. renal, hepatic, pulmonary, and others). Also, for convenience and practicality, most drug assays are obtained from plasma, and accordingly, reflect the plasma concentration of the respective drug rather than "total body concentration." Therefore, both the terminology and the concept of "plasma drug clearance" should be used in place of "total body drug clearance;" nevertheless, both terms are frequently used interchangeably. The concept of plasma clearance (Clp) is described by the following expression:

$$Clp = Clr + Clnr$$

where Clr and $CLnr$ represent renal and nonrenal clearances, respectively.

The renal clearance of a drug is determined not only by its rate of glomerular filtration but also by the net effect of tubular modulation (i.e. tubular secretion and/or reabsorption of the drug). Unbound drugs and their metabolites are usually freely filtered by the glomerulus, with their elimination being thus determined by their apparent volume of distribution, glomerular filtration rate, and tubular reabsorption. In general, the kidneys do not readily clear drugs that have a large volume of distribution and/or are extensively bound in tissue. Likewise, drugs that are highly protein-bound are not cleared by glomerular filtration because of poor filterability; however, they may be substantially cleared by proximal tubular secretion. Obviously, with progressive renal failure, the capacity for filtration and tubular secretion is lost. Furthermore, because the plasma clearance of such a wide variety of pharmaceutical agents is affected by renal failure, the physician must have access to a comprehensive source regarding drug dosing guidelines in renal failure. Fortunately, there are a number of excellent publications available for this purpose (253–256). For drug dose-adjustments in SCI patients with renal insufficiency (assuming the serum creatinine is stable), the GFR can be estimated, preferably from the measurement of creatinine clearance or from the clearance of an exogenously administered radionuclide. Alternatively, the GFR can be estimated using the empiric formula developed by Cockcroft and Gault along with the appropriate correction factors for paraplegia and quadriplegia, which are (84,85):

- (In males) GFR = (140−age in years) × (wgt in kg) ÷ 72 × (serum Cr in mg/dL)
- (In females) GFR = value for males × 0.85
- (In paraplegia) GFR = value for males × 0.60
- (In quadriplegia) GFR = value for males × 0.40

Regarding the administration of drug loading doses in patients with renal insufficiency, in general, a similar loading dose equivalent as that administered to patients with normal renal function can be safely given in renal failure in situations requiring the rapid achievement of therapeutic drug levels. If the loading dose of the drug is not known, it can be calculated using the following formula:

$$\text{Loading dose} = Vd \times IBW \times Cp$$

where Vd is the apparent volume of distribution of the drug (in liters/kg), IBW refers to the patient's ideal body weight (in kg), and Cp repre-

sents the desired steady state plasma concentration of the drug. However, in SCI patients with reduced muscle mass, we recommend using the measured body weight (in kg) rather than IBW.

There are basically two methods by which maintenance drug dosing can be accomplished in renal failure patients. The first is to administer a smaller dose at standard dose intervals, and the second method is to administer the standard dose at prolonged intervals. In the first method, the appropriate dose reduction (or fractional dose) can be calculated using the following formula:

$$Df = t\,{\textstyle\frac{1}{2}}\ \text{normal} \div t\,{\textstyle\frac{1}{2}}\ \text{renal failure}$$

where Df is the fractional dose, $t\,\frac{1}{2}$ *normal* is the elimination half-life of the drug with normal renal function, and $t\,\frac{1}{2}$ *renal failure* is the elimination half-life of the drug with renal insufficiency. If it is deemed advantageous to maintain normal dosing intervals (i.e. when administering a drug with a narrow therapeutic range and short plasma half-life) the amount of drug per dose can be estimated by the following expression:

$$\text{Dose in Renal Impairment} = \text{Normal Dose} \times Df$$

However, when prolonged dose intervals are more advantageous, either for convenience or in cases where the drug has a broad therapeutic range and long plasma half-life, the dosing interval can be estimated using the following expression:

$$\text{Dose Interval in Renal Impairment} = \text{Normal Dose Interval} \div Df$$

Moreover, when drug toxicity is correlated with high trough levels (i.e. aminoglycosides), long dosing intervals are beneficial in reducing toxicity. Additionally, various combinations of drug dose reduction and interval prolongation have been successfully used in patients with renal insufficiency.

In summary, the approach to drug therapy in SCI patients with renal insufficiency should begin with an estimation of residual renal function. This can be accomplished by several methods designed to estimate GFR, including the measurement of creatinine clearance, the use of clearance measurements from exogenously administered radionuclide markers, or the use of the Cockcroft and Gault formula with appropriate modifications for paraplegia and quadriplegia (85,257,258). Once the degree of renal insufficiency is known, a number of sources can be referred to for drug dosing guidelines in renal failure, including the *Physicians Desk Reference* (253–256). Alternatively, drug-dosing schedules can be derived or modified using the formulas and concepts provided herein. Moreover, particularly when toxicity is an issue, the appropriate measurements of plasma or serum drug levels should be utilized in the determination of dosing schedules.

An additional consideration in dialysis patients is that some drug removal may occur during dialysis, necessitating further dosing adjustments. In fact, substantial amounts of certain drugs can be removed from plasma, especially with hemodialysis. This occurs mainly by diffusion, where the drug or its metabolites cross the dialysis membrane, from plasma to dialysate, along a concentration gradient. However, a number of factors function to minimize drug removal by dialysis. These include the molecular size of the drug/metabolite, the degree of protein binding, the apparent volume of drug distribution, the rate at which the drug/metabolite is transported between plasma and other fluid compartments, and the extent to which the drug/metabolite is eliminated from the body by nonrenal mechanisms. Consequently, the removal from plasma of a drug/metabolite by hemodialysis is not very efficient under the following circumstances: 1) when the molecular mass (i.e. drug/metabolite) exceeds 500 daltons; 2) when protein binding exceeds 90 percent; 3) when the apparent volume of distribution is large (i.e. Vd of drug/metabolite > 1 liter/kg body weight); 4) when the distribution of the drug from plasma to other body compartments occurs rapidly; or 5) when extensive tissue binding occurs.

The hemodialysis clearance of a drug/metabolite can be estimated by the following formula:

$$Cl_{HD} = Cl_{urea} \times \frac{60}{MWdrug}$$

where Cl_{HD} and Cl_{urea} are the dialysis clearances of the drug and urea, respectively; and MWdrug is the molecular weight of the respective drug. Therefore, for a drug/metabolite to undergo substantial clearance by hemodialysis (in the range of 15 to 100 ml/min), it must be: 1) relatively small (i.e. MW < 500 daltons); 2) essentially confined to plasma or in ready equilibrium with plasma; and 3) present in sufficient concentration (unbound to protein). This added capacity for drug removal by dialysis patients is expressed by the following:

$$Clp = Clr + Clnr + Cld$$

where *Clp* represents total plasma (drug/metabolite) clearance, *Clr* and *Clnr* refer to renal and nonrenal clearance, respectively, and *Cld* represents drug/metabolite clearance by dialysis. With respect to hemodialysis, drug/metabolite clearance may be increased with the use of high efficiency, high flux dialyzers in conjunction with high dialysate and blood flow rates.

Regarding drug removal in patients undergoing peritoneal dialysis, the same basic principles applicable in hemodialysis also apply here. Therefore, as a general rule, if a drug/metabolite is cleared with hemodialysis, it will also be cleared with peritoneal dialysis. However, with peritoneal dialysis drug/metabolite clearance is far less efficient. For specific recommendations regarding drug dosing in both hemodialysis and peritoneal dialysis patients, the reader is referred to sources 253 through 256.

Regarding pharmacologic therapy in SCI-ESRD patients, it is important to acknowledge that our understanding of pharmacokinetics in the setting of renal failure and dialysis is essentially based on data from studies involving able-bodied patients with renal insufficiency. To further complicate matters, SCI-ESRD patients as a group are both unique and heterogeneous, and accordingly the possibility exists that additional factors are present in this population with unforeseen, and therefore, unpredictable pharmacokinetic modulating effects. Therefore, the validity of basing recommendations regarding the use of pharmacologic agents in SCI-ESRD on data extrapolated mainly from studies in able-bodied ESRD patients and supported only by a relatively limited direct clinical experience is questionable. Moreover, the virtual absence of hard data in this area demonstrates the need for studies designed to systematically evaluate pharmacokinetics and pharmacodynamics in SCI patients with renal insufficiency.

REFERENCES

1. Tribe CR, Silver JR. *Renal Failure in Paraplegia.* London, England: Pittman Medical, 1969. Pp. 35–90.
2. Ditunno JF, Jr., Formal CS. Chronic spinal cord injury. *N Engl J Med* 1994;330(8): 550–556.
3. DeVivo MJ, Black KJ, Stover SL. Causes of death during the first 12 years after spinal cord injury. *Arch Phys Med Rehabil* 1993;74(3): 248–254.
4. Whiteneck GG, Charlifue SW, Frankel HL, Fraser MH, Gardner BP, Gerhart KA, Kirshnan KR, Menter RR, Nuseibeh I, Short, DJ, et al. Mortality, morbidity, and psychosocial outcomes of persons spinal cord injured more than 20 years ago. *Paraplegia* 1992;30(9):617–630.
5. Vaziri ND. Pathophysiology of end-stage renal disease in spinal cord injury. *Mt Sinai J Med* 1993;60(4):302–304.
6. Barton CH, Vaziri ND, Gordon S, Tilles S. Renal pathology in end-stage renal disease associated with paraplegia. *Paraplegia* 1984;22(1): 31–41.
7. Vaziri ND, Mirahmadi MK, Barton CH, Eltorai I, Gordon S, Byrne C, Paul MV. Clinicopathological characteristics of dialysis patients with spinal cord injury. *J Am Paraplegia Soc* 1983;6(1):3–6.
8. Dalton JJ Jr, Hackler RH, Bunts RC. Amyloidosis in the paraplegic; Incidence and significance. *J Urol* 1965;65:553–555.
9. Malament M, Friedman M, Pschibul F. Amyloidosis of paraplegia. *Arch Phys Med Rehabil* 1964;46:406–411.
10. Wall BM, Huch KM, Mangold TA, Steere EL, Cooke CR. Risk factors for development of proteinuria in chronic spinal cord injury. *Am J Kidney Dis* 1999;33(5):899–903.
11. Lehmann KG, Lane JG, Piepmeier JM, Batsford WP. Cardiovascular abnormalities accompanying acute spinal cord injury in humans: incidence, time course and severity. *J Am Coll Cardiol* 1987;10(1):46–52.
12. Silver JR. Immediate management of spinal injury. *Br J Hosp Med* 1983;29(5):412, 414, 417 passim.
13. Kopaniky DR. Pathophysiology of spinal cord disruption and injury. In *Physiologic Basis of Modern Surgical Care.* St. Louis: CV Mosby, 1988. P. 789.
14. Nikakhtar B, Vaziri ND, Khonsari F, Gordon S, Mirahmadi MD. Urolithiasis in patients with spinal cord injury. *Paraplegia* 1981;19(6): 363–366.
15. Grundy DJ, Rainford DJ, Silver JR. The occurrence of acute renal failure in patients with neuropathic bladders. *Paraplegia* 1982;20(1): 35–42.
16. Burr RG. Calculosis in paraplegia. *Int Rehabil Med* 1981;3(3):162–167.
17. DeVivo MJ, Fine PR, Cutter GR, Maetz HM. The risk of renal calculi in spinal cord injury patients. *J Urol* 1984;131(5):857–860.
18. Colice GL. Neurogenic pulmonary edema. *Clin Chest Med* 1985;6(3):473–489.
19. de la Torre JC. Spinal cord injury: review of basic and applied research. Spine 1981;6(4): 315–335.
20. Marion D. *Trauma,* 2nd ed. Norwalk, Connecticut: Appleton & Lange, 1991. Pp 261–275.
21. Barkin M, Herschorn S, Comisarow R. *Early Management of Spinal Cord Injury.* New York: Raven Press, 1982. Pp 273–278.
22. McGuire EJ, Ohl D, Wang S, Noll F, Vasher E. *Spine Trauma.* Philadelphia: W.B. Saunders Company, 1998. Pp 630–638.
23. Lloyd LK. New trends in urologic management of spinal cord injured patients. *Cent Nerv Syst Trauma* 1986;3(1):3–12.
24. Freeman LW. The metabolism of calcium in patients with spinal cord injury. *Ann Surg* 1949;149:177.
25. Minaire P, Pilonchery G, Leriche A. Hyperuricosuria and urinary lithiasis in paraplegic patients (author's transl). *Sem Hop* 1981; 57(33–36):1409–1412.
26. Vaziri ND, Nikakhtar B, Gordon S. Hyperoxaluria in chronic renal disease associated with spinal cord injury. *Paraplegia* 1982;20(1): 48–53.

27. Burr RG, Nuseibeh I. Biochemical studies in paraplegic renal stone patients. 1. Plasma biochemistry and urinary calcium and saturation. *Br J Urol* 1985;57(3):269–274.

28. Burr RG, Nuseibeh I, Abiaka CD. Biochemical studies in paraplegic renal stone patients. 2; Urinary excretion of citrate, inorganic pyrophosphate, silicate and urate. *Br J Urol* 1985;57(3):275–278.

29. Kohli A, Lamid S. Risk factors for renal stone formation in patients with spinal cord injury. *Br J Urol* 1986;58(6):588–591.

30. Trop CS, Bennett CJ. Autonomic dysreflexia and its urological implications: a review. *J Urol* 1991;146(6):1461–1469.

31. Comarr AE. Autonomic dysreflexia (hyperreflexia). *J Am Paraplegia Soc* 1984;7(3):53–57.

32. Lindan R, Joiner E, Freehafer AA, Hazel C. Incidence and clinical features of autonomic dysreflexia in patients with spinal cord injury. *Paraplegia* 1980;18(5):285–292.

33. Perkash I. Problems of decatheterization in long-term spinal cord injury patients. *J Urol* 1980;124(2):249–253.

34. Gillenwater JY. *Campbell's Urology*, 6th ed. Baltimore: W.B. Saunders, 1992. Pp. 499–532.

35. Klahr S. *Current Therapy in Nephrology and Hypertension*, 3rd ed. St. Louis: Mosby-Year Book, 1992. Pp. 81–87.

36. Wilson D, Klahr S. *Diseases of the Kidney*, 5th ed. Boston: Little Brown, 1993. Pp. 657–687.

37. Reyes AA, Martin D, Settle S, Klahr S. EDRF role in renal function and blood pressure of normal rats and rats with obstructive uropathy. *Kidney Int* 1992;41(2):403–413.

38. Purcell H, Bastani B, Harris KP, Hemken P, Klahr S, Gluck S. Cellular distribution of H(+)-ATPase following acute unilateral ureteral obstruction in rats. *Am J Physiol* 1991;261(3 Pt 2):F365–376.

39. Maynard FM, Dionko A. Clean intermittent catheterization in the management of the neurogenic bladder of traumatic spinal cord injured patients: a critical review. *Abstracts Digest Sixth Annual Scientific Meeting, American Spinal Injury Association*, May 8–11, New Orleans, 1980.

40. The prevention and management of urinary tract infections among people with spinal cord injuries. National Institute on Disability and Rehabilitation Research Consensus Statement. January 27–29, 1992. *J Am Paraplegia Soc* 1992;15(3):194–204.

41. Noll F, Russe O, Kling E, Botel U, Schreiter F. Intermittent catheterization versus percutaneous suprapubic cystostomy in the early management of traumatic spinal cord lesions. *Paraplegia* 1988;26(1):4–9.

42. Scheible W, Talner LB. Gray scale ultrasound and the genitourinary tract: a review of clinical applications. *Radiol Clin North Am* 1979;17(2): 281–300.

43. Brandt TD, Neiman HL, Calenoff L, Greenberg M, Kaplan PE, Nanninga JB. Ultrasound evaluation of the urinary system in spinal-cord-injury patients. *Radiology* 1981; 141(2):473–477.

44. Rao KG, Hackler RH, Woodlief RM, Ozer MN, Fields WR. Real-time renal sonography in spinal cord injury patients: prospective comparison with excretory urography. *J Urol* 1986; 135(1):72–77.

45. Ozer MN, Shannon SR. Renal sonography in asymptomatic persons with spinal cord injury: a cost-effectiveness analysis. *Arch Phys Med Rehabil* 1991;72(1):35–37.

46. Beck F, Thurau K, Getraunthaler G. *The Kidney: Physiology and Pathophysiology*, 2nd ed. New York: Raven Press, 1992. P. 3157.

47. Tanner GA, Steinhausen M. Tubular obstruction in ischemia-induced acute renal failure in the rat. *Kidney Int Suppl* 1976;6:S65–73.

48. Myers BD, Moran SM. Hemodynamically mediated acute renal failure. *N Engl J Med* 1986; 314(2):97–105.

49. Molitoris BA. *Acute Renal Failure*, 3rd ed. New York: Churchill-Livingstone, 1993. P. 1.

50. Bonventre JV. Mechanisms of ischemic acute renal failure [clinical conference]. *Kidney Int* 1993;43(5):1160–1178.

51. Bock HA. Pathogenesis of acute renal failure: new aspects. *Nephron* 1997;76(2):130–142.

52. Thadhani R, Pascual M, Bonventre JV. Acute renal failure [see comments]. *N Engl J Med* 1996;334(22): 1448–1460.

53. Lightner DJ. Contemporary urologic management of patients with spinal cord injury. *Mayo Clin Proc* 1998;73(5):434–438.

54. Atkinson PP, Atkinson JL. Spinal shock. *Mayo Clin Proc* 1996;71(4):384–389.

55. Zipnick RI, Scalea TM, Trooskin SZ, Sclafani SJ, Emad B, Shah A, Talbert S, Haher T. Hemodynamic responses to penetrating spinal cord injuries. *J Trauma* 1993;35(4):578–582.

56. Kuhlemeier KV, McEachran AB, Lloyd LK, Stover SL, Tauxe WN, Dubovsky EV, Fine PR. Renal function after acute and chronic spinal cord injury. *J Urol* 1984;131(3):439–445.

57. Palmer BM, Henrich WL. *Diseases of the Kidney*, 6th ed. Boston: Little, Brown and Company, 1997. Pp 1167–1188.

58. Kirschenbaum MA, Shah GM. *Textbook of Nephrology*, Vol I, 3rd ed. Baltimore: Williams and Wilkins, 1995. Pp. 940–946.

59. Smith WL. Prostanoid biosynthesis and mechanisms of action. *Am J Physiol* 1992;263(2 Pt 2): F181–191.

60. vIchikawa I, Pfeffer JM, Pfeffer MA, Hostetter TH, Brenner BM. Role of angiotensin II in the altered renal function of congestive heart failure. *Circ Res* 1984;55(5):669–675.

61. Henrich WL, Berl T, McDonald KM, Anderson RJ, Schrier RW. Angiotensin II, renal nerves, and prostaglandins in renal hemodynamics during hemorrhage. *Am J Physiol* 1978;235(1): F46–51.

62. Zipser RD, Hoefs JC, Speckart PF, Zia PK, Horton R. Prostaglandins: modulators of renal function and pressor resistance in chronic liver disease. *J Clin Endocrinol Metab* 1979;48(6): 895–900.

63. ter Wee PM, Donker AJ. Pharmacologic manipulation of glomerular function. *Kidney Int* 1994;45(2):417–424.

64. Bridoux F, Hazzan M, Pallot JL, Fleury D, Lemaitre V, Kleinknecht D, Vanhille P. Acute renal failure after the use of angiotensin-converting-enzyme inhibitors in patients without renal artery stenosis. *Nephrol Dial Transplant* 1992;7(2):100–104.

65. Badr KF, Ichikawa I. Prerenal failure: a deleterious shift from renal compensation to decompensation. *N Engl J Med* 1988;319(10):623–629.

66. Henrich WL. *The Kidney*, 2nd ed. New York: Raven Press, 1992. Pp. 3289–3304.

67. Foote EF, Halstenson CE. New therapeutic agents in the management of hypertension: angiotensin II-receptor antagonists and renin inhibitors. *Ann Pharmacother* 1993;27(12): 1495–1503.

68. Niwa T, Maeda K, Shibata M. Urinary prostaglandins and thromboxane in patients with chronic glomerulonephritis. *Nephron* 1987;46(3):281–287.

69. Cantley LG, Spokes K, Clark B, McMahon EG, Carter J, Epstein FH. Role of endothelin and prostaglandins in radiocontrast-induced renal artery constriction. *Kidney Int* 1993;44(6): 1217–1223.

70. Altman RD, Perez GO, Sfakianakis GN. Interaction of cyclosporine A and nonsteroidal anti-inflammatory drugs on renal function in patients with rheumatoid arthritis. *Am J Med* 1992;93(4):396–402.

71. Brater DC, Anderson SA, Brown-Cartwright D, Toto RD. Effects of nonsteroidal antiinflammatory drugs on renal function in patients with renal insufficiency and in cirrhotics. *Am J Kidney Dis* 1986;8(5):351–355.

72. Cannon PJ. Prostaglandins in congestive heart failure and the effects of nonsteroidal anti-inflammatory drugs. *Am J Med* 1986;81(2B): 123–132.

73. Toto RD. Renal insufficiency due to angiotensin-converting enzyme inhibitors. *Miner Electrolyte Metab* 1994;20(4):193–200.

74. Smith RD, Chiu AT, Wong PC, Herblin WF, Timmermans PB. Pharmacology of nonpeptide angiotensin II receptor antagonists. *Annu Rev Pharmacol Toxicol* 1992;32:135–165.

75. Fillastre JP, Godin M. *Oxford Textbook of Clinical Nephrology*, 2nd ed. Oxford: Oxford University Press, 1995. Pp. 2645–2657.

76. Shuler CO, Bennett W. *Textbook of Nephrology*, Vol. I, 3rd ed. Baltimore: Williams and Wilkins, 1995. Pp. 930–946.

77. Bennett WM. Mechanisms of aminoglycoside nephrotoxicity. *Clin Exp Pharmacol Physiol* 1989; 16(1):1–6.

78. Humes HD. Aminoglycoside nephrotoxicity [clinical conference]. *Kidney Int* 1988;33(4): 900–911.

79. Kaloyanides GJ, Bosmans JL, DeBroe ME. *Diseases of the Kidney*, Vol. II, 6th ed, Boston: Little, Brown and Company, 1997. Pp. 1115–1151.

80. Feig PU, Mitchell PP, Abrutyn E, Brock SM, Carney WR, Graeber CW, Horak E, Lyons RW, Maher JF. Aminoglycoside nephrotoxicity: a double blind prospective randomized study of gentamicin and tobramycin. *J Antimicrob Chemother* 1982;10(3):217–226.

81. Kahlmeter G, Dahlager JI. Aminoglycoside toxicity—a review of clinical studies published between 1975 and 1982. *J Antimicrob Chemother* 1984;13 Suppl A:9–22.

82. Daschner FD, Just HM, Jansen W, Lorber R. Netilmicin versus tobramycin in multi-centre studies. *J Antimicrob Chemother* 1984;13 Suppl A:37–45.

83. Smith CR, Maxwell RR, Edwards CQ, Rogers JF, Lietman PS. Nephrotoxicity induced by gentamicin and amikacin. *Johns Hopkins Med J* 1978; 142(3):85–90.

84. Cockcroft DW, Gault MH. Prediction of creatinine clearance from serum creatinine. *Nephron* 1976;16(1):31–41.

85. Mirahmadi MK, Byrne C, Barton C, Penera N, Gordon S, Vaziri ND. Prediction of creatinine clearance from serum creatinine in spinal cord injury patients. *Paraplegia* 1983;21(1):23–29.

86. Patel R, Savage A. Symptomatic hypomagne-

semia associated with gentamicin therapy. *Nephron* 1979;23(1):50–52.

87. De Broe ME, Verbist L, Verpooten GA. Influence of dosage schedule on renal cortical accumulation of amikacin and tobramycin in man. *J Antimicrob Chemother* 1991;27 Suppl C: 41–47.

88. De Broe ME, Giuliano RA, Verpooten GA. Choice of drug and dosage regimen: two important risk factors for aminoglycoside nephrotoxicity. *Am J Med* 1986;80(6B):115–118.

89. Gilbert DN. Once-daily aminoglycoside therapy. Antimicrob *Agents Chemother* 1991;35(3): 399–405.

90. Verpooten GA, Giuliano RA, Verbist L, Eestermans G, De Broe ME. Once-daily dosing decreases renal accumulation of gentamicin and netilmicin. *Clin Pharmacol Ther* 1989;45(1): 22–27.

91. Levinson ME. New dosing regimens for aminoglycoside antibiotics. *Ann Intern Med* 1992, 117: 693.

92. Prins JM, Buller HR, Kuijper EJ, Tange RA, Speelman P. Once versus thrice daily gentamicin in patients with serious infections [see comments]. *Lancet* 1993;341(8841):335–339.

93. Maddux MS, Barriere SL. A review of complications of amphotericin B therapy: recommendations for prevention and management. *Drug Intell Clin Pharmacol* 1980;14:177.

94. Medoff G, Kobayashi GS. Strategies in the treatment of systemic fungal infections. *N Engl J Med* 1980;302(3):145–155.

95. Heyman SN, Stillman IE, Brezis M, Epstein FH, Spokes K, Rosen S. Chronic amphotericin nephropathy: morphometric, electron microscopic, and functional studies. *J Am Soc Nephrol* 1993;4(1):69–80.

96. Sawaya BP, Briggs JP, Schnermann J. Amphotericin B nephrotoxicity: the adverse consequences of altered membrane properties [editorial]. *J Am Soc Nephrol* 1995;6(2):154–164.

97. Bean B, Aeppli D. Adverse effects of high-dose intravenous acyclovir in ambulatory patients with acute herpes zoster. *J Infect Dis* 1985; 151(2):362–365.

98. Burgess JL, Birchall R. Nephrotoxicity of amphotericin B, with emphasis on changes in tubular function. *Am J Med* 1972;53(1):77–84.

99. Barton CH, Pahl M, Vaziri ND, Cesario T. Renal magnesium wasting associated with amphotericin B therapy. *Am J Med* 1984;77(3): 471–474.

100. Barbour GL, Straub KD, O'Neal BL, Leatherman JW. Vasopressin-resistant nephro-genic diabetes insipidus: a result of amphotericin B therapy. *Arch Intern Med* 1979;139(1):86–88.

101. Mattie H, Craig WA, Pechere JC. Determinants of efficacy and toxicity of aminoglycosides [see comments]. *J Antimicrob Chemother* 1989;24(3): 281–293.

102. Swan SK, Bennett WM. *Acute Renal Failure*, 3rd ed. New York: Churchill Livingstone, 1993. P. 357.

103. Janknegt R, de Marie S, Bakker-Woudenberg IA, Crommelin DJ. Liposomal and lipid formulations of amphotericin B. *Clin Pharmacokinet* 1992;23(4):279–291.

104. Ringden O, Andstrom E, Remberger M, Svahn BM, Tollemar J. Safety of liposomal amphotericin B (AmBisome) in 187 transplant recipients treated with cyclosporin. *Bone Marrow Transplant* 1994;14(Suppl 5):S10–14.

105. Moreau P, Milpied N, Fayette N, Ramee JF, Harousseau JL. Reduced renal toxicity and improved clinical tolerance of amphotericin B mixed with intralipid compared with conventional amphotericin B in neutropenic patients [see comments]. *J Antimicrob Chemother* 1992; 30(4):535–541.

106. Grunfeld JP, Klienknecht D, Droz D. Diseases of the Kidney, Vol. II, 6th ed, Boston: Little, Brown and Company, 1997. Pp. 1331–1352.

107. Richet G, Sraer JD, Kourilsky O, Kanfer A, Mignon F, Whitworth J, Morel-Maroger L. Renal puncture biopsy in acute renal insufficiency. *Ann Med Interne (Paris)* 1978;129(6-7): 445–447.

108. Cameron JS. Allergic interstitial nephritis: clinical features and pathogenesis. *Q J Med* 1988; 66(250):97–115.

109. Hamburger J, Richet G, Crosnier J. *Nephrology*, Vol. 2. Philadelphia: W.B. Saunders 1968. Pp. 1014–1036.

110. Cameron JS. Immunologically mediated interstitial nephritis: primary and secondary. *Adv Nephrol Necker Hosp* 1989;18:207–248.

111. Ten RM, Torres VE, Milliner DS, Schwab TR, Holley KE, Gleich GJ. Acute interstitial nephritis: immunologic and clinical aspects. *Mayo Clin Proc* 1988;63(9):921–930.

112. Mignon F, Mery JP, Mougenot B, Ronco P, Roland J, Morel-Maroger L. Granulomatous interstitial nephritis. *Adv Nephrol Necker Hosp* 1984;13:219–245.

113. Cacoub P, Deray G, Le Hoang P, Baumelou A, Beaufils H, de Groc F, Rousselis F, Jouanneau C, Jacobs C. Idiopathic acute interstitial nephritis associated with anterior uveitis in adults [see comments]. *Clin Nephrol* 1989;31(6):307–310.

114. Pamukcu R, Moorthy V, Singer JR, Hong R, Simpson DP. Idiopathic acute interstitial nephritis: characterization of the infiltrating cells in the renal interstitium as T helper lymphocytes. *Am J Kidney Dis* 1984;4(1):24–29.

115. Bender WL, Whelton A, Beschorner WE, Darwish MO, Hall-Craggs M, Solez K. Interstitial nephritis, proteinuria, and renal failure caused by nonsteroidal anti-inflammatory drugs: immunologic characterization of the inflammatory infiltrate. *Am J Med* 1984;76(6): 1006–1012.

116. Colvin RB, Fang LST. *Renal Pathology with Clinical and Functional Correlations*, Vol. 1. Philadelphia: Lippincott, 1989. P. 728–776.

118. Grussendorf M, Andrassy K, Waldherr R, Ritz E. Systemic hypersensitivity to allopurinol with acute interstitial nephritis. *Am J Nephrol* 1981; 1(2):105–109.

119. Warren DJ, Leitch AG, Leggett RJ. Hyperuricaemic acute renal failure after epileptic seizures. *Lancet* 1975;2(7931):385–387.

120. Hande KR, Garrow GC. Acute tumor lysis syndrome in patients with high-grade non-Hodgkin's lymphoma [see comments]. *Am J Med* 1993;94(2):133–139.

121. Kjellstrand CM, Cambell DC, von Hartitzsch B, Buselmeier TJ. Hyperuricemic acute renal failure. *Arch Intern Med* 1974;133(3):349–359.

122. Weinstein L, Madoff MA, Samet CM. The sulfonamides. *N Engl J Med* 1960;263:793.

123. Carbone LG, Bendixen B, Appel GB. Sulfadiazine-associated obstructive nephropathy occurring in a patient with the acquired immunodeficiency syndrome. *Am J Kidney Dis* 1988; 12(1):72–75.

124. Abelson HT, Fosburg MT, Beardsley GP, Goorin AM, Gorka C, Link M, Link D. Methotrexate-induced renal impairment: clinical studies and rescue from systemic toxicity with high-dose leucovorin and thymidine. *J Clin Oncol* 1983;1(3):208–216.

125. Brigden D, Rosling AE, Woods NC. Renal function after acyclovir intravenous injection. *Am J Med* 1982;73(1A):182–185.

126. Winek CL, Shingleton DP, Shanor SP. Ethylene and diethylene glycol toxicity. *Clin Toxicol* 1978; 13(2):297–324.

127. Karlson-Stiber C, Persson H. Ethylene glycol poisoning: experiences from an epidemic in Sweden [see comments]. *J Toxicol Clin Toxicol* 1992;30(4):565–574.

128. Cramer BC, Parfrey PS, Hutchinson TA, Baran D, Melanson DM, Ethier RE, Seely JF. Renal function following infusion of radiologic contrast material: a prospective controlled study. *Arch Intern Med* 1985;145(1):87–89.

129. Taliercio CP, Vlietstra RE, Fisher LD, Burnett JC. Risks for renal dysfunction with cardiac angiography. *Ann Intern Med* 1986;104(4): 501–504.

130. Brezis M, Epstein FH. A closer look at radiocontrast-induced nephropathy [editorial] [see comments]. *N Engl J Med* 1989;320(3):179–181.

131. Margulies K, Schirger J, Burnett J, Jr. Radiocontrast-induced nephropathy: current status and future prospects. *Int Angiol* 1992; 11(1):20–25.

132. Davidson CJ, Hlatky M, Morris KG, Pieper K, Skelton TN, Schwab SJ, Bashore TM. Cardiovascular and renal toxicity of a nonionic radiographic contrast agent after cardiac catheterization: a prospective trial. *Ann Intern Med* 1989;110(2):119–124.

133. Barrett BJ, Carlisle EJ. Metaanalysis of the relative nephrotoxicity of high- and low-osmolality iodinated contrast media. *Radiology* 1993;188(1): 171–178.

134. Barrett BJ, Parfrey PS, Vavasour HM, McDonald J, Kent G, Hefferton D, O'Dea F, Stone E, Reddy R, McManamon PJ. Contrast nephropathy in patients with impaired renal function: high versus low osmolar media. *Kidney Int* 1992;41(5):1274–1279.

135. Manske CL, Sprafka JM, Strony JT, Wang Y. Contrast nephropathy in azotemic diabetic patients undergoing coronary angiography. *Am J Med* 1990;89(5): 615-20.

136. Parfrey PS, Griffiths SM, Barrett BJ, Paul MD, Genge M, Withers J, Farid N, McManamon PJ. Contrast material-induced renal failure in patients with diabetes mellitus, renal insufficiency, or both: a prospective controlled study [see comments]. *N Engl J Med* 1989;320(3):143–149.

137. Krumlovsky FA, Simon N, Santhanam S, del Greco F, Roxe D, Pomaranc MM. Acute renal failure: association with administration of radiographic contrast material. *JAMA* 1978;239(2): 125–127.

138. Berkseth RO, Kjellstrand CM. Radiologic contrast-induced nephropathy. *Med Clin North Am* 1984;68(2):351–370.

139. D'Elia JA, Gleason RE, Alday M, Malarick C, Godley K, Warram J, Kaldany A, Weinrauch LA. Nephrotoxicity from angiographic contrast material: a prospective study. *Am J Med* 1982; 72(5):719–725.

140. Bakris GL, Burnett JC, Jr. A role for calcium in radiocontrast-induced reductions in renal hemodynamics. *Kidney Int* 1985;27(2):465–468.

141. Neumayer HH, Junge W, Kufner A, Wenning A. Prevention of radiocontrast-media-induced nephrotoxicity by the calcium channel blocker nitrendipine: a prospective randomized clinical trial. *Nephrol Dial Transplant* 1989;4(12): 1030–1036.

142. Fischer RP, Reed II RL, Yatsu JS. *Complication of Trauma*,1st ed. New York: Churchill Livingstone 1993. Pp. 41–60.

143. Morris JA, Jr., Mucha P, Jr., Ross SE, Moore BF, Hoyt DB, Gentilello L, Landercasper L, Feliciano DV, Shackford SR. Acute posttraumatic renal failure: a multicenter perspective. *J Trauma* 1991;31(12):1584–1590.

144. Shin B, Mackenzie CF, Cowley RA. Changing patterns of posttraumatic acute renal failure. *Am Surg* 1979;45(3):182–189.

145. Tonnesen AS. *Critical Care Practice*. Philadelphia: W.B. Saunders, 1991. P. 242.

146. Ward MM. Factors predictive of acute renal failure in rhabdomyolysis. *Arch Intern Med* 1988; 148(7):1553–1557.

147. Curry SC, Chang D, Connor D. Drug- and toxin-induced rhabdomyolysis. *Ann Emerg Med* 1989;18(10):1068–1084.

148. Honda N. Acute renal failure and rhabdomyolysis. *Kidney Int* 1983;23(6):888–898.

149. Knochel JP. *The Kidney in Systemic Disease*, 2nd ed. New York: Wiley, 1976. Pp. 263–284.

150. Hadjis T, Grieff M, Lockhat D, Kaye M. Calcium metabolism in acute renal failure due to rhabdomyolysis. *Clin Nephrol* 1993;39(1):22–27.

151. Better OS, Rubinstein I, Winaver J. Recent insights into the pathogenesis and early management of the crush syndrome. *Semin Nephrol* 1992;12(2):217–222.

152. Better OS, Stein JH. Early management of shock and prophylaxis of acute renal failure in traumatic rhabdomyolysis [see comments]. *N Engl J Med* 1990;322(12):825–829.

153. Tribe CR, Silver JR. *Renal Failure in Paraplegia*. London: Pitman Medical, 1969. Pp. 13–89.

154. Hackler RH. A 25-year prospective mortality study in the spinal cord injured patient: comparison with the long-term living paraplegic. *J Urol* 1977;117(4):486–488.

155. Borges PM, Hackler RH. The urologic status of the Vietnam war paraplegic: a 15-year prospective followup. *J Urol* 1982;127(4):710–711.

156. Price M. Some results of a fifteen year vertical study of urinary tract function in spinal cord injured patients: a preliminary report. *J Am Paraplegia Soc* 1982;5:31–35.

157. DeVivo MJ, Kartus PL, Stover SL, Rutt RD, Fine PR. Cause of death for patients with spinal cord injuries. *Arch Intern Med* 1989;149(8): 1761–1766.

158. Imai K, Kadowaki T, Aizawa Y, Fukutomi K. Problems in the health management of persons with spinal cord injury. *J Clin Epidemiol* 1996; 49(5):505–510.

159. Lamid S. Long-term follow-up of spinal cord injury patients with vesicoureteral reflux. *Paraplegia* 1988;26(1):27–34.

160. Vaziri ND, Cesario T, Mootoo K, Zeien L, Gordon S, Byrne C. Bacterial infections in patients with chronic renal failure: occurrence with spinal cord injury. *Arch Intern Med* 1982; 142(7):1273–1276.

161. Kincaid-Smith PS, Bastos MG, Becker GJ. Reflux nephropathy in the adult. *Contrib Nephrol* 1984;39:94–101.

162. Hall MK, Hackler RH, Zampieri TA, Zampieri JB. Renal calculi in spinal cord-injured patient: association with reflux, bladder stones, and Foley catheter drainage. *Urology* 1989;34(3):126–128.

163. Claus-Walker J, Campos RJ, Carter RE, Vallbona C, Lipscomb HS. Calcium excretion in quadriplegia. *Arch Phys Med Rehabil* 1972;53(1): 14–20.

164. Kuhlemeier KV, Huang CT, Lloyd LK, Fine PR, Stover SL. Effective renal plasma flow: clinical significance after spinal cord injury. *J Urol* 1985;133(5):758–761.

165. Vaziri ND, Bruno A, Mirahmadi MK, Golji H, Gordon S, Byrne C. Features of residual renal function in end-stage renal failure associated with spinal cord injury. *Int J Artif Organs* 1984; 7(6):319–322.

166. Barton CH, Vaziri ND, Gordon S, Eltorai I. Endocrine pathology in spinal cord injured patients on maintenance dialysis. *Paraplegia* 1984;22(1):7–16.

167. Eschbach JW. The anemia of chronic renal failure: pathophysiology and the effects of recombinant erythropoietin [clinical conference]. *Kidney Int* 1989;35(1):134–48.

168. Vaziri ND. *Current Dialysis Therapy*. Philadelphia: Hanley and Belfus, 1986. Pp. 158–161.

169. Vaziri ND, Byrne C, Mirahmadi MK, Golji H, Nikakhtar B, Alday B, Gordon S. Hematologic features of chronic renal failure associated with spinal cord injury. *Artif Organs* 1982;6(1):69–72.

170. Vaziri ND, Winer RL, Alikhani S, Danviryasup K, Toohey J, Hung E, Gordon S, Eltorai I, Paule P. Antithrombin deficiency in end-stage renal disease associated with paraplegia: effect of hemodialysis. *Arch Phys Med Rehabil* 1985;66(5): 307–309.

171. Vaziri ND, Winer RL, Alikhani S, Toohey J, Paule P, Danviryasum K, Gordon S, Eltorai I. Extrinsic and common coagulation pathways in end-stage renal disease associated with spinal cord injury. *Paraplegia* 1986;24(3):154–158.

172. Vaziri ND, Winer RL, Toohey J, Danviriyasup K, Alikhani S, Eltorai I, Gordon S, Paule P. Intrinsic coagulation pathway in end-stage renal disease associated with spinal cord injury treated with hemodialysis. *Artif Organs* 1985;9(2): 155–159.

173. Vaziri ND, Patel B, Gonzales AE, Winer RL, Eltorai I, Gordon S, Danviryasup K. Protein C abnormalities in spinal cord injured patients with end-stage renal disease. *Arch Phys Med Rehabil* 1987;68(11):791–793.

174. Block GA, Hulbert-Shearon TE, Levin NW, Port FK. Association of serum phosphorus and calcium × phosphate product with mortality risk in chronic hemodialysis patients: a national study. *Am J Kidney Dis* 1998;31(4): 607–617.

175. Rostand SG, Sanders C, Kirk KA, Rutsky EA, Fraser RG. Myocardial calcification and cardiac dysfunction in chronic renal failure. *Am J Med* 1988;85(5): 651–657.

176. Massry SG, Smogorzewski M. Mechanisms through which parathyroid hormone mediates its deleterious effects on organ function in uremia. *Semin Nephrol* 1994;14(3):219–231.

177. Lowrie EG, Lew NL. Death risk in hemodialysis patients: the predictive value of commonly measured variables and an evaluation of death rate differences between facilities. *Am J Kidney Dis* 1990;15(5):458–482.

178. Wills MR, Savory J. Aluminium poisoning: dialysis encephalopathy, osteomalacia, and anaemia. *Lancet* 1983;2(8340):29–34.

179. Alfrey AC, Hegg A, Craswell P. Metabolism and toxicity of aluminum in renal failure. *Am J Clin Nutr* 1980;33(7):1509–1516.

180. Koch KM. Dialysis-related amyloidosis [clinical conference]. *Kidney Int* 1992;41(5):1416–1429.

181. Rostand SG, Brunzell JD, Cannon RO, Victor RG. Cardiovascular complications in renal failure [editorial]. *J Am Soc Nephrol* 1991;2(6):1053–1062.

182. Ventura SC, Garella S. The management of pericardial disease in renal failure. *Semin Dial* 1990;3:21.

183. Parfrey PS, Harnett JD, Barre PE. The natural history of myocardial disease in dialysis patients. *J Am Soc Nephrol* 1991;2(1):2–12.

184. Lazarus JM, Lowrie EG, Hampers CL, Merrill JP. Cardiovascular disease in uremic patients on hemodialysis. *Kidney Int Suppl* 1975(2):167–175.

185. Pahl MV, Vaziri ND, Gordon S, Tuero S. Cardiovascular pathology in dialysis patients with spinal cord injury. *Artif Organs* 1983;7(4): 416–419.

186. Fairshter RD, Vaziri ND, Gordon S. Frequency and spectrum of pulmonary diseases in patients with chronic renal failure associated with spinal cord injury. *Respiration* 1983;44(1):58–62.

187. Gore RM, Mintzer RA, Calenoff L. Gastrointestinal complications of spinal cord injury. *Spine* 1981;6(6):538–544.

188. Fealey RD, Szurszewski JH, Merritt JL, DiMagno EP. Effect of traumatic spinal cord transection on human upper gastrointestinal motility and gastric emptying. *Gastroenterology* 1984;87(1):69–75.

189. Kewalramani LS. Neurogenic gastroduodenal ulceration and bleeding associated with spinal cord injuries. *J Trauma* 1979;19(4):259–265.

190. Kiwerski J. Bleeding from the alimentary canal during the management of spinal cord injury patients. *Paraplegia* 1986;24(2):92–96.

191. Adams PL, Rutsky EA, Rostand SG, Han SY. Lower gastrointestinal tract dysfunction in patients receiving long-term hemodialysis. *Arch Intern Med* 1982;142(2):303–306.

192. Ala-Kaila K, Paronen I, Paakkala T. Increased incidence of duodenitis in chronic renal failure. *Ann Clin Res* 1988;20(3):154–157.

193. Avram MM. High prevalence of pancreatic disease in chronic renal failure. *Nephron* 1977; 18(1):68–71.

194. Milito G, Taccone-Gallucci M, Brancaleone C, Nardi F, Cesca D, Boffo V, Casciani CU. The gastrointestinal tract in uremic patients on long-term hemodialysis. *Kidney Int Suppl* 1985;17: S157–160.

195. Meshkinpour H, Vaziri N, Gordon S. Gastrointestinal pathology in patients with chronic renal failure associated with spinal cord injury. *Am J Gastroenterol* 1982;77(8):562–564.

196. Marcuard SP, Weinstock JV. Gastrointestinal angiodysplasia in renal failure. *J Clin Gastroenterol* 1988;10(5):482–484.

197. Gilmore PR. Angiodysplasia of the upper gastrointestinal tract. *J Clin Gastroenterol* 1988; 10(4):386–394.

198. Posner GL, Fink SM, Huded FV, Dunn I, Calderone PG, Joglekar SS. Endoscopic findings in chronic hemodialysis patients with upper gastrointestinal bleeding. *Am J Gastroenterol* 1983;78(11):720–721.

199. Mills B, Zuckerman G, Sicard G. Discrete colon ulcers as a cause of lower gastrointestinal bleeding and perforation in end-stage renal disease. *Surgery* 1981;89(5):548–552.

200. Mannucci PM, Remuzzi G, Pusineri F, Lombardi R, Valsecchi C, Mecca G, Zimmerman TS. Deamino-8-D-arginine vasopressin shortens the bleeding time in uremia. *N Engl J Med* 1983;308(1):8–12.

201. Livio M, Mannucci PM, Vigano G, Mingardi G, Lombardi R, Mecca G, Remuzzi G. Conjugated estrogens for the management of bleeding associated with renal failure. *N Engl J Med* 1986; 315(12):731–735.

202. Diamond S, Emmet M, Henrich W. Bowel infarction: a common occurrence in dialysis patients (abstract). *Kidney Int* 1986;29:212.

203. Bartolomeo RS, Calabrese PR, Taubin HL. Spontaneous perforation of the colon: a potential complication of chronic renal failure. *Am J Dig Dis* 1977;22(7):656–657.

204. Diamond SM, Emmett M, Henrich WL. Bowel infarction as a cause of death in dialysis patients. *JAMA* 1986;256(18):2545–2547.

205. Popli S, Daugirdas JT, Ing TS. Dialysis ascites [editorial]. *Int J Artif Organs* 1980;3(5):257–258.

206. Harnett JD, Parfrey PS, Kennedy M, Zeldis JB, Steinman TI, Guttmann RD. The long-term outcome of hepatitis B infection in hemodialysis patients. *Am J Kidney Dis* 1988;11(3):210–213.

207. Da Porto A, Adami A, Susanna F, Calzavara P, Poli P, Castelletto MR, Amici GP, Teodoni T, Okolicsanyi L. Hepatitis C virus in dialysis units: a multicenter study. *Nephron* 1992;61(3): 309–310.

208. Malaguti M, Capece R, Marciano M, Arena G, Luciani MP, Striano M, Biagini M. Antibodies to hepatitis C virus (anti-HCV): prevalence in the same geographical area in dialysis patients, staff members, and blood donors. *Nephron* 1992; 61(3):346.

209. Conway M, Catterall AP, Brown EA, Tibbs C, Gower PE, Curtis JR, Coleman JC, Murray-Lyon IM. Prevalence of antibodies to hepatitis C in dialysis patients and transplant recipients with possible routes of transmission [see comments]. *Nephrol Dial Transplant* 1992;7(12): 1226–1269.

210. Eijgenraam FJ, Donckerwolcke RA. Treatment of iron overload in children and adolescents on chronic haemodialysis. *Eur J Pediatr* 1990; 149(5):359–362.

211. Simon P, Meyrier A. Drug-induced liver cytolysis in hemodialyzed patients. *Kidney Int* 1979;15: 453.

212. Silver SM, DeSimone JA, Jr., Smith DA, Sterns RH. Dialysis disequilibrium syndrome (DDS) in the rat: role of the "reverse urea effect." *Kidney Int* 1992;42(1):161–166.

213. Bregman H, Daugirdas JT, Ing TS. *Handbook of Dialysis*, 2nd ed. Boston: Little Brown and Company, 1994. Pp. 149–168.

214. Alvestrand A. Protein metabolism and nutrition in hemodialysis patients. *Contrib Nephrol* 1990; 78:102–118.

215. Blagg CR. Importance of nutrition in dialysis patients [editorial]. *Am J Kidney Dis* 1991;17(4): 458–461.

216. Blumenkrantz MJ, Kopple JD, Gutman RA, Chan YK, Barbour GL, Roberts C, Shen FH, Gandhi VC, Tucker CT, Curtis FK, Coburn JW. Methods for assessing nutritional status of patients with renal failure. *Am J Clin Nutr* 1980;33(7):1567–1585.

217. Mirahmadi MK, Barton CH, Vaziri ND, Gordon S, Penera N. Nutritional evaluation of hemodialysis patients with and without spinal cord injury. *J Am Paraplegia Soc* 1983;6(2):36–40.

218. Hostetter TH, Olson JL, Rennke HG, Venkatachalam MA, Brenner BM. Hyperfiltration in remnant nephrons: a potentially adverse response to renal ablation. *Am J Physiol* 1981;241(1):F85–93.

219. Meyer TW, Anderson S, Rennke HG, Brenner BM. Reversing glomerular hypertension stabilizes established glomerular injury. *Kidney Int* 1987;31(3):752–759.

220. Lafayette RA, Mayer G, Park SK, Meyer TW. Angiotensin II receptor blockade limits glomerular injury in rats with reduced renal mass. *J Clin Invest* 1992;90(3):766–771.

221. Mirahmadi MK, Vaziri ND, Ghobadi M, Nikakhtar B, Gordon S. Survival on maintenance dialysis in patients with chronic renal failure associated with paraplegia and quadriplegia. *Paraplegia* 1982;20(1):43–47.

222. Stacy WK, Falls WF, Hussey RW. Chronic hemodialysis of spinal cord injury patients. *J Am Paraplegia Soc* 1983;6(1):7–9.

223. Vaziri ND, Bruno A, Byrne C, Mirahmadi MK, Nikakhtar B, Gordon S, Zeien L. Maintenance hemodialysis in end-stage renal disease associated with spinal cord injury. *Artif Organs* 1982; 6(1):13–16.

224. Ethier JH, Lindsay RM, Barre PE, Kappel JE, Carlisle EJ, Common A. Clinical practice guidelines for vascular access. Canadian Society of Nephrology. *J Am Soc Nephrol* 1999;10 Suppl 13:S297–305.

225. Bander SJ, Schwab SJ. Central venous angioaccess for hemodialysis and its complications. *Semin Dial* 1992;5:121–128.

226. Schillinger F, Schillinger D, Montagnac R, Milcent T. Post catheterisation vein stenosis in

haemodialysis: comparative angiographic study of 50 subclavian and 50 internal jugular accesses. *Nephrol Dial Transplant* 1991;6(10):722–724.

227. Raja RM. *Handbook of Dialysis*. Boston: Little, Brown and Company, 1994. Pp. 53–77.

228. Harland RC. Placement of permanent vascular access devices: surgical considerations. *Adv Ren Replace Ther* 1994;1(2):99–106.

229. Lazarus JM, Denker BM, Owen Jr WF. *The Kidney*, Vol. II, 5th ed. Philadelphia: W.B. Saunders Company, 1996. pp. 2424–2506.

230. Hoen B, Paul-Dauphin A, Hestin D, Kessler M. EPIBACDIAL: a multicenter prospective study of risk factors for bacteremia in chronic hemodialysis patients. *J Am Soc Nephrol* 1998; 9(5):869–876.

231. Vaziri ND. Long-term haemodialysis in spinal cord injured patients. *Paraplegia* 1984;22(2): 110–114.

232. Vaziri ND, Lopez G, Nikakhtar B, Gordon S, Penera N. Peritoneal dialysis in renal failure associated with spinal cord injury. *J Am Paraplegia Soc* 1984;7(4):63–65.

233. Vinay P, Prud'Homme M, Vinet B, Cournoyer G, Degoulet P, Leville M, Gougoux A, St-Louis G, Lapierre L, Piette Y. Acetate metabolism and bicarbonate generation during hemodialysis: 10 years of observation. *Kidney Int* 1987;31(5): 1194–1204.

234. Mastrangelo F, Rizzelli S, Corliano C, Montinaro AM, De Blasi V, Alfonso L, Aprile M, Napoli M, Laforgia R. Benefits of bicarbonate dialysis. Kidney Int Suppl 1985;17: S188-93.

235. Himmelfarb J, Ault KA, Holbrook D, Leeber DA, Hakim RM. Intradialytic granulocyte reactive oxygen species production: a prospective, crossover trial. *J Am Soc Nephrol* 1993;4(2): 178–186.

236. Loughrey CM, Young IS, Lightbody JH, McMaster D, McNamee PT, Trimble ER. Oxidative stress in haemodialysis. *Qjm* 1994; 87(11):679–683.

237. Toborek M, Wasik T, Drozdz M, Klin M, Magner-Wrobel K, Kopieczna-Grzebieniak E. Effect of hemodialysis on lipid peroxidation and antioxidant system in patients with chronic renal failure. *Metabolism* 1992;41(11):1229–1232.

238. Schulman G, Fogo A, Gung A, Badr K, Hakim R. Complement activation retards resolution of acute ischemic renal failure in the rat. *Kidney Int* 1991;40(6):1069–1074.

239. Harris KP, Schreiner GF, Klahr S. Effect of leukocyte depletion on the function of the postobstructed kidney in the rat. *Kidney Int* 1989; 36(2):210–215.

240. Schiffl H, Lang SM, Konig A, Strasser T, Haider MC, Held E. Biocompatible membranes in acute renal failure: prospective case-controlled study [see comments]. *Lancet* 1994; 344(8922):570–572.

241. Hakim RM, Wingard RL, Parker RA. Effect of the dialysis membrane in the treatment of patients with acute renal failure [see comments]. *N Engl J Med* 1994;331(20):1338–1342.

242. Burkart JM, Nolph KD. *The Kidney*, Vol. II, 5th ed. Philadelphia: WB Saunders Company, 1996. Pp. 2507–2575.

243. Duckworth WC, Jallepalli P, Solomon SS. Glucose intolerance in spinal cord injury. *Arch Phys Med Rehabil* 1983;64(3):107–110.

244. Blumenkrantz M. *Handbook of Dialysis*, 2nd ed. Boston: Little, Brown and Company, 1994. πp. 374–400.

245. Kaupke CJ, Vaziri ND. Nutritional implications of erythropoietin therapy in dialysis patients. *Semin Dial* 1992;5:254.

246. Mitch WE, May RC, Maroni BJ, Druml W. Protein and amino acid metabolism in uremia: influence of metabolic acidosis. *Kidney Int* Suppl 1989;27:S205–207.

247. Ziegler TR, Rombeau JL, Young LS, Fong Y, Marano M, Lowry SF, Willmore DW. Recombinant human growth hormone enhances the metabolic efficacy of parenteral nutrition: a double-blind, randomized controlled study. *J Clin Endocrinol Metab* 1992;74(4):865–873.

248. Goldstein DJ, Strom JA. Intradialytic parenteral nutrition: evolution and current concepts. *J Renal Nutr* 1991;1:9.

249. Descombes E, Hanck AB, Fellay G. Water soluble vitamins in chronic hemodialysis patients and need for supplementation. *Kidney Int* 1993; 43(6):1319–1328.

250. Vanwyck DB. Iron dextran in chronic renal failure. *Semin Dial* 1991;4:112–114.

251. Anderson RJ, Gambertoglio JG, Schrier RW. *Clinical Use of Drugs in Renal Failure*. Springfield, Illinois: Charles C. Thomas, 1976.

252. Aronoff GR, Erbeck KM. *Principles and Practice of Dialysis*. Baltimore: Williams and Wilkins, 1994. Pp. 89–97.

253. Cutler RE, Forland SC, St John Hammond, PG. *Textbook of Nephrology*, Vol. 2, 3rd ed. Baltimore: Williams and Wilkins, 1995. Pp. 1597–1625.

254. Shuler C, Golper TA, Bennett WM. *The Kidney*, Vol. II, 5th ed. Philadelphia: W.B. Saunders Company, 1996. Pp. 2653–2752.

255. Aronoff GR, Erbeck K, Brier ME. *Principles and Practice of Dialysis*, 2nd ed. Baltimore: Williams and Wilkins, 1999. P. 125.

256. Aronoff GR, Berns JS, Brier ME, Golper TA, Morrison G, Singer I, Swan SK, Benner WM. *Drug Prescribing in Renal Failure*, 4th ed. Philadelphia: American College of Physicians, 1999.

257. Gaspari F, Mosconi L, Vigano G, Perico N, Torre L, Virotta G, Bertcchi C, Remuzzi G, Ruggenenti P.: Measurement of GFR with a single intravenous injection of nonradioactive iothalamate. *Kidney Int* 1992;41(4):1081–1084.

258. Sanger JJ, Kramer EL. Radionuclide quantitation of renal function. *Urol Radiol* 1992;14(2): 69–78.

9 Nonoperative Management of Cervical Instability

RUSSELL W. NELSON, MD
ELLEN LEPPEK, MS, BS, PA-C
DANIEL A. CAPEN, MD

CERVICAL SPINE TRAUMA CREATES instability of the spinal column and injury to the spinal cord or serious threat of cord damage and paralysis in many patients. Surgical intervention is often required, either awake under local anesthesia (1) or under general anesthesia with cord monitoring. However, many patients are successfully treated with nonsurgical methods. The goals of the treatment of spine trauma remain protection of the neural elements and realignment of the spine to avoid further injury in both emergent and long-term care (2). Any excessive movement can cause worsening by creating or exacerbating a spinal cord injury (SCI).

EMERGENCY CARE

Medical or paramedical personnel give initial care at the scene of the injury. Spine immobilization by board, sandbag, orthosis, or manual traction serves to initially immobilize the patient. Neutral spine alignment is achieved as the first phase of care (Fig. 9-1). The process of initial care is a risk period for the spine with rapid transport to the hospital, because many of these patients have multisystem injuries that divert attention from the spine.

Life-threatening injury must be treated from initial assessment to transport, but establishing intravenous access, cardiac monitoring, airway management, and long-bone fracture care all must be done and can place the spine at risk without appropriate attention. Modern emergency field technicians are expert in dealing with this and can often apply tongs if needed and reduce iatrogenic injury.

Once the patient is in the emergency area full treatment can begin with accurate evaluation of all injuries. Spine radiographs, spine CAT or MRI, complete neurologic assessment, and evaluation of potentially life-threatening injury can be done. After stabilization of cardiac, respiratory, abdominal and craniofacial injuries, the spine can be addressed. Since Nickel, et al. (3) introduced external skeletal immobilization, there have been many modifications of materials and devices. Nonsurgical treatment often begins in the emergency department after diagnosis of instability is made. Early skeletal traction application permits use of a hospital bed or roto-rest type bed to prevent skin injury and to facilitate complete pulmonary ventilation.

DIAGNOSIS

Accurate diagnosis of instability is critical in selecting treatment by surgery or nonoperative methods. The neurologic status is the other

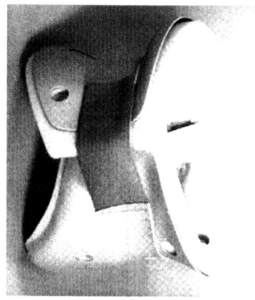

FIGURE 9-1 Standard transportation orthosis applied in the field. This permits safe transport. The Philadelphia-type collar is also utilized post surgery.

important information needed to formulate a treatment plan designed to achieve an optimal outcome. Serial neurologic examinations must be performed to classify the injury. Accurate diagnosis of cord injury type cannot be done until emergence from spinal shock. All cord syndromes are described in the *Standards for Neurological and Functional Classification of Spinal Cord Injury* (4).

Various skeletal systems of classification are reliable. At Rancho Los Amigos, we rely upon the Allen–Ferguson classification of instability (5). The system provides information on location and extent of instability based upon radiographic findings. Identification of fracture pattern allows the surgeon to plan appropriate treatment for the instability. Expected acute and chronic instability are identified by placing the injury in one of the six categories: vertical compression, compressive flexion, distractive flexion, compressive extension, distractive extension, and lateral flexion. Ligament injury frequently prevents successful nonsurgical care, but primary bony injury may be successfully treated in various types of immobilization devices, as in Fig 9-2.

Nelson et al. (6) documented a large series of SCI cases at Rancho that had failure of halo-vest care with persistent instability. The injury types with skeletal fracture, such as those shown in Fig. 9-3, and the vertical compression type injury, frequently healed with halo-vest care for 3 months.

Many cases can require nonsurgical stabilization for the initial treatment due to life-imperiling conditions. Also, quadriparesis and quadriplegia failure of gastrointestinal, urinary, and pulmonary systems can cause extensive delay in the performance of surgery. The surgeon must be able to manage instability nonsurgically until surgery can be tolerated.

HALO-VEST APPLICATION AND USE

The advances in lightweight materials have made the halo-vest more tolerable, but only when properly placed. Garfin (7) has outlined the importance of correct halovest application. The standard pin placement for the skull fixation is the critical point of halo application. Pin intolerance, pain, and pin tract infections can result from inappropriate initial application of the device.

Placement of the halo ring caudad to the biparietal diameter of the skull is critical. Avoidance of the temporalis muscle is also necessary. The cosmetic deficit from halo pins into the forehead above the eyebrows is minimal after the scar formation has matured. After the halo is applied, an appropriate well-molded and padded vest with attachments can provide for semirigid immobilization sufficient to allow for bony healing. As documented in numerous studies, there is some motion at all cervical segments in the halovest because of the difficulty in obtaining complete rigid immobilization (8). In most cases this motion is tolerated for the 3-month halo use required for successful bone healing.

Complications of Halo-vest Immobilzation

In 179 patients treated by halovest immobilization, there were definitive complications report-

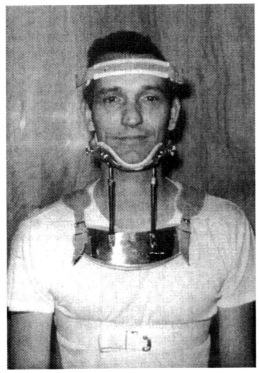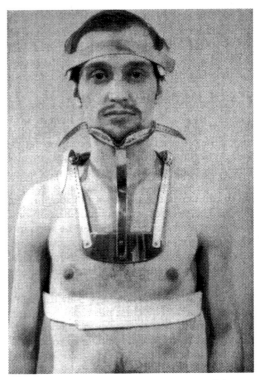

FIGURE 9-2   Semirigid orthosis for odontoid fracture or upper cervical injury. For safe and successful use, maximum patient compliance is required.

ed. Pin loosening and pin infection were the most frequently seen complications in the highest percentage. Some scarring was noted in long-term follow-up after pin loosening and pin infection. Skin pressure sores in multiple areas were noted as a frequently seen complication as well.

The presence of severe complications such as nerve injury and dural puncture was minimal. No deaths occurred. In the series of Garfin et al. (9) and Nelson et al. (10), the overall complication rates approached 20 percent.

Indications for Halo-vest Usage

In a patient with an intact neurologic system the option of surgical versus nonsurgical treatment must be presented. Avoidance of potential neurologic complications is always an important factor in decision-making. In our series, at least a 50 percent success rate with halo treatment is noted. In the majority of cases, a 90 percent or

greater success rate is recorded. The choice of avoidance of surgery is not irrational in this patient group.

We recommend, on the basis of our experience, that surgery can be avoided if the fracture classification fits the profile of patients successfully treated in a halovest and if the neurologic system is totally intact.

The other obvious candidate for halovest usage is the systemically unstable patient. In many cases, the initial period after cervical spinal cord trauma and spinal cord injury is accompanied by a high incidence of systemic illness and complications such as pneumonia, urinary tract infection, and cardiovascular instability. Because of the nature and origin of most spinal cord trauma, there are frequently associated injuries that also prevent early surgery. In many instances surgery for spinal stabilization cannot be performed and the halovest treatment must be utilized. If after 3 months of immobilization there is still documented instability or

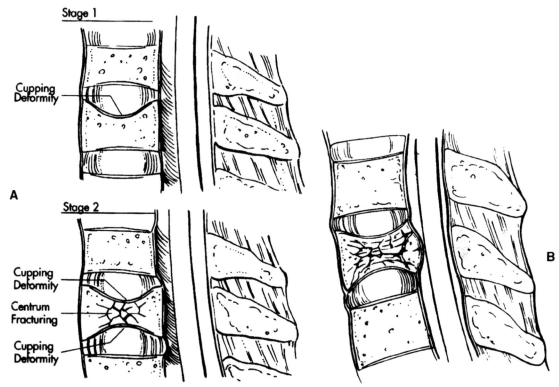

FIGURE 9-3 Allen Classification of Vertical Compression injury illustrates significant bony comminution, which enhances nonsurgical healing.

excessive motion in the cervical spine, surgery can then be considered. Halovest immobilization may be selected after anterior cervical spine decompression and fusion when there is documented accompanying posterior ligamentous instability (most often compression flexion lesions).

In some patients, immediate surgery will be required for spinal cord decompression. In these patients a second procedure, in which posterior wiring or plating and fusion or utilization of the halo-vest for 3 months to allow for graft incorporation, will be necessary to provide complete stabilization. For these patients the halovest is protection against graft dislodgment and development of kyphotic deformity secondary to the posterior ligamentous instability (11). Odontoid fracture is also successfully treated in a vest unless it is Type II fracture where nonunion is frequently observed without surgery (Fig. 9-4).

Contraindications to the Utilization of the Halo-vest

In some purely ligamentous injuries such as distraction flexion 1 and distraction flexion 2 injuries (formerly known as facet dislocations, unilateral and bilateral), there is total ligamentous instability and insufficient bony injury to permit healing. Utilization of the halo for 3 months in cases such as these often results in failure of achievement of bony union. Ligamentous injuries do best with posterior wiring and fusion and surgical stabilization. If identification of a primary ligamentous injury can be made, early surgical stabilizations are the treatment of choice.

In some combined head trauma and spinal cord injured patients, when an unstable skull fracture is present, a contraindication exists for the utilization of a halovest. This cannot provide the appropriate skeletal fixation without compromise of the fracture healing of the skull, and

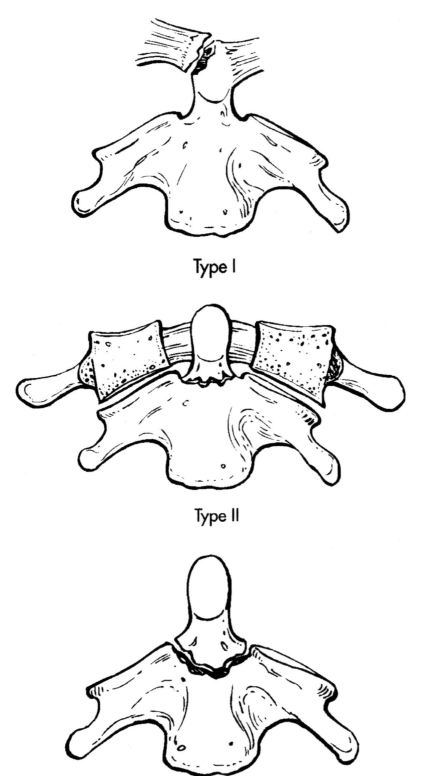

Type I

Type II

Type III

FIGURE 9-4 Odontoid injury can be treated with halo-vest, except Type II where loss of blood supply makes nonunion likely and surgery necessary.

in many cases with massive head trauma there is no bony base that is stable enough to allow for fixation. These cases obviously require alternative forms of treatment, including surgery.

The most obvious situation in which prolonged halovest immobilization is contraindicated is when there is a documented instance of bone and disc compressing the cervical spinal cord combined with documented worsening of neurologic function. These patients will not have improvement of neurologic function created or produced by halo immobilization. If initial traction has been applied and documented bone and disc are still present in the canal, surgical decompression is indicated. When neurologic function deteriorates, this treatment is indicated immediately.

ALTERNATIVE CERVICAL BRACING

Recognizing that not all patients can tolerate a halo, there are several devices available to provide some restriction of cervical motion during the healing period. None provide rigid immobilization, but the proper use can result in stabilization (9). The Somi brace, the Philadelphia collar, and others do prevent excessive rotation, flexion, and extension. They all require patient compliance but are all generally well tolerated. Complications of brace use are usually mild and easily treatable. The authors prefer the Philadelphia collar for most cases of postsurgical immobilization and for upper cervical injuries that are minimally unstable, because it is effective for restriction of motion (10).

CONCLUSION

Nonoperative treatment is clearly suited for many situations, with the halo-vest being the primary treatment of choice. Alternative semi-rigid orthotic devices can also be employed to immobilize the spine. Careful patient selection is of great importance for a successful outcome when considering nonoperative, definitive treatment of cervical instability. When appropriate identification of fracture class is made, the surgeon can utilize the halo based upon results of

recent research. With the use of the halo-vest, Bucholz and Cheung documented an overall failure rate of 15 percent. For distractive flexion injury, they found loss of reduction in 37 percent of all patients (12). Except for distractive flexion and compressive flexion type III injuries, the halovest immobilization is successful in over 90 percent of other fracture types. Bucci et al. had a 40 percent incidence of spinal instability following immobilization in a halo orthosis, with more than half of these subsequently requiring operative stabilization (13). Ligamentous injuries also heal poorly in the halo-vest.

It is acknowledged that primary anterior bone comminution is required to effectively create a stimuli for callous formation and thereby create a significant healing environment. This is present in most fracture types other than those that only involve ligamentous injuries. If care is taken in initial application of the halo and if nursing and rehabilitation management includes detailed attention to potential skin problems, patients can usually tolerate 3 months of vest immobilization while participating in active rehabilitation. Newer materials that are radiopaque also do not interfere with appropriate study of the cervical spinal canal.

Although surgical management is emphasized in most training programs and remains the primary form of treatment of cervical spine instability, the treating surgeon must be familiar with utilization of the halovest because it is extremely successful when appropriately applied.

REFERENCES

1. Zigler J, Waters R, Capen D, et al. Posterior cervical fusion under local anesthesia. *Spine* 1987; 12:206–208.
2. Beatson TR. Fractures and dislocations of the cervical spine. *J Bone Joint Surg* 1963; 45B:21.
3. Nickel VL, Perry J. Garrett A, Heppenstall M. The halo a spinal skeletal traction fixation. *J Bone Joint Surg* 1968; 50–A: 1400.
4. American Spinal Cord Injury Association. Standards for Neurological and Functional Classification of Spinal Cord Injury, Revised. Chicago, Illinois: *American Spinal Cord Injury Association*, 1992.

5. Allen BL Jr, Ferguson RL, Lehmann TR, O'Brien RP. A mechanistic classification of closed indirect fractures and dislocations of the lower cervical spine. *Spine* 1982; 7:1.

6. Nelson RW, Capen DA, Garland D, Waters RL. Halo-vest stabilization of cervical spine fractures and dislocations: a series review and long term follow-up. AAOS Presentation, Annual Meeting. Atlanta, 1984.

7. Garfin SR, Botte MJ, Waters RL, Nickel BL. Complications in the use of the halo fixation device. *J Bone Joint Surg* 1986; 68A:320.

8. Akins V, Eismont FJ. *Comparison of Four Cervical Motions.* Tampa, Florida: Orthopaedic Society, Oct. 20, 1994.

9. Kostuik JP. Indications for the use of the halo immobilization. *Clin Orthop* 1981; 154:46–50.

10. Fisher SV, Bowar JF, Awad EA, et al. Cervical orthoses effect on cervical spine motion: roentgenographic and goniometric method of study. *Arch Phys Med Rehabil* 1977; 58:109–115.

11. Johnsson RM, Hart DL, Simmons EF, et al. Cervical orthoses: a study comparing their effectiveness in restriction cervical motion in normal subjects. *J Bone Joint Surg* 1977; Am 59: 332–329.

10 Management of Peripheral Vascular Disease in the Spinal Cord Injured Patient

BOK Y. LEE, MD, FACS
MARCELO C. DASILVA, MD
LEE E. OSTRANDER, PhD

THE CARDINAL SIGNS of peripheral arterial disease, which include intermittent claudication, rest pain, numbness, and coldness of the limbs, are absent in the spinal cord injured population. The physician, thus, faces the difficult challenge of identifying the patient with peripheral arterial disease at risk of development of gangrene in the absence of signs and symptoms. Additionally, the spinal cord injured patient is at high risk of developing venous disease in the form of venous thrombosis due to venous stasis. Fortunately for the physician responsible for the care of the spinal cord injured patient, a number of simple, noninvasive diagnostic techniques are available in screening for peripheral vascular disease (1–3).

PERIPHERAL ARTERIAL DISEASE

Early detection and treatment of peripheral arterial disease often result in significant improvement of the patient's condition as well as prevention of limb loss by amputation.

Doppler Ultrasound

When peripheral arterial disease is assessed in the spinal cord injured patient, Doppler ultrasonography is typically used for the determination of two parameters: 1) segmental limb systolic pressures and 2) ankle systolic blood pressure relative to brachial systolic blood pressure (reported as an ankle/brachial systolic pressure ratio known as the *ischemic index*).

The ankle systolic pressure is obtained by placing a standard blood pressure cuff proximal to the ankle with the Doppler probe over the posterior tibial or dorsalis pedis artery (Fig. 10-1). The blood pressure cuff is gradually inflated until the blood flow signal disappears, but not exceeding 200 mmHg. If the blood flow signal is still present at 200 mmHg, the blood vessel is deemed incompressible. The blood pressure cuff is then slowly deflated until the blood flow signal is again audible. This systolic pressure is compared with the arm systolic pressure obtained in the standard manner utilizing the stethoscope. A normal ABI is 1.0 or greater; values less than 1.0 are suggestive of peripheral arterial insufficiency. The lower the ABI, the

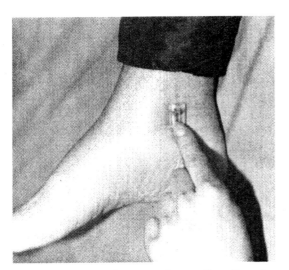

FIGURE 10-1 Technique of recording Doppler ultrasound waves.

more severe the disease. The exception is patients with diabetes mellitus, in whom arteries are calcified, which produces a falsely elevated ankle systolic arterial blood pressure.

The use of segmental limb systolic blood pressures can provide for localization and partial quantification of the arterial obstruction. The Doppler systolic blood pressure is measured at the ankle as three cuffs placed at the upper thigh, above the knee, and at the mid-calf are inflated and deflated (Fig. 10-2). Segmental systolic

pressure reading at the upper thigh and above the knee are particularly important for distinguishing between aortoiliac, femoropopliteal, and combined disease. Normal thigh systolic blood pressure is about 30 mmHg or more above the brachial systolic pressure; the above-the-knee, mid-calf, and ankle systolic pressures normally show a pressure gradient distally, with ankle systolic pressure approximating the brachial systolic blood pressure. The presence of extreme pressure drops between segments indicates occlusive disease between the segments.

Photoplethysmography

The technique of photoplethysmography is particularly advantageous for the detection of small-vessel disease. With the placement of a standard blood pressure cuff at the ankle or metatarsal area and the photoplethysmograph (PPG) probe located on the ventral surface of the toes, the point at which the pulsatile photoplethysmographic waveform returns as the cuff is slowly deflated indicates the ankle or metatarsal pressure (Fig. 10-3). The technique can be used to evaluate the blood supply of each digit and is particularly beneficial for the patient with gangrenous involvement of the toes when a decision has to be made about amputation.

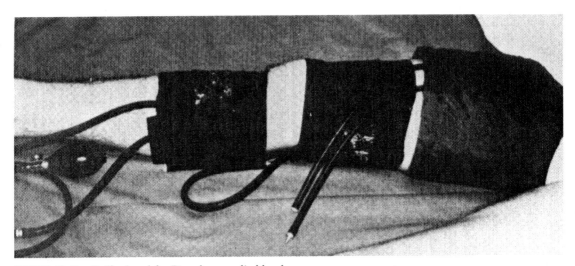

FIGURE 10-2 Cuffs placed for Doppler systolic blood pressure measurements.

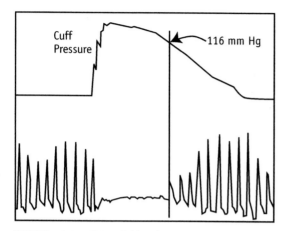

FIGURE 10-3 Digital blood pressure measurement on the toe with an ankle blood pressure cuff.

TABLE 10-1 Techniques for Detecting Microembolization

Segmental Doppler Systolic Pressures

	Right	Left
Brachial	122	112
High thigh	128 (1.1)	114 (1.02)
Above knee	128 (1.1)	118 (1.05)
Calf	126	90
Posterior tibial	124 (1.0)	100 (0.89)
Dorsal pedis	116 (0.95)	106 (0.95)

Photoplethysmograph Pressures at TOES

Toes	Right Ankle/Metatarsal	Left Ankle/Metatarsal
1	72/55	75/64
2	74/20	74/69
3	75/80	46/55
4	105/25	83/64
5	104/54	80/37

Sensitivity in detecting pulses can be influenced by the wavelength of the photons used for photoplethysmography, with evidence that the use of green light can improve sensitivity (4). In the presence of a good metatarsal pressure, a surgeon should feel relatively confident about obtaining primary wound healing with amputation of the involved digit. The technique is also useful in detecting microembolization from an aneurysm or atheromatous plaque: Doppler segmental limb pressure may be normal down to the ankle, but the photoplethysmograph shows decreased metatarsal pressure caused by microembolization (Table 10-1).

Impedance Plethysmography

The technique of arterial impedance plethysmography is concerned with the detection of blood volume change in the limb. A constant high-frequency current is formed between two circumferential electrodes positioned on the limb (Fig. 10-4); resultant voltages are measured between two inner electrodes, and impedance waveforms are generated (Fig. 10-5). The impedance changes are due to segmental volume fluctuation. The shape of the waveform depends on a number of physiologic factors, such as the magnitude of ventricular contraction, blood vessel and limb tissue elasticity, and proximal and distal resistance. In a normal subject, the imped-

ance waveform is characterized by a steep systolic rise, a narrow peak, and a dicrotic of occlusive disease distal to the measured segment; there is a prolongation of the waveform acceleration and deceleration and a rounded peak. Proximal to an obstruction, the acceleration may be relatively normal; the peak, however, will be rounded and the deceleration portion of the curve prolonged.

ASSESSMENT OF THE MICROCIRCULATION

Increased attention is being paid to evaluating the microcirculation for assessments of tissue viability and wound healing potential. Four techniques that have generated considerable interest are transcutaneous oximetry, photon reflectance oximetry, cutaneous fluorometry, and cutaneous pressure photoplethysmography.

Transcutaneous Oximetry

The measurement of oxygen partial pressure transcutaneously ($TcPO_2$), originally devised for use in pediatric intensive care, has been used primarily in assessing the optimal level of amputation. Details of the technique are available else-

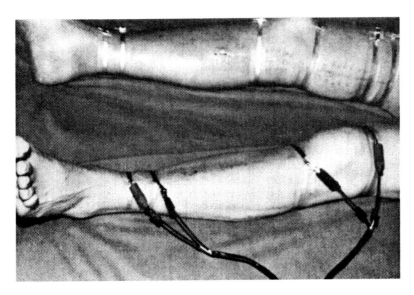

FIGURE 10-4 Electrode placement for impedance plethysmography.

where (5,6). Basically, a suitable current is applied between two polarographic electrodes composed of a platinum cathode and a silver anode immersed in an electrolyte and sealed by a semipermeable membrane. The current that results from the electrochemical reduction of oxygen in the electrolyte is proportional to the partial pressure of oxygen. Heating in the electrode creates conditions of hyperemia by local heating to temperatures between 43°C and 45°C. The heat produced also alters the structure of the skin and enhances the skin's permeability to gases (7). These factors produce a $TcPO_2$ value that approximates the partial pressure of oxygen in arterial blood. A number of additional factors influence the measurement of $TcPo_2$ reading: blood perfusion, skin metabolism, the structure of the microcirculation, the consumption of oxygen by the electrode, the response time of the electrode, the tissue temperature profile, and the physiologic effects of hyperthermia.

In normal adult skin, $TcPo_2$ measurements are subject to considerable variation; at a level of 10 cm below the knee, $TcPo_2$ measurements have been reported to vary from 40 mmHg (8) to 100 mmHg (9). In elderly subjects, a normal $TcPo_2$ below the knee is about 60, $\pm$ 10 mmHg, and should be about 10 mm Hg higher above the knee and about 10 mmHg lower at the foot; in

young subjects, normal $TcPo_2$ is about 5 mmHg to 15 mmHg higher than seen in elderly subjects (10).

In patients with vascular disease, a significant gradient in $TcPo_2$ is seen as one measures distally on the leg, similar to the gradient seen in segmental Doppler systolic blood pressure measurements. The presence of mild ischemia may produce a $TcPo_2$ gradient similar to that seen in normal individuals, but in the presence of severe ischemia, an above-knee-to-foot $TcPo_2$ gradient of greater than 30 mmHg has been reported (2). The reduced $TcPo_2$ in ischemic limbs results primarily from the reduced arterial blood pressure and not a reduction in tissue $TcPo_2$ (10).

The transcutaneous measurement of oxygen partial pressure is simple and convenient, and, in contrast to segmental Doppler systolic blood pressure measurements, the measurement is not influenced by the calcification of arteries seen in diabetic patients (11,12).

Photon Reflectance Oximetry

Measurement of the oxygen deficiency deep within the limb is possible with photon reflectance methods (13,14). These methods utilize the physics of photon transport through biological tissue in the visible and near-infrared wavelengths. Two methods have been applied

Peripheral Impedance

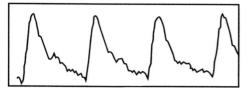

Acceleration = 3.61 Ohm/sec
Accel Time = 136 Msec
Deceleration = 2.04 Ohm/sec
Decel Time = 181 Msec
Peak Height = 307.3 Mohms

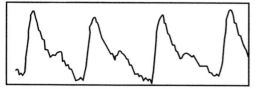

Acceleration = 1.94 Ohm/sec
Accel Time = 136 Msec
Deceleration = 0.94 Ohm/sec
Decel Time = 209 Msec
Peak Height = 171.2 Mohms

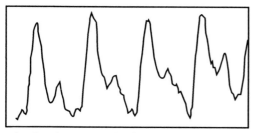

Acceleration = 0.68 Ohm/sec
Accel Time = 158 Msec
Deceleration = 0.502 Ohm/sec
Decel Time = 185 Msec
Peak Height = 69.2 Mohms

FIGURE 10-5 Impedance plethysmographic waveforms.

clinically to photon reflectance measurements. In the first, which is time-resolved, photons are injected at the surface; those photons that take the longest time to return to a nearby measurement location are more likely to have reached deeper tissue layers. Measurement of these photons leads to information about oxygen in the deeper tissue layers. In the space-resolved approach, photons that exit at greater distance from the injection point are more likely to have reached deeper tissue layers. Although photon attenuation increases with depth in both meth-

ods, photons are measurable that may have traveled to a depth approaching 1.5 cm beneath the surface of the skin. Data from normals and subjects with intermittent claudication (IC) can be monitored before, during, and after exercise. Differences in reflectance between normals and IC are generally consistent with expected physiologic differences.

Cutaneous Fluorometry

Cutaneous fluorometry has been shown useful in predicting the viability of skin flaps (15) and assessing ischemia (16). Administered intravenously, fluorescein is delivered to all perfused areas and diffuses into the extracellular fluid. When illuminated with ultraviolet light or blue light, adequately perfused areas fluoresce yellow-green. Originally judged qualitatively, the advent of quantitative measurements with a fluorometer has enhanced the usefulness of the technique. The device transmits blue light to excite the fluorescein and monitors the fluorescence from the fluorescein-stained tissue via a fiberoptic light guide. The instrumentation provides a quantitative measurement both of dye uptake and elimination by the perfused areas. Serial documentation is possible by subtracting residual fluorescence existing from a previous injection. The distribution of fluorescein dye correlates highly with gradations of skin perfusion and, ultimately, skin viability (17).

Perfusion is determined by analysis on the basis of the kinetics of dye wash-in and wash-out from body tissues. Wash-in provides a more rapid measurement of perfusion, provided that the readings are compensated for skin color. This is done by normalizing all fluorometric readings with those readings before dye infusion. Although the wash-out method provides absolute perfusion data unaffected by color, measurements are obtained more slowly, and the results can be distorted by poor kidney function.

The quantitative wash-in measurement, expressed in dye fluorescence units, is commonly reported as a percentage of the value obtained from a well-perfused region. In normal persons, a mean dye fluorescence index of about 77 is obtained. There is a trend toward increasing index values as one proceeds distally from above the knee to the toes (18). This gradient, however, has not been found to be significant. Discriminant analysis has established a dye fluorescence index of 40 for predicting skin viability; indexes greater than 42 accurately predict viability, and indexes less than 38 accurately predict failure of an amputation to heal.

The use of fluorescein is relatively safe. Slow administration of a relatively low concentration dilute dose in resting patients is associated with fewer side effects than seen following a more rapid injection, a larger dose, or both (18).

Cutaneous Pressure Photoplethysmography

An additional technique that has recently been used is cutaneous pressure photoplethysmography (19,20), which is based on localized perfusion pressure in cutaneous tissue. The instrumentation incorporates both pressure and photoplethysmographic monitoring devices within a hand-held probe. An infrared light source in the probe illuminates the surface of the skin, and light reflected back to the probe is modulated by changes in the volume of blood within the illuminated region. With increasing pressure, a level is reached at which pulsations cease. As pressure is reduced, the pressure at which pulsation returns is taken as the cutaneous perfusion pressure. It has been established that patients with cutaneous photoplethysmography pressures over 50 mmHg at the dorsum of the foot achieve primary healing of their amputations (20). In one study, this test was able to predict skin healing in patients after amputation for peripheral vascular disease, whereas other tests—including Doppler pressures—were not predictive (21).

PERIPHERAL VENOUS DISEASE

The spinal cord injured patient is at particularly high risk of developing venous thrombosis of the lower extremity. Loss of movement in the lower extremity produces venous stasis because calf muscle movement no longer pumps venous blood proximally. Undetected and untreated, venous thrombosis can precipitate pulmonary emboli, an event associated with a high mortality rate.

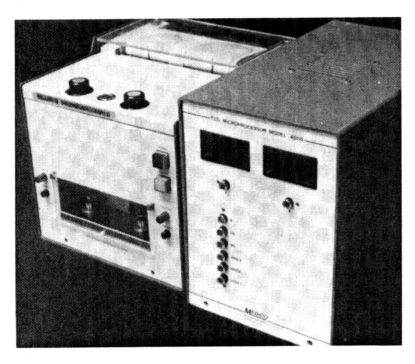

FIGURE 10-6 The thromboelastigraph for measuring blood coagulation dynamics.

Coagulation Dynamics

The role of blood coagulation is an important factor in peripheral vascular disease. Hypercoagulability, particularly when associated with the venous stasis characteristic of the spinal cord injured patient, is a major causative factor in the development of deep venous thrombosis. Monitoring coagulation dynamics is a necessity. The technique of *thromboelastography* provides a measurement of dynamic changes in the viscosity and elastic properties of a blood clot. The *thromboelastogram* provides a permanent graphic documentation of the various phases of the coagulation process.

Two types of instrumentation are available. In both, a piston is lowered into the patient's blood, which has been placed in a rotating cuvette (Fig. 10-6). Initially, the blood is liquid and does not move the piston. The piston begins to rotate with the cuvette as the first fibrin strands begin to form. In the mechanical-optical system, the moving piston deflects a light source directed at light-sensitive film that begins to show a divergence of the original straight line into two curved lines corresponding to the oscillation of the cuvette. In the direct-writing system, the oscillations of the cuvette are transferred to a stylus that prints the thromboelastogram on heat-sensitive paper.

In the *native whole blood thromboelastogram* (Fig. 10-7), the first value obtained is the *r* time, or reaction time, in minutes (30 sec = 1 mm).

This is the initial straight line of the tracing and represents the time from the initial drawing of the blood to the formation of the first fibrin strands. A normal *r* time is 8 to 12 minutes (16 to 24 mm). Alterations of production of plasma thromboplastin constituents or clotting factors XII, XI, IX, and VIII (first-stage factors of the intrinsic pathway) affect the *r* time. A shortened *r* time indicates hypercoagulability that can be associated with thrombosis, postoperative trauma, shock, or first-stage disseminated intravascular coagulation. A prolonged *r* time can be associated with an inherited defect in thromboplastin production such as hemophilia, or an acquired defect, such as those seen during anticoagulation therapy.

The second value is the *k* value, which is the time from the initiation of the clot (the end of the *r* time) to a predefined level of clot strength, the point at which the diverging curved lines are 20 mm apart. The *k* value is a measure of the rapidity of clot development; a normal value is 4 to 8 minutes. The *k* value is responsive for measuring intrinsic plasma and platelet factors and is nonresponsive to prothrombin complex factors; it is prolonged in association with coagulation defects such as intrinsic factor deficiency, circulating anticoagulants, thrombocytopenia, and qualitative platelet defects; and is shortened in association with hypercoagulability.

The maximum amplitude, *ma*, which is the maximum distance between the two diverging

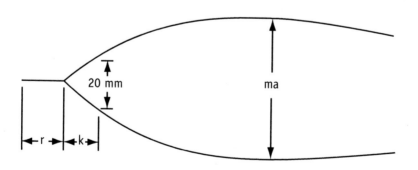

r = reaction time (8–12 minutes)
k = coagulation time (4–8 minutes)
ma = maximum amplitude (50 mm)

FIGURE 10-7 The native whole blood thromboelastogram.

lines, is a direct function of the maximum dynamic properties of fibrin and platelets; it is representative of the stiffness or strength of the clot. A normal *ma* value is approximately 50 mm. The maximum amplitude is affected by the dynamic properties of fibrin calcium, fibrin stabilizing factor, and platelet formation. A decreased *ma* is associated with thrombocytopenia, dextran therapy, anticoagulation therapy, qualitative platelet defects, and decreased fibrinogen levels. An increased *ma* is seen in hypercoagulability.

In *celite-activated thromboelastography*, the patient's blood is "activated" with celite, a chemical additive. Celite-activated thromboelastography (Fig. 10-8) involves a comparison between two simultaneous tracings: one normal and one celite-activated sample. The first two measurements obtained are the *R* and *RC* values, expressed in millimeters as the distance from the first mark to a point where the diverging lines are 2 mm apart. *RK* and *RKC* values are a combination of the *r* and *k* values of native whole blood thromboelastography. *Ma* and *MaC* are identical to the maximum amplitude of the native whole blood thromboelastography. The

angle, a parameter unique to the celite-activated technique, is indicative of the rate of clot stiffening and reflects the rate and quality of developing fibrin and platelet aggregates. The measurements obtained from celite activated thromboelastography are analyzed using the following equation:

$$Y = A_1 + A_2 + R + A_3RK \pm A_4Ma$$
$$+ A_5A + A_6RC + A_7RKC$$
$$-t- A_8MaC + A_9AC$$

where:

$A_1 = -55.55$ $A_4 = -0.03816$ $A_7 = +1.966$
$A_2 = +0.386$ $A_5 = -0.1639$ $A_8 = +0.17321$
$A_3 = -0.508$ $A_6 = +2.088$ $A_9 = +0.877$

A *Y* value between -5 and $+1.5$ is normal; greater than $+2$ is indicative of hypercoagulability, and less than -5 is indicative of hypocoagulability. In native whole blood thromboelastography, hypercoagulability is characterized by a shortened *r* time and *k* value and an increased *ma*. This is indicative of a rapidly forming clot that develops a high degree of stiffness.

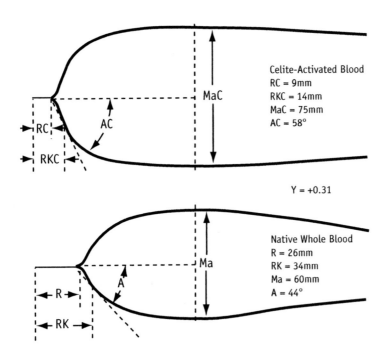

Celite-Activated Blood
RC = 9mm
RKC = 14mm
MaC = 75mm
AC = 58°

Y = +0.31

Native Whole Blood
R = 26mm
RK = 34mm
Ma = 60mm
A = 44°

FIGURE 10-8 The comparison of simultaneous tracings for celite-activated thromboelastography.

Hypocoagulability is characterized by a prolonged r time and k value and a decreased ma, indicative of a slow-forming clot that attains a low degree of stiffness. Such a tracing would be obtained during heparin therapy.

Impedence Plesthysmography

This noninvasive test measures the changes in the electrical conductivity of the leg caused by obstruction of venous outflow. The technique noninvasively quantitates venous capacitance and venous outflow. From the impedance plethysmogram (Fig. 10-9), one can measure the increase in venous volume following inflation of a pneumatic cuff placed around the lower thigh. The maximum venous outflow is measured as the decrease in volume during the first three seconds following release of the occluding cuff. Alternatively, the venous capacitance can be calculated and used with the maximum venous outflow to score the patient's venous hemodynamics (Fig. 10-9). The mathematical relationships for impedance plethysmography are (22):

where:

$$Z_0 = \frac{\rho L}{A} = \frac{\rho L^2}{V}$$

$$\Delta Z_0 = \frac{-\rho L^2}{V^2} \Delta V$$

Z_0 = baseline impedance (ohms)
ΔZ_0 = change in impedance with V
ΔV = change in volume (cc)
ρ = resistivity of limb (150 ohm cm)
L = distance between measuring electrodes (cm)
A = cross-sectional area of limb (cm^2)
V = A • L (cc)

Dividing the above equation for ΔZ_0 by that for Z_0 and by the time interval ΔT, yields the change in blood volume per unit time and per unit volume of tissue:

$$\frac{\Delta V / \Delta T}{V} = \frac{-\Delta Z_0 / Z_0}{\Delta T} \; ml/sec/cc$$

Multiplying by 6000 converts to the conventional reflux units of ml/min/100 cc tissue. If the initial test results are abnormal or equivocal, the test should be repeated three times in succession, with the best result of the tests being used for interpretation. This test will not detect the presence of hemodynamically insignificant thrombi or small isolated calf thrombi. The presence of extensive collateral formation or recanalization of a long-standing clot may lead to a false-negative result.

Impedance plethysmography can also be used to differentiate primary from secondary varicose

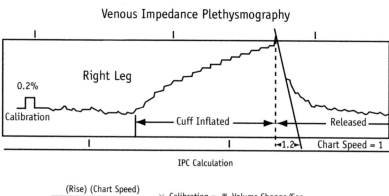

FIGURE 10-9 Tracings and calculations for venous impedance plethysmography.

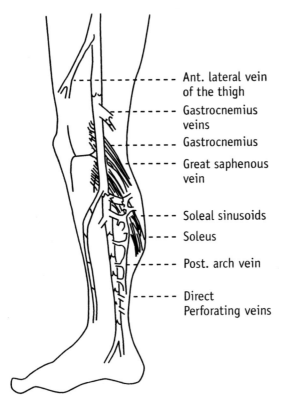

Ant. lateral vein of the thigh

Gastrocnemius veins

Gastrocnemius

Great saphenous vein

Soleal sinusoids

Soleus

Post. arch vein

Direct Perforating veins

FIGURE 10-10   The venous system has two separate reservoirs, one within the calf muscle and the other within the subcutaneous tissue.

veins and quantitate venous reflux. We can consider the venous system as two separate venous reservoirs, one within the calf muscle and the other within the subcutaneous (Fig. 10-10). These reservoirs communicate through numerous perforating veins, including the long and short saphenous veins. The saphenous veins, however, are unique in that they empty directly into the major deep veins with no direct communication with the veins within the calf muscle pump. The out-flow tract of the calf muscle is the popliteal vein.

Contraction of the calf muscle normally forces blood only into the popliteal/femoral vein. Upon relaxation, the pressure is higher and blood is forced into the deep system through communicating veins.

In the case of valvular incompetency of the long saphenous vein, there is retrograde blood flow during exercise, although the valves in the

communicating veins and the pump outflow tract within the calf muscles are normal. The calf pump can compensate for the superficial reservoir with only a minor degree of insufficiency. Clinically, this is reflected as varicose veins, mild aching pain in the legs, and slight edema of the ankle.

In the case of incompetent valves in the communicating veins, blood is forced directly into the superficial veins during muscle contraction. Thus, the pressure in the superficial veins does not fall during exercise, and the symptoms are more serious: ankle edema, skin pigmentation, eczema, and sometimes ulceration of the skin overlying the incompetent communicating veins.

With stenosis or valvular incompetence in the outflow tract, the calf pump is unable to empty during calf muscle contraction. The high pressure generated within the pump causes dilation of the communicating veins and secondary valvular incompetence. If there is obstruction in the outflow tract, pressures may rise during exercise, producing severe symptoms: constant aching pain, venous claudication, skin pigmentation, eczema, lipodermatosclerosis, ulceration, and, in rare cases, fibrous ankylosis of the ankle joint.

To differentiate primary from secondary varicose veins, the patient's legs are placed in a dependent position with impedance electrodes attached to the calf; a pneumatic boot is placed over the calf, inflated to 60 mmHg, allowed to stabilize, and then rapidly released. The test is repeated with a tourniquet placed above the knee to occlude the superficial venous system. The initial test done, without the tourniquet, provides a measure of total venous reflux; the second, with the tourniquet in place, provides a measure of deep venous reflux. By subtracting the deep venous reflux value from total venous reflux, one obtains a measure of the superficial venous reflux. Normal venous reflux refilling time is less than 20.0 ml/min/100 cc. A patient's varicosities are designated as primary if application of the tourniquet reduces the reflux to within normal range (less than 20 ml/min/100 cc) and designated as secondary if the reflux value is abnormal (greater than 20 ml/min/100 cc) both with and without the tourniquet.

Phleborheography

This technique is based on the fact that rhythmic respiration causes variations in venous pressure and volume, and that such variations can be recorded from the lower extremity. Air-filled cuffs are placed around the thorax and at several levels of the lower extremity to apply compression and record transmitted impulses. An absence of significant reduction in the waveform size indicates the presence of an acute episode of deep vein thrombosis. In the presence of a long-standing thrombus, the waveforms are present but are typically smaller and have a rounded peak as opposed to normal. Distal compression gives momentary pooling of the blood in the presence of deep venous thrombosis. By examination of the baseline for recordings taken at different levels, the location of a thrombus can be identified. In normal persons, calf compression causes a fall in the baseline. The technique is highly sensitive for detecting proximal vein thrombosis.

Radioactive Fibrinogen Uptake

This technique is perhaps the most sensitive test for the detection of a developing thrombus or one that is extending or lysing. Briefly, radio-labeled fibrin is injected into a peripheral vein and then incorporated into the developing thrombosis. The radioactive fibrin thus incorporated into the developing clot can be detected noninvasively. After administration, the first screening is done at 2 hours to allow for the removal of any denatured fibrinogen and for equilibrium between intravascular and extravascular fibrinogen. The screening can then be done every 24 hours. Radioactivity counts from the lower extremities are expressed as a percentage of the radioactivity count obtained over the heart. The percentage should remain relatively constant because radioactivity should be washed out of the heart and lower extremities at the same rate. Realistically, however, there is a slight increase that should not exceed 2 percent per day as a result of the greater rates of extravascular fibrinogen in the leg than in the heart. Deep venous thrombosis is determined to be present if there is a 20 percent or more increase in radioactivity at the same position on two different days.

This technique is not specific for the presence of deep venous thrombosis. Increased radioactivity counts are also seen in the presence of superficial thrombophlebitis, hematoma, ulceration, arthritis, cellulitis, or fractures and wounds. The technique does not detect the presence of thrombus in the groin or pelvic areas because of the high background radioactivity of the bladder.

Doppler Ultrasonography

This technique monitors the velocity of blood flow in the veins. A spontaneous signal should be obtained from all patent deep veins of the leg. The technique's accuracy depends heavily on the skill and experience of the technician. The velocity patterns of the lower extremity's veins reflect the periodic changes in intra-abdominal pressure caused by breathing. Velocity flow signals that vary with breathing and are interrupted by a deep breath indicate vein patency proximal to the probe. When the flow is unchanged by a deep inspiration, the vein proximal to the probe is obstructed. Deep venous occlusion can cause the flow velocity signal in the superficial veins to be greatly increased compared with the contralateral limb.

In the normal, patent vein, compression of the extremity distal to the probe produces an increased velocity signal. An increased flow signal is seen with release of the compression. With placement of the Doppler probe over the popliteal vein, compression proximal to the probe causes blood flow toward the probe if the venous valves are incompetent. With the probe positioned over the posterior tibial vein during compression of the calf muscles, a back-and-forth flow velocity signal is seen with compression and release in the presence of incompetent venous valves. Flow reversal in the femoral vein can be detected during quiet respiration when the patient is tilted head-up; with the probe over the saphenous vein, back-and-forth reflux sounds can be detected in the presence of incompetent valves by running the finger distally over the course of the vein.

Tissue Mechanical Pressure Measurement

Vascular diseases can produce characteristic changes in the mechanical condition of the limb. These changes can be seen by measuring the bulk viscoelastic properties of the limb. A platform of large surface area rests lightly on the surface of the skin and serves as a reference for tissue displacement. A centrally located indenter is used to apply pressure, and both pressure and displacement are recorded directly above a limb compartment. The observed pressure–volume displacement relationship shows both elastic and viscous components. The increase in compartmental pressure becomes higher, and the bulk limb tissue becomes more nearly pure elastic. The use of matched sites provides controls by which to account for differences among subjects in fat content and muscle tone.

The pressure–volume displacement curves show a hysteresis (i.e. a phase difference), which is characteristic of energy storage. In a study of 18 limbs with pitting edema, the degree of hysteresis was significantly greater than in normals. The conclusion is that mechanical indentation of the limb provides diagnostic information about fluid accumulation in tissue in the presence of pitting edema, as well as in the presence of the *compartment syndrome.*

In the compartment syndrome, swelling within a limb due to hemorrhage, edema, or other pathology of soft tissue is constrained within an anatomic space whose walls consist of fascia. The ischemia resulting from the pressure creates a progressive cycle of swelling, further ischemia, and tissue damage. Diagnosis and monitoring of pressures in the compartment is frequently done by insertion of a Wick or Stryker catheter directly into the compartment, because clinical signs are unreliable in predicting catastrophic tissue damage.

Compartment syndrome is encountered in traumatic injuries of the limbs and in surgical treatment of large-vessel disease utilizing vascular grafts (i.e., *revascularization compartment syndrome*). It can also be induced by strenuous training in young adults. Permanent neuromuscular damage and possible loss of a limb can occur when diagnosis and treatment are delayed. Surgical fasciotomy is a treatment that requires accurate diagnosis because the treatment poses risks of infection and healing problems. Direct pressure measurements are invasive and add to patient risk and discomfort. The noninvasive approach to monitoring compartment syndrome provides a possible alternative in monitoring and tracking pressure changes.

REFERENCES

1. Rutherford RB. *Vascular Surgery*, 2nd ed. Philadelphia: W.B. Saunders, 1984.
2. Greenhalgh RM. *Diagnostic Techniques and Assessment Procedures in Vascular Surgery.* Orlando, Florida: Grune & Stratton, 1985.
3. Bernstein EF. Noninvasive *Diagnostic Techniques in Vascular Disease.* St. Louis: C.V. Mosby, 1985.
4. Ostrander LE, Cui W, Lee BY. The clinical use of green light photoplethysmography. *Surgical Forum*, American College of Surgeons 1989; 40:520–522.
5. Hebrank DR. Noninvasive transcutaneous oxygen monitoring, a review. *J Clin Eng* 1981; 6:41.
6. Rooke TW. The use of transcutaneous oximetry in the noninvasive vascular laboratory. *Int Angiol* 1992; 11:36–40.
7. Spence VA, McCollum PT. Evaluation of the ischemic limb by transcutaneous oximetry. In McGreenhalgh RM, ed., *Diagnostic Techniques and Assessment Procedures in Vascular Surgery.* Orlando, Florida: Grune & Stratton, 1985. Pp. 331–341.
8. Franyeck UK, Talke P, Bernstein EF, et al. Transcutaneous PO_2 measurements in health and peripheral arterial occlusive disease. *Surgery* 19892; 91:156–163.
9. Mustapha NM, Redhead RG, Jam SK, et al. Transcutaneous partial oxygen pressure assessment of the ischemic lower limb. *Surg Gynecol Obstet* 1983; 156:582–584.
10. Eickoff JH, Engell HC. Transcutaneous oxygen tension ($TcPO_2$) measurements on the foot in normal subjects and in patients with peripheral

vascular disease admitted for vascular surgery. *Scand J Clin Lab Invest* 1981; 41:743–748.

11. Wyss CR, Masten FS, Simmins CW, Burgess EM. Transcutaneous oxygen tension measurements on limbs of diabetic and nondiabetic patients with peripheral vascular disease. *Surgery* 1984; 95:339–346.

12. Karanfiliam RG, Lynch TG, Zirul VT, et al. The value of laser Doppler velocimetry and transcutaneous oxygen tension determination in predicting healing of ischemic forefoot ulcerations and amputations in diabetic and nondiabetic patients. *J Vasc Surg* 1986, 4:511–516.

13. Kooijman HM, Hopman MT, et al. Near infrared spectroscopy for noninvasive assessment of claudication. *J Surg Res* 1997; 72:1–7.

14. Lee BY, Ostrander LE, et al. Noninvasive quantification of muscle oxygen in subjects with and without claudication. *J Rehabil Res Dev* 1997; 34:44–51.

15. McCraw JD, Meyers B, Shanklin KD. The value of fluorescein in predicting the viability of arterialized flaps. *Plast Reconstr Surg* 1977; 60:710–719.

16. Lowry K. Evaluation of peripheral vascular disease using intraarterial fluorescein. *Am Surg* 30:35–39.

17. Silverman DG, Noran KJ, Brousseau DA. Serial fluorometric documentation of flourescein dye delivery. *Surgery* 1985; 97:185–192.

18. Silverman DG, Roberts A, Reilly CA, et al. Fluorometric quantification of low-dose fluorescein delivery to predict amputation site healing. *Surgery* 1987; 101:335–341.

19. Lee BY, Thoden WR, Madden JL, McCann WJ. Cutaneous pressure photoplethysmography: a new technique for noninvasive evaluation of peripheral arterial disease. *Cont Surg* 1984; 25:39–43.

20. Lee BY, Ostrander L, Thoden WR, Madden JL. Use of cutaneous pressure plethysmography in managing peripheral vascular occlusive disease. *Cont Surg* 1987; 30:58–67.

21. van den Broek, TA, Dewars, BJ, et al. A multivariate analysis of determinants of wound healing in patients after amputation for peripheral vascular disease. *Eur J Vasc Surg* 1990; 4:291–295.

22. Webster JG. Measurement of flow and volume of blood. In *Medical Instrumentation*. Boston: Houghton-Mifflin, 1978. Pp. 421.

11 Deep Venous Thrombosis in Spinal Cord Injured Patients

BOK Y. LEE, MD
MARCELO C. DASILVA, MD
LEE E. OSTRANDER, PhD

DEEP VENOUS THROMBOSIS (DVT) and pulmonary embolism (PE) are major health problems and result in significant mortality and morbidity. In the United States, it is estimated that DVT and PE are associated with 300,000 to 600,000 hospitalizations yearly and up to 50,000 deaths each year (1). The spinal cord injured patient is at particularly high risk for the development of DVT (2–6). In these patients, the loss of the active calf muscle pump in the paralyzed limbs significantly reduces blood flow. The blood volume is unsteady; the vascular tone is abnormal and directly dependent upon local and regional stimulation and the capacity of the vascular system to adjust to such conditions as muscular exercise; and thermoregulation is lost (7). The consequent sluggishness of venous return is further exacerbated by the hypercoagulability associated with spinal cord injury (3). When coupled with the pressure exerted by the bed on the calf muscles, this sluggishness puts the bedridden spinal cord injured patient at high risk for the development of DVT.

Reports on the incidence of DVT in the spinal cord injured patient during the first few weeks following injury vary widely. Similar variance is seen with the incidence of PE. Just as reports in the literature differ as to the incidence of DVT from the particular institutions, the incidence also varies among patients at any one study site. Watson found an 81 percent incidence of DVT in 431 spinal cord injured patients with complete lesions versus 8 percent in patients with incomplete lesions (5). Similarly, patients with dorsal lesions had a 23 percent incidence of DVT compared with 12 percent in patients with cervical lesions. Watson also found that the onset of DVT was 1 month following the injury to the spinal cord in a large majority of patients (72 percent). The incidence of DVT dropped off precipitously after 1 month to 12 percent at 2 months after injury, and 14 percent at 3 months after injury. More importantly, PE occurred at the same time as the deep vein thrombosis (i.e., the PE occurred without warning) in 45 percent of patients. At 1, 2, 4, and 8 weeks after diagnosis of the deep vein thrombosis, the incidence of PE was 14, 18, 14, and 9 percent, respectively. A significant reduction in mortality from PE has not been seen in spite of available therapy. It is readily apparent that the best treatment of PE is prophylaxis prevention of DVT (1).

PATHOGENESIS OF DEEP VENOUS THROMBOSIS

Three factors contribute to the development of DVT: venous stasis, hypercoagulability, and vessel injury, and in the case of bedridden spinal cord patients, one may add pressure on the calf muscles (Fig. 11-1).

Venous Stasis

Normal blood flow through a vessel has a physiologic antithrombotic effect by: 1 diluting locally activated clotting factors; 2 renewing circulating natural inhibitors of the clotting mechanisms; and 3 limiting red blood cell aggregation, thus maintaining normal blood viscosity (9). In the presence of venous stasis, both volume and velocity of flow are decreased. Although the precise mechanism of the formation of a thrombus due to venous stasis is uncertain, it is clear that once thrombus formation is initiated, the thrombus develops rapidly, grows, and may extend into the lumen of the vessel, promoting further stasis.

Immobility is the most common precipitating factor in the development of venous thrombosis.

In patients undergoing surgery, clearance time for leg veins is shown to be significantly slower in anesthetized patients than in awake patients (10). The parallel to spinal cord injured patients is obvious. In the lower extremities, the deep veins are embedded in the thick calf muscles, which are surrounded by the strong crural fascia. This arrangement enables the calf to function as a pump during contraction of the calf muscles. The contraction of the calf muscles compresses the veins, emptying them proximally into larger veins. Thus, repetitive contraction results in an emptying of the deep veins. The absence of the calf muscle pump activity in an immobile patient promotes the development of venous stasis, platelet aggregation, and activation of the coagulation system.

Hypercoagulability

The concept of hypercoagulability is not well understood (8). In patients undergoing surgery, postoperative changes in platelets, coagulation cascade proteins, and fibrinolytic activity have been identified as factors that may lead to thrombosis (11). Similar changes have also been noticed in nonsurgical patients with thrombosis, but a cause-and-effect relationship has not been established (9). Functionally, hypercoagulability can be divided into two categories: *tissue injury* and *impaired defense mechanism* (8). Tissue injury initiates thrombosis by activating the coagulation cascade. Impaired tissue defense facilitates thrombosis. This includes deficiency of AT-III, protein C and S, anticardiolipin antibody, and lupus antibodies and factor V Leiden, as well as the presence of defective plasminogen or a low fibrinolytic response; estrogen; and impaired blood flow (8).

Vessel Injury

The endothelium of the blood vessels is important to preventing thrombus formation because it contains several antithrombotic substances, such as tissue plasminogen activator, prostacyclin, and a number of glycosaminoglycans (9).

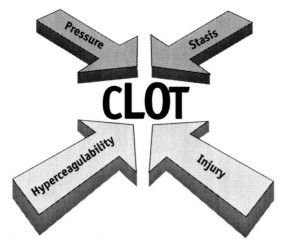

FIGURE 11-1   Pathogenesis of DVT.

TABLE 11-1 Guidelines for the Prevention of Thromboembolism in Spinal Cord Injury. Clinical Decision.

Level of Risk	Motor Incomplete	Motor Complete	Motor Complete With Other Risk*
Intensity Prophylaxis			
Low	Compression hose Compression boots +	Compression hose Compression boots +	Compression hose Compression boots +
Intermediate	UH+: 5000 U q 12 h to high normal aPTT++;or LMWH+++: 30mg bid ±	UH+: Dose adjusted to high nPTT++; or LMWH+: 30mg bid	UH+:Dose adjusted
High	–	–	IVC filter
Duration of Prophylaxis			
	Compression boots: 2 weeks; Anticoagulants: while in hospital for ASIA class D and up to 8 weeks for ASIA class C	Compression boots: 2 weeks; Anticoagulants: at least 8 weeks discharge from rehabilitation	Compression boots: 2 weeks; Anticoagulants: 12 weeks or until

*Poor pulmonary reserve, obesity
Adapted from Consortium for Spinal Cord Medicine. Clinical Practice Guidelines: Prevention of Thromboembolism in Spinal Cord Injury. *Spinal Cord Medicine*, February 1997. Pp. 1–20.

Damage to the endothelium resulting in the exposure of the subendothelium provides stimulus for thrombus formation as platelets adhere, aggregate, and release the contents of their secretory granules—leading to thrombin formation, local activation of coagulation factors, and clot formation (12).

Prevention of Deep Venous Thrombosis

A number of methods are available for the prevention of DVT, including adjusted-dose heparin, low-dose heparin, warfarin, dextran, external pneumatic compression, and pressure-gradient elastic stockings. The National Institute of Health Consensus Development Conference on the Prevention of Venous Thrombosis and Pulmonary Embolism, however, reported that external pneumatic compression and pressure gradient elastic stockings are "the methods of choice" for prophylaxis in patients with head injury and acute spinal cord injury (1). External pneumatic compression is recommended over stockings, however, because pressure-gradient stockings have not been adequately studied and "must be carefully fitted if they are to have prophylactic merit" (1). Indeed, external pneumatic compression is recommended for use in most high-risk patient groups.

Our own work using external pneumatic compression (13–16) shows it to be most effective in preventing postoperative DVT in surgical patients as well as the recognized high-risk group of patients undergoing hip replacement or hip fracture repair (16).

In September 1994, the Paralyzed Veterans of America (PVA) developed guidelines for prevention of thromboembolism in the spinal cord injured patient (22). The primary goals of these guidelines were to:

1. Provide a rationale for implementation of thromboprophylaxis
2. Make available to health care providers current knowledge and expert consensus regarding safe and effective prophylaxis measures

3. Encourage providers to re-examine their practice patterns and to individualize treatment based on patient characteristics
4. Stimulate future research regarding thromboprophylaxis for spinal cord injury
5. Improve outcomes for patients with spinal cord injury by decreasing the frequency thromboembolism and its complication.

The clinical practice guidelines made recommendations regarding mechanical methods of prophylaxis of thromboembolism based on patients' level of risk (Table 11-1). Compression hose or pneumatic devices should be applied to the legs of all patients for the first 2 weeks following injury. Compression devices should be inspected for proper placement and underlying skin injuries with every nursing shift. Insertion of a vena cava filter is indicated in SCI patients who failed anticoagulant prophylaxis or who have a contraindication to anticoagulation, such as active or potential bleeding not amenable to local control. Filter placement should also be considered in SCI patients with complete motor paralysis due to a high cervical cord injury (C2, C3), patients with poor cardiopulmonary reserve (COPD), or in those with documented thrombus in the inferior vena cava despite anticoagulant prophylaxis.

The guidelines recommend that prophylaxis with either low molecular weight heparin or adjusted-dose unfractionated heparin should be initiated within 72 hours after SCI, except in cases of active bleeding, evidence of head injury, or coagulopathy. Anticoagulants should be continued until hospital discharge in patients with incomplete injuries and for 8 weeks in patients with uncomplicated complete motor injury. Patients with complete motor injury and other risk factors (e.g., lower extremity fractures, history of thrombosis, cancer, heart failure, obesity, age over 70) should receive anticoagulation therapy for 12 weeks or until discharge from rehabilitation.

Protocol for Use of External Pneumatic Compression

Before the use of external pneumatic compression, the patient is screened using venous impedance plethysmography to determine the patency of the venous system. The recording of a positive impedance plethysmogram, indicating the possible presence of pre-existing thrombosis, is a contraindication to the use of the system. Resolution of the pre-existing thrombosis is required before using external pneumatic com-

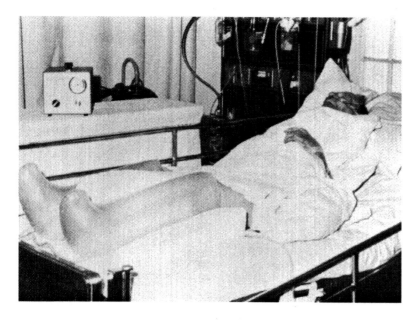

FIGURE 11-2 The external pneumatic compression system in use. The system is fitted to the patient by a technician, who ensures the proper functioning of the system.

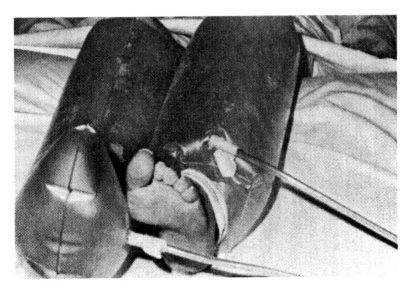

FIGURE 11-3 The external pneumatic compression system consists of an easily portable pneumatic compressor and paired, double-walled inflatable plastic boots or sleeves.

pression. The external pneumatic compression system is fitted to the patient (Fig. 11-2) by a technician, who ensures the proper functioning of the system. During continuous use, the nursing staff can remove the system for routine skin care. If the system is discontinued for more than 30 minutes, an impedance plethysmography should be obtained before the system is replaced.

Operation of the System. The external pneumatic compression system is completely noninvasive and designed to reduce the risk of DVT by simulating calf muscle contraction. The system (Fig. 11-3) consists of a portable pneumatic compressor and paired, double-walled inflatable plastic boots or sleeves. The system's pneumatic compressor provides a rhythmic cycle of inflation and deflation that yields an intermittent compression of the calf muscle. While the system is inflated, the patient's leg floats comfortably on an evenly distributed cushion of air. The controls of the system's pneumatic compressor consist of a single on/off switch and a dial to control the inflation pressure. During operation, there is a standard 12 sec compression and 48 sec decompression cycle. An inflation pressure of 40 to 45 mmHg is found to produce sufficient emptying of the calf veins. The system operates with any air source of 35 to 136 psi. The effectiveness

of the system is caused by both mechanical and biological effects.

Mechanical Effect of External Pneumatic Compression. We have shown external intermittent pneumatic compression to cause a pulsatile component to venous blood flow in mimicking calf muscle contraction (13). In studies on canines and primates, intraoperative electromagnetic flow meter studies have shown pulsatile flow in the canine femoral vein (Fig. 11-4A) and in primate inferior vena cava (Fig. 11-4B) that coincides with the 12 sec compression phase of the cycle. Similar results have been recorded in humans (Fig. 11-4C). During a major abdominal surgical procedure, an electromagnetic flow probe placed around the inferior vena cava (with the external pneumatic compression system on the lower extremities) recorded a pulsatile component in the venous flow with little or no net increase in the mean venous return.

Biochemical Effect of External Pneumatic Compression. A study by Hill et al. (17) found that the protection against DVT produced by external pneumatic compression was not apparent in patients with malignancies. This suggests that other factors contribute to the system's prophylactic effect. A subsequent study by Allenby et al. (18) found an increase in fibrinolytic activity to be associated with the use of external

Canine Study—Augmentation of Venous Flow during Boot Inflation

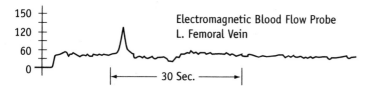

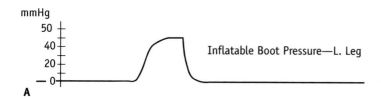

A

Primate Study—Augmentation of Venous Flow during Boot Inflation

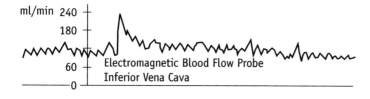

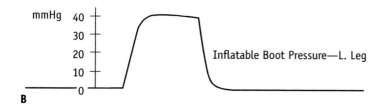

B

Augmentation of Venous Flow during Surgical Boot Inflation

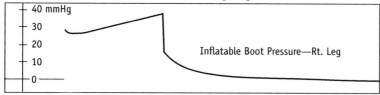

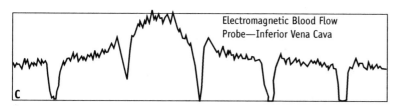

C

FIGURE 11-4 Experimental studies in the canine (A), primate (B), and human (C) using intraoperative electromagnetic flowmetry show external pneumatic compression to impart a pulsatile component to venous blood flow.

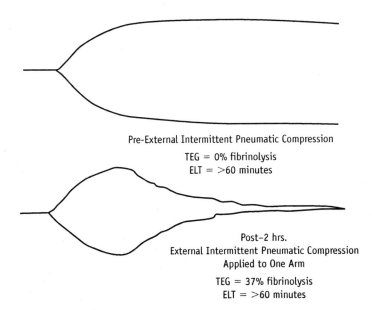

Pre-External Intermittent Pneumatic Compression
TEG = 0% fibrinolysis
ELT = >60 minutes

Post-2 hrs.
External Intermittent Pneumatic Compression
Applied to One Arm
TEG = 37% fibrinolysis
ELT = >60 minutes

FIGURE 11-5 Studies using thrombo-elastography show external pneumatic compression to enhance the naturally occurring fibrinolytic activity of the venous system.

pneumatic compression. Using thromboelastography (Fig. 11-5), we have quantitatively demonstrated enhanced fibrinolytic activity with external pneumatic compression (19). In 50 patients who had external pneumatic compression applied to one arm for 2 hours, 62 percent showed a quantitative increase in fibrinolytic activity ranging from 8 to 116 percent (mean ± s.d. = 245 ± 286 percent). It is possible that external pneumatic compression, by means of its producing a transient period of venous occlusion and/or simulating calf muscle exercises, causes a release of plasminogen activators into the blood stream (18–19).

REFERENCES

1. Consensus Conference: prevention of venous thrombosis and pulmonary embolism. *JAMA* 1986; 256:744–749.
2. Perkash A, Prakash V, Perkash I. Experience with the management of thromboembolism in patients with spinal cord injury: Part I. Incidence, diagnosis, and role of some risk factors. *Paraplegia* 1978; 16(3):322–31.
3. Todd JW, Frisbie JH, Rossier AB, Adams DF, Als AV, Armenia RJ, Sasahara AA, Tow DE. Deep venous thrombosis in acute spinal cord injury: a comparison of 125I fibrinogen leg scanning, impedance plethysmography, and *venography*. Paraplegia 1976; 14(1):50–57.
4. Van Hove E. Prevention of thrombophlebitis in spinal injury patients. *Paraplegia* 1978; 16(3): 332–335.
5. Watson N. Venous thrombosis and pulmonary embolism in spinal cord injury. *Paraplegia* 1978–1979; 16:113–121.
6. Watson N. Anti-coagulant therapy in the prevention of venous thrombosis and pulmonary embolism in the spinal cord injury. *Paraplegia* 1978; 16(3):265–269.
7. Bidart Y, Maury M. The circulatory behaviour in complete chronic paraplegia. *Paraplegia* 1973; 11(1):1–24.
8. Wessler S. Prevention of venous thromboembolism: rationale, practice, and problems. Prevention of Thromboembolism and Pulmonary Embolism, National Institute of Health Consensus Development Conference, March 24–26, 1986. Pp. 15–18.
9. Peterson CW. Venous thrombosis: an overview. *Pharmacotherapy* 1986; 6 (4 Pt 2): S12–17.
10. Lewis CE Jr., Mueller C, Edwards WS. Venous stasis on the operating table. *Am J Surg* 1972; 124(6):780–784.
11. Bergquist D. *Postoperative Thromboembolism: Frequency, Etiology, Prophylaxis.* New York: Springer-Verlag, 1983. Pp. 35–50.
12. Baumgartner HR, Muggli R, Tschopp TB, Turitto VT. Platelet adhesion, release and aggregation in flowing blood: effects of surface properties and platelet function. *Thromb Haemost* 1976; 35(1):124–138.
13. Lee BY, Madden JL, Trainor FS, Kavner D, Dratz HM, Ejercito E. Detection and prevention

Deep Venous Thrombosis in Spinal Cord Injured Patients | **147**

of deep vein thrombosis in the general surgical patient. In Madden JL, Hume M, ed., *Venous Thromboembolism*. New York: Appleton-Century-Crofts, 1976. Pp. 61–90.

14. Lee BY, Thoden WR, Trainor FS, Kavner D. Noninvasive evaluation of peripheral arterial disease in the geriatric patient. *J Am Geriatr Soc* 1980; 28(8):352–360.

15. Lee BY, Trainor FS, Kavner D, Madden JL, Dratz HM, Ejercito EM. Noninvasive prevention of thrombosis of deep veins of the thigh using intermittent pneumatic compression. *Surg Gyn Obstet* 1976; 142(5):705–714.

16. Lee BY, Sarabu MR, Thoden WR, et al. Intermittent pneumatic compression in the prevention of deep vein thrombis is following hip replacement of fracture. *Contemp Orthoped* 1980; 1:585–588.

17. Hills NH, Pflug JJ, Jeyasingh K, Boardman L, Calnan JS. Prevention of deep vein thrombosis by intermittent pneumatic compression of calf. *Br Med J* 1972; 1(793):131–135.

18. Allenby F, Boardman L, Pflug JJ, Calnan JS. Effects of external pneumatic intermittent compression on fibrinolysis in man. *Lancet* 1973; 2(7843):1412–1414.

19. Lee BY, Thoden WR, Sarabu MR. Fibrinolytic activity of intermittent pneumatic compression. *Contemp Surg* 1981; 18:77–79, 82, 86.

20. Gore RM, Mintzer RA, Calenoff L. Gastrointestinal complications of spinal cord injury. *Spine* 1981; 6(6):538–544.

21. Miller LS, Staas WE Jr., Herbison GJ. Abdominal problems in patients with spinal cord lesions. *Arch Phys Med Rehabil* 1975; 56(9): 405–408.

22. Consortium for Spinal Cord Medicine. Clinical Practice Guidelines: Prevention of Thromboembolism in Spinal Cord Injury. *Spinal Cord Medicine*, February 1997. Pp. 1–20.

12 Acute Abdomen in Spinal Cord Injured Patients

BOK Y. LEE, MD
MARCELO C. DASILVA, MD
LEE E. OSTRANDER, PhD
WILLIAM BOND, MD

A GREAT CHALLENGE EXISTS in the diagnosis of an acute abdomen in spinal cord injured (SCI) patients. Typical findings of an acute intra-abdominal process may be missing or misleading. Because of delayed diagnosis and misdiagnosis, the mortality rate is 10 to 15 percent in these patients (1).Diagnosis and management is based on an understanding of the level of spinal cord injury and whether this is complete (no movement or sensation below the level of injury) or incomplete. Recently, diagnostic laparoscopy, a minimally invasive procedure to help in the diagnosis of peritonitis, has been introduced. By way of example, we present 20 cases from our last 25 years of experience of abdominal surgery in SCI patients.

The presentation of SCI patients suffering from acute intra-abdominal disease is different from that of patients with an intact neuroaxis. SCI patients represent a substantial patient population, with an estimated 200,000 paraplegics in the U.S. in 1989. This number is compounded by approximately 50 cases per 1 million population per year. Acute abdomen in SCI patients carries mortality rates reported from 5 to 15 percent. In our series, the mortality rate is 4 per-cent, representing one death in 25 cases. The classic signs and symptoms of acute abdomen in SCI patients are significantly different from those in non-SCI patients, delaying the diagnosis by 1 to 4 days.

In a recent review of 1,300 patients with SCI over a period of 14 years, 12 (< 1 percent) patients presented with an acute abdomen. Seven (0.5 percent) events occurred during the initial admission, ranging from 10 days to 9 months from injury, and five (0.3 percent) occurred during the readmission of "chronic" SCI patients. Four were in the acute stage 10 to 30 days from injury. All patients in this study presented with peptic ulcer perforations. The remainder of patients had intestinal obstruction, appendicitis, or peritonitis. Therefore, the diagnosis of acute abdomen in SCI patients requires the use of multiple, time-consuming, and expensive diagnostic studies.

LEVEL OF INJURY

There are three major levels of injury to the spinal cord. Within these regions there may be variations of somatic and autonomic innervations.

Completeness of the injury may mean that typical findings are absent or modified; incomplete lesions usually produce a response more likely to lead to localization and a timely diagnosis.

Lesions below T11 and T12 spare the splanchnic outflow tract, with the abdominal wall skin and musculature innervations usually left intact. In such patients, the presentation of abdominal disease is the same as in patients with an intact spinal cord (2). Lesions of the lower thoracic cord from T10 to T12 interrupt somatic sensation below the level of injury. Visceral sensations, however, may enter the posterior root and travel several levels above this cord injury, using the sympathetic chain, or they may travel an accessory vagal pathway. Usually, innervations of the abdominal wall, bladder, and distal colon undergo extensive alteration. High cord lesions above T5 block both the splanchnic outflow tract and impulses involving the abdominal wall muscles and skin.

SIGNS AND SYMPTOMS

In the initial injury period, spinal shock causes an absence of reflexive activity below the cord lesion. There may be a paucity of signs and symptoms. Flaccid paralysis of the abdominal wall muscles may completely mask peritonitis, and shock is often the initial presentation of a perforated or gangrenous lesion (1). A high index of suspicion must be maintained during the period of spinal shock to avoid the high mortality associated with a delay in diagnosis.

After the period of spinal shock, reflexive arcs are reestablished below the level of injury. A number of signs and symptoms must be borne in mind, especially for high cord lesions above T5. Anorexia, nausea, and a vague feeling of being unwell are early clues of possible abdominal involvement. The patient feels "restless" (1,2). Abdominal pain is described as dull and not localized. This is believed to be caused by slow conduction velocities of unmyelinated class C fibers of distal-to-injury reflex area. In contrast, pain associated with radiculopathy is described as sharp, burning, and often bilateral, with pin-

prick hypersensitivity. Referred pain may be based on innervations that share a common embryologic origin. The diaphragm can refer pain to the neck and shoulder (Fig. 12-1), the stomach to the intrascapular area, the spleen to the shoulder, the appendix to the umbilicus, the kidney to the testes, the ureter to the inner thigh, and the bladder to the perineum (8).

Abdominal distention with dilated loops of bowel is common in spinal cord injured patients. Unless there is progression or other signs and symptoms, distention alone may not be of great significance. Increased spasticity of the abdominal wall muscle may make palpation of the abdomen difficult or impossible. Although tenderness is usually absent, it may herald a perforated bladder of viscus or other emergency event. Abdominal masses, when palpable, may be due to chronic constipation. Even neurogenic bowel dysfunction can cause problems involving distention and discomfort that mimic an acute abdomen. Diarrhea

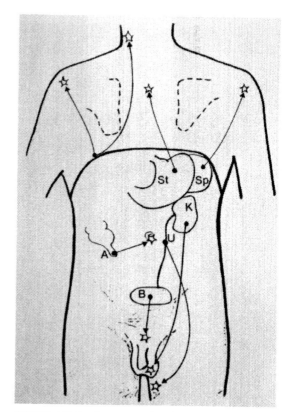

FIGURE 12-1 Patterns of referred pain from the diaphragm.

and urinary incontinence may be reflexive activities of an abdominal process, via reflexive arcs to the bladder and distal colon. Reflexive activity causes a rise in pulse, respiration rate, and blood pressure. These alone are frequently seen in the stabilized spinal cord injured patient without surgical pathology. Autonomic hyperreflexia is mostly associated with abdominal emergencies in patients with high cord lesions above the splanchnic outflow tract (1). Bladder, bowel, and peritoneal reflexive arcs cause transient hypertension with or without bradycardia. Patients usually complain of a severe headache. Although a nonsurgical cause, such as distended bladder, is more common, this can be an important clue if other symptoms and signs are present.

Fever may simply be a response to ambient conditions, such as a thermostat-controlled airbed. A high, spiking fever above 39°C usually indicates a genitourinary infection, although lower ranges of fever may be associated with abdominal events (5,6). "Quadriplegic fever" almost always has a definite cause (1,5).

Initial laboratory studies of the spinal cord injured patient with a possible acute abdomen usually include CBC with differential, serum chemistries, and urine studies. These are most helpful if baseline studies are available. Chest radiographs, flat plate of the abdomen, and intravenous pyelogram (IVP) have also proved quite useful as part of the initial work-up, allowing differentiation among abdominal, genitourinary, or supradiaphragmatic pathology (3,7). Cleansing of the bowel using cathartics or enemas is not needed before initial IVP studies. Chronic constipation and impaction makes evaluation difficult and sometimes dangerous.

ILLUSTRATIVE CASES

Case 1

This 30-year-old male incomplete quadriplegic at the C6 level presented with a one-day history of nausea. Bowel sounds were hyperactive, the abdomen was distended, and a dull pain was localized to the right lower quadrant. Vital signs included pulse rate of 90 bpm, temperature of 99.4°F, and blood pressure of 124/84 mmHg (the patient's usual blood pressure was 105/70 mmHg). An ilioconduit procedure had been performed several years earlier. That night, the patient vomited his supper and complained of a very severe headache. Digital disimpaction was unproductive for stool. A flat plate radiograph of the abdomen was ordered and showed a small bowel obstruction. An emergency exploratory laparotomy with lysis of adhesions was performed. The postoperative course was unremarkable.

Case 2

This 54-year-old male complete paraplegic at the level of T8 presented with flaccid paralysis in the lower extremities. During the night, his temperature spiked to 104°F, and he complained of back pain radiating to the right lower inguinal area. On physical examination, the left flank was tender to percussion. The white blood count was 31,000 per/cm³, urinalysis found more than 100,000 organism of *Proteus*, and radiographs revealed left ureteral renal calculi. Retrograde studies confirmed left ureteral obstruction. An emergency ureterolithotomy was performed. The postoperative course was uncomplicated. ·

Case 3

This 52-year-old male complete paraplegic at the level of T7 had been followed for several months for ischemic colitis. He suffered from loose bowel movements, abdominal pain, and rectal bleeding. Although a diversionary transverse colostomy was performed, it did not solve these problems. Follow-up barium enema studies showed a persistent "thumbprint" pattern in the left colon. A left hemicolectomy was performed with an uneventful recovery.

Case 4

This 53-year-old man had incomplete paraplegia at the level of L2 with severe peripheral vascular disease. Primarily, he had a left above-knee

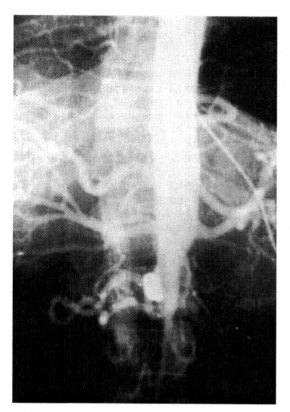

FIGURE 12-2 Aortogram demonstrating occlusion of the distal aorta with a meandering artery.

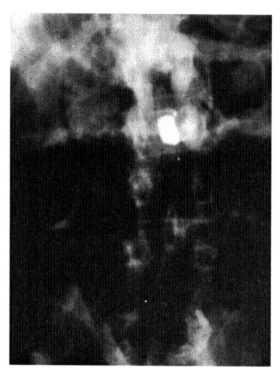

FIGURE 12-3 The left colon is not visualized.

amputation for gangrene, axillofemoral bypass, and right above-knee amputation. An aortogram at the time demonstrated occlusion of the distal aorta with a meandering artery (Fig. 12-2). Two nights postoperatively, his temperature rose to 102 °F with a pulse of 120 bpm. He complained of diffuse abdominal pain without localization; bowel sounds were hyperactive; there was no nausea, vomiting, or diarrhea. Plain abdominal radiographs showed dilated loops of small bowel. The left colon was not visualized (Fig. 12-3). Laboratory studies were significant for a mild elevation in creatinine kinase (CK). The white blood count was 6100/cm³, with an unremarkable differential. The urinalysis showed an acute infection. On the third postoperative night, he became hypothermic to 96.6°F and hypotensive with blood pressure down to 90/40 mmHg from his usual 150/90 mmHg. The pulse was 80 bpm and described as irregular.

Initial treatment consisted of nasogastric suction and intravenous fluid replacement. Differential diagnosis included postoperative ileus, small or large bowel obstruction, or mesenteric vascular thrombosis. With decreasing return of gastric secretions, a trial clamping of the gastric tube was done. Air appeared in the left colon on radiograph by this time. The patient tolerated this well and the tube was removed. Two days later, his abdomen was again distended and even tympanitic. Gastric suction was reinstated.

Although a barium enema was attempted, it was unsuccessful as a result of fecal impaction. Colonoscopy was performed; large amounts of stool were visualized but no obstruction was seen. Flatus reappeared after this. The abdominal pain resolved and enemas finally yielded positive results. Several days later the gastric suction was discontinued. A regular diet was tolerated thereafter, and his usual bowel care was resumed. At this time, gallbladder series and upper GI series were obtained with normal findings.

Case 5

This 66-year-old male incomplete paraplegic at the level of T10 was admitted for surgical reconstruction of a right ischial pressure sore. A superiorly based gluteus maximus myocutaneous flap was used to close the defect under general anesthesia. On the second postoperative night, the patient's temperature rose to 103.4°F. Panculture (blood, urine, sputum, and wound cultures) identified *Proteus* in the urine, and the same species was found in preoperative cultures. Rapid defervescence came about with selected postoperative antibiotic treatment. By the third postoperative day, the patient complained of general malaise. The fourth postoperative day saw the onset of mild, left lower quadrant pain. For the next three days, the patient's abdomen became progressively distended with hyperactive bowel sounds. However, there was never guarding or rebound or episodes of nausea and vomiting. Concurrent with this was postoperative atelectasis. Although breath sounds were diminished, the lungs sounded clear. A chest radiograph on the sixth postoperative day revealed pleural effusion requiring thoracentesis. The effusions did not recur, and with intense respiratory therapy the patient's postoperative atelectasis quickly improved.

Laboratory studies during this time showed a white blood count between 9.8 and 9.6 thousand per/cm^3. Repeated sputum and blood cultures were negative. Vital signs were consistent with preoperative baseline values, except for mild tachypnea and fever. Bowel care and enema were given on the seventh postoperative day in the face of the progressive abdominal distention. This produced evacuation of large amounts of stool with abdominal decompression.

DISCUSSION

A total of 20 spinal cord injured patients were reviewed for this study. Acute cholecystitis occurred most commonly, followed by perforated viscus and bowel obstruction (Table 12-1).

Cholecystitis has been reported without any signs and symptoms (1,2,5). Because of this, cholelithiasis in the spinal cord injured patient is an indication for cholecystectomy in these patients. If the procedure is uncomplicated, an incidental appendectomy should be carried out. All of our four patients presented with abdominal pain. For three patients, this was a chronic problem of several months' duration. The diagnosis of cholecystitis was made when gallbladder study was included as part of the radiological examination of the gastrointestinal tract. The fourth patient presented with right upper quadrant pain of sudden onset. He was a T8 complete paraplegic whose abdominal wall spasm made the physical examination difficult. However, rebound tenderness was present over the gallbladder. An abdominal ultrasonographic examination showed gallstones; the patient underwent open cholecystectomy.

Abdominal adhesions are the most common cause of small bowel obstruction in patients with previous abdominal surgery. This is also true for spinal cord injured patients. This population usually has several abdominal procedures, such as those for diversion of urine and stool. This was the presentation of Case 1. The severe headache most likely represented an autonomic dysreflexia crisis secondary to intestinal obstruction. A prompt work-up indicated the need for exploratory laparotomy and lysis of adhesions. The other patient with small bowel obstruction in our series also underwent a lysis of adhesions;

TABLE 12-1 Acute Abdominal Procedures in Spinal Cord Injured Patients: A 25-Year Experience

Lesions	No. of Patients
Acute cholecystitis	4
Perforated viscus	3
Bowel obstruction	2
Lower GI bleeding	2
Bowel volvulus	1
Abdominal aortic aneurysm	1
Pyelonephritis	1
Ureterolithiasis	2
Ischemic colitis	1
Dolichocolon	2
Metastatic carcinoid tumor	1
Total	20

diverting colostomy and ilioconduit had been performed previously to aid in healing severe decubitus ulcers. No hernias were seen in this series. Elective repair is indicated to avoid the risk of overlooked strangulation.

Appendicitis did not occur on our series. However, Charney et al. reported five cases of acute appendicitis. All patients had perforations with abscess formation and high cord injuries. Delay in diagnosis in this series ranged from 3 days to 3 weeks (1). Dollfus et al. reported one abscess (5000 ml) from a perforated appendix. A high index of suspicion helped arrive at early intervention in four other cases (8). The one appendectomy performed in our series was done incidentally in the course of an exploratory laparotomy. This patient had severe abdominal pain and rectal bleeding, necessitating multiple transfusions. Although barium enema and upper GI series suggested regional enteritis, no significant pathology was found at time of surgery. The patient, a T10 incomplete paraplegic, recovered uneventfully.

Urologic surgical case presentations, as represented by Case 2, were consistent with those in the literature previously cited. All these patients had high spiking fevers, suggesting genitourinary pathology. Intravenous pyelograms demonstrated ureteral calculi. Lithotomies were performed in two cases. In the third case, perinephric and periureteral abscesses were found in addition to a ureteral stone, requiring additional drainage.

Bowel obstruction in the spinal cord injured patient is frequently due to fecal impaction. The signs and symptoms of abdominal distention warrant a surgical consultation. Colon pathology in this series ranged from ischemic colitis (Case 3) to sigmoid volvulus, perforated diverticulum, and dolichocolon. Surgical management in these cases was straightforward after the pathology was defined and documented. More frequently, feces may obstruct the colon. Case 4 illustrates an extensive work-up that stopped just short of exploratory laparotomy.

In the postoperative period of myocutaneous flap reconstruction, it is desirable to put the bowel at rest. This is done through diet and enemas preoperatively, then diet and an anticathartic regimen postoperatively. Because of this, some abdominal distention is usually seen after surgery. The patient in Case 5 presented with a rapid onset of abdominal distention in such a postoperative period. Also, this patient had previous abdominal exploration, putting him at risk of adhesions.

The management of fecal impaction in such a postoperative period is further complicated by the fact that the patient is on airbed. Colonoscopy and radiologic studies are usually not bedside procedures. Transferring the patient out of the airbed places the flap at risk for dehiscence, infection, and pressure necrosis.

In Case 5, a high spiking fever provided the clue to a urologic source. An entire genitourinary work-up in the month before the patient's admission, including cystoscopy and intravenous pyelogram, had demonstrated normal upper and lower tracts. Urinalysis with culture identified the urinary tract infection. This was treated with appropriate antibiotics.

With colonoscopic decompression of the colon, bowel function returned and the patient's condition improved. In contrast, another 23-year-old C7 quadriplegic, still in spinal shock 3 weeks after his initial injury, presented with distention but with no other signs or symptoms. Abdominal radiograph showed free air. At emergency laparotomy, the stomach was perforated. An omental patch was used to close the defect, and the patient recovered uneventfully.

Another quadriplegic was admitted in septic shock with abdominal distention. Rapid work-up showed a bowel obstruction. At laparotomy, an internal hernia and anterior cecal wall perforation were found and repaired with reduction and cecostomy. He died 3 weeks postoperatively of septic complications.

Another consultation for abdominal pain and distention demonstrated a pulsatile abdominal mass. A lumbar arteriogram demonstrated a leaking abdominal aortic aneurysm (Fig. 12-4). The specimen shows the leak in the posterior wall (Fig. 12-5). This was resected uneventfully (Fig. 12-6).

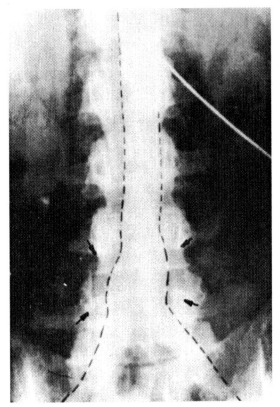

FIGURE 12-4 Lumbar arteriogram demonstrates a pulsatile abdominal mass.

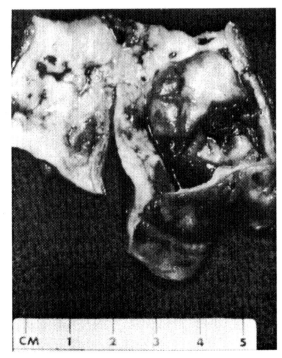

FIGURE 12-5 Leak in posterior wall.

When the diagnosis of acute abdomen is entertained through physical examination and history, it normally requires the use of multiple, time-consuming, and expensive diagnostic studies (9). The diagnosis of gangrenous cholecystitis, perforated viscus (appendix), pancreatic or intraperitoneal abscess, diverticulitis, cholangitis, strangulated bowel, uncontrolled bleeding and peritonitis, or sickle cell crisis may not be so straightforward in SCI. A complete blood work (CBC) with differential may be helpful, but it also may be elevated in stress states or depressed such as in immunocompromised (HIV) patients or in patients undergoing immunossuppresion. Serum amylase and liver function tests may also be elevated because of other conditions, such as transient bowel or liver ischemia caused by a low flow state. Therefore, in SCI patients, laboratory tests can be misleading, and radiological studies, such as CT-scans, and contrast studies may

be helpful. Abdominal ultrasonography, in the decision-making process of evaluating an acute abdomen, provides a definite diagnosis in 25 percent of the cases, hemorrhage of unknown origin (44 percent) or septicemia from an undetected focus (39 percent) (10).

Diagnostic and therapeutic laparoscopy has a low mortality and low morbidity, and provides a correct diagnosis in 93 to 100 percent of the cases (11,12). We described the use of a 2mm laparoscope in six patients with signs and symptoms of acute abdomen in the critical care setting. The 2mm laparoscopy revealed one patient with acute diverticulitis and one patient with ruptured ovarian cyst, two patients had negative laparoscopy. Two patients with acute appendicitis underwent laparoscopic appendectomy with the 2mm laparoscope.

CONCLUSION

A total of 20 cases of acute abdomen in spinal cord injured patients seen over the past 25 years are presented. One patient admitted in septic

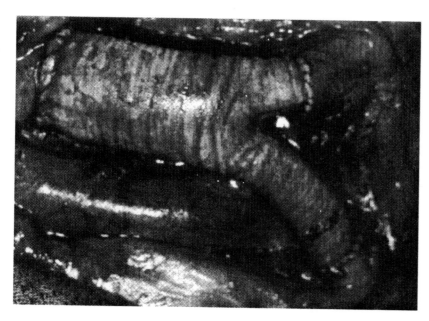

FIGURE 12-6 Resection of leak in the posterior wall.

shock died postoperatively of multisystem organ dysfunction syndrome (MODS). The mortality rate of 5 percent is consistent with other reported rates of 10 to 15 percent. Types of surgery included biliary, aorta, gastric, colonic, genitourinary, and lysis of adhesions. In the stabilized spinal cord injured patient, delay in surgery is to be avoided. Early clues of fever, pain anorexia, and dysreflexia deserve work-up. Laboratory values are best interpreted against baselines. Genitourinary problems may not only mimic the acute abdomen but may also be coexistent with it (4).

It is clear that SCI patients suffering from acute intra-abdominal disease present a diagnostic challenge. Nevertheless, with the introduction of laparoscopy, it is now possible to diagnose these conditions in a timely and accurate manner, minimizing the morbidity and mortality rates, which are higher in this cohort of patients.

Finally, it is imperative to know the level of spinal cord injury and whether it is complete. Patients with incomplete lesions tolerate early exploratory laparotomy much better than they do a delayed diagnosis with catastrophic sequelae (1–8).

The question that most surgeons have to answer is whether the SCI patient with laboratory and radiographic evidence of acute abdomen requires abdominal exploration. Diagnostic and therapeutic laparoscopy has shown to have a low mortality and morbidity rate, providing a correct diagnosis in 93 to 100 percent of the cases. This procedure can help the surgeon to make the diagnosis of acute abdomen, and thus aid in critical management decisions. DaSilva et al. has described the use of the 2mm laparoscope in patients in a critical care setting with acute abdomen. The pathologies encountered in this population were as varied as those found in our SCI patients. The use of the 2 mm laparoscope in the critical care setting, for both diagnosis and therapy, is a pioneering effort that can easily be applied to diagnostic challenges presented to those assessing spinal cord injured patients in whom intraabdominal pathology is suspected. The presentation of the SCI patient suffering from acute intra-abdominal disease is different from that of the patient with an intact neuroaxis. The delay in diagnosis and treatment of the acute abdomen in these patients may have horrific outcomes. Awareness of the often subtle signs and symptoms manifested by SCI patients is essential for timely diagnosis. Those charged with the care of such patients must be vigilant in pursuing the source of any suggestive signs and symptoms, even in the presence of known "benign" urinary tract disease. The 2-mm laparoscope offers another safe and minimally invasive diagnostic and or therapeutic tool in the care of SCI patients.

REFERENCES

1. Charney KJ, Juler GL, Comarr AE. General surgery problems in patients with spinal cord injuries. *Arch Surg* 1975; 110(9):1083–1088.
2. Juler GL, Eltorai IM. The acute abdomen in spinal cord injury patients. *Paraplegia* 1985; 23(2):118–123.
3. Miller LS, Staas WE Jr, Herbison GJ. Abdominal problems in patients with spinal cord lesions. *Arch Phys Med Rehabil* 1975; 56(9):405–408.
4. O'Hare JM. The acute abdomen in spinal cord injury patients. Proceedings of the Annual Clinical Spinal Cord Injury Conference 1966. Pp. 113–117.
5. Sugarman B, Brown D, Musher D. Fever and infection in spinal cord injury patients. *JAMA* 1982; 248(1):66–70.
6. Greenfield J. Abdominal operations on patients with chronic paraplegia. *Arch Surg* 1949; 1077–1087.
7. Ingberg HO, Prust FW. The diagnosis of abdominal emergencies in patients with spinal cord lesions. *Arch Phys Med Rehabil* 1968; 49(6):343–348.
8. Dollfus P, Holderbach GL, Husser JM, Jacob-Chia D. Proceedings: must appendicitis be still considered as a rare complication in paraplegia? *Paraplegia* 1974; 11(4):306–309.
9. Geis WP, Kim HC. Use of laparoscopy in the diagnosis and treatment of patients with surgical abdominal sepsis. *Surg Endosc* 1995; 9 (2):178–182.
10. Lerch MM, Riehl J, Buechsel R, Kierdorf H, Winkeltau G, Matern S. Bedside ultrasound in decision making for emergency surgery: its role in medical intensive care patients. *Am J Emerg Med* 1992; 10(1):35–38.
11. Navez B, d'Udekem Y, Cambier E, Richir C, de Pierpont B, Guiot P. Laparoscopy for management of nontraumatic acute abdomen. *World J Surg* 1995; 19(3):382–386.
12. Connor TJ, Garcha IS, Ramshaw BJ, Mitchell CW, Wilson JP, Mason EM, Duncan TD, Dozier FA, Lucas GW. Diagnostic laparoscopy for suspected appendicitis. *Am Surg* 1995; 61(2):187–189.

13 Surgical Stabilization in Cervical Spine Trauma

DANIEL A. CAPEN, MD
ELLEN M. LEPPEK, BS, PA-C

THE CERVICAL SPINE FUNCTIONS as a mobile connection of the skull to the trunk. Motion in flexion, rotation, tilt, and extension permit positioning of sight, sound, and speech organs in multiple planes. The cervical region is, however, subjected to many high-energy forces when injured. Falls, sports injuries, and vehicular trauma comprise the majority of accidental causation. Civilian violence also represents an increasing percentage of total spine injury causation, although these injuries often penetrate without destabilizing the spine. The unstable cervical spine is a challenge to the surgeon with or without neurologic injury.

Traumatic instability of the cervical spine must be treated by reduction of deformity, decompression of neural elements, and maintenance of alignment during the healing of skeletal tissue (1). The goals of surgical stabilization include ability to participate in rehabilitation, an environment for optimal neural recovery, and restoration of as much spinal function without pain as possible. Surgical management has been shown by Ducker et al. to provide rigid immobilization and favorable clinical results (2). With emergency diagnosis there also has been documented improvement with high-dose methylprednisolone given within 8 hours of injury (3).

UPPER CERVICAL INJURY

Nonfatal injury to the occipital-cervical spine requires surgical treatment when ligament injury is present. The craniocervical junction provides an extremely wide range of motion through ligamentous connections of the atlas and axis. The facets are horizontal to facilitate rotation, and the odontoid process of C2 provides primary transitional stability. Injury to skeletal structures with no neural deficit may reach successful outcome by nonsurgical orthotic immobilization (see Chapter 9 on nonsurgical care). However, unstable ligament injury with or without neurologic injury frequently needs internal fixation and arthrodesis to stabilize the spine.

Classification systems, such as the Orthopedic Trauma Association spine trauma system (4) or the Allen Classification (5), help define cases in need of surgery. All systems emphasize surgical treatment to stabilize injury that is both acutely and chronically unstable. Most of these injuries involve primary injury through ligament and disc (Fig. 13-1). Some injuries, such as Type II odontoid fracture, result in devascularized bone, which acts to prevent fracture healing. Facet fracture-dislocation can also involve insufficient bone frag-

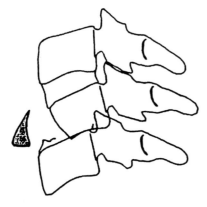

Compression fracture of vertebral body

Rupture of interspinous ligament

A   **Compressive Flexion Injury**

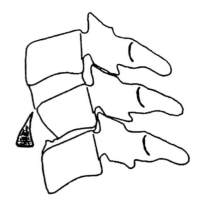
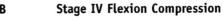

B   **Stage IV Flexion Compression**

C   **Stage V Flexion Compression**

FIGURE 13-1 As seen here, the compressive flexion group of injuries represents largely unstable injuries needing posterior treatment of ligaments and sometimes anterior decompression.

mentation to permit bone healing (Fig. 13-2). These injuries have better results with surgery. The outcome for the individual patient depends on accurate identification of spinal column instability and neurologic injury (Fig. 13-3). The authors utilize the Allen Classification of spinal instability and the American Spinal Injury Association (ASIA) (6) neurologic index for complete presurgical planning. We find this to be a key step to avoid unneeded surgery and inadequate stabilization surgery.

LOWER CERVICAL INJURY

The most frequently encountered instability is middle cervical injury (Fig. 13-4). High- or low-energy trauma destabilizes the spine and often

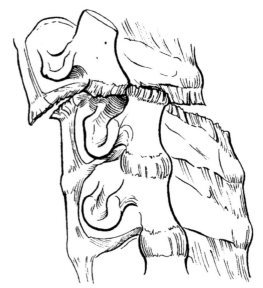

FIGURE 13-2 The facet and disc injury for distractive flexion groups also require posterior surgery.

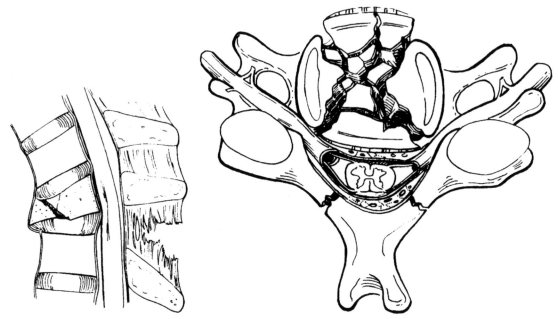

FIGURE 13-3 The use of skeletal and neurologic classification will guide appropriate care to stabilize and decompress for cord or root improvement.

creates partial or complete neural deficit (as described in Chapter 9, some midcervical injury patterns can be treated with halo or other immobilization, but most injuries in this region benefit from stabilization and/or decompression). The surgical approach demands an accurate and complete understanding of instability, neural injury, and overall patient condition. All but a very few cases are treated in the urgent or chronic setting. The indications for emergency surgery are indeed rare. The information provided by several animal studies suggests an inverse relationship between time of compression and recovery (7–9), but no well-controlled studies exist to mandate emergent decompression except in documented neruologic worsening or if the decompression can be done within 8 to 12 hours of injury (10).

Surgery after the first 24 hours to 48 hours but within 10 days may actually have increased systemic complication rates (11,12). Decompressive surgery performed emergently may benefit the recovery process, but always must be accompanied by adequate stabilization to preclude the requirement of a second surgery.

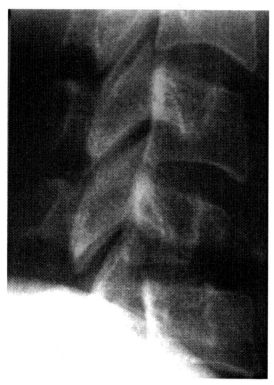

FIGURE 13-4 Radiograph of Cf 4 lesion with canal compromise and ligament injury.

POSTERIOR SURGICAL PROCEDURES

Upper cervical stabilization may be achieved by graft and immobilization or by graft and internal fixation. Occiput to C2 fixation can be done with various wire techniques (13,14), Luque rods (15,16) or sublaminar wires (17) (Figs. 13-5 and 13-6). Screw and plate fixation can fix without passage of wires into the canal, but proper placement of screws is essential to avoid arterial or root injury.

Atlantoaxial fixation by Gallie fusion, Brooks fusion, Halifax clamp, and the Magerl facet screw all stabilize the C1–C2 articulation. The passage of wire is demanding and potential complications can occur. Monitoring by local anesthesia is safest, although this requires a co-operative patient and team (18). Spinal cord monitoring under general anesthesia can also be effective to prevent cord injury.

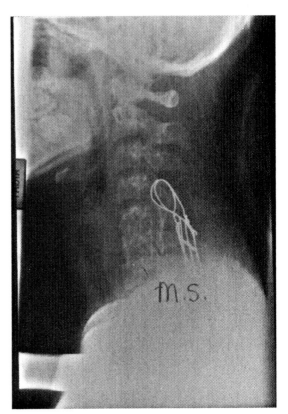

FIGURE 13-6 Posterior wire and fusion technique with modification of upper facet wire placement.

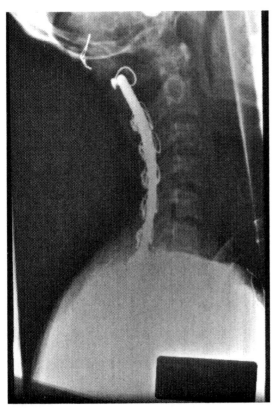

FIGURE 13-5 Luque wire stabilization. Note complete loss of cervical motion capability.

Wiring techniques with a high fusion rate can perform posterior stabilization of the middle cervical spine. Capen et al. (19) followed a large group of patients with Rogers wiring (Fig. 13-7) and nonunion was rare, but fusion extension was prevalent. Posterior plating as described by Anderson (20) is probably the most frequently performed stabilization procedure for limited cervical segment fusion. Fixation can be achieved even with laminar fracture without increasing immobilization. The screw placement is demanding and can injure exiting nerve roots, the vertebral artery, or the cord itself. Intra-articular screw placement results in poor fixation. In the good fixation group, fusion rate is above 90 percent.

Laminaplasty is a decompressive procedure for central cord trauma from extensive canal compromise from degenerative conditions. Fusion is rarely required. Laminectomy is rarely indicated

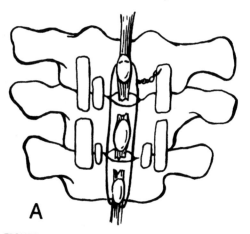
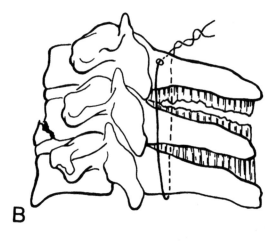

FIGURE 13-7   Classic Rogers wire technique with onlay graft.

and is fraught with extensive complication rates (21), including worsening of neural injury, inadequate decompression, and late deformity, as in (Fig. 13-7).

ANTERIOR CERVICAL PROCEDURES

The primary role of anterior surgery in the cervical spine is for decompression of the spinal canal. Bone and disc fragments are removed

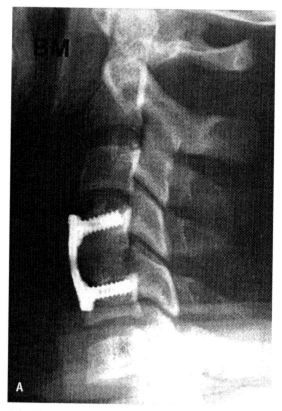
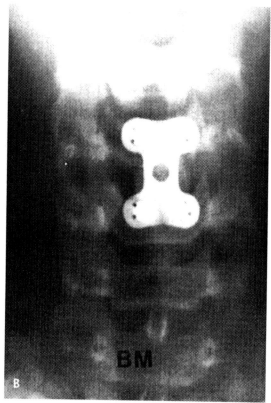

FIGURE 13-8   Anterior decompression, fusion, and plating for complete fixation.

through an anterior approach. Stabilization can be achieved by graft from the iliac crest with semirigid immobilization. Graft must be corticocancellous and fashion-fitted under tension.

The new development by several manufacturers of plating systems allows anterior decompression and fixation of spine segments with reduced post surgical bracing (Fig. 13-8). This permits the surgeon to decompress, fuse, and maintain alignment in most cervical instability patterns. Complications are infrequent and fusion rates are high (22). Most failures, as shown by Kostuick (23), are associated with improper patient selection or poor technique of application. In severe instability, both anterior and posterior stabilization are performed. The standard case from significant destabilizing trauma with severe cord injury often involves posterior stabilization as the initial procedure. After allowing a period of cord recovery the anterior decompression and fusion can take place, understanding that recovery can occur up to 2 years after injury with late decompression of the canal.

The use of anterior plates in the cervical spine can provide stability and a secure graft to prevent dislodgment. The anterior plate is extremely stable in rotation and extension and somewhat stable in flexion. As anterior fixation improves it may become the procedure of choice for all instability, provided reduction can be achieved.

Combined anterior and posterior arthrodesis may permit totally brace-free rehabilitation and can provide secure fixation in the most severe cases of traumatic instability. This can also be utilized in the more severe degenerative and tumor cases, where bone quality does not favor a single stabilization procedure.

CONCLUSION

Surgical intervention can enhance rehabilitation potential and compress rehabilitation time by permitting a brace-free program. Procedures are not without risk, and the total picture of skeletal diagnosis, neurologic diagnosis, and patient condition must be considered prior to performing surgery. If instability and neural compromise is

appropriately diagnosed, and treated, a successful outcome can be achieved.

The authors recommend:

1. Identify neurologic and skeletal injury
2. Plan treatment to optimize recovery
3. Never operate emergently without purpose, especially with laminectomy
4. Stabilize the area that is unstable; that is, anterior or posterior or both.

REFERENCES

1. Slucky AV, Eismont FJ. Treatment of acute injury of the cervical spine. *J Bone Joint Surg* 1994; 76A:1882.
2. Ducker TB. Salman M, Daniell HB: Experimental cord trauma, III: therapeutic effect of immobilization and pharmacologic agents. *Surg Neuro* 1978;10:71.
3. Bracken MB, Shephard MJ, Collins WF. A randomized controlled trial of methylprednisolone or naloxone in treatment of spinal cord injury. *N Engl J Med* 1990;322:1405.
4. Orthopedic Trauma Association. Comprehensive classification of fractures. *Supplement to J Orthop Trauma* 1995.
5. Allen BL, Ferguson RL , et al. A mechanistic classification of closed, indirect fractures and dislocations of the lower cervical spine. *Spine* 1982;7:1.
6. American Spinal Cord Injury Association. Standards for Neurological and Functional Classification of Spinal Cord Injury, Revised. Chicago. Illinois ASIA proceedings, 1992.
7. Bohlman HH. Acute fractures and dislocations of the cervical spine: an analysis of three hundred patients and review of the literature. *J Bone and Joint Surg* 1979;61A:1110.
8. Anderson PA, Bohlman HH. Anterior decompression and arthrodesis of the cervical spine improvement. *J Bone and Joint Surg* 1992;74A:683.
9. Bohlman HH, Anderson PA. Anterior decompression and arthrodesis of the cervical spine: long-term motor improvement. Part I: improvement in incomplete quadriparesis. *J Bone and Joint Surg* 1992;74a:683.
10. Marshall LF, et al. Deterioration following spinal cord injury: a multicenter study. *J Neurosurg* 1987; 66:400.
11. Levi L, et al. Anterior decompression in cervical spine trauma: does timing of surgery affect outcome? *Neurosurgery* 1991;29:216.

12. Schlegel J, et al. Timing of surgical decompression and fixation of acute spinal fractures. *J Orthop Trauma* 1996; 10:323.

13. Wertheim SB, Bohlman HH. Occipitocervical fusion: indications, techniques and long-term results in thirteen patients. *J Bone and Joint Surg* 1987; 69A:833.

14. Ransford AO, et al. Craniocervical instability treated by contoured loop fixation. *J Bone and Joint Surg* 1986; 68B:173.

15. Itoh T, et al. Occipitocervical fusion reinforced by Luque segmental spine instrumentation for rheumatoid diseases. *Spine* 1988; 13:1234.

16. Smith MD, Anderson PA, Grady MS. Occipitocervical arthrodesis using contoured plate fixation technique. *Spine* 1993; 18:1984.

17. Sasso RC, et al. Occipitocervical fusion with posterior plate and screw instrumentation: a long-term follow-up study. *Spine* 1994; 19:2364.

18. Zigler J, Rockowitz N, Capen D, Nelson R, Waters R. Posterior cervical fusion using local anesthesia: the awake patient as the ultimate spinal cord monitor. *Spine* 1987; 12:206-208.

19. Capen DA, Waters RL, Garland D. A comparative analysis of anterior and posterior cervical fusions. *Clin Ortho and Rel Res* 1985; 186:229.

20. Anderson PA, et al. Posterior cervical arthrodesis with AO reconstruction plates and bone graft. *Spine* 1991; 16 suppl: S72–79.

21. Capen DA, Nelson RW, Zigler JE. Decompressive laminectomy in cervical spine trauma: a review of early and late complications. *Contemporary Ortho* 1987; 17:21.

22. Garvey TA, Eismont FJ, Roberti LF. Anterior decompression, structural bone grafting, and Caspar plate stabilization for unstable spine fractures and dislocations. *Spine* 1992; 17:S431.

23. Kostuick JP, Connolly PJ, Esses SI. Anterior cervical plate fixation with titanium hollow screw plate system. *Spine* 1993; 18:1273.

14 Management of Neurogenic Dysfunction of the Bladder

INDER PERKASH, MD

NEUROANATOMY, NEUROPHYSIOLOGY, AND CRITICAL CONTROL MECHANISMS FOR CONTINENCE

THE SPINAL CORD CARRIES messages to and from the brain to accomplish voluntary control over micturition; injuries and diseases of the central nervous system therefore result in some loss of control over voiding. Bladder function also differs according to the level of lesion in the spinal cord. The micturition reflex center or detrusor reflex center has been localized in the pontine mesencephalic reticular formation in the brainstem. The center has interconnections to and from frontal lobes and other areas in the cortex and subcortical areas (1). The reticular spinal tracts are in close proximity to the pyramidal tracts in the lateral columns of the spinal cord. Efferent axons from the pontine micturition center connect to the detrusor motor nuclei located in the spinal 2, 3, and 4 segments, in the sacral gray matter of the spinal cord. Sacral 3 and 4 have major innervation to and from the detrusor muscle through the pelvic parasympathetic nerves. The sacral 2 spinal segment has a major innervation to the external urethral sphincter through the pudendal nerves. Intracranial lesions above the pons result in a hyperreflexic bladder,

and those below the pons but above the conus produce detrusor sphincter dyssynergia. Lesions in the conus can lead to detrusor areflexia. This is illustrated in Figure 14-1.

Peripheral Components of Voiding

The essential components of bladder voiding are bladder musculature, bladder-neck mechanism, urethra, striated periurethral, and pelvic floor musculature. The bladder wall consists of involuntary plain muscles not well defined in layers, but which continue into the bladder neck, where they tend to be oriented in two layers. The inner longitudinal muscle continues into the urethra, and the external longitudinal muscle merges with the striated periurethral sphincter around the prostate in males. In females, it continues into the striated external urethral sphincter. However, there is some definition of a third layer near the bladder neck, where the middle layer of detrusor muscle seems to be prominent and forms a bladder neck that is seen as an internal sphincter in a cystoscopic examination. The striated muscle component of the urethra consists of pelvic floor musculature and periurethral extension of striated muscle between the urogenital diaphragm and the apex of the prostate.

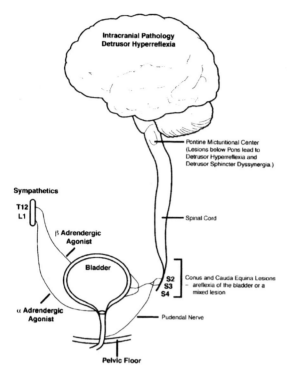

FIGURE 14-1 Bladder innervation and neurologic bladder dysfunctions following different levels of injury in the nervous system.

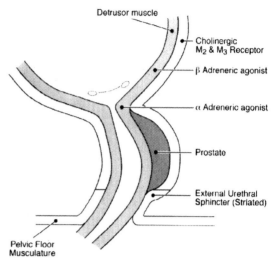

FIGURE 14-2 Saggittal section showing the relationship and extent of striated and plain muscles in the male urethra around the prostate. Anteriorly, the prostate has been omitted to show the likeness of it to the female urethra. Distribution of the autonomic receptors in the bladder and bladder neck are also depicted.

This is illustrated in Figure 14-2. The female urethra and the posterior urethra in the male essentially resemble each other except for the presence of the prostate in the male urethra, which partly displaces the homogeneous anatomic configuration seen in the female urethra, as seen anteriorly in Figure 14-2. Recent histochemical and electron microscopic studies show a well-developed circular smooth muscle extension from the bladder into the urethra to the entrance of the ejaculatory ducts in males and a rather less developed extension in females. Furthermore, the distribution of sympathetic nerve fibers in the smooth muscle coat is sparse in females in comparison with the male bladder neck region. This finding provides evidence for the necessity of preventing retrograde ejaculation in the male.

Bladder Innervation

The detrusor muscle forming the bladder wall extends into the posterior urethra and is innervated with three sets of nerves—parasympathetic, sympathetic, and somatic. Figure 14-3 illustrates the bladder innervation.

Parasympathetic Innervation.
The detrusor muscle in the bladder wall is richly supplied with parasympathetic nerves, which arise from sacral 2, 3, and 4 segments in the spinal cord. They are cholinergic, with ganglion cells located in the bladder wall. This innervation is so profuse that nearly every smooth muscle is individually supplied by one or more cholinergic nerve fibers. These nerves are both motor and sensory to the bladder wall. The third sacral nerve root has the major innervation to the detrusor muscle. Activation of the parasympathetic system releases acetylcholine from postganglionic nerves, which in turn excites various muscarinic receptors. Although pharmacological M1–M5 subtype receptors have been defined (22), receptor binding and molecular biology

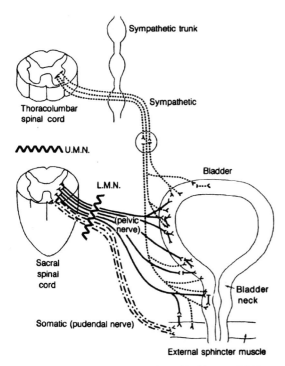

FIGURE 14-3   Innervation of the bladder. (U.M.N. = Upper motor neuron, L.M.N. = lower motor neuron.) (From Perkash I. Neuromuscular disorders of the bladder. In Friedland GW, Filly R, Govis ML, Gross D, Kempson R L, Korobkin M, Thurber BD, and Walter J, eds., *Uroradiology an Integrated Approach*. London: Churchill Livingstone, 1983. Pp. 1291–1316).

studies suggest that the human bladder is endowed with the M2 and M3 subtypes of receptors (23). It is believed that M2 receptors (indirectly), and M3 receptors (directly), mediate the main part of the bladder contraction.

Sympathetic Innervation.   Preganglionic sympathetic neurons originate in the intermedio lateral gray column of the spinal cord from spinal segments T10–L2. Sympathetic stimulation releases norepinephrine at the receptor sites. The bladder wall is essentially supplied with beta adrenergic agonist fibers, which on stimulation produce relaxation of the bladder wall. On the other hand, the bladder neck is innervated heavily with alpha agonist fibers. Their stimulation results in the closure of the bladder neck. The male bladder, as compared to that of a female, shows a predominance of alpha adrenergic innervation much needed for prevention of ret-

rograde ejaculation during sexual activity. When the sympathetic nerves are stimulated, the smooth muscles of the prostate, seminal vesicles, and ejaculatory ducts contract, resulting in ejaculation. The bladder neck also simultaneously contracts thereby preventing semen from entering into the bladder. Mixing urine with spermatozoa reduces their mobility.

External Urethral Sphincter.   The striated urinary sphincter is located in the lower half of the prostatic urethra. This is under voluntary control and is innervated by pudendal nerve. A majority of the innervation is from the S2 spinal segment. The toe plantar flexors also have S1 and S2 innervation. The preservation of toe planter flexors gives a clue to an intact external urethral sphincter following spinal cord injury.

Micturition Reflex and Normal Voiding

The local reflex arc originating in the bladder wall with sacral 2, 3, and 4 nuclei in the conus produces bladder contraction. The cortical centers provide for adequate voluntary control on voiding with a variety of positive and negative feedback loops. Spinal cord micturition reflex is segmentally controlled to achieve perfect control on voiding. Any sudden activity such as jumping, coughing, or straining reflexes leads to the contraction of the striated external urethral sphincter that prevent leakage of urine, and thus continence is maintained. Only an attempted voiding with a volitional control would therefore produce voiding with a relaxed external urethral sphincter. Thus, spinal guarding reflex becomes pathologic in spinal cord lesions below the pons and leads to detrusor sphincter dyssynergia, where with each bladder contraction there is a simultaneous contraction of the external urethral sphincter. It seems that the micturation center is located in the brainstem in the pontine mesencephalic area. Lesions below the pontine center result in detrusor sphincter dyssynergia. This is helpful in maintaining continence in spinal cord injured patients who empty their bladder with intermittent catheterization.

Bladder Physiologic Studies

Neurologic lesions of the central nervous system produce certain distinct neurologic dysfunctions. Bladder physiologic studies—such as urodynamic evaluation—are necessary to document the changes in various voiding parameters that may be detrimental to the urologic tract and also impair total renal functions.

Bladder physiologic studies include the *cystometric* (CMG) study, which involves filling the bladder with air or water at body temperature. It also may be carried out with radiographic contrast in the bladder for both voiding cystogram and cystometrogram or combined cinefluoroscopic studies. Similar studies also may be performed using a linear array transrectal probe to provide visualization of the dynamic contraction of the bladder while intravesical pressures are being recorded through a small catheter connected to a strain gauge or a simple manometer.

Cystometric Studies. A French size 7 or 10 triple-lumen catheter (Fig. 14-4) is used to fill the bladder and simultaneously record the pressure. Prior to filling the bladder, the clinician instructs the patient to relax and tell when he or she has a "feeling" of filling and/or has the desire to void. The patient is then instructed to void. A paraplegic or quadriplegic patient cannot stand and void; ambulatory patients are asked to stand and void so that voiding pressures can be determined. In spinal injured patients, suprapubic gentle tapping with the fingers can trigger voiding and thus voiding pressures can be determined.

In normal persons, the first sensation of fullness is usually perceived when the bladder is filled with 100 ml of fluid; there is a desire to void when the bladder is filled with about 300 to 400 ml of fluid. During filling of the bladder, the intravesical pressure is usually around 20 cm water; however, if the bladder is fibrosed, this pressure may rise steeply, and the bladder is then considered noncompliant. Maximum voiding pressures on attempted voiding are noted. Postvoid residuals are checked before and after cystometric examination. In patients with neurogenic bladder dysfunction, about 100 ml of post-void residual is considered acceptable. The cystometric study, thus, is used to assess bladder sensation, compliance, and maximum voiding pressures.

The International Continence Society has classified the detrusor as either normal, hyperreflexic, or hyporeflexic based on the CMG. The hyperactive disorder is characterized by involuntary detrusor contractions that may be spontaneous or provoked by rapid filling. When involuntary detrusor contractions are caused by neurologic disorders, the condition is called *detrusor hyperreflexia*. In the absence of a demonstrable neurological etiology, involuntary detrusor contractions are defined as *detrusor instability*. The absence of a detrusor contraction, particularly in females, during CMG is not considered abnormal

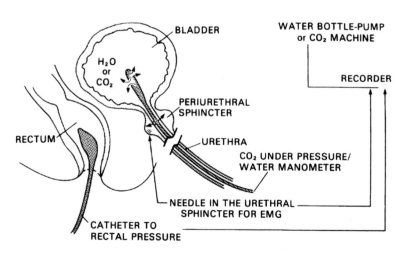

FIGURE 14-4 Method of urodynamic recording of urethral pressure profile, intraabdominal presure, and EMG of external urethral sphincter. (Modified from Ghista, Perkash I, et al. *Advances in Bioengineering* 1978, 19–23; and Constantinou CE. *Urology Digest* March 1977; 13–21).

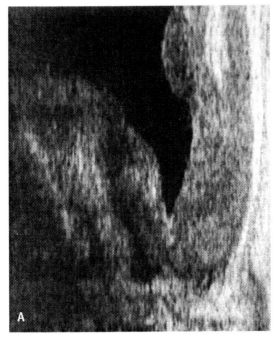
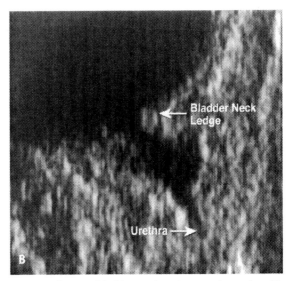

FIGURE 14-5 **A.** Transrectal linear array sonogram that shows wide open bladder neck and prostatic urethra. **B.** Bladder neck ledge in another patient on intermittent catheterization.

unless there are other clinical or urodynamic findings to substantiate the presence of lower motor neuron disease. In patients with spinal cord injury, suprapubic tapping can initiate voiding. It is also important to record blood pressure during the bladder filling, particularly in tetraplegic patients, to find out if patients show a significant rise in B.P. (17) and are thus considered prone to autonomic dysreflexia.

ACT OF MICTURITION (FLOW RATES)

In neurologically impaired patients, such as spinal cord injured patients, suprapubic tapping over the bladder region 15 to 20 times often leads to micturition. It is usually intermittent, which does not give an easily measured flow rate. Intermittent flow rate, however, is indicative of the existence of detrusor sphincter dyssynergia. The dyssynegic urethral sphincter often relaxes intermittently. Patients with spinal cord injury can also be evaluated at the bedside (bedside urodynamics): the bladder is first palpated and then suprapubicly tapped. If, follow-

ing this procedure, the bladder empties easily with a good stream and without the patient becoming dysreflexic, with no significant rise in blood pressure, chances are that the patient is voiding satisfactorily.

Bladder outlet obstruction due to a bladder neck ledge (Fig. 14-5), enlarged prostate, or detrusor sphincter dyssynergia is associated with a diminished uroflow but usually with a sustained detrusor contraction and high intravesical pressure (Fig. 14-6). Alternatively, impaired detrusor contractility is characterized by a diminished flow rate and a low-pressure detrusor contraction that is poorly sustained. Even a normal uroflow may not always exclude bladder outlet or sphincteric obstruction in incomplete spinal cord lesions. Therefore, uroflow is not of great clinical value as a single examination.

ELECTROMYOGRAPHY OF THE EXTERNAL URETHRAL SPHINCTER

Simultaneous cystometrographic study and electromyography (EMG) of the external urethral

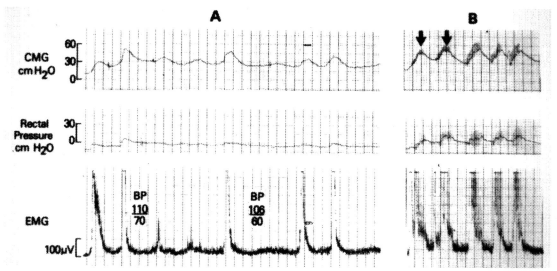

FIGURE 14-6 Simultaneous cystometrogram, EMG external urethral sphincter, and rectal pressures. Tracings A and B show detrusor sphinter dyssynegia where each of the bladder contractions are associated with increased EMG activity of the external urethral sphincter.

sphincter is important to diagnose detrusor external sphincter dyssynergia. A triple-lumen catheter is used to fill the bladder and to record intravesical and intraurethral pressures. The bladder is filled with air or water for cystometric studies (Fig. 14-4). Intra-abdominal pressures are recorded with a rectal balloon, and the EMG activity of the external urethral sphincter is monitored simultaneously either with surface electrodes or coaxial needles in the perineum. In the relaxed state, the normal external sphincter is generally electrically silent, with only infrequent low-amplitude motor units. With progressive bladder filling, there is usually an increase in external urethral sphincter EMG activity, which reaches a maximum just prior to voiding. An increase in EMG activity usually accompanies cough, straining, or body movement. The beginning of a voluntary detrusor contraction is marked by relaxation of the external urethral sphincter in a normal person. When this happens, the sphincter EMG becomes electrically silent, and maximum urethral pressure drops dramatically. Sphincter relaxation persists through the detrusor contraction, and, at the end of voiding, electromyographic activity resumes.

CYSTOUROFLOWMETRY

In cystouroflowmetry multichannel studies use a triple-lumen catheter in the bladder and a rectal catheter to determine rectal pressure, which also indicates abdominal pressure. The bladder is filled with water through one channel. The second channel records pressure through transducers, and the third channel (with a side hole) records urethral pressure. Pressure flow studies provide bladder pressure (Pves) and corresponding urine flow rates (Qura). True detrusor pressure (Pdet) can be determined by subtracting rectal pressure (Pabd) from bladder pressure (Pves).

URETHRAL PRESSURE PROFILOMETRY

The urethral pressure profile (UPP) represents the lateral closure pressure along the length of the urethra. It is usually studied with a multichannel catheter. Profilometry, with a pull-through technique, provides graphic representation of the lateral pressure along the length of the urethra. Currently, the practiced technique has been adapted from Brown and Wickham (2). The functional length of the urethra can be measured. These studies are done with an empty bladder.

For static UPP, one of the holes meant for sensing the pressure is positioned in the middle of the posterior urethra. A triple-lumen catheter typically has a terminal hole 1 cm from the tip for filling the bladder and another side hole at 10 cm to sense the urethral pressure. Other sophisticated techniques using a microtransducer mounted at the tip of the urethral catheter have been used over the simpler and less expensive perfusion catheter systems. These microtransducer catheters are expensive, fragile, and difficult to insert in the male urethra. They also are prone to distortional errors and irritation (9) due to the curvature and length of the transducer catheter. While the bladder is gradually filled for CMG, both intravesical and urethral pressures can be simultaneously recorded. In patients with neurologic lesions of the spinal cord, when the bladder contracts, the rise in urethral pressure, along with increased EMG activity of the external urethral sphincter, is indicative of detrusor sphincter dyssynegia. Figure 14-6 illustrates dyssynergia.

VOIDING CYSTOURETHROGRAPHY AND VIDEOURODYNAMIC TESTING

To perform voiding cystourethrography or videourodynamic testing, the bladder is filled until either an involuntary detrusor contraction occurs, the patient is asked to void voluntarily, or leakage of the infusant occurs at the urethral meatus, which gives a leak pressure. Bladder outlet obstruction is characterized by a high voiding pressure and low flow. If obstruction is suspected but the site of the obstruction is not clear, the combination of radiographic visualization and urethral pressure drop just beyond obstruction may provide a definitive answer.

TRANSRECTAL LINEAR ARRAY SOMOGRAPHY

Bladder neck obstruction is easily visualized via transrectal linear array sonography (15). Secondary bladder neck obstruction due to a ledge in patients with spinal cord injury has been reported (16); recognition of this obstruction is important, because intermittent catheterization may be difficult in these patients. Sonographic voiding cystourethrogram shows bladder neck obstruction due to a ledge (shown as an arrow) posteriorly at the bladder neck in (Figure 14-5B). The ledge is believed to be a complication in patients with detrusor sphincter dyssynegia who are on long-term intermittent catheterization. The presence of a bladder neck ledge invariably leads to difficulty in catheterization with a plain catheter. A coude tip catheter is more effective for intermittent catheterization.

Combined synchronous, ultrasonographic, and urodynamic monitoring is feasible. This study may be done in lieu of a cine radiographic study combined with simultaneous urodynamics. It has been shown that during simple insertion of a catheter, touching the bladder neck ledge can result in bladder contraction and wide-open bladder neck and posterior urethra. It is therefore important to catheterize such patients carefully and not stimulate the bladder neck to produce a bladder-neck stimulated cystometrogram (9). Persistent narrowing of the membranous urethra on ultrasonographic imaging or on voiding cystourethrogram (Figs. 14-5B and 14-7) and elevated detrusor pressure is consistent with detrusor external sphincter dyssynergia (DESD) in a complete suprasacral spinal cord injury. The main advantage of the sonographic study over cine radiographic studies is the lack of radiation exposure for the patients. However, bladder shape, trabeculation, diverticula, and vesicoureteral reflux are difficult to visualize on sonography alone.

NEUROLOGIC-IMPAIRED BLADDER: COMMON CAUSES

Neuromuscular disorders of the bladder may be congenital or acquired. Myelodisplasia is the common congenital cause. Various other causes are shown in Table 14-1.

Central nervous system lesions above the midbrain pontine center are usually associated with detrusor hyperreflexia. Widespread acute vascular cortical lesions may initially be associated with detrusor areflexia, such as following a hemorrhagic stroke. In about 6 percent of patients,

TABLE 14-1   Common Neurologic Disorders Leading to Bladder Dysfunction*

Neurologic Disorder	Usual Type of Dysfunction
Suprapontine lesions	Detrusor hyperreflexia with absent detrusor-sphincter dyssynergy
Delayed CNS maturation (childhood)	Persistence of uninhibited bladder beyond age 2–3. Enuresis later on.
Cerebrovascular accidents	
Multiple sclerosis	Uninhibited bladder (early)
Senile dementia	Uninhibited bladder
Parkinsonism	Uninhibited bladder
Brain tumors	Uninhibited bladder
Lesions below pons (Supraconal lesions)	Usually associated with detrusor sphincter dyssynergia
Spinal cord injuries	Hyperreflexic bladder
Spinal cord neoplasms—primary or secondary	Reflex bladder
Syringomyelia	Reflex bladder
Multiple sclerosis	Hyperreflexic bladder
Spinal cord inflammatory lesions	Hyperreflexic bladder
Prolapsed disc (cervical, thoracolumber)	Hyperreflexic bladder
Conus lesion	Absent detrusor–sphincter dyssynergia
Cauda equina injuries or neoplasms	Areflexic bladder (autonomous bladder)
Acute transverse myelitis	Areflexic bladder (autonomous bladder)
Extensive rectal carcinoma	Areflexic bladder (autonomous bladder)
Following abdominoperineal resection of rectal carcinoma	Areflexic bladder (autonomous bladder)
Perivesical fibrosis following extensive pelvic surgery or trauma	Areflexic bladder (autonomous bladder)
Herniated intervertebral disc (Lumbosacral)	Areflexic bladder (autonomous bladder)
Myelodysplasia and spina bifida	Areflexic bladder (autonomous bladder)
Poliomyelitis	Areflexic bladder (motor-paralytic, sensory intact)
Injury, neoplasms, and herniated disc involving motor nerves to the bladder	Areflexic bladder (motor paralytic, sensory intact)
Diabetes mellitus	Areflexic bladder (sensory paralytic bladder, areflexic due to overdistention)
Tabes dorsalis	Areflexic bladder (sensory paralytic bladder, areflexic due to overdistention)
Guillainn-Barre syndrome	Areflexic bladder

*After Perkash, Reference 15.

detrusor sphincter dyssynergia has also been reported even in cortical and subcortical lesions. All spinal cord lesions above the conus (supraconal lesions) are associated with some degree of detrusor sphincter dyssynergia. In patients with severe pelvic floor muscle spasticity, severe dyssynergia may be associated with intermittent spasticity noticed during simultaneous EMG studies of the external urethral sphincter.

Cauda equina lesions are usually associated with a noncontractile (areflexic) bladder. The bladder is usually large and may be associated with a denervated external urethral sphincter.

THERAPEUTIC DRUGS TO MODULATE NEUROGENIC BLADDER DYSFUNCTION

Bladder Relaxant Drugs

General indications of pharmacologic treatment include reduction of bladder voiding pressures, improvement in voiding, reduction or elimina-

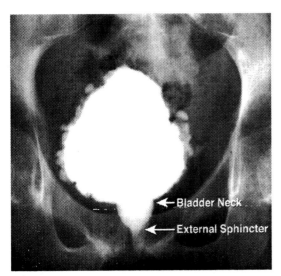

←Bladder Neck

←External Sphincter

FIGURE 14-7 Voiding cystourethrogram shows irregular margin of the bladder, dilated bladder neck, and closed urethra due to detrusor sphincter dyssynergia.

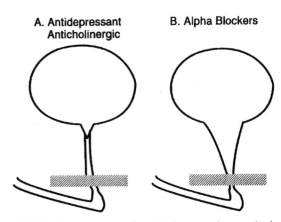

A. Antidepressant Anticholinergic

B. Alpha Blockers

FIGURE 14-8 Action of anticholinergic drugs, which relax bladder, and alpha blockers, which open bladder neck.

tion of reflex incontinence, reduction in frequency of catheterization in patients on intermittent catheterization, and reduction of uninhibited bladder contractions in patients with indwelling catheters. The mechanism of action of these drugs is shown in Table 14-2. Oxybutynine hydrochloride is a moderately potent antimuscarinic agent with a pronounced muscle relaxant activity and has some anaesthetic activity on the bladder as well. Usual oral dose is 2.5 to 5.0 mgm 3 times a day. Most of the side effects are related to antimuscarinic action, with dry mouth the most common complaint. Recently a slow-release tablet seems to result in less oral dryness. Clinical practice should aim at individual titration of drug dosage for a maximum therapeutic effect with minimal side effects. Another drug recently available is tolterodine, which is a competitive muscarinic receptor antagonist. Tolterodine (2 mgm bid) appears to be as effective as oxybutynin (5 mgm tid) with less dryness in the mouth.

Drugs to Improve Voiding

Alpha-adrenoceptor blockers have been widely used to improve voiding in patients with an enlarged prostate and in patients with spinal cord injury. Phenoxybenzamine, a long-acting, powerful nonselective blocker, has frequently been used to improve voiding and control autonomic dysreflexia in spinal cord injured (SCI) patients. The selective alpha 1 adrenoceptor blockers (Fig 14-8), which are clinically used to control hypertension, include prazosin, terazosin, and doxazosin. Table 14-2 shows the pharmacological activities of alpha adrenoceptor blockers available for clinical use.

Bladder Afferents Blocking Drugs

The vanilloide group of drugs, such as capsaicin (8) and resiniferatoxin, have been used with some success in patients with detrusor hyperreflexia due to spinal cord lesions, such as multiple sclerosis and chronic spinal cord injury (20).

MANAGEMENT OF BLADDER FOLLOWING SPINAL CORD INJURY—ACUTE PHASE

Immediately following injury, patients are in a state of shock and are usually on intravenous fluids. There is widespread paralysis of the autonomic nervous system. To prevent overhydration and pulmonary edema, it is important to frequently monitor fluid intake and output, and therefore, they need an indwelling catheter. After the patient is stabilized, usually 1 to 3 weeks after

TABLE 14-2 Mechanism of Action of Various Drugs on the Bladder
Mostly Through the Automatic Nervous System*

Drugs	Alteration in Mode of Action	Bladder Function
Cholinergic drugs Acetylcholine	Physiologic neurotransmitter for bladder contractions.	Increases intravesical pressure and facilitates voiding.
Muscarinic Bethanechol Methacholine	Physiologic neuro transmitter for bladder contractions.	Increases intravesical pressure and facilitates voiding.
Antimuscarinic Ditropan Tolterodine Trospium	Blocks M2 and M3 receptors. Blocks M2 receptors mostly. Blocks M2 receptors mostly.	
Nicotinic Nicotine	Nicotinelike response resembles sympathetic stimulation mediated through release of norepinephrine.	
Anticholinergics	Blockage of endogenous transmitter at post synaptic receptor	Reduces bladder contractility and may lead to urinary retention.
Atropine Propantheline d-Tubocurarine	Atropine blocks muscarinic action and d-tubocurarine blocks nicotinic action of acetyl choline. Propantheline blocks muscarinic action and also has a ganglion-blocking action.	
Reserpine Guanetidine	Essentially adrenergic neuron blocker.	
Phenothiazines Antihistaminics	Mild anticholinergic action.	
Adrenergic Alpha adrenergic Agonist response Phenylephrine Ephedrine	Sympathomimetic response (response mostly on alpha adrenergic receptors).	Increases bladder outlet and urethral pressure.
Imipramine	Action similar to alpha adrenergic stimulation.	
Alpha adrenergic Blockers Phenoxybenzamine Phentolamine Prazosin Terazosin Dexazosin	Sympatholytic response.	Lower bladder outlet and urethral pressures.
Tamsulosinhel	Selective receptor blockage.	
Beta stimulants Isoproterenol Progesterone	Sympathomimetic.	Lower urethral pressure relaxes bladder detrusor muscle.
Beta blockers Propranolol	Sympatholytic.	Increases urethral pressure.
Vanilloid Capsaicin Resiniferat Oxin	Bladder afferent blocking drugs.	Bladder capacity.

*Modified from Perkash I. Neuromuscular disorders of the bladder. In Friedland GW, Filly R, Govis ML, Gross D, Kempson R L, Korobkin M, Thurber BD, and Walter J, eds. *Uroradiology—An Integrated Approach*. London: Churchill Livingstone 1983. Pp. 1291–1316 (15).

injury, he may be placed on intermittent catheterization every 4 hours. This requires restriction of fluid intake to about 1.5 to 2.0 liters in 24 hours. During the acute phase, the sterile technique is used (19), but later, in a home setting, the patient may be catheterized using a clean technique (10), preferably using a clean glove and a clean catheter. The patients are monitored frequently for urinary tract infection and bladder voiding pressures. Patients with voiding pressure over 40 cm water are given anticholinergic drugs to reduce bladder pressures and achieve some degree of continence with intermittent catheterization. Those with autonomic dysreflexia also benefit from anticholinergic drugs. Tetraplegics with poor hand function may be considered for transurethral sphincterotomy and external condom drainage (11). This reduces dependence on a caretaker for intermittent catheterization and also reduces the intensity of autonomic dysreflexia (12). Follow-up urodynamic studies are required in patients on intermittent catheterization (IC) to evaluate voiding pressure so that optimal dosage of the anticholinergic drug is established. Such studies may initially be done 6 to 8 weeks after the start of intermittent catheterization and are repeated with any change in spasticity, repeated urinary tract infections, and frequent episodes of autonomic dysreflexia (13). Patients on IC are actively treated for any symptomatic urinary tract infection.

AUTONOMIC DYSREFLEXIA

Patients with spinal cord lesions above T6 are prone to autonomic dysreflexia, which is associated with a rise in blood pressure and bradycardia. Lesions above T5 lead to sympathetic denervation of the splanchnic bed, which is supplied by the greater splanchnic nerve (T5, T6, T7, T8). Any rise in blood pressure, mostly as a result of visceral activity, such as a full bladder or loaded rectum producing peripheral vasoconstriction, is normally countered by vasodilation in the splanchnic bed through the greater splanchnic nerve. Also, there is slowing of the heart through vagal stimulation. Persons with spinal injuries above T5 do not have control of the splanchnic bed to redistribute excess circulating blood but the heart rate may slow because of the intact vagus nerve. Therefore, in typical patients, autonomic dysreflexia manifests itself as high blood pressure and a slow heart rate. The usual trigger is a full bladder or fecal impaction in the rectum. Occasionally, high bowel impaction or a stone impacted in the ureter evokes dysreflexia. We also have noticed autonomic dysreflexia during extracorporeal shock-wave lithotripsy (5). It is advisable to have patients carry a card indicating that they are prone to dysreflexia.

Mild autonomic dysreflexia is manifested as sweating, an increase in spasticity, and goose pimples with or without any significant rise in blood pressure or fall in pulse rate. The normal systolic blood pressure in the quadriplegic patient is less than 100 mmHg, with a pulse rate around 60 to 65 per minute. Severe autonomic dysreflexia is usually accompanied by a marked rise in systolic blood pressure and a drop in the pulse rate to as low as below 50 per minute.

Management includes raising the head end of the patient, loosening the clothes, and emptying the bladder with a catheter. If the rectum is loaded, it is manually evacuated following insertion of tetracaine ointment (Nupercainal). For acute and emergency management of raised blood pressure secondary to autonomic dysreflexia, Nifedipine, 10 mg either sublingually or swallowed after breaking the capsule, seems ideal. Nitropaste patches are also available for persistent dysreflexia. When dysreflexia develops in the operating room, it is best managed either with Nitroprusside, 0.5 to 10 Ng/kg per minute in the intravenous drip, which can be titrated to reduce the blood pressure immediately; Hydralazine, 5 to 10 mg intravenously or 5 to 20 mg intramuscularly, and repeated if necessary; or other antihypertensive drugs that the anesthetist feels comfortable in using for a particular patient. After the administration of hypotensive drugs, blood pressure may drop precipitously; therefore, patients need careful monitoring.

Long-term management of dysreflexia includes improving bladder drainage with transurethral resection of the sphincter (TURS), transurethral prostatic resection, or the use of alpha blockers such as Prazosin or Terazosin. We have found Prazosin, 1 mg orally every 4 to 6 hours as needed, very useful if the systolic blood pressure is above 130 mmHg after transurethral surgery and also after an acute episode of severe dysreflexia.

CARE OF EXTERNAL COLLECTING DEVICES

During the early phase of injury, patients may have an indwelling catheter connected to a disposable bed bag. It is preferable to use a clean bag every day. Once patients are on intermittent catheterization and are continent, they do not need leg bags. However, return of reflex bladder activity does lead to urinary accidents, and patients must wear an external collecting device connected to a leg bag. Proper placement of the external condom catheter is important because tight tape at the base of the penis may result in skin breakdown and ulceration. There are several commercially available external condoms that do not need an adhesive tape to hold them.

Patients with small, retractile penises may have a problem holding a condom. This is particularly evident in patients who are obese, wherein their retractile penis virtually disappears when they sit up. Such patients may need a penile implant to hold an external condom (6,18).

CARE OF LEG BAGS AND BED BAGS

External or internal indwelling catheters are connected to leg bags or bed bags for urine collection. These bags provide good culture media for the growth of bacteria. It is therefore important to clean the reusable leg bags every day to prevent urinary tract infection. In a controlled in vitro study of various chemical disinfectants for leg bags, it was found that 6 percent household bleach solution was the best to eradicate all bacteria (4). Acetic acid (0.25 percent) and hydrogen peroxide (3 percent) were not as effective. We have therefore recommended the use of 6 per-

cent bleach over the years, with significant reduction in urinary tract infections. After irrigating the leg bag with bleach, it is imperative to clean the bag thoroughly in running water, beacause bleach is a strong oxidizing agent and can hurt the skin.

MANAGEMENT OF URINARY TRACT INFECTION

Urinary tract infection in patients with neurogenic bladder differs from that in normal people (3). The simple criteria of significant numbers of microbials cultured from a urine specimen does not necessarily indicate a significant infection because there is a heavy contamination caused by the collection devices worn by such patients. However, if there is an associated rise in body temperature of 1.5°F or more and or presence of 5 to 10 pus cells per high-power field under the microscope, it necessitates treatment of such infection. Patients on IC need careful monitoring. A significant number of cultured microbial colonies usually require the use of antibiotics or chemotherapeutic agents. Such patients are also encouraged to stay on prophylactic medication such as Macrodantin 50 to 100 mg/day orally or alternating every other month with Malhenamine, 1G 3 times a day.

Followup

Patients usually need a regular 3- to 6-month follow-up during the first year of injury and every year later on. Renal ultrasonography and isotope study (21) provide reasonable information for early detection of hydronephrosis or loss of renal function to necessitate further evaluation and management of such patients.

FEMALE NEUROGENIC BLADDER MANAGEMENT

Ideal urologic management in females, like males, is to be free from indwelling urethral catheter for permanent drainage of the bladder. This may be realistic in male patients but it is difficult to accomplish in females mainly because of anatomic differences and lack of availability of a suitable external collecting device for women. It is therefore important to appreciate that bladder drainage in women with spinal cord injury is different from males. Women with functioning hands can be trained to develop an intermittent catheterization program to empty their bladders less frequently than males. Depending upon their fluid intake, they may need catheterization only three to four times a day, such as an hour after breakfast, 1 to 2 hours after lunch, and 1 to 2 hours after dinner. They may also be helped to increase bladder capacity with a small dose of Oxybutynin, about 2 to 5 mgn two or three times a day. Overall, fewer urologic complications have been reported in the females. Tetraplegic women need an attendant who can also intermittently catheterize them. In the past, however, a majority of these women have relied on indwelling catheters for bladder drainage. The other choices available are permanent implantation of nerve roots stimulators or surgical diversions and/or bladder augmentation.

CONCLUSION

Management of the neurogenic bladder for individuals with spinal cord disease or injuries is still evolving. Freedom from indwelling urethral catheters has become the first choice of management. Intermittent catheterization is the method of choice for bladder drainage. During hospital stay, a sterile technique is preformed to prevent spread of nosocomial resistent infections. However in the home setting, clean technique is preferred. It saves cost and is less cumbersome. Long-term results are not significantly different while using clean or sterile technique in the non-hospital setting. Tetraplegic males and females have to depend on an attendant for intermittent catheterization. In males who can wear an external collecting device, transurethral sphincterotomy seems to be advantageous to free patients from dependence on attendants, reduce incidence of autonomic dysreflexia, and also to reduce incidence of

other urologic complications such as stone disease, hydronephrosis, and other urologic complications. Placement of an indwelling catheter and/or suprapubic cystostomy depends upon individual choice and convenience, motivation, and social situation. Regular yearly follow-up is needed to monitor renal function to predict and prevent urologic complications.

REFERENCES

1. Bradley WE, Teague CT. Spinal cord organization of micturition reflex afferents. *Exp Neurol* 1968; 22:504.
2. Brown M, Wickham JEA. The urethral pressure profile. *Br J Urol* 1969; 41:211.
3. Cardenas DD, Hooton TM. Urinary tract infection in persons with spinal cord injury. *Arch Phys Med Rehabil* 1995; 76:272.
4. Giroux J, Perkash I. In vitro evaluation of current disinfectants for leg bags. *J Am Paraplegia Soc* 1985; 8:13.
5. Kabalin JH, Lennon S, Gill HS, et al. Incidence and management of autonomic dysreflexia and other intraoperative problems encountered in spinal cord injured patients undergoing ESWL without anesthesia on a second generation lithotriptor (abstract). *J Urol* 1992; 147:219A.
6. Kabalin JN, Rosen J, Perkash I. Penile advancement and lengthening in spinal cord injury patients with retracted phallus who have failed penile prosthesis placement alone. *J Urol* 1990; 144:316.
7. Kuhlemeier KV, McEachron AB, Lloyd LK, Stover SL, Fine PR. Serum creatinine as an indicator of renal function after spinal cord injury. *Arch Phys Med Rehabil* 1984; 65:694.
8. Maggi CA. Capsaicin and primary afferent neurons: from basic science to human therapy. *J Auton Nerv Syst* 1991; 33(1):1.
9. Perkash I, Friedland GW. Catheter-induced hyperreflexia in spinal cord injury patients: diagnosis by sonographic voiding cystourethrography. Radiology 1986; 159:453.
10. Perkash I, Giroux J. Clean technique in intermittent catheterization in spinal cord injured patients. *J Urol* 1993;149:1068.
11. Perkash I. Contact laser sphincterotomy: further experience and longer follow-up. *Spinal Cord* 1996; 34:227.
12. Perkash I. Detrusor-sphincter dyssynegia and dyssynegia responses: recognition and rationale for early modified transurethral sphincterotomy

in complete spinal cord injury lesions. *J Urol* 1978 ;120:469.

13. Perkash I. Long-term urologic management of the patient with spinal cord injury. *Urol Clin North Am* 1993; 20:423.

14. Perkash I. Management of neurogenic dysfunction of the bladder and bowel. In Kottke, Lehman, eds., *Krusens Handbook of Physical Medicine and Rehabilitation*, 4th ed. Philadelphia: W.B. Saunders 1990. Pp. 810–832.

15. Perkash I. Neuromuscular disorders of the bladder. In Friedland GW, Filly R, Govis ML, Gross D, Kempson RL, Korobkin M, Thurber BD, Walter J, ed., *Uroradiology—an Integrated Approach*. London: Churchill Livingstone, 1983. Pp. 1291–1316.

16. Perkash I, Friedland GW. Posterior ledge at the bladder neck: the crucial diagnostic role of ultrasonography. *Urol Radiol* 1986; 8:175.

17. Perkash I. Pressor response during cystomanometry in spinal injury patients complicated with detrusor-sphincter dyssynergia. *J Urol* 1979; 121:778–782.

18. Perkash I, Kabalin JN, Lennon S, et al. Use of penile prostheses to maintain external condom catheter drainage in spinal cord injured patients. *Paraplegia* 1992; 30:327.

19. Rhames SF, Perkash I. Urinary tract infections occurring in recently injured spinal cord patients on intermittent catheterization. *J Urol* 1979; 122:669.

20. Szallasi A, Blumberg PM. Vanilloid receptors: new insights enhance potential as therapuetic target. *Pain* 1996; 68:195–208.

21. Tempkin A, Sullivan G, Paldi J, Perkash I. Radioisotope renography in spinal cord injury. *J Urol* 1985; 133:228.

22. Wang P, Luthin GR, Ruggleri MR. Muscarinic acetylcholine receptor subtypes mediating urinary bladder contractility and coupling to GTP biding proteins. *J Pharmacol Exper Ther* 1995; 273:959–966.

23. Yamaguchi O, Shishido K, Tamura K, Ogawa T, Fugimura T, Otsuka A. Evaluation of mRNAs encoding muscarinic receptor subtypes in human detrusor muscle. *J Urol* 1996; 156:1208–1213.

15 Spinal Cord Injury Treatment and the Anesthesiologist

JOSEPH P. GIFFIN, MD
KENNETH GRUSH, MD
PAUL J. DADIC, MD

Currently, on an annual basis, 10,000 patients with spinal cord trauma survive the initial injury to arrive at our nation's hospitals (1), presenting anesthesiologists and other intensive care specialists with a unique responsibility and challenge. The fact that 70 percent of these patients are 19 to 34 years of age (2) makes this an especially poignant problem in terms of lost human potential as well as the urgency to preserve whatever function remains and restore as much lost function as possible.

Although the mortality for these patients remains high, approximately 50 percent reported in 1980 (3), recent advances in resuscitation and rehabilitation have resulted in an expanding population of long-term survivors (2,4). Despite continuing disagreement on the advisability of surgical intervention, 78 percent of patients admitted to one spinal injury center with acute spinal cord injury underwent some type of surgical procedure (5). Clearly, there is a need for the anesthesiologist to be familiar with the nature of spinal cord injury and its management.

Consequently, our attention in this discussion is directed toward the acute management of spinal cord injury and the medical sequelae of spinal cord injury that may influence the anesthetic management for diagnostic and surgical procedures. Finally, current concepts of the pathophysiology

of spinal cord injury are discussed with regard to experimental as well as clinical modalities of spinal cord resuscitation that bear some hope for the restoration of useful function.

ACUTE MANAGEMENT OF SPINAL CORD INJURY

Because anesthesiologists are frequently consulted to assist in the management of patients in unstable conditions arriving with severe spinal cord injury in the emergency department, a brief review of the necessary steps in stabilizing such patients follows (6). As in most life-threatening medical emergencies, attention must first be directed to the ABCs (airway, breathing, and circulation). Any comatose and/or multiple trauma patient must be considered to have a cord injury until proved otherwise. First, an airway is established using the jaw thrust technique, while the head and neck are maintained in the neutral position. Absent ventilation after this mandates the initiation of artificial ventilation, either mouth-to-mouth or bag-valve-mask. Inability to ventilate the patient in spite of jaw thrust usually means that a foreign body is occluding the airway; this should be assessed and remedied. Although movement of the neck is contraindicated, asphyxia certainly carries a worse prognosis than cervical cord injury. It is the most common early cause of death (6).

Laryngoscopy and intubation should be carried out as expediently as possible, with the immobilization of the spine maintained. Ventilation should be given to produce a normal minute ventilation (75 to 80 ml/kg). In the breathing patient, supplemental oxygen and intensive observation are indicated.

Once these goals are satisfied, the systemic blood pressure should be supported at normal levels with the judicious administration of intravenous fluids if hypotension is present. Ventilatory and circulatory management of these patients are discussed in greater detail later.

Between 25 to 65 percent of spinal cord injured patients have associated problems, the most common being head, chest, abdominal, and skeletal injuries (7,8). These may complicate ventilatory and circulatory problems resulting from the cord injury, and a high index of suspicion is necessary in evaluating these patients. As soon as feasible, appropriate roentgenographic studies should be completed (including magnetic resonance imaging and computed tomographic scans). Initial laboratory determinations should include complete blood chemistry (CBC), arterial blood gases, serum electrolytes, serum creatinine, and any other study dictated by the individual patient's intrinsic illnesses or associated injuries.

Once the ABCs have been addressed and life-threatening deficits managed, the next priority becomes rapid transport of the patient, with the spine immobilized, to a major trauma center or, when feasible, to an acute cord injury center (7,4). Upon arrival at the hospital, diagnostic studies to determine the extent of injury and whether surgery is indicated are initiated, followed by appropriate medical therapy.

MEDICAL COMPLICATIONS OF SPINAL CORD INJURY AND THEIR MANAGEMENT

Respiratory Complications

Depending on the level and degree of spinal cord injury, respiration may be impaired by paralysis of abdominal, intercostal, diaphragmatic, and accessory muscles of respiration progressively as the site of trauma moves from low thoracic to high cervical or even brainstem levels. Loss of motor function originating at C3 to C5, giving rise to the phrenic nerves, results in diaphragmatic paralysis (major contribution from C4) as well as the loss of intercostal and abdominal motor function. High quadriplegia (C4 or above) results in a severe, life-threatening decrease in all standard measures of respiratory mechanics and dynamics-forced vital capacity (FVC), forced expiratory volume in one second (FEV1), peak inspiratory and expiratory force and flow, and total pulmonary compliance. Only the accessory muscles of inspiration (sternocleidomastoid, scalenes, and trapezius) function during inspiration. Lower rib cage and abdominal paradox is seen as the hemidiaphragms passively respond to the changes in intrathoracic pressure caused by accessory muscle activity. As the upper rib cage expands (less than with intact intercostal muscles), upward diaphragm motion decreases intra-abdominal pressure, resulting in inward movement of it and the lower rib cage. The reverse occurs during expiration. The paradoxical diaphragm motion and its cephalad displacement decrease the efficiency of already diminished muscle activity in effecting gas exchange (9). Tidal volume, inspiratory and expiratory reserve volumes (IRV and ERV), and functional residual capacity (FRC) are critically reduced, while residual volume (RV) is increased (10).

Alveolar hypoventilation results in hypercarbia. Hypoventilation, atelectasis, and airspace collapse associated with the decrease in FRC relative to closing volume produce ventilation–perfusion (V/Q) mismatching and cause hypoxemia. Respiratory function in this case is worst in the supine or Trendelenburg positions, because abdominal contents displace the diaphragm further cephalad, and it improves if other variables (e.g., blood pressure) permit some degree of head and thorax elevation. Global hypoventilation often worsens further during sleep, occasionally progressing to sleep apnea, which has been attributed to diminished carbon dioxide responsiveness (11,12).

Sighing and coughing are essential to maintain alveolar patency and pulmonary toilet. A near-normal inspiratory reserve is required in the former case, while the generation of pressure against a closed glottis and maintenance of flow following glottic opening is essential in the latter. Decreases in IRV, ERV, FVC, peak inspiratory and expiratory force and flow, as well as inability to splint the diaphragm accompanying diaphragmatic, intercostal, and abdominal paralysis cause inability to cough and clear airway secretions or to sigh and diminish atelectasis (13).

Low quadriplegic patients with partial or complete integrity of diaphragmatic innervation have variable diaphragmatic strength. Also, the diaphragms are prevented from achieving their optimal, steeply domed fiber length–tension position at end-expiration because of intercostal and abdominal muscle paralysis; hence, their inspiratory efficiency is impaired. Adding to this effect is the upper rib cage paradoxical *inward* motion during inspiration (lower rib cage and abdominal paradox in high quadriplegics) (13). The resulting decrease in respiratory capacity may produce V/Q mismatching and hypoxemia.

Five months after injury, a group of these patients was found to have a 50 percent decrease in FVC, peak expiratory and inspiratory flow, and inspiratory and expiratory reserve volumes. Decreases in expiratory flow were much less at low lung volumes (at 25 percent of total lung volume, flow was 72 percent of the predicted value) than at higher lung volumes (55 percent of predicted value). This was taken to implicate muscle weakness rather than intrinsic airway disease, airway compression, or decreased lung compliance as the primary cause of the decreased flow rates: normally, initial expiratory flow rate is effort-dependent, whereas late expiratory flow rates are effort-independent and limited by airway compression, which increases resistance proportionately to thoracic pressure. Muscle weakness, therefore, would decrease early expiratory flow as well as end-expiratory resistance. Assuming the Trendelenburg position, by shifting the diaphragms cephalad to a more mechanically advantageous starting fiber length, actually increased IRV and FVC an average of 300 ml (14).

The importance of the extent of diaphragmatic involvement is emphasized by a study comparing quadriplegics having complete cord lesions at the C5 to C6 level, with an average FVC of 1.5 L (24 percent of predicted), to those having complete lesions at C4 with an average FVC of 1.3 L (21 percent of predicted). Four of 11 patients with C5 to C6 lesions required oxygen, but only two required mechanical ventilation. All five patients with C4 lesions received oxygen and were ventilated. Although both groups approximately doubled their vital capacities over the next 3 months and were breathing unassisted, two patients having C4 level lesions displayed postural hypoxemia and hypercarbia (15).

The significance of at least some presence of intercostal muscle activity on EMG was demonstrated by measured decreases in FRC, transpulmonary pressure at FRC, and static expiratory compliance in patients lacking parasternal intercostal EMG activity. These three values remained normal in those who displayed such EMG activity—a finding attributed to a postulated role for tonic inspiratory intercostal activity in helping to determine FRC, which has usually been attributed to passive chest wall recoil balanced against lung compressibility. This increases transpulmonary pressure, increases FRC, maintains alveolar inflation, and improves lung compliance (16). The same investigators have found previously unsuspected participation of the pectoralis major and possibly other muscles during expiration, accounting for the persistence of a small ERV in patients with paralysis of all commonly accepted expiratory muscles (10). Training directed at both expiratory and inspiratory accessory muscles and diaphragms combined with any functional intercostal recovery can result in improved strength and endurance as well as decreased likelihood of fatigue (17).

Although respiration is less compromised in low quadriplegics and paraplegics than in high quadriplegics, those with low lesions are still at risk for hypoventilation, V/Q mismatching, and retention of secretions paralleling the changes in respiratory parameters already outlined. Aside from diaphragmatic and intercostal muscle strength, a key factor in overall respiratory function is the contribution of the abdominal muscles in increasing expiratory pressure directly as well as improving the efficiency of the intercostals in forced expiration or coughing by preventing paradoxical movement of the diaphragm into the abdomen. The importance of abdominal muscle tone in optimizing diaphragmatic position for inspiration has already been discussed. The abdominal weakness or paralysis accounts for the persistence of respiratory complications, especially retained secretions and pulmonary infections seen in some paraplegics with intact diaphragms and intercostal muscles.

Evaluation of the respiratory status of a spinal cord injured patient should be directed toward any obvious signs of hypoxemia or dyspnea, tidal volume, FVC, FEV1, respiratory rate, and minute volume, as well as observation of abdominal and thoracic movement, which should indicate the level of respiratory muscle impairment. Accessory muscle activity can be detected by inspection and careful palpation of the muscles involved or electromyography, as needed. Arterial blood gas analysis should be done as soon as feasible.

Any comatose, apparently apneic, or cyanotic patient or those unable to manage their secretions should be endotracheally intubated as soon as possible, as has usually already been done before arrival at the hospital in severely compromised patients. Immobilization of the spine is essential in preventing extension or completion of an incomplete lesion. In cervical injuries, the head should be maintained in the neutral position (neither flexed nor extended) by *gentle* traction (the aim is *not* reduction) so as to avoid neck movement during intubation. Blind nasotracheal intubation, as well as laryngoscopic or flexible fiberoptic oral or nasal intubation, are all possible and should be chosen on the basis of the ability to accomplish the task both as quickly as possible and without disturbing the existing cervical alignment (18).

A wide selection of laryngoscope blades, endotracheal tube sizes, a fiberoptic laryngo-scope, cricothyroidotomy apparatus, supplemental oxygen, manual and mechanical ventilation equipment, suction apparatus, and other resuscitation equipment and drugs should be available and ready for use. Surgical tracheostomy back-up should also be available. Sedation and/or neuromuscular blockade is not advisable in view of the further respiratory compromise and loss of muscular cervical splinting that they cause. Superior laryngeal nerve block and meticulous topical anesthesia improves patient tolerance when time and airway status permit their use. The distinct possibility of sinus arrest or complete heart block resulting from unopposed vagovagal reflexes following pharyngeal and tracheal stimulation in lesions above T4 should be borne in mind and can be prevented by 20 mcg/ks of atropine administered intravenously (19–22). Some investigators question this practice as rarely needed and prefer treatment with atropine on an occurrence basis. Although tracheostomy is rarely needed acutely, once the indications for anterior cervical fusion have been excluded, early tracheostomy provides greater patient comfort and makes eating, talking, and pulmonary toilet easier in those patients who will require prolonged mechanical support.

Once intubation has been accomplished, ventilatory assistance is indicated in patients displaying an elevated $PaCO_2$ or a borderline PaO_2 in the face of maximal sustainable ventilatory efforts. Spontaneously breathing intubated patients with adequate ventilation should be given supplemental oxygen; continuous positive airway pressure (CPAP) may be added incrementally to normalize FRC, thus reducing atelectasis and V/Q mismatching, while improving compliance and lessening the work of breathing. Frequent respiratory assessment is mandatory, especially in view of the frequent cephalad extension of injuries that can occur in the acute period.

No mode of ventilation is inherently superior (13), although synchronized intermittent mandatory ventilation (SIMV) has the theoretical advantages of greater hemodynamic stability and continuing exercise of functional muscles.

Positive end expiratory pressure (PEEP) may be added for considerations already mentioned. The recent introduction of variable pressure support ventilation, in which all spontaneous breaths can be supported at any desired pressure level and synchronized with variable frequency mandatory machine breaths, combines many of the advantages of SIMV with the security of controlled or assist-control ventilation in terms of compensating for potential muscle fatigue. In the exclusively pressure-support mode, fine tuning of muscle work load is possible for training and weaning purposes.

In cases of complete lesions above C3, alternatives to chronic positive pressure ventilation include radiofrequency electrophrenic stimulation in patients with damaged phrenic nuclei but intact phrenic nerves (23), or intermittent negative pressure ventilation in an iron lung when the phrenic nerves are interrupted. Chronic subtotal diaphragmatic dysfunction can be managed by means of a rocking bed, chest cuirass, or pneumobelt (9).

Respiratory complications are the most common cause of death in acute spinal cord injury, with pneumonia being the most important after anoxic death at the time of injury (6,24). In patients with chronic, stabilized conditions, respiratory infections decrease and cause less than 10 percent of the febrile episodes. The importance of aggressive pulmonary toilet in addressing this problem was evidenced by a 33 percent decrease in prolonged ventilation as a result of such measures as careful monitoring of pulmonary function, vigorous chest physical therapy, and early bronchoscopy and lavage if lobar collapse develops as shown by chest roentgenographs (25). Any fever accompanied by leukocytosis or physical and/or radiographic evidence of pneumonitis should be aggressively treated.

Cardiovascular Complications

The hemodynamic sequelae of spinal cord injury follow a sequential pattern beginning at the moment of injury. First, it has been well documented experimentally (26) that for 3 to 4 minutes following spinal cord compression, a sudden drastic increase in systolic blood pressure, between 200 and 250 mmHg, occurs. This has been attributed both to an early thoracic sympathetic outflow and to a later, adrenally mediated secretion of catecholamines (27). The possible role of this abrupt pressor response in augmenting the extent of hemorrhagic necrosis and releasing possible mediators of secondary injury is discussed later in this chapter, in the section on pathophysiology.

Experimental cord injury has also been shown to result in transient but significant increases in intracranial pressure, blood–brain barrier permeability, brain water, and extravascular lung water with a marked decrease in cerebral blood flow (28). This investigation verified the extreme increase in blood pressure (to a mean of 225 mmHg), which lasted for 6 minutes, and also showed increases in pulmonary artery pressure, pulmonary capillary occlusion pressure, central venous pressure, and cardiac output. However, the intracerebral and pulmonary changes occurred before the cardiovascular changes were fully developed. This, along with the fact that phentolamine pretreatment sufficient to prevent the cardiovascular changes did not prevent the brain and lung events, seems to support independent but causally linked mechanisms producing both processes. At any rate, this work is compatible with the clinically observed susceptibility to pulmonary (29) and cerebral edema seen during the resuscitation of spinal cord injured patients and reinforces the advisability of early hemodynamic monitoring to guide fluid management in these patients.

Because spinal cord injured patients rarely reach medical attention within minutes of their injury, acute hypertension is rarely, if ever, observed. Most patients manifest varying degrees of hypotension. This phase, commonly called *spinal shock*, features hypotension, bradycardia, decreased total peripheral resistance, low or normal central venous pressure, and normal or elevated cardiac output (29). Orthostatic and other pressor reflexes are diminished or absent, and thermoregulation is lost. At the same time, somatic and visceral motor and sensory loss below the level of the lesion is observed. The extent of these changes is a result of the level of the cord injury. Injuries at or above T1 may result in mean blood pressures as low as 40 mmHg. The observed bradycardia may be due to unopposed vagal tone secondary to loss of the cardiac accelerator fibers (T1 to T4), but many believe that the Bainbridge reflex, caused by a fall in right atrial and central venous pressures, is a more important contributing factor, because bradycardia is seen with lesions below T4. The critical level above which significant hypotension will be manifested is T6 to T7.

This phase of spinal shock may last days to weeks but is more abbreviated than the period of skeletal muscleflaccid paralysis. Unfortunately, no one has delineated the point at which the sympathetic neurons regain their functional ability, now autonomous from higher control; but it is clear that they do regain some tonic activity as well as the ability for reflex reaction as evidenced by the unpredictable onset of potentially catastrophic sympathetic reflex spasticity.

Alterations in cardiovascular function during the subacute and chronic phases of spinal cord injury feature the persistence of a slightly low to normal blood pressure and pulse rate in most patients, punctuated by episodes of severe hypertension in up to 85 percent of patients with lesions at or above T6. These hypertensive spasms are triggered by day-to-day stimuli—most often distention of a hollow viscus, such as bladder or rectum. Other stimuli—including temperature, contractions of labor, and surgery—may be particularly potent (30). The tendency toward reflex hypertension is called *autonomic hyperreflexia*. Its symptoms include facial paresthesias, nasal congestion, severe headache, dyspnea, nausea, and blurred vision. Typical diagnostic signs are vasoconstrictive pallor, sweating, piloerection below the level of the lesion (31), vasodilation, and flushing above the lesion site, accompanied by bradycardia and severe hypertension (32). Subarachnoid and retinal hemorrhages have been observed, which eventuate in syncope, convulsions, and finally death if the hypertension continues unabated (30).

The neuroanatomic correlates of this syndrome include stimuli arising from somatic or visceral receptors, which cause afferent impulses that follow their normal course via the posterior columns and spinothalamic tracts. Spinal cord section prevents these impulses from reaching the brain, but they do synapse with cells of the intermediolateral gray matter, giving rise to efferent sympathetic discharges. Normally these reflexes are localized in nature, but after spinal cord injury they tend to involve most of the sympathetic system below the level of the lesion. The usual homeostatic inhibitory impulses from higher centers following the initial arrival of the afferent impulses are never triggered. Intense, unabated somatic and visceral muscle contractions, arteriolar spasm, sweating, and piloerection are caused by the unchecked sympathetic reflexes below the cord lesion. Above the cord lesion, the hypertension caused by the arteriolar spasm and adrenal secretion activates carotid sinus and aortic arch baroreceptors, as well as other CNS reflexes, to cause vagally induced bradycardia as well as generalized vasodilation. These measures, however, are insufficient to prevent the hypertension when the lesion is above the origin of the splanchnic sympathetic outflow (T4 to T6). The time at which spastic autonomic or somatic reflex activity supersedes spinal shock and flaccid paralysis is difficult to predict and may occur 1 to 3 weeks or more after injury (32).

Cardiac arrhythmias and electrocardiographic abnormalities may also contribute to cardiovascular risk in these patients. In monkeys, acute, midthoracic spinal cord compression, besides producing hypertension, also usually results in sinus or nodal bradycardia. Moreover, this initial response often precedes the pressor response. The initial bradyarrhythmias are followed by premature atrial and ventricular contractions, A-V dissociation, or ventricular tachycardias. Atropine prevents the bradycardia, whereas propranolol prevents the delayed ventricular tachyarrhythmias (33). The electrocardiogram frequently shows ST-T wave changes variously interpreted as left ventricular strain pattern or consistent with subendocardial ischemia (13,34). Similar arrhythmias have been reported in 75 percent of autonomic hyper-reflexia episodes (31). The potential for severe bradycardia, heart block, and even cardiac arrest pursuant to tracheal stimulation in these patients has already been noted (19–21).

Management of these cardiovascular problems is dictated by the physiologic alterations that produce them. In the case of hypotension, a conservative approach is usually indicated, the urgency of treatment being proportional to the degree of hypotension and the symptomatology (CNS, cardiac, renal, and the like) produced. The etiology of the hypotension is usually a decreased venous return following sympathetic denervation, which causes increased venous capacitance as well as some degree of decreased arteriolar tone. However, cautious addition of volume is indicated in view of decreased cardiac reserve. This deficit in ability to accommodate excess volume is a natural consequence of the inability to further increase venous capacitance as the venous reservoir becomes full. Central venous pressure increases relatively little, until the point when volume equals capacity, and then rises abruptly. On the other hand, left ventricular and left atrial pressures increase proportionately with filling volume, and such indices as pulmonary capillary occlusion pressure (PCOP) provide an early measure of volume status before CVP finally rises equivalently. Furthermore, sympathetically mediated reflex increases in heart rate and contractility are not possible in the event of lesions above T1 (35). Finally, the possibility of altered pulmonary capillary permeability to water during the acute phase of spinal cord injury, as discussed, may play a role in the observed susceptibility to pulmonary edema during resuscitation of these patients, as occurred in 44 percent of patients in one series (29).

In view of these findings, early use of pulmonary artery catheters in monitoring fluid resuscitation during spinal shock would seem prudent. Not only are filling pressures and volume status readily assessable, but cardiac output and total peripheral resistance (TPR) can also be measured and manipulated if they are found to contribute to the hypotension. One clinical investigator (36) has used pulmonary arterial hemodynamic monitoring to categorize three groups of spinal cord injury patients. Rapid fluid infusion (50 ml/min in 250 ml increments), leg raising, or military antishock trousers (MAST) were used to increase central volume. One group of patients displayed a 3 to 4 mmHg rise in PCOP, which settled to a level 2 mmHg above control, with concomitant increases in cardiac output. A second group showed similar increases in PCOP, which then returned to baseline, with no net change in cardiac output. The third group showed progressive increases in PÇOP and no change or a fall in cardiac output. He interpreted these findings as indicating adequate volume loading in the first instance, the need for more volume in the second group, and excessive volume and/or an indication for inotropic support in the last group. These guidelines seem appropriate in optimizing filling pressures at the lowest value yielding adequate cardiac output and perfusion pressures.

If, in spite of volume loading, cardiac output and mean arterial pressure are such that spinal cord and other organ hypoperfusion seems likely, inotropic support is indicated. One study compared the efficacy of either dopamine or transfusion in raising mean arterial pressure and augmenting SCBF in rats. Although both yielded improvements in these two variables, transfusion alone was better than dopamine alone (37). The demonstration that naloxone-mediated increases in systemic blood pressure and spinal cord blood flow may be mediated by augmented endogenous plasma dopamine levels in the systemic circulation also suggests that this inotrope may be used when indicated without adversely affecting the potential for spinal cord recovery (38).

The management of autonomic hyperreflexia is problematic in conscious patients, because the offending stimulus is not perceived, and headache or other symptoms of an already severely elevated blood pressure is usually the first clue that an episode is in progress. The aim in chronic spinal cord injured patients is, therefore, to avoid known stimuli through such measures as regular self-catheterization. Persistent attacks may require surgical or chemical ablation of the afferent pathways initiating the reflex through such measures as sacral neurotomy, dorsal rhizotomy, and use of subarachnoid phenol or alcohol. Pharmacological regimens investigated for preventing or treating autonomic hyperreflexia include ganglionic blockers (trimethaphan, hexamethonium, pentolinium), catecholamine depleters (guanethidine), alpha-adrenergic blockers (phentolamine, phenoxybenzamine) and direct-acting vasodilators (nitroprusside). Unfortunately, many of the studies were small, lacked controls, or featured concomitant use of anesthetics. Consequently, comparison of the various drugs is difficult. Unpleasant side effects have also limited their usefulness. Finally, the ability to control visceral and somatic muscle spasms is not achieved when blood pressure is controlled only by adrenergic blockers or direct-acting vasodilators. Basically, any treatment regimen for an acute episode that controls the arteriolar spasm and arrhythmias while maintaining cardiac output is acceptable.

Attempts at the prevention of autonomic hyperreflexia during surgery and anesthesia have met with more success. Schonwald et al. (39) reported a series of 219 patients with spinal cord injuries. Of those patients with lesions at or above T5, 33 percent underwent general anesthesia with halothane (37 cases) or enflurane (12 cases), and none of these developed autonomic hyperreflexia or arrhythmias. Of nine patients in this group receiving nitrous oxide–narcotic anesthesia, two developed intraoperative hyperreflexia. In 97 cases of spinal anesthesia with tetracaine, no attacks occurred, but one lidocaine spinal anesthetic apparently wore off before the end of urological surgery, resulting in autonomic hyperreflexia. The author noted the level of injury as a major factor influencing the technical ease and feasibility of lumbar subarachnoid block, with low levels of injury resulting in failure in three of 19 patients, most likely as a result of previous spinal surgery or traumatic distortion of the anatomy.

It should be borne in mind that successes in preventing hyperreflexia intraoperatively are not infrequently reversed by episodes occurring in the recovery room as the patient recovers from anesthesia; therefore, continued intensive monitoring and such measures as temperature regulation and bladder or bowel evacuation should be routine.

Significant arrhythmias, such as ventricular tachycardia, are usually attendant to episodes of autonomic hyperreflexia and can likewise be prevented by adequate anesthetic depth or neural blockade in the surgical patient, or the other modalities discussed previously for day-to-day prophylaxis. Any life-threatening tachyarrhythmia that occurs in spite of prophylactic measures should be treated with beta-adrenergic blockers (concurrent alpha-adrenergic blockade is mandatory if significant hypertension is present) or other indicated antiarrhythmics. The baseline high vagal tone of these patients should be kept in mind and atropine and pacemaking capability should be available if the combination of vagal tone and antiarrhythmic therapy results in sinus arrest, heart block, or too slow a rate to support adequate cardiac output. The potential need for atropine to treat the vagal reflexes attending tracheal stimulation should be anticipated (22).

Genitourinary Complications

Acute renal failure, although uncommon, may occur in spinal cord injured patients as a result of hypotension, dehydration, sepsis, use of nephrotoxic drugs, acute obstruction, associated kidney trauma, and other influences. During the chronic phase of spinal cord injury, renal failure becomes a progressively more important cause of death, accounting for 20 to 75 percent of mortality (24). In one series, renal failure caused only 4.5 percent of all deaths in patients surviving only 2 years but caused 60 percent or more of deaths among those surviving more than 10 years. Overall, renal failure is the factor producing death in 36 percent of all spinal cord injured patients (32). Pyelonephritis, amyloidosis, and hypertension were the most commonly identified proximate causes of death (24).

Urinary retention, more often a problem in the flaccid lower motor neuron bladder than in the spastic upper motor neuron type, predisposes the patient to autonomic reflexes and cystitis. Vesicoureteral reflux may result from this cause as well as neurogenic causes; repetitive ascending pyelonephritis occurs, leading eventually to secondary renal and adrenal amyloidosis and insufficiency. Neuropathic bladder outflow obstruction often contributes to the problem. Renal calculi tend to be recurrent in these patients. They are most often of the triple-phosphate variety associated with urease-producing bacteria (e.g., *Proteus* spp.); however, some investigators believe that hypercalciuria may play a limited role (24). A large proportion of surgery in chronic spinal cord injured patients is devoted to cystoscopy, urological invasive diagnostic studies, stone removal, lithotripsy, and urinary drainage or diversion procedures.

Urinary tract infections are a persistent problem. One autopsy series found a 90 percent incidence of genitourinary disease including acute and chronic pyelonephritis (65 percent), cystitis (74.5 percent), nephrolithiasis (11.8 percent), and other genitourinary infections (39.2 percent). Another pathological study reported secondary amyloidosis in almost all specimens with an average post-injury survival of 12 years (32). Prophylactic drug regimens have not been successful in substantially decreasing bacteriuria and bacteremia. Intermittent bladder catheterization seems to result in fewer infections and fewer instances of urolithiasis and renal dysfunction when compared with indwelling catheterization (at the expense of considerable time and equipment), but conclusive prospective studies are lacking (24).

Renal insufficiency causes disturbances of the fluid and electrolyte, cardiovascular, and other systems. Hyponatremia, hypoproteinemia, hypocalcemia, increased extracellular and total body water, hypertension, and congestive heart failure may all be caused or exacerbated. These, as well as altered drug clearance, are clearly of concern to the anesthesiologist, and careful evaluation of renal function is a must. The avoidance of potentially nephrotoxic drugs is obviously advisable.

Proteinuria is usually the earliest sign of renal dysfunction, although it is qualitative rather than quantitative (32). Serum creatinine studies may be misleading in view of the decrease in muscle mass seen in chronic quadriplegics. Although intravenous pyelography allows excellent visualization of the upper urinary tract, it is limited by potential allergic reactions, discomfort during the procedure and preparation, potential nephrotoxicity of the contrast material, cumulative radiation, and the fact that significant functional impairment may precede detectable anatomic alterations. Renal scintigraphic determination of effective renal plasma flow seems to be a sensitive indicator of renal dysfunction and also correlates with the presence of calculi and altered renal architecture; it may be used for serial follow-up of these patients and in determining the need for an intravenous pyelogram (40,41).

Sexual dysfunction is the usual finding in these patients. Male patients suffer from impotence and decreased or absent ability to achieve orgasm and ejaculation. Infertility is frequent; abnormal spermatocytes are seen. The effects are more pronounced the higher the lesion, and no underlying endocrinologic cause has been found. Female patients have altered sexual function on the basis of sensory and motor deficits, although normal menses usually resume within 1 to 3 months of the injury (24). Female fertility seems to be unimpaired, although premature labor and delivery are more common. Sensory loss may make labor unknown to the mother, predisposing to delivery under unfavorable conditions. Weekly examination after 32 weeks of gestation is advised, and bedrest is indicated if any effacement is detected. Autonomic hyperreflexia is a major threat. It may be triggered by bowel or bladder stimuli as well as labor itself. Induction of labor has also been associated with a high risk of hyperreflexia and is relatively contraindicated. Spinal, epidural, and even general analgesia and anesthesia seem to decrease hyperreflexive episodes effectively (42,43).

Abnormal Response to Depolarizing Muscle Relaxants

Of great importance to the anesthesiologist is the massive translocation of intracellular potassium from skeletal muscle to the extracellular space following the administration of a depolarizing muscle relaxant such as succinylcholine. This phenomenon may occur as early as 3 days after injury and is thought to result from the denervation process of overgrowth and spread of cholinergic nicotinic receptors to include extrajunctional sarcolemma. This results in supersensitivity to depolarizing agents, whereby the entire affected muscle mass depolarizes synchronously and releases large amounts of potassium into the circulation (44).

A number of important points should be emphasized. First, the magnitude of potassium release is more a function of the amount of muscle mass affected than of the amount of drug given: 20 milligrams of succinylcholine have been noted to result in a serum potassium concentration of 13.6 meg/L (45). Also, the causative overgrowth of receptors may well occur before spasticity replaces flaccid muscle paralysis. Finally, pretreatment with a "defasciculating" dose of nondepolarizing relaxants does not reliably block the occurrence of significant hyperkalemia. Because the precise onset of supersensitivity is unpredictable, depolarizing agents should be avoided in all spinal cord injured patients.

Should the inadvertent administration of succinylcholine occur, electrocardiographic changes progress from atrial conduction disturbances to prolonged PR interval (> 7 mEq/L), tall peaked T waves (7 to 9 mEq/L), progressive widening and aberration of the QRS complex (> 6 to 7 mEq/L), and finally to sinusoidal ventricular complexes and ventricular fibrillation when serum potassium concentration exceeds 12 to 14 mEq/L.

Pharmacologic treatment includes sodium bicarbonate (44 to 88 mEq) and glucose-insulin (1 to 2 units per 5 gm of dextrose) administration to shift potassium intracellularly, as well as calcium (0.5 to 1 gm) to antagonize the membrane effects of potassium. Hyperventilation may also be employed acutely. If circulation fails, CPR is, of course, mandatory to support cellular metabolism (which will resequester the potassium in 10 to 15 minutes) as well as to circulate resuscitative drugs.

Altered Thermoregulation

Temperature regulation is impaired for a number of reasons (46). Afferent information to the hypothalamic thermoregulatory center is interrupted. Sympathetic denervation causes cutaneous vasodilation, which increases heat loss. Also, inability to shiver or sweat limits the ability to increase or decrease body temperature, respectively. Spinal cord injured patients, therefore, become relatively poikilothermic. Efforts to avoid both hypothermia and hyperthermia are necessary. The use of a heating–cooling mattress, variable operating room temperatures, the adjustment of ventilator circuit temperature and humidity, and intravenous fluid temperatures tailored to the situation allow either a raising or a lowering of body temperature as indicated.

Other Systemic Alterations

Spinal cord injury produces alterations in a number of other systems, the more salient of which will be summarized here. Several recent reviews detail and discuss these and other sequelae in more detail (13,24). Besides the changes in fluid and electrolyte status caused by the occurrence of renal insufficiency, hypercalcemia and hypercalciuria have been observed in the early stages of spinal cord injury. This phenomenon occurs most often in young male patients, seems to result from calcium release from denervated (flaccid) muscle and possibly from bone stores, and occurs in the first year with a peak around 10 weeks after injury. It is more common in higher level injuries, and serum sodium and parathyroid hormone levels are normal (47). When hypercalcemia is severe, symptoms include anorexia, nausea and vomiting, abdominal pain, polyuria, constipation, dehydration, psychosis, depressed mental status, and eventually coma. Shortening of the QT interval is seen on the electrocardiogram. Hypertension and ventricular arrhythmias may occur. Treatment includes rehydration with saline, potent diuretics, glucocorticoids, and if necessary, calcitonin. In contrast, long-term spinal cord injured patients develop osteoporosis as a result of increased calcium loss and, especially in the case of supervening renal failure, become hypocalcemic.

The skin of denervated areas becomes atrophic and susceptible to pressure sores. Underlying bone is at risk of osteomyelitis. In addition, pathologic fractures often result from the osteoporosis. Skeletal muscle spasticity or contractures complicate skin and general patient care and make surgical positioning difficult.

Heterotopic calcification occurs below the level of injury in 50 percent of patients, primarily involving the proximal two joints of the upper and lower extremities. Alkaline phosphatase is elevated, and acute inflammation may be apparent at the involved site. Commencing weeks to months after injury, the process usually stabilizes within $1\frac{1}{2}$ years and may vary from asymptomatic to a debilitating condition that decreases range of motion (24).

Average metabolic rates are usually depressed after injury, but catabolism and hypoproteinemia can occur acutely, especially when infection occurs. Increased protein and caloric intake can overcome this tendency.

Endocrine function is usually normal when assessed, with two possible exceptions. A number of investigators have documented moderate glucose intolerance, often with hyperinsulinemia, suggesting relative resistance to endogenous insulin (glucagon levels were normal) (48). Also, the potential for adrenal insufficiency after steroid therapy should be considered.

Hematologic studies show anemia in 52 percent of patients with normal kidney function, which may be either normocytic hypochromic in nature (56 percent) or normochromic (32 percent). Possible causes for these anemias include increased plasma water in response to augment-

ed venous capacity, significant pressure sores, and chronic or severe urinary tract infections.

The digestive system is affected as well. Gastrointestinal bleeding may occur acutely in up to 20 percent of patients. Gastric distention, ileus, and nonspecific liver dysfunction with a normal serum bilirubin are common complications—usually occurring during the first week after injury and resolving over several weeks, although occasionally persisting longer. Pancreatitis also occurs, but it is unknown if this is related to the cord injury per se. Diagnosis of these and other intra-abdominal emergencies may be difficult as a result of altered sensation. Vomiting may occur without pain or nausea. The newly described syndrome of gastroduodenal motor dysfunction, possibly secondary to loss of adrenergic inhibitory control, features altered motility, pain, and vomiting. It is seen in certain spinal cord injury cases and responds to low doses of adrenergic agonists such as ephedrine (49). Gastric and bowel distention and the tendency toward vomiting in most of these disorders warrants a high index of suspicion and preparation for airway protection on the part of the anesthesiologist. The distention itself may hinder ventilatory ability.

Last but not least, chronic pain is a problem in many of these patients. It can cause and reinforce the tendency toward depression that is often present. Proper management of pain and psychosocial support have proved essential for adaptation and rehabilitation of the patient.

ANESTHETIC MANAGEMENT OF PATIENTS WITH SPINAL CORD INJURY

In view of the high percentage of spinal cord injured patients with associated injuries, the anesthesiologist may be required to care for these patients during initial diagnostic procedures, during emergency operations aimed at managing life-threatening trauma elsewhere in the body (e.g., closed head injury, hemorrhage), for emergency spinal decompression, or for other procedures (e.g., urological, plastic) during the more chronic phase of injury. The foregoing discussion of acute and chronic derangements in systemic function provides the basis for rational and safe anesthetic management as well as daily care of these patients.

Acutely, maintenance of normal acid–base and blood gas parameters, as well as adequate spinal cord perfusion pressures, is paramount in importance. Experimental work in cats has suggested that there is no therapeutic advantage of either hypercarbia or hypocarbia over normocarbia in terms of both neurologic recovery and histological tissue preservation. Although not statistically significant, mortality and tissue preservation results suggested that hypocarbia may be less harmful than hypercarbia in the acute post-injury period (50). Consequently, it seems prudent to maintain $PaCO_2$ in the 35 to 40 mmHg range. Management of closed head injury with increased intracranial pressure takes precedence in this area ($PaCO_2$ maintained between 25 and 30 mmHg).

Hypoxemia must be prevented by careful attention to minimizing significant physiologic shunting, which is suggested by the inability to maintain a $PaCO_2$ greater than 60 mmHg with an FIo_2 of 50 percent. Possible contributing causes such as hemothorax or pneumothorax, pulmonary embolization of fat or thrombi, foreign body or gastric content aspiration, and noncardiogenic pulmonary edema should be searched for and either excluded or treated appropriately. PEEP may be required to decrease shunting and increase oxygenation once pneumothorax or other reversible causes of hypoxemia have been excluded. However, the possible negative effect of PEEP on cardiac output and intracranial pressure must be considered. In case the patient is not already intubated and this is necessary, it should be carried out as during acute resuscitation, with caution used in avoiding neck displacement, managing airway reflexes, avoiding aspiration, and with the capability of treating severe vagal bradycardia or arrest.

Cardiovascular management, as discussed already, most frequently requires judicious repletion of intravascular volume to restore normal venous return and filling pressures.

However, it should be recalled that three of 19 patients in the study cited on volume loading in the acute post-injury period actually showed decreased cardiac output and progressive increase in PAOP. This required decreasing or eliminating halothane or other myocardial depressants or even the use of an inotrope (36). During the phase of spinal shock, lasting anywhere from 3 days to 6 weeks (average of 3 weeks), the advantages of pulmonary artery catheter monitoring are obvious in maintaining hemodynamics and avoiding pulmonary edema (22). Also, when it is employed, it allows quantitation of shunt and monitoring of the respiratory and hemodynamic effects of PEEP.

In choosing fluids for perioperative resuscitation and maintenance, the use of glucose-containing solutions is questionable. Recent investigations have documented deleterious effects of the hyperglycemia resulting from dextrose infusion on the neurological outcome after cerebral (50a) and spinal cord (50b) ischemia. In the latter study, Drummond and Moore showed that mild to moderate increases of plasma glucose averaging only 40 mg/dl tripled the incidence of paraplegia in rabbits subjected to transient spinal cord ischemia following aortic occlusion (nine of 10 dextrose-treated animals as compared with three of 10 control animals). The authors considered end products of hypoxic glucose metabolism, such as lactate (which has experimentally verified adverse effects on physiologic and histologic outcome after cerebral ischemia), to be the most likely mechanism by which enhanced glucose availability could worsen tolerance to ischemia. However, this was not elucidated by the study design. Of note was the lack of correlation between the magnitude of plasma glucose elevation and the extent of neurologic injury. This result was thought to possibly be attributable to differences in intracellular glucose availability not reflected by extracellular concentration, perhaps as a result of varying insulin effect. In light of these findings, routine use of dextrose containing fluids, as part of initial resuscitation, or perioperatively in cases in which the development or worsening of spinal cord ischemia is possible, should be confined to those instances in which a definite medical indication exists and close monitoring and control of plasma glucose is possible. The data were not sufficient to recommend that an already elevated plasma glucose be lowered emergently when encountered intraoperatively, keeping in mind that electrolyte, neuromuscular, and other potential systemic alterations are also necessary, with management as already outlined.

Of relevance for surgery during the acute phase of spinal cord injury or for any procedure that might feasibly result in new or worsened injury, Cole and coworkers (50c) recently investigated the effect of various anesthetic regimens on the susceptibility to ischemic SCI on anesthetized rats in a controlled, blinded fashion. Of the three agents investigated—halothane, fentanyl/nitrous oxide, and subarachnoid lidocaine—all increased the duration of ischemia required to produce spinal cord injury. No one agent was relatively more favorable or deleterious than the others in terms of final neurologic outcome. Possible mechanisms for this protective effect, while not clear at present, may include depression of spinal cord metabolism, effects on SCBF, alterations in endogenous catecholamine levels, alteration of opiate receptor activity, or interaction with other potential mediators of secondary SCI (e.g., prostaglandins). Hence, although anesthetics have not been shown to play a role in treating spinal cord injury, in this model the anesthetized state using the aforementioned agents seems to provide some degree of protection against its occurrence.

As noted by Schonwald et al. (39) and Lampert (43), both a sufficiently deep general anesthetic technique, employing halothane or enflurane, and regional anesthesia (subarachnoid or epidural) effectively prevented episodes of autonomic hyperreflexia. An alternative when surgical considerations require high spinal levels (above T5) is subarachnoid block followed by light general anesthesia, with endotracheal intubation and controlled ventilation.

A study in dogs (51) showed consistent statistically significant increases in lumbosacral spinal cord blood flow with a lesser, nonsignificant tendency toward increases in thoracic and cervical cord flow after subarachnoid tetracaine, as long as mean arterial pressure remained 100 mmHg or more. The favorable effect was blocked by the addition of epinephrine to the tetracaine; in fact, a nonsignificant tendency toward decreased thoracic and cervical cord flows actually occurred. Hence, spinal anesthesia may improve cord blood flow, and vasoconstrictors should not be added to the anesthetic.

Although spinal or epidural anesthetics have been considered hemodynamically unpredictable in these patients (32), baseline hemodynamic stability as well as ablation of autonomic hyperreflexia has been verified by many other workers (39,42). One recent study (52) showed such stability of cardiac output, stroke volume, and heart rate during cystoscopy that it was actually impossible to determine from the data alone when bladder distention and emptying had occurred. Also, no ephedrine was required during the study. These authors emphasized the importance of judicious choice of the anesthetic dosage and attention to intravascular volume as factors contributing to the recorded stability. A note of caution is warranted in patients with spinal subarachnoid block of cerebrospinal fluid circulation because a 14 percent incidence of neurological deterioration after removal of cerebrospinal fluid or from delayed leakage through the puncture sites has been reported (53). Continuous intra-arterial and pulmonary arterial or central venous pressure monitoring allows safe management of any of these techniques as well as the detection and management of hyperreflexive breakthroughs.

The obstetrical management of women with spinal cord injury during labor and delivery or cesarean section, as mentioned, is complicated by the possibility of autonomic hyperreflexia, threatening both the mother and the fetus. Although many anesthesiologists think that epidural anesthetics in these circumstances, while not needed for analgesia, are indicated for and are effective in preventing hyperreflexive episodes (42,54–56), others fear hypotension as a potential complication. In our personal practice, epidural anesthesia with careful titration of drug dosage and maintenance of normal cardiac filling pressures is used if not otherwise contraindicated by the obstetric condition.

Techniques based on nitrous oxide, oxygen, and narcotics seem less recommendable in light of their failure to prevent hyperreflexia in two of nine patients. Regardless of the technique employed, direct-acting arteriolar dilators (e.g., nitroprusside), alpha-adrenergic blockers (e.g., phentolamine), and antiarrhythmics (e.g., lidocaine, propranolol, and esmolol), new antihypertensives (e.g., labetalol and nifedipine), and atropine should be readily available (39). The need to avoid succinylcholine is reiterated; however, the new short-acting nondepolarizing agents make this constraint clinically feasible, because they are a reasonable alternative.

The increased utilization of extracorporeal shock wave lithotripsy (ESWL) and the incidence of nephrolithiasis in spinal cord injured patients prompts consideration of the proper anesthetic management for ESWL in such patients. Five traumatic quadriplegic patients were studied during ESWL performed without either general or regional anesthesia (57). Although some increase in blood pressure was noted in all patients, it was transient or mild in most; however, in two patients the increase was sufficient to warrant therapy for the hypertension. An effort to avoid hydronephrosis and bladder distention was made by catheterization, ureteral stents, or percutaneous nephrostomies in most patients. Two patients with intact pinprick sensation in the skin overlying the impact area received field blocks (50 to 60 ml of 0.25 percent bupivacaine). All of the patients received incremental intravenous doses of diazepam (2.5 mg) and fentanyl (25 μg). Total doses ranged from 25 to 200 μg of fentanyl and from 5 to 15 mg of diazepam. Because none of the patients demonstrated other signs or symptoms of autonomic hyperreflexia, they concluded that the hypertension was probably caused by another etiology, such as the translocation of blood from the peripheral to the central vascular compart-

ment. They conclude that ESWL may be safely performed using their methodology without risking possible morbidity from general or spinal anesthesia.

There are a number of problems with this study. First, the number of patients is small and without a control group. Second, the lack of hemodynamic monitoring leaves their explanation for the central vascular overload suppositional. The etiology of autonomic hyperreflexia would have been supported by measurement of serum catecholamines during the procedure, because increased serum norepinephrine, but not epinephrine, has been found during hyperreflexive episodes (58). Until the results of further controlled studies are available, it may be advisable to utilize an anesthetic prophylactic technique with appropriate safeguards.

In the case of incomplete spinal cord lesions, somatosensory-evoked potentials (SSEP) and motor-evoked potentials (MEP) can be useful in monitoring cord function (see below). This is true during surgery to relieve cord compression or to correct spinal deformity as well as during the acute phase of spinal cord injury, when neurologic status may progressively worsen. Of possible value during surgery in patients with incomplete lesions is the observation that etomidate improved the SSEP in patients receiving neuroleptanesthesia by increasing the latency and increasing the amplitude of the short latency cortical responses (59). A 0.3 to 0.5 mg/kg bolus of etomidate followed by a continuous infusion of 0.01 to 0.05 mg/kg/min was used. Areas of potential concern that should be resolved include the possibility that the improved amplitude may be associated with etomidate's tendency to produce myoclonic activity and its ability to produce adrenocortical suppression for 8 to 24 hours. The clinical significance of these two drug properties when etomidate is used on a short-term basis remains to be documented, in contrast to the known adrenal insufficiency (which required treatment and influenced mortality) when the drug was employed for more prolonged sedation in a critical care setting. Further study is needed before there will be widespread acceptance of this technique. However, when SSEP monitoring is considered essential but is technically nonreproducible, etomidate may provide the solution. Another recent report (60) suggests that the use of lower than usual stimulus presentation rates (1.1 to 2.1 Hz, as compared with 5.1 Hz) resolved problems similar to those found in the first study and may provide an acceptable alternative solution.

PATHOPHYSIOLOGY

Spinal cord trauma results in both primary and secondary injuries. The primary injury, if severe enough, results in functional or anatomic disruption of the cord at the scene of the accident with a correspondingly dismal prognosis. The uniformly encountered anatomic and histologic findings associated with such primary injury include direct neurilemmal and neuronal disruption and/or destruction, petechial hemorrhages, gross hematomyelia, or even total cord transection—a rare event. The areas rendered nonviable by this primary insult develop cavitating necrosis and ultimately glial scar formation.

The observation that areas of the spinal cord not immediately destroyed by traumatic force subsequently undergo progressive hemorrhagic necrosis, edema, and inflammation at a rate proportional to the severity of the lesion has produced the concept of a secondary injury, perhaps mediated and propagated by mechanisms distinct from the initial mechanical deformation.

The extension of the lesion from the initial gray matter involvement to include the white matter is preceded by endothelial damage with platelet adhesion, platelet aggregation, microvascular occlusion, and embolization of microthrombi. On a macroscopic scale, corresponding vascular stasis, decreased spinal cord blood flow, and ischemia are noted. Axonal degeneration (hydropic and then granular), myelinolysis, cell necrosis, inflammatory infiltrate, and neuronophagia ensue. A striking feature is the finding of intra-axonal calcium hydroxyapatite crystals and mitochondrial calcification. Similar degenerative changes have been observed following in vivo exposure of rat spinal cords to calcium or calcium in the presence of an ionophore (61).

Biochemical events coinciding with this process of progressive autodestruction include a massive translocation of calcium from the extracellular to the intracellular space; decreased $Na+$, $K+$-ATPase activity; the loss of intracellular potassium; activation of phospholipase A_2 leading to arachidonic acid release and its metabolism to lipid peroxides (via free radical attack), prostaglandins (via cyclo-oxygenase), or leukotrienes (via lipoxygenase); increase in total thromboxane A_2, as well as its ratio to prostacyclin; the degradation of axonal and myelin proteins by neutral proteinases; the failure of energy metabolism and protein synthesis; and hypoxia and lactic acidosis (61,62).

The tantalizing aspect of this wealth of biochemical data is that it is possible to organize these events into a positive feedback cascade mechanism activated by the release of certain catalysts from the blood and their initial intracellular flux, caused by the endothelial and neuronal membrane disruption at the initial site of maximal tissue trauma. Calcium (63), in addition to bradykinin, thrombin, and ferrous ion (62), has been cast in such a role. Another investigator (64) made a case for norepinephrine. The basic scheme of such a secondary injury hypothesis is an activation of membrane phospholipase A_2, yielding arachidonic acid, lipid peroxides, free radicals, prostaglandins (mostly thromboxane), and leukotrienes. These can account for membrane lipid destruction, microcirculatory thrombosis and stasis, vasogenic edema, ischemia, and chemotaxis. Calcification of mitochrondria and other intracellular sites secondary to influx through damaged membranes should have obvious deleterious effects on cellular energy metabolism and maintenance of integrity and function. $Na+$, $K+$-ATPase has been shown to be phospholipid dependent and very susceptible to free radical attack and lipid peroxidation (64); this enzyme is needed to maintain normal cellular volume and ion content, membrane potential, and cellular function. Finally, the neutral proteinase, which is the predominant source of increased proteolytic activity in experimental spinal cord injury, is calcium activated (63).

The feasibility of such secondary injury mechanisms is supported by a number of additional observations. The time course of change in tissue concentration of the various proposed mediators closely matches that of the histologic biochemical, and physiologic processes already described above. In the case of calcium, neurologic deficit scores have also been shown to be proportional to the extent of calcium influx, the rise in phospholipase-generated metabolites, vascular damage, and increased tissue water content (65). In addition, exposure of the spinal cord to calcium chloride solution results in similar prostaglandin (thromboxane) generation, proteolysis, and morphologic changes in proportion to the solution molarity (63).

Finally, Faden and his coworkers have demonstrated an increase in the endogenous opioid *kappa* receptor agonist dynorphin, as well as an increase in receptor binding capacity after experimental spinal cord injury in rats that correlates closely with neurologic dysfunction. No change in *mu* or *delta* receptor binding was found. Because intrathecal dynorphin A, but not other opiate agonists, can produce drug-related hindlimb paralysis in the rat, it has been postulated that this opioid system may contribute to the pathophysiology of secondary spinal cord injury (66,67).

However, caution must be exercised in equating close correlation with causation, and further investigation continues. Nevertheless, what has been clearly documented is that in the period following primary spinal cord injury, a progressive decrease in spinal cord blood flow occurs, resulting in marked ischemia associated with a morphologic and biochemical cascade, as detailed above (68). The fact that this sequence may not begin for more than 1 hour, or in some cases as much as 4 hours, after the primary injury suggests the possibility of pharmacological intervention to prevent or alter the ischemic sequence (69).

The normal mean spinal cord blood flow of 40 to 50 ml/100 gm/min is partitioned in a ratio of 3:1 between gray and white matter, respectively (70). Autoregulation of spinal cord blood flow between 60 and 150 mmHg has been demonstrated in rats (71). Spinal cord blood flow has been shown to vary in direct proportion (1:1) with $PaCO_2$ (72). Although conflicting results have been reported as mentioned (73), the preponderance of researchers agree that total spinal cord blood flow decreases significantly from 1 to 4 hours after subtotal experimental injury, with most of the decrease occurring in the central cord region (68).

Spinal cord injury in cats has been shown to abolish autoregulation with the onset of ischemia (74). This would be expected to render the spinal cord susceptible to increased hemorrhage and edema in the face of significantly increased blood pressure, as has been shown experimentally in cats (75). Such a hypertensive phase has been documented for 3 to 4 minutes after experimental spinal cord injury (26,27). Spinal shock, in which endorphin-mediated parasympathetic stimulation has been implicated, decreases spinal cord blood flow in the absence of autoregulation.

Also, vasoconstriction of resistance vessels more readily results in ischemia. Such vasoconstriction may be secondary to some of the mediators already mentioned: a preponderance of thromboxane A_2 over prostacyclin, PGF_2, and slow-reacting substance of anaphylaxis (61). Although the originally proposed increase in spinal cord catecholamines (as a cause of ischemia and hemorrhagic necrosis) (76,77) has not been verified by subsequent investigators, norepinephrine has been shown to significantly reduce spinal cord blood flow when the cord–blood barrier had been disrupted (78). More recent investigations already mentioned have described a number of membrane-damaging factors, operating by way of free radical attack and lipid peroxidation, that may disrupt the cord–blood barrier and that correlate with cord edema. Norepinephrine has been shown capable of activating similar membrane-lipid peroxidation (64). Of interest is the finding that acute ethanol intoxication (blood level of 100 mg/dl) worsens spinal cord hemorrhage and the extent of anatomical damage and impairs recovery of function (79). Possible reasons for this include the direct effects on neuronal conduction, vascular congestion, and increased permeability (altered blood–cord barrier), increased lactate production, increased free radical peroxidation catalyzed by iron, and toxic aldehyde metabolite effects.

On a gross physiologic scale, spinal cord impulse transmission, as assessed by evoked potentials, disappears immediately with complete transection and after a variable delay period in less severe lesions. Somatosensory-evoked potentials (SSEPs) studied in humans distinguished complete anatomic lesions with little or no possibility of recovery from those in patients with complete or incomplete functional deficits but could not predict the degree of functional deficit (80). On the other hand, motor-evoked potentials (MEPs) or corticomotor-evoked potentials (CMEPs) have been shown in both rat and cat dynamic spinal cord injury models to be more sensitive indicators of the onset of injury (81) as well as good predictors of the extent of tissue damage and prognosis for functional recovery (82,83).

RESUSCITATIVE MODALITIES IN SPINAL CORD INJURY

A number of pharmacological and physical measures have been employed in an effort to limit the progression of secondary spinal cord injury and yield improved neurologic recovery. Spinal cord injury may abolish normal autoregulation, causing spinal cord blood flow and blood volume to vary directly with perfusion pressure. Spinal cord perfusion pressure must be maintained close to the middle of the normal autoregulatory range of 60 to 150 mmHg by cautious restoration of a normal circulating blood volume (see Cardiovascular Complications, earlier in this chapter). In addition, glucocorticoids and hyperosmolar agents have frequently been used to decrease posttraumatic edema and increase spinal cord blood flow.

Mannitol draws fluid from the interstitial into the intravascular space and then promotes a net loss of fluid via osmotic diuresis. It has been shown to reduce edema following traumatic canine spinal cord injury (84). In view of the initially low central venous pressures in the acute phase after spinal cord injury and the limited cardiac reserve, allowance must be made for the initial rise and then fall in venous return caused by mannitol.

In a canine model, improved functional recovery after spinal cord injury has been demonstrated with dexamethasone therapy (85). Better recovery of SSEPs and partial restoration of extracellular calcium concentration have been shown in cats receiving 15 to 30 mg/kg of methylprednisolone 45 minutes after spinal cord contusion (86). Others have found less axonal degeneration using morphometric analysis when the same steroid dose was given to rats after spinal cord injury (87). Nonetheless, the multicenter, double-blind randomized clinical trial in humans sponsored by the National Acute Spinal Cord Injury (NASCIS) Study Group failed to find any improvement in motor or sensory neurologic function 1 year after injury as a result of two levels of methylprednisolone therapy (88).

Several cautionary comments regarding interpretation of this study are pointed out by the authors themselves. First, the animal studies may not accurately duplicate conditions of human spinal cord injury, not to mention interspecies differences in anatomy, physiology, or biochemistry. Second, both study arms, 100 mg or 1000 mg initial boluses of methylprednisolone followed by the same dose daily (four divided doses) for 10 days, used doses below the 15 to 30 mg/kg range used in the most successful animal studies. Third, there was no placebo control; the two steroid regimens were compared with each other and then with historic outcome data. Finally, only 12 percent of the patients started treatment within 3 hours of injury and another 20 percent between 3 and 6 hours after injury; the remainder entered the study up to 48 hours after their injury. For these reasons, further investigation is warranted before steroids are determined not to be useful, especially when given earlier and in larger doses.

In view of the potential shortcomings in this study (NASCIS1), the same group of investigators completed a second study (NASCIS2) (88a), which added placebo-controlled and naloxone therapeutic arms to the original study design. The study was carried out in a prospective, randomized, double-blind manner. The study groups received one of three drug regimens: methylprednisolone plus naloxone placebo, naloxone plus methylprednisolone placebo, or methylprednisolone placebo plus naloxone placebo. Each drug or placebo was administered through separate intravenous sites by separate pumps. Methylprednisolone was administered in a bolus dose of 30 mg/kg followed by a maintenance infusion of 5.4 mg/kg/hr, while naloxone was administered in a bolus dose of 5.4 mg/kg followed by a maintenance infusion of 4.0 mg/kg/hr. Both bolus doses were given over a 15-minute period followed in 45 minutes by the maintenance infusion for 23 hours.

As compared with NASCIS1, NASCIS2 found that treatment with the higher 30 mg/kg regimen improved sensory and motor function as evaluated 6 weeks and 6 months after injury. This effect was statistically significant only when treatment was initiated within 8 hours of injury. On the other hand, naloxone failed to influence outcome. The naloxone regimen employed was essentially identical to that employed in the Phase I study, reinforcing its negative conclusions and suggesting the need for evaluation of a higher-dose regimen.

It should be noted, however, that the NASCIS1 study excluded patients with severe associated injuries. Another investigation found that spinal cord injured patients with severe multiple trauma had more than a threefold increase in infections, which often involved multiple organisms and foci, when they received steroid therapy for CNS trauma (4 to 20 mg of dexamethasone every 6 hours). All of the septic deaths occurred in steroid-treated patients (89).

Although NASCIS2 (88a) revealed no increase in septic complications or overall morbidity and mortality and the steroid regimen used was different, a vigilant attitude with regard to possible increased susceptibility to sepsis is still warranted.

The area of opiate antagonist therapy is currently a subject of heated research and debate. Following the demonstration that the opiate antagonist naloxone improved arterial pressure and survival in hemorrhagic and septic shock, investigators studied its effect in spinal shock and in enhancing recovery from spinal cord injury (38).

Intravenous naloxone has effectively prevented or reversed spinal shock in rat and cat cervical cord transection models—significantly increasing mean arterial pressure (MAP), increasing respiratory rate, and decreasing hypothermia (90,91). Also, naloxone in doses of 2 to 20 mg/kg has been shown to yield significant improvement in SSEPs (92) and neurologic function (93).

Although these and many other animal studies supported naloxone's effectiveness, a human Phase I clinical trial of naloxone was less encouraging. This trial showed some clinical improvement only with the highest loading dose of 5.4 mg/kg (IV) followed by continuous hourly infusion of 75 percent of this amount for 23 hours; however, the results fell short of statistical significance. The mortality rate was not greater than expected in similar injuries, but awareness of pain was significantly increased. A possible contributing factor limiting success may be the average interval of 6.6 hours from admission until the start of therapy (94). Further clinical trials are needed. However, a number of animal researchers have recently challenged the effectiveness of naloxone (95–97).

A potentially significant effect of rialoxone therapy in patients undergoing general anesthesia was reported. The patient had received the 5.4 mg/kg regimen mentioned in the preceding paragraph 30 minutes before a stabilization procedure of the thoracolumbar spine was performed. Fentanyl (25 µg/kg), isoflurane (2 to 3.5

percent), thiopental (700 mg), diazepam (10 mg), morphine (15 mg), and sufentanil (0.5 μg/kg) were used during and immediately after surgery to manage hypertension and hyperventilation. This resistance to normally effective anesthetic doses was attributed to an antianalgesic and analeptic effect of the naloxone treatment (98).

Experimental work on the possible sites and mechanisms of action of opiate antagonists has been reviewed (38). Briefly summarized, evidence indicates that naloxone interacts stereospecifically at a central site to inhibit opiate receptor mediated stimulation of the parasympathetic nervous system in achieving improvement of MAP and SCBF. A central outpouring of beta-endorphin following spinal cord injury has been found at the time of cord ischemia, and naloxone may antagonize its effects.

In addition, naloxone elevates peripheral dopamine levels 300 to 400 percent, partially contributing to the hemodynamic effects of naloxone after spinal cord injury. Other catecholamine levels remain unaltered. It is postulated to be an indirect effect, possibly mediated by the central parasympatholysis.

Finally, because naloxone is effective only in dose orders of magnitude greater than those required for *mu* receptor agonist reversal, it is possible that it is acting as a receptor, perhaps the *kappa* receptor, for which it has marginal affinity. Naloxone and a specific *kappa* receptor antagonist have prevented experimental cord damage induced by dynorphin, a κ receptor agonist (see above). In fact, some evidence exists that naloxone acts through nonopioid mechanisms, involving its ability to inhibit membrane damage by free radical-induced lipid peroxidation, act as an antioxidant, modulate calcium fluxes, and increase cyclic-AMP activation of prostaglandins.

Thyrotropin-releasing hormone (TRH), in addition to stimulating release of TSH from the anterior pituitary, is thought to act as a partial physiologic, not pharmacologic, opiate antagonist. It seems to reverse the behavioral and autonomic effects of opiates without antagonizing their analgesic effects. TRH has also improved recovery following experimental spinal cord injury (98a).

Methylprednisolone sodium succinate, alpha-tocopherol (vitamin E), selenium (cofactor of glutathione peroxidase), and DMSO have been shown to be experimentally beneficial in ameliorating spinal cord injury, perhaps as a result of their shared ability to act as antioxidants or reducing agents in scavenging free radicals and interrupting lipid peroxidation reactions (62). Protease inhibitors such as leupeptin have shown promise experimentally (99).

Finally, it should be noted that new physiotherapeutic measures show promise in preserving and enhancing function remaining after spinal cord injury, and initial investigation of chemical and physical stimulation of axonal regeneration is showing some promising results. Functional neuromuscular stimulation has been used to create or enhance knee extension and bicycle ergometer exercises. However, limitation in skeletal strength, the deteriorated condition of the muscles, and lack of cardiopulmonary and other system adjustments to exercise have limited its success. Strength and endurance gains have been made, but relatively easy fatigability remains a problem (100).

Recent studies have demonstrated potential effectiveness of GM-1 ganglioside (101) and a combination of triethanolamine and cytosine arabinoside (102) to markedly stimulate axonal growth in spinal cord transected rats. Continuously applied weak electrical fields achieved similar results in guinea pigs (103). A series of investigations has shown that peripheral nerve grafts or central nervous system implants derived from the embryonal neuraxis can stimulate axonal outgrowth and may prove useful in repairing disrupted intraspinal circuits (104).

Currently, much of this work has proved to be of limited clinical utility. Nevertheless, understanding and new directions for research, as well as more effective application of existing knowledge, are advancing at an unprecedented and encouraging pace. Prompt initiation of currently accepted therapy or experimental protocols in a specialized care center holds the most hope for preserving or restoring function.

Acknowledgments

The authors wish to thank Grune & Stratton for permission to use information previously published in *Seminars in Anesthesia* Vol. VI, No. 4 December 1987, pp. 246–259.

In addition, special thanks go to James E. Cottrell, MD, for editorial assistance, and to Adriene Daviger for preparation of the manuscript.

REFERENCES

1. Kalsbeek WD, McLaurin RL, Harris BSH, III. The national head and spinal cord injury survey: major findings. *J Neurosurg* 1980; 53:519.
2. Eisenberg MG, Tierney DO. Changing demographic profile of the spinal cord injury population: implications for health care support systems. *Paraplegia* 1985; 23:335.
3. Kraus JF. A comparison of recent studies on the extent of the head and spinal cord injury problem in the United States. *J Neurosurg* 1980; 53:535.
4. Green BA, Eismont FJ, O'Heir JT. Spinal cord injury—a systems approach: prevention, emergency medical services, and emergency room management. *Crit Care Clin* 1987; 3:471–493.
5. Woolsey, RM. Rehabilitation outcome following spinal cord injury. *Arch Neurol* 1985; 42:116.
6. Greenberg J, Geisler FH. Management of traumatic spine injuries and acute paralysis. *Neurologic Emergencies* 2nd ed., 1990. Pp. 167.
7. Albin MS. Resuscitation of the spinal cord. *Crit Care Med* 1978; 6:270.
8. Soderstrom CA, McArdle DQ, Ducker TB, et. al. The diagnosis of intra-abdominal injury in patients with cervical cord trauma. *J Trauma* 1983; 23:l061–1065.
9. Luce JM, Culver BH. Respiratory muscle function in health and disease. *Chest* 1982; 81:82.
10. DeTroyer A, Estenne M, Heilporn A. Mechanism of active expiration in tetraplegic subjects. *N Engl J Med* 1986; 314:740.
11. Davis JN, Goldman M, Loh L. Diaphragm function and alveolar hypoventilation. *Q J Med* 1976; 177:87.
12. Heros RC. Spinal cord compression. In Ropper AH, et al., eds, *Neurological and Neurosurgical*

Intensive Care. Baltimore, Md.: University Park Press, 1982. Pp. 231–248.
13. Luce JM. Medical management of spinal cord injury. *Crit Care Med* 1985; 13:126.
14. Forner JV, Llombart RL, Valledor MCV. *The flow-volume loop in tetraplegics.* Paraplegia 1977–78; 15:245.
15. Ledsome JR, Sharp JM. Pulmonary function in acute cervical cord injury. *Am Rev Respir Dis* 1981; 124:41.
16. De Troyer A, Heilporn A. Respiratory mechanics in quadriplegia: the respiratory function of the intercostal muscles. *Am Rev Resp Dis* 1980; 122:591.
17. Gross D, Ladd HW, Riley EJ. The effect of training on strength and endurance of the diaphragm in quadriplegia. *JAMA* 1980; 68:27.
18. Suderman VS, Crosby ET, Lui A. Elective oral tracheal intubation in cervical spine injured patients. *Can J Anaesth* 1991; 38:785–789.
19. Welphy NC, Mathias CJ, Frankel HL. Circulatory reflexes in tetraplegics during artificial ventilation and general anesthesia. *Paraplegia* 1975; 13:172.
20. Winslow EBJ, Lesch M, Talano JV, et al. Spinal cord injuries associated with cardiopulmonary complications. *Spine* 1986; 11:809–812.
21. Abd AG, Braun, NMT. Management of life life-threatening bradycardia in spinal cord injury. *Chest* 1989; 95:701–702.
22. Mackenzie CF, Ducker TB. Cervical cord injury. In Matjasko J, Katz J, eds., *Clinical Controversies in Neuroanesthesia and Neurosurgery.* Orlando, Florida: Grune & Stratton, 1986.
23. Glenn WWL, Holcomb BEE, McLaughlin AJ. Total ventilatory support in a quadriplegic patient with radiofrequency electrophrenic respiration. *N Engl J Med* 1972; 286:513.
24. Sugarman B. Medical complications of spinal cord injury. *Quart J Med* 1985; 54:3.
25. McMichan JC, Michel L, Westbrook PR. Pulmonary dysfunction following traumatic quadriplegia. *JAMA* 1980; 243:528.
26. Rawe SE, Perot PL. Pressor response resulting from experimental contusion injury to the spinal cord. *J Neurosurg* 1979; 50:58.
27. Young W, DeCrescito V, Tomasula JJ. The role of the sympathetic nervous system in pressor responses induced by spinal injury. *J Neurosurg* 1980; 52:473.
28. Albin MS, Bunegin L, Wolf S. Brain and lungs at risk after cervical spinal cord transection: intracranial pressure, brain water, blood–brain barrier permeability, cerebral blood flow, and extravascular lung water changes. *Surg Neurol* 1985; 24:191.

29. Meyer GL, Berman IR, Doty DB. Hemodynamic responses to acute quadriplegia with or without chest trauma. *J Neurosurg* 1971; 34:168.

30. Kurnick NB. Autonomic hyperreflexia and its control in patients with spinal cord lesions. *Ann Intern Med* 1956; 44:678.

31. Kendrick WW, Scott JW, Jousse AT. Reflex sweating and hypertension in traumatic transverse myelitis. *Treatment Serv Bull* (Ottawa) 1953; 8:437.

32. Desmond J. Paraplegia: problems confronting the anaesthesiologist. *Can Anaesth Soc J* 1970; 17:435.

33. Evans DE, Kobrine AI, Rizzoli HV. Cardiac arrhythmias accompanying acute compression of the spinal cord. *J Neurosurg* 1980; 52:52.

34. Quimby CA, Williams RN, Greifenstein FE. Anesthetic problems of the acute quadriplegic patient. *Anesth Analg* 1973; 52:333.

35. Troll GF, Dohrmann GJ. Anaesthesia of the spinal cord-injured patient: cardiovascular problems and their management. *Paraplegia* 1975; 13:162.

36. MacKenzie, CF, Shin B, Krishnaprasad D, et al. Assessment of cardiac and respiratory function during surgery in patients with acute quadriplegia. *J Neurosurg* 1985; 62:843.

37. Dolan EJ, Tator CH. The effect of blood transfusion, dopamine, and gamma hydroxybutyrate on posttraumatic ischemia of the spinal cord. *J Neurosurg* 1982; 56:350.

38. Hamilton AJ, Black PM, Carr DB. Contrasting actions of naloxone in experimental spinal cord trauma and cerebral ischemia: a review. *Neurosurgery* 1985; 17:845.

39. Schonwald G, Fish KJ, Perkash I. Cardiovascular complications during anesthesia in chronic spinal cord injured patients. *Anesthesiology* 1981; 55:550.

40. Kuhlemeier KV, Huang CT, Lloyd LK. Effective renal plasma flow: clinical significance after spinal cord injury. *J Urol* 1985; 133:758.

41. Kuhlemeier KV, Lloud LK, Stover SL. Long-term follow-up of renal function after spinal cord injury. *J Urol* 1985; 134:510.

42. Verduyn WH. Spinal cord injured women, pregnancy and delivery. *Paraplegia* 1986; 24:231.

43. Lambert DH, Deane RS, Mazuzan JE. Anesthesia and the control of blood pressure in patients with spinal cord injury. *Anes Analg* 1982; 61:344348.

44. Gronert GA, Theye RA. Pathophysiology of hyperkalemia induced by succinylcholine. *Anesthesiology* 1975; 43:89.

45. Tobey RE. Paraplegia, succinylcholine and cardiac arrest. *Anesthesiology* 1970; 32:359.

46. Cheshire DJE, Coats DA. Respiratory and metabolic management in acute tetraplegia. *Paraplegia* 1965; 3:178–181.

47. Claus-Walker J, Carter RE, Campos RJ. Hypercalcemia in early traumatic quadriplegia. *J Chronic Dis* 1975; 28:81.

48. Duckworth WC, Jallepalli P, Solomon SS. Glucose intolerance in spinal cord injury. *Arch Phys Med Rehabil* 1983; 64:107.

49. Sninsky CA, Martin JL, Mathias JR. Effect of lidamidine hydrochloride, a proposed alpha2-adrenergic agonist in patients with gastroduodenal motor dysfunction. *Gastroenterology* 1983; 84:1315.

50. Ford RWJ, Malm DN. Therapeutic trial of hypercarbia and hypocarbia in acute experimental spinal cord injury. *J Neurosurg* 1984; 61:925.

50a. Lanier WL, Stangland KJ, Scheithauer BW, Milde JH, Michenfelder JD. The effects of dextrose infusion and head position on neurologic outcome after complete cerebral ischemia in primates: examination of a model. *Anesthesiology* 1987; 66:39.

50b. Drummond JC, Moore SS. The influence of dextrose administration on neurologic outcome after temporary spinal cord ischemia in the rabbit. *Anesthesiology* 1989; 70:64.

50c. Cole, DJ, Shapiro HM, Drummond JC, et al. Halothane, fentanyl, nitrous oxide, and spinal lidocaine protect against spinal cord injury in the rat. *Anesthesiology* 1989; 70:967.

51. Kozody R, Palahniuk RJ, Cumming MO. Spinal cord blood flow following subarachnoid tetracaine. *Can Anaesth Soc J* 1985; 32:23.

52. Barker I, Alderson J, Lydon M. Cardiovascular effects of spinal subarachnoid anaesthesia. *Anaesthesia* 1985; 40:533.

53. Hollis PH, Malis LI, Zappulla RA. Neurological deterioration after lumbar puncture below complete spinal subarachnoid block. *J Neurosurg* 1986; 64:253.

54. McCunniff DE, Dewan D. Pregnancy after spinal cord injury: letter to the editor. *Obstet Gynecol* 1984; 63:757.

55. Spielman FJ. Parturient with spinal cord transection: complications of autonomic hyperreflexia: letter to the editor. *Obstet Gynecol* 1984; 64:147.

56. McGregor JA, Meevusen J. Autonomic hyperflexia: a mortal danger for spinal cord-damaged women in labor. *Am J Obstet Gynecol* 1985; 151:330–333.

57. Spirnak PJ, Bodner D, Udayashankar S. Extracorporeal shockwave lithotripsy in traumatic quadriplegic patients: can it be safely performed without anesthesia? *J Urol* 1988; 139:18.

58. Mathias CJ, Christensen NJ, Corbett JL, et al. Plasma catecholamines during paroxysmal neurogenic hypertension in quadriplegic man. *Circ Res* 1976; 39:204.

59. Sloan TB, Ronai AK, Toleikis RJ. Improvement of the intraoperative somatosensory evoked potentials by etomidate. *Anesth Analgesia* 1988; 67:582.

60. Schubert A, Drummond JC, Garfin SR. The influence of stimulus presentation rate on the cortical amplitude and latency of introperative somatosensory-evoked potential recordings in patients with varying degrees of spinal cord injury. *Spine* 1987; 12:969.

61. Banik NL, Hogan EL, Hsu CY. Molecular and anatomical correlates of spinal cord injury. *CNS Trauma* 1985; 2:99.

62. Anderson DK, Demediuk P, Saunders RD. Spinal cord injury and protection. *Ann Emerg Med* 1985; 14:816.

63. Hogan EL, Hsu CY, Banik NL. Calcium-activated mediators of secondary injury in the spinal cord. *CNS Trauma* 1986; 3:175.

64. Kurihara M. Role of monamines in experimental spinal cord injury in rats: relationship between Na+, K+-ATPase and lipid peroxidation. *J Neurosurg* 1985; 62:743.

65. Hsu CY, Hogan EL, Gadsden KM Sr. Vascular permeability in experimental spinal cord injury. *J Neurosci* 1985; 70:275.

66. Faden AI, Molineaux CJ, Rosenberger JG. Increased dynorphin immunoreactivity in spinal cord after traumatic injury. *Regulatory Peptides* 1985; 11:35.

67. Krumins SA, Faden AI. Traumatic injury alters opiate receptor, binding in rat spinal cord. *Ann Neurol* 1986; 19:498.

68. Sandler AN, Tator CH. Review of the effect of spinal cord trauma on the vessels and blood flow in the spinal cord. *J Neurosurg* 1976; 45:638.

69. Senter HJ, Venes JL. Altered blood flow and secondary injury in experimental spinal cord trauma. *J Neurosurg* 1978; 49:569.

70. Rivlin AS, Tator CH. Regional spinal cord blood flow in rats after severe cord trauma. *J Neurosurg* 1978; 49:844.

71. Hickey R, Albin MS, et al. Autoregulation of spinal cord blood flow: is the cord a microcosm of the brain? *Stroke* 1986; 17:1183.

72. Griffiths IR. Spinal cord blood flow in dogs. Part 2: the effect of the blood gases. *J Neurol Neurosurg Psych* 1973; 36:42.

73. Kobrine AI, Doyle TF, Martins AN. Local spinal cord blood flow in experimental traumatic myelopathy. *J Neurosurg* 1975; 42:144.

74. Senter HJ, Venes JL. Loss of autoregulation and posttraumatic ischemia following experimental spinal cord trauma. *J Neurosurg* 1979; 50:198.

75. Rawe SE, Lee WA, Perot PL. The histopathology of experimental spinal cord trauma: the effect of systemic blood pressure. *J Neurosurg* 1978; 48:1002.

76. Osterholm JL, Matthews GJ. Altered norepinephrine metabolism following experimental spinal cord injury. Part 1: relationship to hemorrhagic necrosis and post-wounding neurological deficits. *J Neurosurg* 1972; 36:386.

77. Osterholm JL, Matthews GJ. Altered norepinephrine metabolism following experimental spinal cord injury. Part 2: protection against traumatic spinal cord hemorrhagic necrosis by norepinephrine synthesis blockade with alpha methyl tyrosine. *J Neurosurg* 1972; 36:395.

78. Crawford RA, Griffiths IR, McCulloch J. The effect of norepinephrine on the spinal cord circulation and its possible implications in the pathogenesis of acute spinal trauma. *J Neurosurg* 1977; 47:567.

79. Anderson TE. Effects of acute alcohol intoxication on spinal cord vascular injury. *CNS Trauma* 1986; 3:183.

80. Chabot R, York DH, Watts C. Somatosensory evoked potentials evaluated in normal subjects and spinal cord-injured patients. *J Neurosurg* 1985; 63:544.

81. Levy W, McCaffrey M, York D. Motor evoked potential in cats with acute spinal cord injury. J Neurosurg 1986; 19:9.

82. Levy WJ, McCaffrey M, Hagichi S. Motor evoked potential as a predictor of recovery in chronic spinal cord injury. *Neurosurg* 1987; 20:138.

83. Simpson RK, Baskin DS. Corticomotor evoked potentials in acute and chronic blunt spinal cord injury in the rat: correlation with neurological outcome and histological damage. *Neurosurgery* 1987; 20:131.

84. Parker AJ, Park RD, Stowater JL. Reduction of trauma-induced edema of spinal cord in dogs given mannitol. *Am J Vet Res* 1973; 34:1355.

85. Kuchner EF, Hansebout RR. Combined steroid and hypothermia treatment of experimental spinal cord injury. *Surg Neurol* 1976; 6:371.

86. Young W, Flamm ES. Effect of high-dose corticosteroid therapy on blood flow, evoked potentials, and extracellular calcium in experimental spinal injury. *J Neurosurg* 1982; 57:667.

87. Iizuka H, Iwasaki Y, Yamamoto T. Morphometric assessment of drug effects in experimental spinal cord injury. *J Neurosurg* 1986; 65:92.

88. Bracken MB, Shepard MJ, Hellenbrand KG, et al. Methylprednisolone and neurological function 1 year after spinal cord injury: results of the National Acute Spinal Cord Injury Study. *J Neurosurg* 1985; 63:704.

88a. Bracken MB, Shephard MJ, Collins WF, et al. A randomized, controlled trial of methylprednisolone or naloxone in the treatment of acute spinal cord injury. *N Engl J Med* 1990; 322:1405.

89. DeMaria EJ, Reichman W, Kenney PR. Septic complications of corticosteroid administration after central nervous system trauma. *Ann Surg* 1985; 202:248.

90. Holaday JW, Faden AI. Naloxone acts at central opiate receptors to reverse hypotension, hypothermia, and hypoventilation in spinal shock. *Brain Res* 1980; 189:295.

91. Holaday JW, Faden AI. Spinal shock and injury: experimental therapeutic approaches. *Adv Shock Res* 1983; 10:95.

92. Flamm ES, Young W, Demopoulos HB. Experimental spinal cord injury: treatment with naloxone. *Neurosurgery* 1982; 10:227.

93. Faden AI, Jacobs TP, Holaday JW. Opiate antagonist improves neurologic recovery after spinal injury. *Science* 1981; 211:493.

94. Flamm ES, Young W, Collins WF. A phase I trial of naloxone treatment in acute spinal cord injury. *J Neurosurg* 1985; 63:390.

95. Haghighi SS, Chehrazi B. Effect of naloxone in experimental acute spinal cord injury. *Neurosurgery* 1987; 20:385.

96. Wallace MC, Tator CH. Failure of naloxone to improve spinal cord blood flow and cardiac output after spinal cord injury. *Neurosurgery* 1986; 18:428.

97. Wallace MC, Tator CH. Failure of blood transfusion or naloxone to improve clinical recovery after experimental spinal cord injury. *Neurosurgery* 1986; 19:489.

98. Benthuysen JL. Naloxone therapy in spinal trauma: anesthetic effects. *Anesthesiology* 1987; 66:238.

98a. Faden AI, Jacobs TP, Holaday, JW. Thyrotropin-releasing hormone improves neurologic recovery after spinal cord trauma in cats. *N Engl J Med* 1981; 305:1063.

99. Iwasaki Y, Iizuka H, Yamamoto, TY. Alleviation of axonal damage in acute spinal cord injury by a protease inhibitor: automated morphometric analysis of drug effects. *Brain Res* 1985; 347:124.

100. Glaser RM. Physiologic aspects of spinal cord injury and functional neuromuscular stimulation. *CNS Trauma* 1986; 3:49.

101. Bose B, Osterholm JL, Kalia M. Ganglioside-induced regeneration and reestablishment of axonal continuity in spinal cord-transected rats. *Neuroscience Letters* 1986; 63:165.

102. Guth L, Barrett CP, Donati EJ. Enhancement of axonal growth into a spinal lesion by topical application of triethanolamine and cytosine arabinoside. *Exp Neurol* 1985; 88:44.

103. Borgens RB, Blight AR, Murphy DJ. Transected dorsal column axons within the guinea pig spinal cord regenerate in the presence of an applied electric field. *J Comp Neurol* 1986; 250:168.

104. Reier PJ. Neural tissue grafts and repair of the injured spinal cord. *Neuropathol Appl Neurobiol* 1985; 11:81.

16 The Role of Electrical Stimulation in Management of Spinal Cord Injured Patients

E. B. MARSOLAIS, MD, PhD
R.J. TRIOLO, PhD
R. KOBETIC, MS
S. NANDURKAR, MD

THE FOOD AND DRUG ADMINISTRATION (FDA) has recently approved several devices using electrical stimulation for treatment of spinal cord injured patients. These devices, including the implantable FreeHand® system for control of hand grasp in quadriplegic patients; the implantable Vocare® system for control of bladder and bowel function; and the Parastep®, which uses surface muscle stimulation for standing and walking in paraplegia, have been successfully transferred to clinical practice and are now commercially available. New versions of these devices are also being developed to improve current function and to provide additional functions, such as arm reaching for a hand grasp system. An implantable system for exercise and standing is undergoing through clinical trials and should be available in the near future. Feasibility has been demonstrated for other more complex implantable systems for walking in paraplegia with and without braces, and prototypes are being developed. This chapter reviews the state of exercise, standing, and walking systems using electrical stimulation.

BASIC PRINCIPLES OF ELECTRICAL STIMULATION

The direct stimulation of muscle fibers requires a threshold more than 100 times higher than that of a nerve (1). Therefore, the application of electrical stimulation described in this chapter provides muscle contraction through excitation of nerves and is based on the premise that lower motor neurons of the target muscles are intact. Electrical stimulation can be applied to the surface of the body (2) or internally using either percutaneous intramuscular electrodes (3,4) or implanted intramuscular (5), epimysial (6,7), epineural (8), or nerve cuff (9) electrodes. However, the intensity of stimulus diminishes with distance from the electrode. Therefore, surface stimulation is less likely to activate deeper motor neurons, such as those innervating the iliopsoas muscle (10), and less specific than implanted electrodes that are placed near the motor point. When an electrical current of sufficient amplitude and duration is applied to the nerve, it causes a change in the nerve membrane potential, resulting in generation and propagation of an action potential. The larger diameter axons of the alpha motor neurons have the lowest threshold to electrical stimulation and are recruited first, followed by the smaller diameter fibers such as C pain fibers (11). The larger muscle fibers, which have a fast response and generate a high level of forces and fatigue quickly, are recruited before the smaller, slow-response, and more fatigue-resistant fibers (1). This recruitment order is the reverse of what naturally occurs in the intact nervous system and places limitations on those functional uses requiring extended activity, such as standing, and consistent repeatable responses, such as walking. The limitations are further amplified by the disuse atrophy following muscle paralysis that tends to convert muscle fibers to the fast-twitch, fast-fatiguing type (12). In addition, the fast-twitch fibers are smaller in diameter, thus producing lower forces. Therefore, to prepare paralyzed muscles for functional use, they must first undergo electrical exercise conditioning. It has been shown that chronic electrical stimulation results in changes in the metabolic makeup of muscle fibers from fast-twitch glycolytic (or type II), to slow-twitch oxidative, (or type I), fibers, which have a high capacity for oxidative metabolism and are fatigue resistant (13).

SYSTEM-LEVEL OVERVIEW OF FNS TECHNOLOGY

Functional neuromuscular stimulation (FNS), also known as functional electrical stimulation (FES), refers to the activation and coordination of a number of muscles to obtain a useful, purposeful movement from an otherwise paralyzed limb. This is contrasted to stimulation solely for exercise or other purely therapeutic purposes. In these applications, neuromuscular electrical stimulation serves as the basis of a *neural prosthe-* *sis* because it replaces the missing function of the efferent motor pathways interrupted by injury or disease.

All FNS systems intended to provide motor function share several common elements. The fundamental components of a neural prosthesis for motor function are represented schematically as solid lines in Figure 16-1. First, the user of an FNS system must have a way to communicate his or her intent to the device to select, activate, or directly control the resulting limb movement. This *command input* can take any number of forms, from simple switch closures and timer settings to more complicated sequences of EMG activity from muscles still under volitional control (14–20). Once the user delivers a command to the system, the device must process the input, which could be interpreted differently depending on the prior history of stimulation, the current state of the device, or the status of the limb. After the *command processor* unambiguously recognizes the intent of the user, the neural prosthesis must take action. The *control processor* selects the appropriate channels (corresponding to the nerves or muscles required to effect the intended motion) as well as the relative timing, intensity, and frequency of stimulation. These parameters are then used by the *stimulus delivery* subsystem to create the stimulation waveforms and deliver current to the nerves. These components of the system include cables, leads, and electrodes that interface with the body. Optional features of a motor prosthesis are indicated by the dotted lines in Figure 16-1. The user can be made aware of what the system is doing through *cognitive feedback* of the state of the device via direct observation, displays, warning lights, or audio tones. The majority of clinically applied FNS systems operate *open loop*; that is, they are unresponsive to the environment and do not automatically correct for errors that arise between the intended and actual motions of the limbs. Sensors have been employed experimentally to feed the state of the biological system (joint angles, contact forces, etc.) back to the controller. Such *closed loop* systems require sensors to provide output feedback and a *sensor*

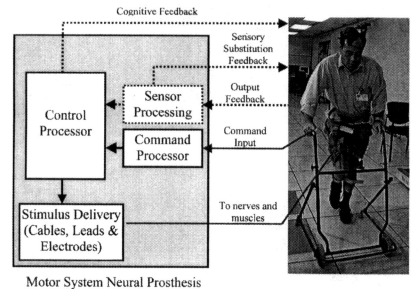

Cognitive Feedback

Sensory Substitution Feedback

Output Feedback

Command Input

To nerves and muscles

Control Processor

Sensor Processing

Command Processor

Stimulus Delivery (Cables, Leads & Electrodes)

Motor System Neural Prosthesis

FIGURE 16-1 Basic motor system neural prosthesis. Dotted lines indicate optional components for advanced control. Components of such systems can be implanted if communication channels are maintained with external components via radio-frequency links.

processor to monitor the actions of the limbs and allow the control processor to adjust stimulus levels automatically without conscious input from the user. Finally, the user can be informed of the orientation and state of his body (rather than the state of the device) through *substitute sensory feedback*. In this scheme, the closed loop sensor signals are used to modulate tactile stimulation to sensate areas or provide other indications of the status of the limbs and joints and their interaction with the environment (21,22).

Various portions of the neural prosthesis depicted in the shaded region of Figure 16-1 can be made implantable. FNS systems can be completely external, in which case no foreign material is introduced into the body and only the stimulating current crosses the skin boundary. When subsystems are implanted (for example, the electrodes and/or stimulus delivery circuitry), communication must be maintained with those parts of the system remaining outside of the body. This can be done by direct percutaneous connection or via a radio frequency (RF) transmission. In the latter case, nothing crosses the skin except electromagnetic energy, reducing the likelihood of infection present with percutaneous connections and improving the convenience of donning and doffing over completely external systems. Implanting components of the

system requires additional circuitry (RF transmitters and receivers) to complete the communication pathways indicated by the arrows in Figure 16-1, and may increase the complexity of the design. As a consequence of the required surgery, implantable systems offer the advantage of placing the stimulating electrodes in close proximity to nerves, thus greatly increasing the selectivity and efficiency of activation while reducing the current required.

INTERFACING WITH THE NERVOUS SYSTEM: ELECTRODE AND LEAD TECHNOLOGY

Electrodes for FNS applications are classified according to the location of their stimulating surfaces. They are usually designed to activate nerves in the periphery and fall into three broad classes: surface electrodes applied to the skin, muscle-based electrodes, and nerve-based electrodes. Alternatively, lead wires connecting the electrodes to the stimulus-generating circuitry are described by the course they take and the tissues through which they pass. Electrode leads can be classified as external, percutaneous, or implanted. All surface electrodes use external leads, while muscle- and nerve-based electrodes are connected to either percutaneous or implanted lead wires.

Surface electrodes deliver electrical charge to the motor nerve transcutaneously. They are applied to the surface of the skin over the *motor point*, the location exhibiting the best contraction from the target muscle at the lowest levels of stimulation. These low-threshold regions occur approximately one-third the distance between origin and insertion of the muscle and are likely to be associated with the location of a major branch of a motor nerve. Transcutaneous stimulation with surface electrodes offers several distinct advantages: 1) the electrodes are generally easy to apply and remove; 2) the stimulation technique is noninvasive and therefore reversible (i.e., the position of the electrodes can be readily changed to elicit optimal stimulated responses); 3) the use of surface electrodes can be easily learned and applied in the clinic; and 4) neuromuscular stimulators and surface electrodes are relatively inexpensive and commercially available. Stimulation with surface electrodes is the most widely used technique for therapeutic applications.

Despite their apparent convenience when applied individually in small numbers, surface electrodes for transcutaneous stimulation have several disadvantages: 1) they tend to activate any nerve beneath them, making it difficult to selectively stimulate a single isolated muscle; 2) daily doffing and donning can complicate use, especially if electrode positions vary slightly from day to day, producing different stimulated responses; and 3) multiple electrode systems rapidly become impractical as the number of muscles (and stimulus channels), required for function increases to six or more (23). In this situation, donning, doffing, and connecting multiple electrodes becomes cumbersome. In addition, the skin offers substantial resistance to the flow of electrical current. Removing oils, hair, or dead skin cells by cleaning or shaving the skin can reduce skin resistance and improve current delivery to the deeper nerves but may also irritate the skin. Precautions also must be taken to ensure good electrical contact of the electrode with the skin through some highly conductive medium or electrolytic gel. As with all applica-

tions of electricity, the potential exists for a burn if a large portion of a surface electrode loses contact with the skin, creating an area of high charge density. Large currents may be required to drive sufficient charge through the skin and intervening tissues between the electrode and the peripheral nerve, thus decreasing the efficiency of surface stimulation. In many cases, cutaneous pain receptors are excited as current passes through these tissues, and patients with preserved or heightened sensation may find it difficult to tolerate surface stimulation at the levels required to produce a motor response. Surface electrodes also may irritate the skin in certain individuals (2).

Muscle-based electrodes bypass the high resistance of the skin and cutaneous sensory fibers. Because their stimulating surfaces lie closer to the motor nerve branches of the desired muscles, they provide a means to produce contractions more efficiently (with small currents) and more selectively than surface electrodes. After recovery from implantation, stimulation can also be more comfortable because more of the muscle can be recruited without eliciting the sensation of pain from the cutaneous fibers. For these reasons, muscle-based electrodes are preferable for many functional applications of FNS that require independent control of several isolated muscles. The stimulating tips of *intramuscular electrodes* reside within the muscle tissue itself and generally include a barbing mechanism to snare the tissue to resist movement until encapsulation occurs. Depending on their intended application, intramuscular electrodes are designed to be introduced either percutaneously (3,4,24) or in an open surgical procedure (5,6). In addition to their selectivity, low current requirements, and ease of implantation, intramuscular electrodes allow access to deep nerves that are difficult to approach surgically. When used with percutaneous leads, they can also be removed easily and provide a means for producing strong repeatable contractions on either an acute or longer-term basis. Early movement away from the target nerve within the first 6 weeks post-implantation (before encapsulation is complete) can result in altered stimulated responses and is the most frequently observed failure mode of these devices (25). *Epimysial electrodes* are sutured directly to the epimysium or fascia to eliminate this early movement and provide immediate and permanent fixation. Because they require surgery, they are used almost exclusively with implantable leads and stimulators. Figure 16-2 shows examples of two designs of muscle-based electrodes developed at Case Western Reserve University in Cleveland, Ohio (5,6).

Nerve-based electrodes have more intimate contact with the peripheral nerve and therefore require even less current than muscle-based electrodes to produce a contraction. They take the form of *epineural electrodes*, which are sutured to the connective tissue on either side of a motor nerve; *cuff electrodes*, which envelope the nerve; and *intrafasicular* or *intraneural electrodes*, which are still laboratory-based investigational tools. Epineural and nerve cuff designs have both been employed as stimulating electrodes in FNS systems to restore motor function in spinal cord injury and stroke (8,9). Cuff electrodes have also been configured to record from afferent nerves in attempts to utilize the natural sensors in the body to provide feedback signals to control and adjust the stimulation (26). Nerve cuff electrodes have been widely used in humans for phrenic pacing or to stimulate the peroneal nerve to produce dorsiflexion and correct foot-drop in individuals with hemiplegia.

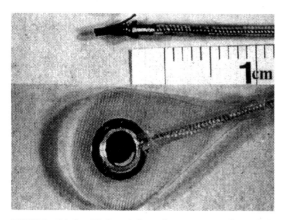

FIGURE 16-2 Epimysial and intramuscular electrodes developed at CWRU.

Electrodes are connected to stimulating or recording circuitry through lead wires. *Percutaneous leads* are designed to connect chronically indwelling intramuscular and epimysial electrodes to circuitry external to the body while maintaining a barrier to infection. The leads are made of multiple strands of stainless steel insulated in Teflon that are helically wound to form a thin, flexible cable of small enough diameter for the tissue to heal around as it exits the skin. The helical configuration converts bending motions to torsional stresses in the coils of the lead, providing mechanical resistance to fracture due to metal fatigue. Alternately, the leads can be coiled around a central core of suture material or wound a second time to form a "compound helix" which offers additional flexibility near the critical stimulating tip (4). The open coils also promote tissue growth and assist with fixation. A thin layer of endothelial cells proliferates around the coils near the skin surface at sufficient depth to provide a barrier to infection. Because of their small diameter, helically coiled percutaneous leads from multiple electrodes can exit the skin in relatively high densities. These electrodes are then connected to an external stimulator.

Although they facilitate donning and doffing of neural prosthesis by eliminating the need to apply individual electrodes, and simplify connecting to other electronic components, percutaneous leads require continual attention from the user. They must be cleaned, dressed, and properly inspected and maintained. These leads are subject to breakage at areas of high shear stress, such as where they cross fascial planes. Although they can remain functional for years without infection or complication, percutaneous leads are usually reserved for acute applications and are generally not recommended for long-term clinical use.

Implanted leads can be of larger dimensions than percutaneous lead wires because they need to be more robust and resistant to failure, and are not required to cross the skin. One popular configuration consists of two Teflon-insulated stranded stainless steel cables wound in tandem with each other (27). The redundant conductor assembly is then enclosed in an elastomer sheath to prevent in-growth, provide mechanical stability, and allow the leads to slide through the tissues between the electrode and the implanted stimulating circuitry. To promote serviceability and allow repair or revision of implanted FNS systems, provisions have been made in several designs to isolate system subcomponents from each other via high reliability implantable connectors (28). *In-line connectors* permit the surgical removal and repositioning of individual electrodes with minimal dissection and without extensive exposure of larger implanted circuit packages. These designs reduce the risk of infection and minimize the likelihood of damage to other implanted components during maintenance procedures. Implantable electronic components can also be designed as *passive devices* that derive their power from the RF signals providing communication channels to external command or control processors. Systems utilizing this configuration eliminate the need for additional surgery to replace internal batteries.

THERAPEUTIC APPLICATIONS OF LOWER EXTREMITY FNS

Exercise and Cycling

Lower extremity FNS can be an effective exercise modality for persons paralyzed by SCI. Progressive resistance knee-extension exercise utilizing electrical stimulation of the quadriceps can reverse or prevent disuse atrophy, improve appearance, and promote circulation (29). The mechanisms of these changes appear to be peripheral, rather than central, adaptations and include fiber type conversion (fast to slow-twitch), increased concentration of metabolic enzymes, hypertrophy, and higher capillary density (30–32).

Protocols similar to voluntary high-resistance weight training have been found to be effective with FNS in individuals with spinal cord injuries (33–35). Two to four sessions per week, consisting of a small number of sets (typically three) of multiple repetitions (10 to 30) of weighted leg-lift exercises with FNS, can result in significant increases in quadriceps strength, endurance, and mass if the applied resistance is progressively increased over the training period to maintain overload on the muscles. Initial resistance should be low (less than 2 kg), and contractions should be slow (2 to 5 per minute) to assure safety and allow adequate habituation to FNS. As performance improves, the resistance can progress slowly (e.g., 0.5 kg increments) to a maximum of approximately 15 kg (or one-quarter body weight) without adverse effects. Once this level has been achieved, the number of repetitions per set can be increased for further gains in endurance.

Although it can promote substantial peripheral changes in the paralyzed muscle, strength and endurance training of this type will not elicit marked central cardiopulmonary responses (36). Stationary bicycle ergometers were developed to address this need and promote cardiovascular fitness in persons with spinal cord injuries. Cycle ergometers utilizing computer-controlled surface stimulation to the quadriceps, hamstrings, and gluteal groups are commercially available for use in the home or clinic environments and can be prescribed by a physician. Contractions are coordinated with the actions of the pedals by sensing the shaft position and velocity and adjusting the stimulus timing and intensity accordingly. Up to 50 revolutions per minute can be achieved with some systems, corresponding to 300 contractions per minute when gluteal, hamstring, and quadriceps muscles are activated.

Much of the work in the physiologic responses to lower extremity cycling exercise with FNS has been conducted at the Institute for Rehabilitation Research and Medicine at Wright State University in Dayton, Ohio. Exercise protocols typically consist of three sessions per week, each comprised of a series of 30 minutes of uninterrupted cycling separated by rest periods of 10 minutes. Initial power output is set at 0 watts (not resisted) until an entire 30-minute period can be achieved without fatigue. Resistance at subsequent sessions is increased to produce increments in power output of 6.1 watts until the limit of the ergometer is reached (42.7 watts). These exercises induce aerobic metabolic and cardiopulmonary responses, as well as favorable central and peripheral hemodynamic responses (37,38). Chronic cycling in this manner has been shown to produce significant physiologic and psychologic benefits, including increased dimension and thickness of cardiac muscle (39); elevated HDL levels (suggesting reduced risks of coronary heart disease); enhanced immunoreactivity (40); improved scores on depression, self-image, and mood indices (41); and reduced incidence of pressure sores and kidney and bladder infections. These effects may take months to years of regular exercise to manifest themselves.

Cardiovascular fitness training can be further enhanced by adding voluntary arm cranking to the FNS-generated leg cycling exercise program (29,42). Studies at Wright State suggest that combining lower extremity FNS and voluntary exercise provide superior cardiopulmonary training than either mode alone. This may be caused by the larger muscle mass utilized by exercising both upper and lower extremities simultaneously, as well as the enhanced venous return provided by the cyclic contractions of the limbs.

Improved Tissue Viability and Prevention of Pressure Sores

A major physiologic complication arising following paralysis by SCI is the development of pressure sores (also known as decubitus ulcers, ischemic sores, pressure ulcers, and bedsores). Sustained loading produced by prolonged maintenance of the same seated or lying posture restricts blood flow and occludes lymph vessels, limiting the available oxygen available and preventing removal of toxic metabolic products. These conditions lead to cell necrosis and tissue breakdown, resulting in a pressure sore. This significant secondary complication of SCI is known to be a multifactorial process. Extrinsic factors are related to the physical conditions at the subject–support interface and soft tissue biomechanics. Intrinsic factors concern the health

and physiologic profile of the individual. Electrical stimulation can simultaneously impact several intrinsic and extrinsic factors that contribute to the risk of pressure sores.

Blood flow is the major intrinsic factor in pressure sore development affected by SCI. Following SCI there is a decrease in sympathetic nervous activity leading to reduced systemic vascular resistance and generalized vasodilation, particularly after cervical spinal injury. Thus, both systolic and diastolic blood pressures are decreased. The measurement of tissue blood flow provides an indirect assessment of tissue viability, which is dependent upon adequate nutrient supply to the soft tissues. Transcutaneous oxygen levels in supine SCI subjects are significantly lower than in normal controls (43), and there is evidence that SCI impairs the ability to respond to applied pressure (44,45). FNS has been shown to increase blood flow and vascularity of muscle tissue, thus improving tissue viability and resistance to pressure sore development. Long-term stimulation converts fast-twitch Type II muscle fibers, predominant in atrophied muscle, to slow-twitch Type I fibers (46). Mean fiber diameter therefore decreases in stimulated muscles, shortening the diffusion pathway of oxygen and nutrients to the fiber center. These effects combine to significantly increase capillary density, as well as aerobic capacity and fatigue resistance (47). Increases in muscular vascularization can begin as early as 4 days after initiating long-term low-frequency electrical stimulation (48,49). Skin blood flow also increases with FNS exercise. Electrical stimulation has been observed to improve cutaneous tissue oxygen levels in both able-bodied controls and persons with diabetes (50,51). Levine and co-workers found that surface stimulation of the gluteus maximus increased regional blood flow in both able-bodied subjects and volunteers with SCI (52). These increases in blood flow above baseline levels can be maintained for more than 15 minutes after removal of FNS (45). These reports suggest that electrical stimulation improves the overall tissue viability of paralyzed muscle and skin.

The primary extrinsic factor in the development of pressure sores is externally applied pressure. In particular, nonuniform pressures, such as those occurring in the region of bony prominence with reduced soft tissue coverage, cause tissue distortion and tend to collapse the regional vasculature. The interface pressure required to occlude blood flow over hard sites, such as bony prominences, is roughly half that required in soft sites (53). Furthermore, a large body build improves pressure distribution at the support interface (54). These findings provide indirect evidence to support the hypothesis that increased muscle bulk in the gluteal region after exercise with FNS improves the pressure distribution at the buttock–cushion interface. Reduction of peak pressures over bony prominences due to increased muscle mass and seating support areas will result in a decreased risk of pressure sore formation. Periodic muscular contractions produced by stimulation can produce postural variation, thus alleviating prolonged applied pressures.

FUNCTIONAL NEUROMUSCULAR STIMULATION FOR STANDING

Functional neuromuscular stimulation can provide individuals paralyzed by thoracic or low cervical spinal cord injuries with the ability to perform many activities that were previously impossible or difficult from the wheelchair, including standing, transfers, and simple mobility functions such as side and back stepping (55–57). Preliminary clinical trials of lower extremity neuroprostheses for standing clearly indicate that continuous open-loop stimulation of the trunk, hip, and knee extensors allows people with paraplegia to overcome physical obstacles (23), negotiate architectural barriers (58), and exert a greater control over their environment by affording them the ability to reach and manipulate objects that are otherwise inaccessible from the wheelchair (59,60).

Paralysis from spinal cord injury is a debilitating and costly condition that compromises the ability to work, engage in social or leisure activities, pursue an education, or participate in other activities usually associated with an independent and productive lifestyle. Complications resulting from SCI can lead to recurrent, lengthy, and expensive hospitalizations. Long periods of immobility can cause degenerative changes of almost every major organ system including the bones and joints, bowel and bladder, heart, lungs, and skin. For example, persons unable to stand or transfer are almost four times as likely to develop pressure sores than other disabled individuals (61,62) and are at increased risk of other immobility-related diseases (63). The increased muscle bulk and improved perfusion from exercise and standing with FNS may reduce the risk of developing pressure sores and positively impact the overall health of persons with SCI. Exercise and weight bearing with FNS can improve cardiovascular fitness (64) and reduce osteoporosis (65) without adversely affecting the insensate joints (66). Standing with FNS can postpone or prevent the medical complications associated with immobility and improve the functional independence of people with spinal cord injuries by providing a means to exercise and assume an upright posture.

A standing neuroprosthesis may have significant functional benefits for individuals with low cervical or thoracic injuries. Standing with FNS is an option to the wheelchair and provides a means to negotiate architectural barriers that obstruct access to physical places or life opportunities. Users can reach objects from high shelves, gain entry to places inaccessible from the wheelchair, and participate in social or work situations on eye level with their peers. FNS not only provides the ability to stand independently, it can also facilitate an assisted transfer by raising, supporting, and lowering an individual under the power of his or her own stimulated muscles. A standing neuroprosthesis may be particularly valuable for elderly individuals with frail or weak spouses incapable of assisting with conventional transfers or young adults who depend on aging parents. This is a growing segment of the SCI population, because these individuals can now expect to live near-normal life spans of close to 75 years. The presence of a spinal cord injury compounds the impact of the physical limitations imposed by the natural aging process and further increases the importance of a standing neuroprosthesis for preserving personal mobility.

There are currently between 177,000 and 195,000 people with spinal cord injuries in the United States, and between 30 and 40 new cases occur per million people per year (67–69). Standing neuroprostheses would be indicated for about 25 percent of the SCI population at large—approximately 50,000 persons. Medical complications, such as peripheral nerve damage, cardiac abnormalities, and other contraindications to FNS may be present in as many as 50 percent of the population targeted for lower extremity neuroprostheses (70), further reducing the number of potential users to approximately 25,000. A conservative estimate of the potential clinical impact of lower extremity FNS systems by Jaeger et al. (71) places the user population somewhere between 10,000 and 22,000 individuals, representing 5 to 11 percent of all individuals with SCI.

Standing with FNS has been achieved with relatively simple systems consisting of two to six channels of continuous surface stimulation (16,72,73). Surface electrodes can be easily applied and removed without invasive procedures, although daily variation in electrode placement can adversely affect the repeatability of the stimulated responses. Nevertheless, multi-channel surface stimulation systems have been successful at producing standing and stepping movements in people with SCI in both laboratory and clinical settings (74–76). Lower extremity FNS systems employing percutaneous intramuscular electrodes have also been successful in providing lower extremity functions to individuals with paraplegia (77,78). Persons with SCI using 16 or fewer channels of percutaneous intramuscular stimulation can perform simple mobility and one-handed reaching tasks while standing (58,79). The advantages of percutaneous intramuscular electrodes include improved repeatability and selectivity of responses, access to

anatomically deep muscles, and low current requirements. Percutaneous approaches to most muscles of the lower extremities have been defined, allowing the generation of more complex movements than with surface stimulation alone (80). More recently, totally implanted pacemaker-like neuroprostheses for standing after SCI have undergone feasibility and initial clinical testing. Exercise and standing have been reported with a cochlear implant modified to deliver 22-channels of stimulation (81), and a 12-channel system for activation of the L2–S2 motor roots has been applied to a handful of volunteers (82). Alternative systems of distributed single-channel micromodular implants are also under development (83). For long-term clinical application, implanted systems such as these provide major advantages over surface and percutaneous stimulation including improved convenience, cosmesis, reliability, and repeatability (84).

In our laboratory, implantable systems for standing have been undergoing successful clinical testing since 1992. Figure 16-3 shows an individual with complete motor and sensory mid-thoracic paraplegia using the implanted standing system. The implanted components of this system include an eight-channel receiver–stimulator (27) and epimysial (85) and surgically–implanted intramuscular (86) electrodes, pictured in Figure 16-4. In a single surgical procedure, epimysial electrodes are installed bilaterally in the quadriceps, hamstrings, and gluteus maximus, while intramuscular electrodes are inserted at the lumbar spinal roots to activate the erector spinae muscles. A system-level diagram of the standing system and a composite radiograph showing the internal components of the neuroprosthesis is provided in Figures 16-5 and 16-6. Continuous stimulation to the extensor musculature braces the body against collapse, while the hands are used for balance (87). Stepping can be achieved with 16 channels of stimulation through the addition of a second implant to activate the hip flexors and ankle dorsiflexors (88,89). To date, a total of 11 surgically implanted neuroprostheses for standing or stepping have been successfully installed

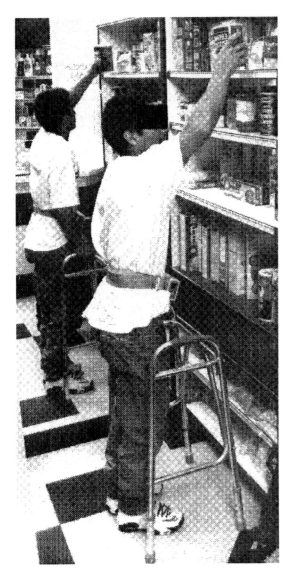

FIGURE 16-3 Standing with continuous stimulation to the trunk, hip, and knee extensors with an eight-channel implanted neuroprosthesis. Balance must be maintained by one extremity on an assistive device.

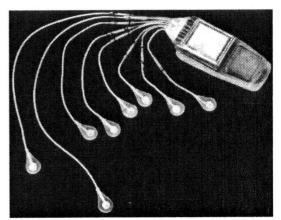

FIGURE 16-4 CWRU/VA Eight-Channel Implanted Receiver/Stimulator (IRS-8) showing epimysial electrodes and in-line connector.

by our team and are now approaching widespread clinical use.

All lower extremity FNS systems still require assistive devices, such as crutches, walkers, or additional bracing, to provide supplemental support or allow the upper extremities to inject the corrective forces necessary to maintain a stable upright posture. The magnitudes of these corrective forces can be quite small—on the order of 10 percent of body weight or less (90). They can be produced routinely by a single extremity without undue exertion (91), freeing the other hand to perform reaching tasks or other functions, as illustrated in Figure 16-7. Still, relying on an assistive device for balance restricts activities with FNS to one-handed tasks and requires users of FNS systems to carry assistive devices with them at all times to be able to stand spontaneously. It also limits working environments to those containing a counter, desk, or another appropriately sturdy waist-high support surface. However, the functional limitations imposed by using one hand for balance are more burdensome than the necessity of finding environments with adequate supports. Bimanual activities are prohibitively difficult or impossible with current open-loop FNS systems, regardless of the presence or absence of the appropriate surfaces on which to hold.

FNS can readily generate the muscle forces and joint moments required for rising from a chair into standing *posture* with minimal assistance from the upper extremities. Producing the postural corrections necessary to maintain *balance* in the presence of intrinsic (voluntary motions) or extrinsic (unanticipated environmental perturbations) destabilizing disturbances, however, remains a major challenge to the designers of FNS systems. Practical and robust control systems to provide *standing bal-*

ance (i.e., the maintenance of standing posture), even for the brief periods typically required for completing simple reaching activities, has been an elusive goal.

BIOMECHANICAL EVALUATIONS OF STANDING WITH FNS

Over the past 15 years, we have been collecting data regarding the responses of paralyzed muscle to electrical stimulation. We have been able to achieve standing up, upright stance, and controlled sitting by activating the major muscles of the lower limbs with surgically implanted epimysial electrodes, chronically indwelling intramuscular electrodes with percutaneous leads, and surface electrodes (92). The muscles targeted for stimulation to achieve standing and balance are illustrated in Figure 16-8. The rectus abdominis, erector spinae, and quadratus lumborum (not pictured) can be stimulated to control the trunk and stabilize the pelvis; the iliopsoas (iliacus and psoas major) can be activated via an intramuscular electrode at the lumbar roots for hip flexion. Hip extension can be generated by stimulation of the gluteus maximus, the hamstrings, and the posterior portion of the adductor magnus. Knee extension can be achieved with an electrode near the femoral nerve, which excites the entire quadriceps muscles or activates the individual vasti. We prefer-

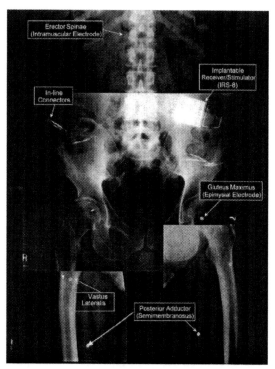

FIGURE 16-6 Radiograph of implanted components.

entially target the vastus lateralis and vastus intermedius separately for the option of generating knee extension without hip flexion. Medial-lateral stability can be controlled with bilateral stimulation of the gluteus medius. We have also implanted intramuscular electrodes in both the long and short heads of the biceps femoris for the option of coupling knee and hip extension or providing isolated knee flexion. At the ankle, significant plantarflexion moments can be generated with the gastrocnemius and soleus, while dorsiflexion can be obtained from activation of the tibialis anterior and peroneals. All these muscles are accessible with either epimysial, intramuscular, or surface electrodes.

The strength and endurance of electrically activated paralyzed muscles are often significantly less than maximal volitional contractions due to the changes in cross-sectional area and metabolism that follow SCI. These factors can be modified with appropriate exercise. Table 16-1 presents the average isometric moments obtained with FNS in well-conditioned subjects in our laboratory. These stimulated responses

8-Channel Standing/Transfer System

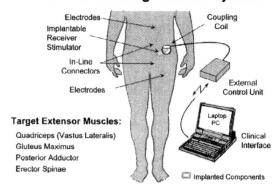

FIGURE 16-5 System diagram of standing neuroprosthesis.

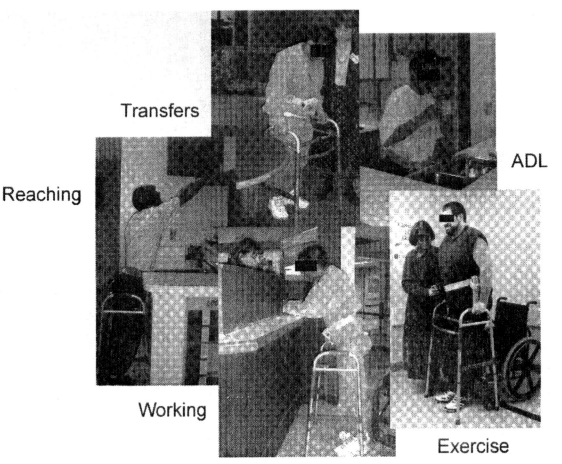

Reaching

Transfers

Working

ADL

Exercise

FIGURE 16-7 Representative functional activities possible while standing with an eight-channel implanted neuroprosthesis.

exceed those measured during the sit-to-stand transition and quiet standing by Kralj and Bajd et al. (16). Although somewhat less than exhibited by able-bodied individuals, they are still substantial and fall within the limits identified for lower extremity functional activities in computer simulation studies. Our experimental and analytical work indicates that the strength and endurance of stimulated muscle may be sufficient to make the postural corrections required to maintain balance. Without adequate hip extension moment, however, corrections to disturbances in the sagittal plane are difficult to generate. We have found that activating the erector spinae muscles tends to stabilize the pelvis and enhance the effectiveness of the hip extensors. Simultaneously activating the erector spinae can increase the hip extension moment generated by the hamstrings by as much as 10 Nm. This indicates that activation and control of the paraspinals, and other trunk muscles, are critical to the maintenance of erect posture in

TABLE 16-1 Average Isometric Joint Moments with FNS

Function	Moment (Nm)	Position
Trunk Extension	70	0°
Hip Extension	63	45° Hip Flexion
Hip Abduction	44	0°
Hip Adduction	30	0°
Knee Extension	80	45° Knee Flexion
Ankle Plantarflexion	55	15° Dorsiflexion
Ankle Dorsiflexion	15	15° Plantarflexion

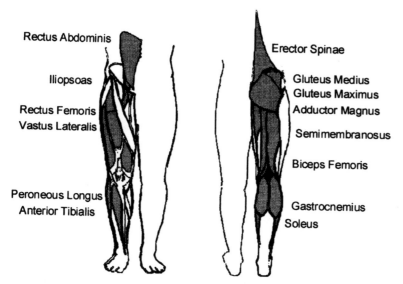

Rectus Abdominis

Iliopsoas

Rectus Femoris
Vastus Lateralis

Peroneous Longus
Anterior Tibialis

Erector Spinae

Gluteus Medius
Gluteus Maximus
Adductor Magnus

Semimembranosus

Biceps Femoris

Gastrocnemius
Soleus

FIGURE 16-8 Candidate muscles for postural control accessible to FNS by surface, intramuscular, or implanted electrodes.

the presence of internal or external disturbances.

Fatigue is commonly observed in chronically stimulated muscle. The force generated during a muscular contraction decays rapidly over several minutes and then maintains a nearly constant lower level. In standing trials with continuous stimulation, elapsed standing time is primarily limited by losses of balance or fatigue of the hip extensor muscles, rather than fatigue of the knee extensors. Figure 16-9 illustrates a typical isokinetic (30 deg/sec) moment profile showing the onset and time course of fatigue during cyclic stimulation of the quadriceps. Well-conditioned

individuals can maintain more than 50 percent of maximal muscle output during continuous stimulation (93). Properly conditioned quadriceps muscle can support the weight of the body and prevent collapse during quiet standing for sufficient periods of time (2 to 10 minutes) to complete many activities of daily living, including transfers, reaching, and other tasks involving use of one hand. This suggests that attention should be focused primarily on the *ankle*, *hip*, and *trunk* to provide balance, reject disturbances, and improve stability for short periods during which the hands can be used functionally, rather than on the knees to merely extend quiet standing duration.

The distribution of support forces between upper and lower extremities while standing with continuous stimulation is measured as part of our routine clinical protocols. The upper extremity corrective forces required for balance with open-loop stimulation can be quite small, on the order of the weight of the arms themselves, as illustrated in Figure 16-10. This is not true for all users of currently available standing neuroprostheses, who exhibit a great deal of variability in their standing performance. This fact motivated a series of investigations into the biomechanical and functional characteristics of basic standing systems using continuous stimulation.

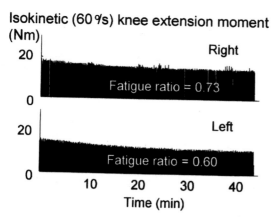

Isokinetic (60 °/s) knee extension moment
(Nm)

20
Right
Fatigue ratio = 0.73

0

20
Left
Fatigue ratio = 0.60

0

10   20   30   40

Time (min)

FIGURE 16-9 Quadriceps fatigue during cyclic stimulation (1:3 duty cycle). Ratio of final to initial momemt (fatigue ratio) indicates endurance.

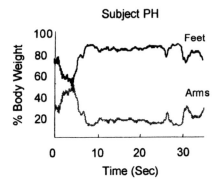

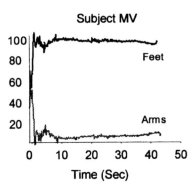

FIGURE 16-10 Distribution of body weight during standing with continuous stimulation. Support is provided primarily by the legs, with small corrections by the upper extremities.

The support forces imposed on the arms while upright depend on many variables, including postural alignment and the stimulated moment produced at the joints. To determine the relationships between these quantities, the isometric strengths of the stimulated hip extensor muscles (gluteus maximus, semimembranosus, and posterior portion of adductor magnus) were measured on a dynamometer for subjects with multiple chronically indwelling percutaneous intramuscular electrodes. Subjects then stood with continuous stimulation to the quadriceps while activation of the hip extensors was altered in a manner similar to that applied while on the dynamometer. Hip angle was monitored by a goniometer, arm forces were measured by strain gauge instrumented parallel bars (94,95), and forces on the feet were recorded with a biomechanics platform while hip extension moment varied. The experimental set-up is illustrated in Figure 16-11A. Increasing stimulated hip extension consistently decreases the vertical support forces placed on the upper extremities, and the same hip extension moment is more effective at decreasing the forces on the arms at more erect standing postures. Figure 16-11B summarizes these findings and presents data from two standing subjects. The dashed lines represent the decrease in arm forces as a function of hip flexion angle predicted by a static sagittal plane mechanical model. At more erect postures (5 and 10 degrees of hip flexion), small amounts of active stimulated hip extension moment produce large decreases in arm support forces. At more flexed postures (15 to 25 degrees), much more

hip extension is required to reduce the arm support forces by similar amounts (96,97). These results indicate that strong stimulated hip extension and the ability to assume an erect posture will be prerequisites for advanced control methods to provide postural corrections to destabilizing events.

Aside from use of the upper extremities and an assistive device, the only mechanism to stabilize posture in continuous stimulation systems is to co-contract agonist–antagonist muscle groups. We performed a theoretical analysis of the open-loop control scheme typically used in the clinical setting to determine which properties of stimulated muscle were most important to stability and whether an optimal level of co-activation could be specified (98–100). The effects of co-activation and muscle model parameters were evaluated based on the ability of a pair of modified Hill-type muscles acting on single-segment inverted pendulum to resist external disturbances. The results indicate that system performance is strongly influenced by intrinsic muscle length dependencies. The slope of the moment–angle (length–tension) curve significantly affected system performance in terms of peak angular displacement in response to a fixed disturbance. In contrast, the slope of the moment–velocity (force–velocity) curve had relatively little effect on the ability to maintain the desired position. Muscle gain (peak isometric force) also strongly influenced system performance by determining muscle stiffness at a given operating point.

Our analysis further indicated that a certain co-activation level is needed to stabilize the

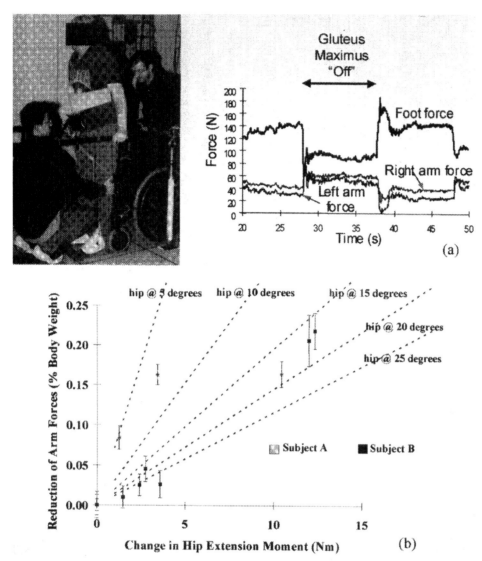

FIGURE 16-11 Effects of stimulated hip extension moment on arm support. Subject standing (a) with FNS on a force platform in instrumented parallel bars (left) as stimulation is altered to the hip extensors (right). Arm support decreases with increasing hip extension at faster rates when subjects are more erect (b).

musculoskeletal system in the presence of a specific disturbance, but increasing co-activation over this level may not substantially improve stability. High co-activation levels cause rapid muscle fatigue, and low co-activation levels compromise stability. We used this trade-off to define a cost function to optimize the level of co-activation for a specific task, based on the relative importance of system performance or fatigue to the neuroprosthesis user. For example, a low level of co-activation may be most appropriate

while standing quietly, and a higher level may be desirable while reaching for an object or preparing for an anticipated disturbance. This technique can provide the user of an FNS system with the ability to adjust co-activation parameters in a task-dependent manner.

CLINICAL EVALUATIONS OF STANDING

We have constructed a clinical evaluation of standing function based upon the ability to acquire, move, and release objects of various sizes and weights while standing with FNS. The Functional Standing Test extends the Jebsen Test of Hand Function (101,102), a standard upper extremity evaluation in the horizontal plane, to include a vertical dimension. The results from applying this test in standing were significantly different than in sitting, indicating that it was sensitive to changes in postural demand. Standing performance with open-loop FNS was comparable to results obtained in knee-ankle-foot orthoses (KAFOs) for all activities but within able-bodied limits only for those subtasks involving the manipulation of small, light objects. The most difficult subtasks with FNS involved moving large and heavy objects, which would normally be manipulated with two hands. FNS users changed their posture in preparation for these tasks by exerting increased forces upon the parallel bars. These results suggest that a mechanism to produce automatic postural corrections may decrease the reliance on the contralateral extremity for balance and facilitate bimanual activities.

The metabolic energy cost associated with quiet standing with continuous FNS is less than three times the basal metabolic rate during able-bodied standing (103) and close to twice that of standing with knee-ankle-foot orthoses. This is a level comparable to tub bathing, piano playing, or fishing (104) and is due primarily to the stimulated activity of the lower extremity musculature, rather than from upper extremity exertion. Control strategies that minimize high levels of continuous stimulation when not absolutely required to prepare for, or respond to, a change in postural demand must be considered to keep energy expenditures at reasonable levels.

LOWER EXTREMITY NEUROPROSTHETIC APPLICATIONS OF FNS FOR WALKING

Surface Stimulation for Stepping

Pioneering work in the application of surface stimulation for restoring standing and walking function to individuals with complete and incomplete spinal cord injuries was conducted in the 1970s and 1980s in Ljubljana, Slovenia. The techniques developed by Kralj, Bajd et al (18,19,105) continue to be employed in many laboratories and clinics around the world. Using as few as two surface stimulation channels per leg, standing and reciprocal walking is produced by activation of the quadriceps muscles and the triggering of a flexion withdrawal reflex. A pair of surface electrodes is placed over the quadriceps on the anterior thigh. A second pair of electrodes is located distally over the dermatomes of the peroneal, sural, or saphenous sensory nerves. Standing is achieved by simultaneously activating the quadriceps bilaterally in response to a command input, such as the simultaneous depression of switches on the handles of a rolling walker or crutches. A stride is produced by maintaining activation to the quadriceps of the stance leg while initiating a flexion withdrawal in the contralateral limb. Depression of the crutch or walker mounted switch on the swing leg stimulates the afferent sensory fibers and triggers a spinal reflex arc that causes hip, knee, and ankle flexion. To complete the reaching phase of the stride, activation of the knee extensors on the swinging leg is initiated while the reflex is still active and flexing the hip. The stimulus producing the flexion reflex is then removed, leaving the user in double-limb support once again with bilateral quadriceps stimulation. Some paralyzed subjects have been reported to walk at speeds approaching one quarter of normal and ascend a curb or step with surface stimulation (18).

Trunk extension is usually achieved passively by adopting a C-curve posture. Alternatively, two additional stimulus channels have been used to activate the gluteal muscles to extend the hips (19,106). Complicating issues with this system include active flexion generated by the rectus femoris when the quadriceps are stimulated with surface electrodes. This makes erect standing difficult and results in an anterior pelvic tilt with compensatory lordosis or excessive weight on the arms to maintain an upright posture. Not all patients exhibit a flexion-withdrawal reflex that is strong or repeatable enough to be used for stepping. Because it is a mass flexion pattern resulting from synergistic activity of a group of muscles triggered by a single stimulus, the swing limb motion is difficult to control. Reflex stepping can be effective in well-selected individuals, although it tends to be jerky and inconsistent. The reflex also habituates with repeated activation, limiting the number of steps that can be taken at one time.

The Slovenian group has fitted surface stimulation systems to more than 50 patients with several years follow-up (17) and has developed extensive prescriptive criteria for individuals with various neurological deficits (16). Patients with incomplete injuries are first evaluated for conventional orthoses alone before adding FNS. Individuals with high-level injuries are considered for combinations of orthoses and stimulation, and persons with mid- to low-level paraplegia are candidates for the surface FNS system without orthoses. These systems and implementation procedures have been successfully transferred to clinical practice, and a commercially available surface stimulation system (Parastep by Sigmedics, Inc., Northfield, Illinois) for standing and stepping has received FDA approval (107,108).

Currently, standing and walking with any form of FNS is not possible without the use of assistive devices such as crutches or a rolling walker for balance. Methods to modulate stimulation automatically in response to postural disturbances detected by sensors during standing and walking are being investigated to minimize the necessity of upper extremity support to maintain posture and balance (21,109,110). However, such "closed loop" control systems are still experimental and have not yet been incorporated into the designs of portable stimulators or completely implantable devices. Continuous preprogrammed "open loop" stimulation may have immediate clinical applications for standing for periods sufficient to complete transfer or reaching tasks and stepping for short distances in the vicinity of the wheelchair to avoid physical obstacles or architectural barriers.

APPLICATION OF SURFACE FES TO INCOMPLETE SCI PARAPLEGIC AND TETRAPLEGIC PATIENTS

Because of improved motor vehicular safety and better early care, there is an increasing number of SCI patients with incomplete injury (111). With the help of FES, many of these can become functional walkers because some of their motor, sensory, and proprioception function has been preserved. After using FES strengthening of knee extensors, three different groups of patients were identified (112). The first group included those in whom voluntary and stimulated response was improved. The second group gained strength in stimulated response only, and in the third, no improvement in either stimulated or voluntary response was noted. With about 50 Nm of knee extension moment under voluntary control, no assistance by FES was needed for walking during stance. In some patients an exaggerated extensor tone provided safe standing, but they were unable to initiate a step. In those patients, bilateral peroneal stimulators were found useful to inhibit extensor tone and help initiate a step (113). Thus, four groups of patients were identified for application of FES. The least affected could stand and needed only unilateral peroneal stimulation to elicit flexion response for stepping after undergoing strengthening of the knee and hip extensors (114). Others needed bilateral step initiation. In most, one leg was completely paralyzed although the other was sufficiently strong to allow safe standing. This group of patients needed unilateral stimulation of knee extensors and afferent stimulation for step initiation. The last group required at least bilateral knee extensor control and step initiation.

The drawback of using afferent stimulation is habituation of the flexion response and a diminished hip flexion after first few steps (114). In some, where quadriceps spasticity interfered with stepping, FES exercise reduced quadriceps tone while increasing voluntary muscle strength. When needed, hip abductors, hamstrings, and trunk extensors were included in stimulation patterns (115). The voluntary strength improvement was also noted with FES in hip flexors and extensors, when the patient had the minimal manual muscle grade of 2. The result was increased stride length and reduced physiological cost index during walking (115).

FNS–ORTHOTIC HYBRID SYSTEMS

One method to overcome the disadvantages of standing and walking systems that rely exclusively on surface stimulation involves combining FNS with conventional bracing (116–120). The advantages of orthoses lie primarily in their ability to constrain the motions of the joints, reduce the degrees of freedom of movement, and provide mechanical stability. For static activities such as quiet standing, individuals with paraplegia can assume a stable posture with little or no muscular exertion by locking the knees of a brace and hyperextending the hips, thus avoiding the fatigue associated with continuous stimulation. FNS is quite effective at introducing large impulsive forces into the biomechanical system through activation of large lower extremity muscles, which reduce the upper extremity exertion required for walking in conventional braces. Combining FNS and bracing in a hybrid orthosis takes advantage of the positive aspects of each technology and minimizes the potential shortcomings.

In 1972, Tomovic, Vukobratovic, and Vodovnik described the Hybrid Actuator for orthotic systems. The concept was that the anatomic joint would be controlled internally by means of FNS or externally by means of a hypothetical three-state joint actuator incorporated onto an exoskeletal brace. This work initiated the development of hybrid orthotics. The braces may reduce the possibility of joint injury and provide a convenient mounting site for sensors for force and joint angles. They can provide a backup system should the FNS component of the system fail. In the 1980s, Schwirlich and Popovic (121) and Andrews (122) demonstrated limited functional capability of their systems and used the term "hybrid orthosis" to describe the

combination. Other hybrid combinations have since been reported but remain primarily exercise devices.

The hip-knee-ankle-foot orthosis (HKAFO) hybrid system incorporates feedback control of reciprocal hip flexion and extension. FNS is also applied to the quadriceps to assist in standing and sitting maneuvers. When the patient is standing, the knee joints are locked. More recently, the HKAFO brace has been upgraded using lightweight plastic components with a molded trunk jacket and hip joints that are reciprocally coupled by means of low-friction, push-pull, flexible linear bearings (Bowdenflex, Bowden Controls Ltd., Llanelli, Dyfed, Wales, U.K.). The Strathclyde hybrid uses locked knee joints that reduce ground clearance for the swinging leg and allow only level walking. In 1986, Andrews and Baxendale introduced a new hybrid system that featured a knee control system that continuously monitored the action of the ground reaction force. The next major change was Petrofsky's combination (127) of FNS with the Louisiana State University RGO brace, which has seen further development by Solomonow.

In another approach, the CWRU team has combined eight to 16 channels of percutaneous or implanted electrical stimulation and computer-controlled bracing to provide functional standing and walking to individuals with complete paraplegia. The CWRU prototype allowed free knee operation during part of gait to improve ground clearance while retaining the option to lock the knee (Figure 16-12). One method of combining the advantages of orthoses and FNS that has been tested extensively was developed at Louisiana State University (LSU). Solomonow and colleagues have been developing a practical hybrid system that utilizes an LSU reciprocating gait orthosis (RGO) and a custom-designed surface stimulator (118,119). The LSU-RGO is a passive mechanical HKAFO (123) consisting of solid, custom-molded polypropylene ankle-foot components joined by lateral uprights to lockable knee and hip joints and terminating in a thoracic strap positioned below the axilla.

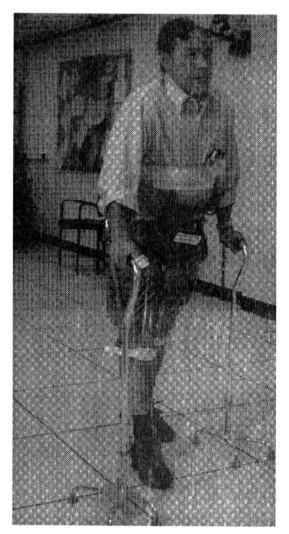

FIGURE 16-12 CWRU hybrid system using 16-channels of percutaneous electrical stimulation combined with modified isocentric reciprocal gait orthosis.

Medial uprights extend from the AFO to the articulated knee and end two-thirds of the way up the medial thigh. The ratcheted knee mechanisms have intermediate stops to allow standing with some knee flexion and are fitted with bail-locks that are engaged automatically upon losing contact with the wheelchair as the user rises. The most important feature of the LSU-RGO is the coupling between the hip joints. Two stainless steel cables inside a low-friction conduit join the hip mechanisms to transmit extension movements on one side to flexion movements on the contralateral side. This reciprocating mechanism

engages automatically when the hips are fully extended upon standing and can be disengaged voluntarily to allow the user to return to the seated position. With knees locked and reciprocating mechanisms engaged, individuals with complete paraplegia can walk by shifting their weight onto the stance limb, pushing up on a walker with their arms, and letting the swing limb advance as the stance limb extends. As with the ratcheted knee joint, intermediate locking positions are possible at the hip, which facilitates walking up ramps. Coupling the hip motions in this manner serves not only to transmit hip extension moments to contralateral flexion (and vice versa); it also prevents bilateral hip flexion and forward leaning of the trunk during quiet standing.

The FNS component of the hybrid system consists of a four-channel surface stimulator and a flexible copolymer electrode cuff that locates and maintains the surface electrodes over the rectus femoris and hamstrings. Because walking is accomplished with the knees locked, stimulating the hamstrings extends the hip and flexes the contralateral hip through the action of the reciprocating mechanism. Conversely, the rectus femoris is used to flex the hip actively, rather than extend the knee, and assist with contralateral hip extension via the reciprocating mechanism. Rectus femoris and contralateral hamstrings are activated simultaneously to initiate a step upon the depression of a walker-mounted switch. Hybrid systems of this type have been fitted to more than 50 patients to date with complete or incomplete thoracic or low-level cervical injuries at LSU and collaborating centers (120).

Similar systems employing a hip-guidance orthosis or alternative reciprocating mechanism have been devised and tested in various centers in North America and Europe (124). Such systems are reliable and offer the additional advantages associated with being relatively simple to implement in clinical environments with orthotic and prosthetic fabricating capacity. Control and stimulation electronics is uncomplicated, and no invasive procedures are necessary. Standing with locked knees allows all stimulation to be removed, which prevents or postpones the onset of fatigue. The orthotic component of these systems may also protect the insensate joints and osteoporotic bones of users with long-standing SCI from possible damage resulting from the loads applied during weight bearing and ambulation. However, the bracing employed by hybrid systems can potentially encumber individuals in the execution of activities of daily living for which they were not designed. For example, locking the knees can hinder the completion of more complex movements useful for personal mobility, such as stair climbing. Similarly, the thoracic component can prohibit lateral bending and trunk rotation while sitting in the wheelchair. The devices are usually worn outside the clothing, and donning, doffing, and cosmetic aspects are similar to conventional braces.

Different joint locks have been incorporated into braces. An early solution was the sliding lock with a metal sleeve on the upper member that slid down over a projection from the lower member, resulting in solid locking of the joint. This required hands-on locking and unlocking of the joint, interrupting other hand functions. Alternatively, the bail lock had a ring behind the knees that looked much like the handle on a pail. The wearer backed into a prospective seating space and pressed the metal projecting handle against the seat. The pressure unlocked the knee joints, letting the individual sit. A controlled-brake orthosis that contains computer regulated friction brakes at the hip and knee has been developed (125,126).

The hybrid orthoses for walking in paraplegia have been motivated primarily by the need to improve hip and trunk stability and forward progression. The simplest hybrid system utilizes a reciprocating gait orthosis for support against gravity via mechanical locks at the joints. Stimulation assists in getting into stance and powering the reciprocal motion during walking (127). The refinement of such systems resulted in brace designs with hip abduction and a ratchet for the knee that allows locking at less than full extension (118). Other hybrid systems use the brace to provide mechanical support only at

certain times in the gait cycle. With the joints passively locked by gravity, stimulation switches off and is only reactivated when the joint becomes unstable. In this way, stimulation duty cycle is reduced and the onset of fatigue can be delayed (128). A third type of hybrid system regulates joint position with a controllable friction brake (125), hand-controlled mechanical joint locks (129), or externally powered joint actuators (130). Follow-up studies on RGO-based hybrid orthoses showed that up to 41 percent of system recipients used it for gait (131), while 66 percent used it for exercise (132), which resulted in a significant decrease in spasticity, total cholesterol, and low density lipids (133).

Implanted Systems for Stepping

Clinicians and researchers at the Veterans Administration Medical Center and Case Western Reserve University in Cleveland, Ohio, have developed systems that utilize implanted electrodes for personal mobility functions such as transfers; standing; one-handed reaching; forward, side, and back stepping; and stair ascent and descent. This approach has involved individual activation of a number of muscles (typically eight or more) rather than the use of synergistic patterns such as the flexion withdrawal reflex, or extensive bracing.

Kobetic and colleagues have synthesized complex lower extremity motions (78) by activating up to 48 separate muscles with chronically indwelling, helically coiled fine wire intramuscular electrodes with percutaneous leads (3,4) under the control of a programmable microprocessor-based external stimulator (134). Users selected one of a series of movement patterns by scrolling through a menu of options, presented on a liquid-crystal display, via switches on a command ring worn on the index finger. Some well-trained subjects were able to walk 300 meters repeatedly at 0.5 m/sec with this system (135). All components were worn by the user, freeing him or her from cabling to a walker or other assistive device. Freely articulating AFOs were used to protect the ligaments and structure of the foot and ankle. The quality of the motions produced by FNS with this system depended on the availability, strength, and endurance of paralyzed muscles; the ability of the therapist or engineer to specify patterns of stimulation for ambulation; and the subject's experience with the device (135).

Because of their ability to activate muscles inaccessible with surface stimulation, intramuscular electrodes with percutaneous leads proved to be valuable tools to simulate the action of completely implanted FNS systems. Researchers in Cleveland utilized these devices to complete three studies essential to proceeding with trials of implanted FNS technology. First, multichannel percutaneous systems were employed to devise a standardized procedure and set of rules for specifying and adjusting patterns of stimulation for reciprocal walking (78). This codified the process of generating stimulus profiles in such a way as to be repeatable by other clinicians or researchers. Next, experiments with subjects with multichannel percutaneous systems defined the minimal muscle set required to achieve stable standing and repeatable stepping (136). This provided a set of primary targets for implantation. Finally, the locations and stimulated responses of intramuscular electrodes with percutaneous leads were used to guide the establishment of the surgical approaches required to access the motor points of the target muscles (137). Cadaver and intraoperative tests confirmed the insight provided by the experience with percutaneous electrodes. To date, these approaches have been used to install surgically implanted lower extremity systems for standing, transfers, and short distance mobility in the vicinity of the wheelchair to seven volunteers with complete thoracic or incomplete low-cervical injuries (89,138).

The implanted components of these systems are illustrated in Figures 16-2 and 16-4. They include an eight-channel receiver-stimulator (Fig. 16-4), a passive pacemaker-like device that receives power and command signals from a wearable external control unit, and epimysial (85) and surgically implanted intramuscular (86)

electrodes. A schematic representation of these components configured to provide standing and standing transfers is presented in Figure 16-5. Epimysial electrodes are installed bilaterally in the vastus lateralis (to achieve knee extension without hip flexion), the semimembranosus (and alternately the posterior portion of the adductor magnus), and the gluteus maximus, while intramuscular electrodes are inserted at the lumbar spinal roots to activate the erector spinae muscles. The entire system can be implanted in a single surgical procedure. A radiograph of such a system installed in one volunteer with complete paraplegia is shown in Figure 16-6. Figures 16-3 and 16-7 show recipients of the implanted standing–transfer system using FNS for standing and performing one-handed reaching tasks to retrieve objects from inaccessible shelves.

Standing and stepping can be achieved without braces for persons with complete paraplegia with 16 channels of stimulation (the four listed above for standing, plus the tibialis anterior, tensor fascia latae, sartorius, and hamstrings bilaterally). These systems rely on two eight-channel devices, as shown in Figure 16-13. Users of the standing systems depicted in Figure 16-5, with complete thoracic level injuries below the level of T4, can have the second implant installed to activate the additional muscles required for walking in a second surgical procedure. Figure 16-14 shows the 16-channel dual-implant system in action.

Other multichannel implanted systems for walking in paraplegia provide standing and swing-through gait (139,140). Exercise and standing functions have been reported with a cochlear implant modified to deliver 22-channels of stimulation to the lower extremities (141) and a 12-channel system for intradural stimulation of the L2–S2 motor roots (82). For long-term clinical applications, implanted pacemaker-like systems such as these provide many major advantages over surface and percutaneous stimulation including improved convenience, cosmesis, reliability, maintenance, and repeatability (84).

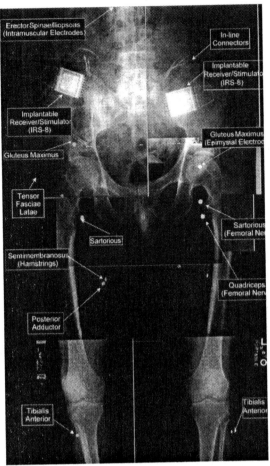

FIGURE 16-13 Composite X-ray of the dual-implant 16-channel FES system. Both IRS-8 devices and all in-line connectors are visible, along with all 14 epimysial electrodes (intramuscular electrodes are not pictured). Note: For clarity, not all electrodes are labeled.

THE POTENTIAL FUNCTIONAL BENEFITS OF FNS

The true value of lower extremity FNS systems in their current forms may lie primarily in their ability to facilitate or provide options for short-duration mobility-related tasks, such as overcoming physical obstacles or architectural barriers in the vicinity of the wheelchair. Exercise, standing, standing transfers, and one-handed reaching are all possible with relatively simple surface or surgically implanted FNS systems without extensive external bracing. The functional impact of lower extremity neuroprosthet-ic applications of FNS on the ability to complete activities of daily living is still an active area of research. It is clear from preliminary work, however, that exercise and standing with FNS can improve tissue viability and overall health, facilitate standing transfers by eliminating the heavy lifting and lowering required by an assistant, and allow selected individuals with SCI to regain access to objects, places, and opportunities impossible or exceedingly difficult from the wheelchair. FNS can augment and extend the function of the wheelchair and may prove to be a valuable option to enhancing the well-being and independence of persons with disabilities. All this can be achieved with reliable implanted components that maximize cosmesis, personal convenience, and long-term use.

From the reports in the literature to date, walking with FNS appears to be a promising form of exercise, rather than an alternative to wheelchair locomotion. The metabolic energy currently required to walk with FNS can be too high to make it a truly practical alternative to the wheelchair for long distance transportation over level surfaces, although this remains a worthwhile and achievable long-term goal. The energy required to operate hybrid systems appears to be less than braces alone but increases rapidly with walking velocity. At slow to moderate speeds, energy consumption for both modes of walking is still less than with FNS alone (64). However, energy consumption for FNS walking decreases as walking speed increases, suggesting that as velocities approach normal the differences between walking modalities will be minimized or reversed (with brace-walking requiring more energy than FNS). Although sustained activities such as walking can be exhausting, the metabolic energy expended for short duration tasks such as standing transfers, reaching, or negotiating environmental obstacles can be easily tolerated. Although locomotion with FNS as transportation may not yet be practical, the technology may eventually prove to be particularly useful for activities such as stair climbing that are impossible from the wheelchair.

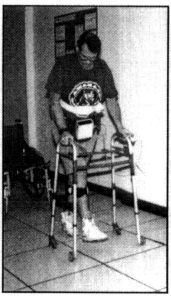 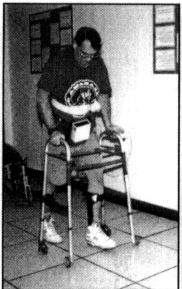 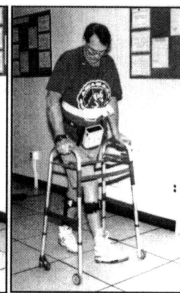

FIGURE 16-14 Stepping function with the dual-implant walking system. Freely articulating orthoses protect the foot and ankle. The subject activates each step by pressing a ring-mounted command switch. Repeated walks in the vicinity of the wheelchair of more than 30 feet are possible.

CLINICAL CONSIDERATIONS

Not all individuals with SCI are well suited for lower extremity FNS because of clinical issues that contraindicate joint mobilization, weight bearing, or the application of electrical currents to the body. Several of the major physical barriers to application of FNS, and possible interventions to address pre-existing conditions, are summarized below. With these issues in mind, the interested clinician can coordinate preparatory treatments and increase the number of individuals with SCI who may benefit from application of FNS technology.

Range of motion must be maintained in ranges commonly accepted for brace prescription. Although stretching is the mainstay of treatment, severe spasticity or equinus deformities may require night splinting. When stretching and splinting fail, early surgical release is essential before bony deformities develop. If releases are performed, muscles that might be utilized for function with electrical stimulation in the future should not be over-lengthened.

Spasticity can interfere with the performance of functional activities with FNS. Exercise with

FNS can provide short-term relief or stronger, but less frequent, involuntary spasms. Pharmacologic treatment should not include neuromuscular blocking agents that may adversely affect the excitability of the peripheral nerve or contractile ability of the muscle and, hence, result in weak, nonfunctional responses to stimulation. Rhizotomies of isolated spastic muscles appear appropriate in theory, although there have been no reports of their use with lower extremity FNS in the SCI population.

Joint instability can be particularly problematic at the hip (66). Acetabular coverage of the femoral head is at a minimum with the hips flexed, so stimulated exercise of the hip adductors and flexors in preparation for walking with FNS should be performed supine rather than while sitting to minimize the risk of hip subluxation. Should subluxation occur, surgical procedures such as soft-tissue releases and bony supplementation are possible. The knee hyperextension commonly seen in females does not seem to be affected by exercise or weight bearing with FNS. The long-term effects of stimulation and the additional demands of ambulation on the insensate joints have yet to be determined, although the acute effects of exercise and mobilization with FNS are encouraging (66). Ankle instability can be easily addressed with several cosmetically acceptable bracing options.

Peripheral denervation is the most frequently observed impediment to the application of FNS (55). Without an intact and excitable peripheral nerve, high stimulating currents or long-duration stimulating pulses are required to activate the muscle tissue directly, which is impractical for functional applications requiring the coordination of many muscles. In the lower extremities, the highest incidence of denervation occurs in individuals with T12–L3 level injuries.

CONCLUSION

Paralysis compromises the ability to work, engage in social or leisure activities, pursue an education, or participate in other activities associated with an independent and productive lifestyle. Complications resulting from SCI can lead to recurrent and costly hospitalization. Long periods of immobility can cause degenerative changes of almost every major organ system including the bones, joints, heart, lungs, and skin. FNS has the potential to postpone or prevent these medical complications and improve the functional independence of people with SCI by providing a means to exercise, stand, and step around barriers that obstruct access to places or life opportunities.

As technology and clinical management of SCI advance, more individuals will be able to take advantage of the functional and therapeutic benefits of FNS. Regular use of FNS can positively impact bone density and joint status, improve cardiovascular fitness, and increase resistance to pressure sores. With increases in longevity because of the advent of antibiotics to treat urinary tract and respiratory infections, the aging sedentary SCI population faces other life-threatening health problems, such as cardiovascular disease. Because manual wheelchair propulsion does not provide a significant exercise effect (142), FNS may also be an effective

mechanism to improve fitness and provide health benefits similar to regular exercise in able-bodied individuals.

Almost one-third of all individuals with paraplegia report needing assistance with activities of daily living, community mobility, or essential transfers (143). FNS can increase independence and address these mobility impairments by improving the ability to stand and maneuver within a wide variety of environments. Although the wheelchair offers a means of efficient transportation over unobstructed level surfaces, it is of limited utility in many environments encountered on a daily basis. Individuals with paraplegia need options negotiating architectural barriers; completing essential daily bed, shower, or toilet transfers; and gaining access to high cabinets, cupboards, or shelves that are difficult or impossible to reach from a wheelchair.

Because of improved motor vehicular safety and better early care there is an increasing number of SCI patients with incomplete injury (111,144). With the help of FNS, many nonambulatory individuals with partial paralysis may become community walkers, because some of their motor, sensory, and proprioceptive functions have been preserved. This offers a potential for brace-free and wheelchair-independent mobility and increased independence.

REFERENCES

1. Mortimer JT. Motor Prostheses. In Brookhart JM, Mountcastle VB, eds., *Handbook of Physiology—The Nervous System II* Bethesda, Maryland: American Physiological Society, 1981. Pp. 155–187.
2. Benton LA, Baker LL, Bowman BR, Waters RL. *Functional Electrical Stimulation: A Practical Clinical Guide*, 2nd ed. Downey, California: Rancho Los Amigos Medical Center, 1981.
3. Marsolais EB, Kobetic R. Implantation techniques and experience with percutaneous intramuscular electrodes in the lower extremities. *J Rehabil Res Dev* 1986; 23:1-8.
4. Scheiner A, Polando G, Marsolasi EB. Design and clinical application of a double helix electrode for functional electrical stimulation. *IEEE Trans Biomed Eng* 1984; 41:425–431.
5. Memberg W, Peckham PH, Keith MW. A sur-

gically implanted intramuscular electrode for an implantable neuromuscular stimulation system. *IEEE Trans Rehabil Eng* 1994; 2:80–91.

6. Grandjean PA, Mortimer JT. Recruitment properties of monopolar and bipolar epimysial electrodes. *Ann Biomed Eng* 1986; 14:53–66.

7. Waters RL, Campbell JM, Nakai R. Therapeutic electrical stimulation of the lower limb with epimysial electrodes. *Clin Orthop and Related Res* 1988; 233:44–52.

8. Holle J, Frey M, Gruber H, Kern H, Stohr H, Thoma H. Functional electrostimulation of paraplegics. Experimental investigations and first clinical experience with an implantable stimulation device. *Orthopaedics* 1984; 7:1145–1160.

9. Waters R, McNeal D, Faloon W, Clifford B. Functional electrical stimulation of peroneal nerve for hemiplegia. *J Bone Joint Surg* 1985; 67:792–793.

10. Stanic U, Acimovic-Janezic R, Gros T, Trnkoczy A, Bajd T, Klajic M. Multichannel electrical stimulation for correction of hemiplegic gait. *Scand J Rehabil Med* 1977; 10:175–192.

11. McNeal R. Analysis of a model for excitation of myelinated nerve. *IEEE Trans Biomed Eng* 1976; 23:329–337.

12. Riley DA, Allin EF. The effects of inactivity, programmed stimulation, and denervation of the histochemistry of skeletal muscle fiber types. *Exp Neurol* 1973; 40:391–398.

13. Peckham PH, Mortimer JT, Marsolais EB. Alteration in the force and fatigability of skeletal muscle in quadriplegia humans following exercise induced by chronic electrical stimulation. *Clinical Orthop* 1976; 114:326–334.

14. Marsolais E, Kobetic R. Functional walking in paralyzed patients by means of electrical stimulation. *Clin Orthop* 1983; 175:30–36.

15. Peckham PH. Functional electrical stimulation: current status and future prospects of applications to the neuromuscular system in spinal cord injury. *Paraplegia* 1987; 25:279–285.

16. Kralj A, Bajd T. *Functional Electrical Stimulation: Standing and Walking After Spinal Cord Injury.* Boca Raton, Florida: CRC Press, 1989.

17. Kralj A, Bajd T. Turk R. Enhancement of gait restoration in spinal injured patients by functional electrical stimulation. *Clin Orthop* 1988; 233:34–43.

18. Kralj A, Bajd T, Turk R, Benko H. Gait restoration in paraplegic patients: a feasibility demonstration using multichannel surface electrode FES. *J Rehab R & D* 1983; 20:3–20.

19. Bajd T, Kralj A, Turk R, Benko H, Sega J. The use of a four-channel electrical stimulator as an ambulatory aid for paraplegic patients. *Physical Therapy* 1983; 63(7):1116.

20. Graupe D. EMG pattern analysis for patient-responsive control of FES in paraplegics for walker-supported walking. *IEEE Trans Biomed Eng* 1989; 36(7):711–719.

21. Chizeck HJ, Kobetic R, Marsolais EB, Abbas JJ, Donner IH, Simon E. Control of functional neuromuscular stimulation systems for standing and locomotion in paraplegics. *Proc IEEE* 1988; 76(9):1155–1165.

22. Crago PE, Chizeck HJ, Neuman M, Hambrecht FT. Sensors for use with functional neuromuscular stimulation. *IEEE Trans Biomed Eng* 1986; 33:256–268.

23. Triolo RJ, Kobetic R, Betz R. Standing and walking with FNS: technical and clinical challenges. In Harris G, ed, *Human Motion Analysis.* New York: IEEE Press, 1996. Pp. 318–350.

24. Handa Y, Hoshimiya N, Iguchi Y, Oda T. Development of percutaneous intramuscular electrode for multichannel FES system. *IEEE Trans Biomed Eng* 1989; 36(7):705–710.

25. Scheiner A, Polando G, Marsolais EB. Design and clinical application of a double helix electrode for functional electrical stimulation. *IEEE Trans Biomed Eng* 1994; 41(5):425–431.

26. Haugland MK, Hoffer JA, Sinkjaer T. Skin contact force information in sensory nerve signals recorded by implanted cuff electrodes. *IEEE Trans Rehabil Eng* 1994;2:18–28.

27. Smith B, Peckham PH, Keith MW, Roscoe DD. An externally powered, multichannel implantable stimulator for versatile control of paralyzed muscle. *IEEE Trans Biomed Eng* 1987; 34(7):499–508.

28. Letechepia JE, Peckham PH, Gazdik M, Smith B. In-line lead connector for use with implanted neuroprostheses. *IEEE Trans Biomed Eng* 1991; 38:707–709.

29. Glaser RM. Functional neuromuscular stimulation: exercise conditioning of spinal cord injured patients. *Int J Sports Med* 1994; 15:142–148.

30. Glaser RM. Physiologic aspects of spinal cord injury and functional neuromuscular stimulation. *Cen Nerv Syst Trauma* 1986; 3:49–62.

31. Glaser RM. Physiology of functional electrical stimulation-induced exercise: basic science perspective. *J Neuro Rehab* 1991; 5: 49–61.

32. Martin TP, Stein RB, Hoeppner PH, Reid DC. Influence of electrical stimulation on the morphological and metabolic properties of paralyzed muscle. *J Appl Physiol* 1992; 72:1401–1406.

33. Faghri PD, Glaser RM, Figoni SF, Miles DS.

Feasibility of using two FNS exercise modes for spinal cord injured patients. *Clin Kinesiol* 1989; 43: 62–64.

34. Gruner JA, Glaser RM, Feinberg SD, Collins SR, Nussbaum NS. A system for evaluation and exercise conditioning of paralyzed leg muscles. *J Rehab R & D* 1983; 20:21–30.

35. Rodgers MM, Glaser RM, Figoni SF, Hooker SP, Ezenwa BN, Collins SR, Mathews T, Suryaprasad AG. Musculoskeletal responses of spinal cord injured individuals to functional neuromuscular stimulation-induced knee extension exercise training. *J Rehab R & D* 1991; 28: 19–26.

36. Figoni SF, Glaser RM, Rodgers MM, Hooker SP, Ezenwa B, Collins SR, Mathews T, Suryaprasad AG, Gupta SC. Acute hemodynamic responses of spinal cord injured individuals to functional neuromuscular stimulation-induced knee extension exercise. *J Rehab R & D* 1991; 28: 9–18.

37. Ragnarsson KT, O'Daniel W. Edgar R. Pollack S. Petrofsky J, Nash MS. Clinical evaluation of computerized functional electrical stimulation after spinal cord injury: a multicenter pilot study. *Arch Phys Med & Rehab* 1988; 69: 672–677.

38. Pollack SF, Axen K, Spielholz N, Levin N, Haas F, Ragnarsson KT. Aerobic training effects of electrically induced lower extremity exercises in spinal cord injured people. *Arch Phys Med & Rehab* 1989; 70:214–219.

39. Nash MS, Bilsker S, Arcillo AE, Issac BS, Botelho LA, Lkose KJ, Green BA, Rountree MT, Shea JD. Reversal of adaptive left ventricular atrophy following electrically stimulated exercise training in human tetraplegics. *Paraplegia* 1991; 29:590–99.

40. Twist DJ, Culpepper-Morgan JA, Ragnarsson KT, Petrillo, Kreck MJ. Neuroendocrine changes during functional electrical stimulation. *Am J Phys Med Rehab* 1992; 71:156–163.

41. Sipski ML, Delisa JA, Schweer S. Functional electrical stimulation bicycle ergometry: patient perceptions. *Am J Phys Med Rehab* 1989; 68:147–149.

42. Hooker SP, Figoni SF, Rodgers MM, Glaser RM, Ezenwa B, Mathews T, Suryaprasad AG, Gupta SC. Metabolic and hemodynamic responses to concurrent voluntary arm crank and electrical stimulation leg cycle exercise in quadriplegics. *J Rehab R & D* 1992; 29:1–11.

43. Ramos MV, Freed MM, Kayne HL. Resting blood pressure in spinal cord injured patients. *SCI Digest* 1981; 3:19–25.

44. Bader DL, Gant CA. Effects of prolonged loading on tissue oxygen levels. In Spence VA, Sheldon CD, eds., *Practical Aspects of Skin Blood Flow Measurements*. London: Biological Engineering Society, 1985.

45. Mawson AR, Siddiqui FH, Biundo JJ Jr. Enhancing host resistance to pressure ulcers: a new approach to prevention. *Prev Med* 1993; 22(3):433–450.

46. Hudlicka O, West D, Kumar S, El Khelly F, Wright AJA. Can growth of capillaries in the heart and skeletal muscle be explained by the presence of an angiogenic factor? *Br J Exp Pathol* 1989; 70(30):237–246.

47. Hudlicka O, Brown M, Cotter M, Smith M, Vrbova G. The effect of long-term stimulation of fast muscles on their blood flow, metabolism and ability to withstand fatigue. *Pflugers Archives* 1977; 369:141–149.

48. Brown M, Cotter M, Hudlicka O, Vrbova G. The effects of different patterns of muscle activity on capillary density, mechanical properties and structure of slow and fast rabbit muscles. *Pflugers Archives* 1976; 361:241–250.

49. Salmons S, Henriksson J. The adaptive response of skeletal muscle to increased use. *Muscle & Nerve* 1981; 4:94–105.

50. Baker LL, Bennetts L, Khalaiabadi M, Sanderson D. Electrical stimulation and cutaneous oxygen supply effect on wound healing. *Physical Therapy* 1983; 63(5):751.

51. Baker LL, Chambers R, Merchant L, Park D, Sokolski D, Toneyama C. The effects of electrical stimulation on cutaneous oxygen supply in normal older adults and diabetic patients. *Physical Therapy* 1986; 66(5):749.

52. Levine SP, Kett RL, Gross MD, Wilson BA, Cederna PS, Juni JE. Blood flow in the gluteus maximus of seated individuals during electrical muscle stimulation. *Arch Phys Med & Rehab* 1990; 71(9):682–686.

53. Seiler WO, Stahelin HB. Skin oxygen tension as a function of imposed skin pressure: implication for decubitus ulcer formation. *J Am Ger Soc* 1979; 27:298–301.

54. Garber S, Krouskop T. Body build and its relationship to pressure distribution in the seated wheelchair patient. *Arch Phys Med & Rehab* 1982; 63:17–20.

55. Jaeger RJ. Lower extremity applications of functional neuromuscular stimulation. *Assistive Technology* 1992; 4(1):19–30.

56. Marsolais EB, Kobetic R. Functional electrical stimulation for walking in paraplegia. *J Bone Joint Surg. (Am)* 1987; 69A:728–733.

57. Marsolais EB, Kobetic R, Chizeck HJ, Jacobs JL. Orthoses and electrical stimulation for walking in complete paraplegia. *J Neuro Rehab* 1991; 5(1–2):13–22.

58. Moynahan M, Mullin C, Cohn J, Burns CA, Halden EE, Triolo RJ, Betz, RR. Home use of a FES system for standing and mobility in adolescents with spinal cord injury. *Arch Phys Med & Rehab* 1996; 77(10):1005–1013.

59. Triolo RJ, Reilley B, Freedman W, Betz R. Development and standardization of a clinical evaluation of standing function. *IEEE Trans Rehab Eng* 1993; 1(1):18–25.

60. Triolo RJ, Eisenhower G, Stabinski T, Wormser D. Inter-rater reliability of a clinical test of standing function. *J Spinal Cord Med* 1995; 18(1):13–21.

61. Bogie KM, Nuseibeh I, Bader DL. New concepts in the prevention of pressure sores. In Frankel HL, ed., *Handbook of Clinical Neurology: Spinal Cord Trauma*, Oxford: Elsevier, 17(61): 347–365, 1992.

62. Berlowitz DR, Wilking SVB. Risk factors for pressure sores: a comparison of cross-sectional and cohort-derived data. *J Am Geriatric Soc* 1989; 37:1043–1050.

63. Harper CM, Lyles YM. Physiology and complications of bed rest. *J Am Geriatr Soc* 1988; 36:1047–1054.

64. Edwards BG, Marsolais EB. Metabolic responses to arm ergometry and functional neuromuscular stimulation. *J Rehab Res and Dev* 1990; 27(2):107–114.

65. Lew RD. The effects of FNS on disuse osteoporosis. *Proceedings of the 10th Annual RESNA Conference*, San Jose, California. Pp. 616-617. June 19–23, 1987.

66. Betz R, Boden B, Triolo RJ, Mesgarzadeh M, Gardner ER, Fife R. Effects of functional neuromuscular stimulation on the joints of adolescents with spinal cord injury. *Paraplegia* 1996; 34:127–136.

67. Harvey C, Rothschild R, Asmann A, Stripling T. New estimates of traumatic SCI prevalence: a survey-based approach. *Paraplegia* 1990; 28:537–544.

68. Stover SL, Fine PR. *Spinal Cord Injury: The Facts and Figures*. Birmingham: The University of Alabama at Birmingham, 1986.

69. Stover SL, Fine PR. The epidemiology and economics of spinal cord injury. *Paraplegia* 1987; 28:225–228.

70. Triolo RJ, Betz RR, Mulcahey MJ, Gardner ER. Application of functional neuromuscular stimulation to children with spinal cord injuries: candidate selection for research applications. *Paraplegia* 1994; 32:824–843.

71. Jaeger R, Yarkony G, Roth E, Lovell L. Estimating the user population of a simple electrical system for standing. *Paraplegia* 1990; 28:505–511.

72. Jaeger RJ, Yarkony GM, Roth EJ. Rehabilitation technology for standing and walking after spinal cord injury. *Am J Phys Med Rehab* 1989, 68(3): 128–133.

73. Yarcony GM, Rothe EJ, Cybulski GR, Jaeger RJ. Neuromuscular stimulation in spinal cord injury: I. Restoration of functional movement of the extremities. *Arch Phys Med & Rehab* 1992;73: 78–86.

74. Jaeger RJ, Yarkony GM, Roth EJ. Standing the spinal cord injured patient by electrical stimulation: refinement of a protocol for clinical use. *IEEE Trans Biomed Eng* 1989; 36(7):720–728.

75. Yarcony GM, Jaeger RJ, Roth E, Kralj A, Quintern J. Functional neuromuscular stimulation for standing after spinal cord injury. *Arch Phys Med & Rehab* 1990; 71:201–206.

76. Graupe D, Kohn K. *Functional Electrical Stimulation for Ambulation by Paraplegics*. Malabar, Florida: Krieger Publishing Co., 1994.

77. Scheiner A, Polando G, Marsolais EB. Design and clinical application of a double helix electrode for functional electrical stimulation. *IEEE Trans Biomed. Engr* 1994, 41(5):425–431.

78. Kobetic R, Marsolais EB. Synthesis of paraplegic gait with multichannel functional neuromuscular stimulation. *IEEE Trans Biomed Engr* 1994; 2(2):66–67.

79. Triolo RJ, Bieri C, Uhlir J, Kobetic R, Scheiner A, Marsolais EB. Implanted FNS systems for assisted standing and transfers for individuals with cervical spinal cord injuries: clinical case reports. *Arch Phys Med & Rehab* 1996; 7(11):1119–1128.

80. Marsolais EB, Kobetic R. Implantation techniques and experience with percutaneous intramuscular electrodes in the lower extremities. *J Rehab R & D* 1986; 23(3):1–8.

81. Davis R, Eckhouse R, Patrick JF, Delehanty A. Computer-controlled 22-channel stimulator for limb movement. *Acta Neurochirurgica, Suppl* 1987; 39:117–120.

82. Rushton DN, Perkins TA, Donaldson N, Wood DE, Harper VJ, Tromans AM, Barr FMD, Holder DS. LARSI: how to obtain favorable muscle contractions. *Proceedings of the Second Annual IFESS Conference (IFESS 97) and Neural Prosthesis: Motor Systems 5 (NP 97)*, Burnaby, British Columbia, Canada. Pp.163–164 16–21 Aug. 1997.

83. Cameron T, Loeb GE, Peck RA. Micromodular implants to provide electrical stimulation of paralyzed muscles and limbs. *IEEE Trans Biomed Eng* 1997; 44:781–790.

84. Kilgore KL, Peckham PH, Keith MW, Thrope GB, Wuolle KS, Bryden AM, Hart RL. An implanted upper extremity neuroprosthesis: a five-patient follow-up. *J Bone Joint Surg (Am)* 1997; 79A: 533–541.

85. Akers JM, Peckham PH, Keith MW, Merritt K. Tissue response to chronically stimulated implanted epimysial and intramuscular electrodes. *IEEE Trans Rehab Eng* 1996; 5(2):207–220.

86. Memberg WD, Peckham PH, Keith MW. A surgically implanted intramuscular electrode for an implantable neuromuscular stimulation system. *IEEE Trans Biomed Eng* 1994; 2(2):80–91.

87. Triolo RJ, Bogie K. Lower extremity applications of functional neuromuscular stimulation after spinal cord injury. *Topics in SCI Rehab* 1999; 5(1): 44–65.

88. Sharma M, Marsolais EB, Polando G, Triolo RJ, Davis JA, Bhadra N, Uhlir J. Implantation of a 16-channel functional electrical stimulation walking system. *Clin Ortho Related Res* 1998; 347:236–242.

89. Kobetic R, Triolo RJ, Uhlir J, Bieri C, Wibowo M, Polando G, Marsolais EB, Davis JA, Ferguson K, Sharma M. Implanted functional electrical stimulation system for mobility in paraplegia: a follow-up case report. *IEEE Trans Rehab Eng* 1999; 7(4):390–398.

90. Barnette N, Lamitie H. A comparison of energy expenditure between KAFO and FNS standing in adolescents with spinal cord injuries. MS Thesis. Department of Physical Therapy: Beaver College, Glenside Pennsylvania 1991.

91. Moynahan M. Postural responses during standing in subjects with spinal-cord injury. *Gait and Posture* 1995; 3:156–165.

92. Kobetic R, Triolo RJ. Muscle selection and walking performance of multichannel FES systems for ambulation in paraplegia. *IEEE Trans Rehab Eng* 1997; 5(1):23–29.

93. Carroll SG, Triolo RJ, Chizeck HJ, Kobetic R, and Marsolais EB. Tetanic responses of electrically stimulated paralyzed muscle at varying interpulse intervals. *IEEE Trans Biomed Eng* 1989; 36 (7):644–653.

94. Jin Z, Kobetic R. Rail supporting transducer posts for three-dimensional force measurement. *IEEE Trans Rehab Eng* 1997; 5(4):380–387.

95. Jin Z, Chizeck HJ. Instrumented parallel bars for three-dimensional force measurement. *J Rehab Res & Dev* 1992; 29(2):31–38.

96. Wibowo MA, Triolo RJ, Uhlir JP, Kobetic R, Kirsch RF. Effects of hip extension moment and posture on arm forces during FNS-induced standing. *J Rehab R & D* (submitted).

97. Wibowo MA, Triolo RJ, Uhlir JP, Kobetic R, Kirsch RF. The effect of stimulated hip extensor moment on the loads imposed on the arms during standing with FES. *Proceedings of the 1998 Annual RESNA Conference*. Pp. 384–366. June 1998.

98. Zhang X, Triolo RJ, Abbas JJ. The effects of co-stimulation and muscle model parameters on FNS system performance. *IEEE Trans Rehab Eng* (submitted).

99. Zhang X, Triolo RJ, Abbas JJ. Task-dependent adjustments to co-stimulation levels in functional neuromuscular stimulation systems. *Proceedings of the IEEE EEMBS*. Atlanta, Georgia. 1999, pp. 658–659.

100. Zhang X, Triolo RJ, Abbas JJ. The effects of co-stimulation map parameters on FNS system performance. *Annals Biomed Eng* October 1998; S133.

101. Jebsen RH, Taylor N, Trieschmann RB, Trotter MJ, Howard LA. An objective and standardized test of hand function. *Arch Phys Med & Rehab* 1969; 50:311–319.

102. Taylor N, Sand PL, Jebsen RH. Evaluation of hand function in children. *Arch Phys Med & Rehab* 1974; 54:129–135.

103. Miller P, Kobetic R, Lew R. Energy costs of walking and standing using functional electrical stimulation. *Proceedings of the 13th Annual RESNA Conference*. Pp. 155–156. Washington DC, 1990.

104. Glaser RM. Physiologic aspects of spinal cord injury and functional neuromuscular stimulation. *Central Nervous System Trauma* 1986; 3(1):49–61.

105. Bajd T, Kralj A, Turk R. Standing up of a healthy subject and a paraplegic patient. *J Biomech* 1982; 15(1):1–10.

106. Isakov E, Mizrahi J, Majenson T. Biomechanical and physiological evaluation of FES-activated paraplegic patients. *J Rehab R & D* 1986; 23:9–19.

107. Graupe D, Kohn K. *Functional Electrical Stimulation for Ambulation by Paraplegics*. Malabar, Florida: Krieger Publishing Co., 1994.

108. Gallien P, Brissot R, Eyssette M, Tell L, Barat M, Wiart L, Petit H. Restoration of gait by functional electrical stimulation for spinal cord injured patients. *Paraplegia* 1995; 33:660–664.

109. Jaeger R. Design and simulation of closed-loop electrical stimulation orthoses for restoration of quiet standing in paraplegics. *J Biomech* 1986; 19(10):825–835.

110. Abbas JA, Chizeck HJ. Feedback control of coronal plane hip angle using functional neuromuscular stimulation. *IEEE Trans Biomed Eng* 1991; 38:687–698.

111. Bedbrook GM. A balanced viewpoint in the early management of patients with *spinal* injuries who have neurological damage. *Paraplegia* 1985; 23:8–15.

112. Bajd T, Kralj A, Turk R, Benko H. FES rehabilitative approach in incomplete SCI patients. RESNA 9th Annual Conference, Minneapolis, Minnesota, 1986. Pp. 316–318.

113. Bajd T, Kralj A, Turk R, Benko H, Sega J. Use of functional electrical stimulation in the rehabilitation of patients with incomplete spinal cord injuries. *J Biomed Eng* 11:96–102.

114. Kralj A, Bajd T, Kvesic Z, Turk R. Electrical stimulation of incomplete paraplegic patients. Proceedings of the REANS 4th Annual Conference. Pp. 226–228. Washington D.C. 1981.

115. Granat MH, Ferguson ACB, Andrews BJ, Delargy M. The role of functional electrical stimulation in the rehabilitation of patients with incomplete spinal cord injury: observed benefits during gait studies. *Paraplegia* 1993; 31:207–221.

116. Andrews B, Baxendale R. A Hybrid orthosis incorporating artificial reflexes for spinal cord damaged patients. *J Physiol* 1988; 198:380.

117. Marsolais EB, Kobetic R, Chizeck HJ, Jacobs JL. Orthoses and electrical stimulation for walking in complete paraplegia. *J Neuro Rehabil* 1991; 5:13–22.

118. Solomonow M, Baratta RV, Hirokawa S. The RGO generation II: muscle stimulation powered orthosis as a practical walking system for paraplegics. *Orthopaedics* 1989; 12:1309–1315.

119. Solomonow M. Biomechanics and physiology of a practical functional neuromuscular stimulation powered walking orthosis for paraplegics. In Stein RB, Peckham PH, Popovic DP, eds., *Neural Prostheses: Replacing Motor Function After Disease or Disability*. New York: Oxford University Press, 1992. Pp. 202–232.

120. Kantor C, Andrews BJ, Marsolais EB, Solomonow M, Lew RD, Ragnarsson KT. Report on a conference on motor prostheses for workplace mobility of paraplegic patients in North America. *Paraplegia* 1993; 31:439–456.

121. Schwirlich L, Popovic D. Hybrid orthosis for deficient locomotion. In *Advances in External Control of Human Extremities* VII. 1984. Pp. 23–32.

122. Andrews BJ, Baxendale RH, Barnett R, Phillips GP, Yamazaki T, Paul JP, Freeman PA. A hybrid orthosis for paraplegics incorporating closed loop control and sensory feedback. *J Biomed Eng* 1988;10:189–195.

123. Douglas R, Larson PF, D'Ambrosia R, McCall RE. The LSU reciprocation gait orthosis. *Orthopedics* 1983; 834–838.

124. McClelland M, Andrews BJ, Patrick JH, Freeman PA. Augmentation of the Oswestry Parawalker orthosis by means of surface electrical stimulation: gait analysis of three patients. *Paraplegia* 1987; 25(1): 32–38.

125. Durfee WK, Hausdorff JM. Regulating knee joint position by combining electrical stimulation with a controllable friction brake. *Ann Biomed Eng* 1990; 18:575–596.

126. Goldfarb M, Durfee WK. Design of a controlled-brake orthosis for FES-aided gait. *IEEE Trans Rehab Eng* 1996; 4(1):13–24.

127. Petrofsky JS, Phillips CA, Douglas R, Larson P. A computer-controlled walking system: the combination of an orthosis with functional electrical stimulation. *J Clin Eng* 1986; 11(2): 121–133.

128. Andrews BJ, Baxendale RH, Barnett R, Phillips GF, Paul JP, Freeman PA. A hybrid orthosis for paraplegics incorporating feedback control. Proceedings of the 9th Symposium of ECHE. Pp. 297–311; 1987.

129. Popovic D, Schwirtlich L. Design and evaluation of the self-fitting modular orthosis (SFMO). *IEEE Trans Rehab Eng* 1993; 1(3): 165–174.

130. Popovic DB. Functional electrical stimulation for lower extremities. In Stein RB, Peckham RH, Popovic DB, eds., *Neural Prostheses, Replacing Motor Function After Disease or Disability*. Oxford University Press, 1992. Pp. 233–251.

131. Franceschini M, Baratta S, Zampolini M, Loria D, Lotta S. Reciprocating gait orthoses: a multicenter study of their use by spinal cord injured patients. *Arch Phys Med Rehab* 1997;78:582–586.

132. Solomonow M, Aguilar E, Reisin E, Baratta RV, Best R, Coetzee T, D'Ambrosia R. Reciprocating gait orthosis powered with electrical muscle stimulation (RGO II). Part I: Performance evaluation of 70 paraplegic patients. *Orthopedics* 1997; 20(4):315–324.

133. Solomonow M, Reisin E, Aguilar E, Baratta RV, Best R, D'Ambrosia R. Reciprocating gait orthosis powered with electrical muscle stimulation (RGO II). Part II: Medical evaluation of 70 paraplegic patients. *Orthopedics* 1997; 20(5): 411–418.

134. Borges G, Ferguson K, Kobetic R. Development and operation of portable and laboratory electrical stimulation systems for walking in paraplegic subjects. *IEEE Trans Biomed Eng* 1989; 36(7):798–800.

135. Kobetic R, Marsolais EB, Samame P, Borges G. The next step: artificial walking. In Rose J, Gamble JG, eds. *Human Walking*, 2nd ed. Baltimore, Maryland: Williams and Wilkins, 1994. Pp. 225–252.

136. Kobetic R, Triolo RJ. Muscle selection and walking performance of multichannel FES systems for ambulation in paraplegia. *IEEE Trans Rehabil Eng* 1997;5:23–29.

137. Sharma M, Marsolasi EB, Polando G, et al. Implantation of a 16-channel functional electrical stimulation walking system. *Clin Orthop* 1998;347:236-242.

138. Triolo RJ, Bieri C, Uhlir J, Kobetic R, Scheiner A, Marsolais EB. Implanted FNS systems for assisted standing and transfers for individuals with cervical spinal cord injuries: clinical case reports. *Arch Phys Med Rehabil* 1996; 77:1119–1128.

139. Brindley GS, Polkey CE, Rushton DN. Electrical splinting of the knee in paraplegia. *Paraplegia* 1979; 16:248.

140. Holle J, Frey M, Gruber H, Kern H, Stohr H, Thoma H. Functional electrostimulation of paraplegics: experimental investigations and first clinical experience with an implantable stimulation device. Orthopaedics 1984; 7:1145–1160.

141. Davis R, MacFarland WC, Emmons SE. Initial results of the Nucleus FES-22-implanted system for limb movement in paraplegia. *Stereotactic & Func Neurosurg* 1994; 63:192–197.

142. Cooper R. Guest editorial:wheelchair research and development for people with spinal cord injury. J Rehab R & D 1998; 35(1):xi.

143. Berkowitz M, Harvey C, Greene C, Wilson S. *The Economic Consequences of Traumatic Spinal Cord Injury.* New York: Demos Press, 1992.

144. Marsolais EB, Scheiner A, Miller PC, Kobetic R, Daly J. Augmentation of transfers for a quadriplegic patient using an implanted FNS system: case report. *Paraplegia* 1994; 32:573–579.

17 Surgical Management of the Upper Limb in Tetraplegia

MICHAEL W. KEITH, MD
EDUARDO GONZALES, MD

THE RECONSTRUCTION OF the upper limb in tetraplegia has emerged as a bright area for surgical and rehabilitative progress during the past decade. As spinal cord injury centers have improved the survival and prospects for a longer and more productive life, persons with spinal injury have asked for greater hand function and greater flexibility in controlling their lives, work, and ambitions. Hand surgeons have responded with innovations refinement, and improvement of traditional techniques. Outcome studies have shown improvement in measures of impairment and activities of daily living (ADL), and reduction in disability.

The opportunity for earlier intervention, prevention of contracture, reduction in spasticity, improvement in dexterity, and greater strength have been the results of concerted efforts by an international group of dedicated surgeons, therapists, and rehabilitationists. This chapter summarizes the traditional and newer approaches to and philosophies of reconstruction and rehabilitation.

CLASSIFICATION OF SPINAL CORD INJURIES

Description of patients with complex dysfunction is important to communication between clinicians and as a means of following clinical progress. Careful examinations over time are needed to demonstrate a plateau of function or to detect the predictable root level improvement seen with complete injuries (1). In incomplete spinal injuries, progress may be unpredictable, and optimistic results can occur with time. With the development of good acute critical care and transport systems, persons with greater injury severity scores are surviving their initial accident. Their additional injuries—including fractures, lower motor neuron lesions, brachial plexus injuries, peripheral nerve injuries, multiple cord injuries, head injuries, and penetrating abdominal and thoracic injuries—produce new challenges to the management of more complex survivors.

Two useful classifications of upper limb impairment have predominated during the past two decades. The scoring system of the American Spinal Injury Association (ASIA) uses unequivocal joint and muscle movements and sensory dermatome representations to classify levels. The scheme is shown in Table 17-1. Strength on manual muscle testing is graded on a 0–5 scale according to the British Medical Research Council (BMRC) (2,3). Grade 3 force was chosen as the reference because grades 4 and 5 are subjective measures that depend upon the examiner's strength in confrontation testing. Sensory exam is rated as absent (0), impaired (1), normal (2), or not testable (NT). The classifica-

TABLE 17-1 ASIA Classification of The Upper Limb in Spinal Cord Injury

Spinal Segment	Functional Group
C5	Elbow Flexors
C6	Wrist Extensors
C7	Elbow Extensors
C8	Finger Flexors
T1	Fifth Finger Abduction

Muscles are graded at Grade 3, antigravity through a full range of motion.

TABLE 17-2 International Classification for Surgery of the Hand in Tetraplegia

"O" for "Oculo." Poor two-point discrimination >10mm requiring visual control. "Cu" for "Cutaneous." Two-point discrimination <10mm.

Group	Motor evaluation (BRMC Grade 4 or stronger):
1	BR brachioradialis (BR)
2	ECRL extensor carpi radialis (longus ECRL)
3	ECRB extensor carpi radialis brevis*
4	PT pronator teres
5	FCR flexor carpi radialis
6	Extrinsic finger extensors
7	Thumb extensor
8	Extrinsic finger flexion
9	Lacks intrinsic only
0	Exceptions

T+ or T− indicates triceps strength at grade 4.

Revised at the 6th International Conference, Cleveland, Ohio, 1999.

*At the time this classification was originally proposed, it was thought that assessment of ECRB strength was possible only at the time of surgery. The New Zealand group headed by Rothwell has pointed out that a groove between the ECRL and ECRB is appreciable on examination of the lateral forearm of a lean person, while they extend the wrist against resistance. This simple observation is known as the "Bean sign" and predicts a strong ECRB.

tion is consistent and reproducible over time by varied examiners. Moberg (4), Zancolli (5,6), Freehafer (7,8), and Lamb (9), among other pioneers in the field, proposed independent classification systems for the tetraplegic upper extremity according to remaining motor function. Total arm muscle strength is related to the level of spinal cord injury.

A compromise classification was adopted at the First International Conference on Surgical Rehabilitation of the Upper Limb in Tetraplegia in Edinburgh, Scotland, in 1978. The International Classification is coding shorthand that describes remaining sensory and motor ability in the forearm and hand. The assignment to one of nine groups is made according to the number of grade 4 muscles under voluntary control below the elbow. Shoulder and elbow function was considered separately. Recently, the classification has been modified at the Sixth International Conference on Tetraplegia in Cleveland, Ohio, to include the presence or absence of triceps function at grade 4 (+ or −) (Table 17-2).

Moberg popularized the static two-point discrimination (TPD) of Weber (1835) (10) and believed that sensory preservation at 10 mm of static two-point discrimination within the C6 dermatome in tetraplegic patients was a useful index of coordination and sensation for motor function in the finger and thumb. The label Cu is for "cutaneous" TPD (less than 10 mm), and O for lesser cutaneous function requiring visual or "ocular" input for control. Motor and sensory evaluations are done for both arms independently because it is common to have asymmetric function.

Many surgeons have adopted the International Surgical Classification because the classification implies the ability to perform tendon transfer surgery in a logical, sequential way. The classification is less useful after reconstructive surgery because new functions are created that do not fit the classification, and index muscles are transferred. It does not reliably describe combined injuries or head injuries in conjunction with spinal cord injury. It must be used in conjunction with other outcome studies to be useful in clinical studies.

Other factors such as the usage patterns, sitting balance, comorbidities, peripheral nerve, and incomplete sensory injuries contribute to the selection of surgical procedures. Persons with high-level injuries have patterns of overuse of antigravity muscles, and shoulder joint function is limited by imbalance. Figure 17-1 is an example of how muscle imbalance proximally limits distal reconstruction to the context of learned hand usage.

PHARMACOLOGICAL STABILITY

Pharmacologic control at a plateau of tolerance and efficacy is important before assigning a muscle grade. Higher levels of effective spasmolytic agents, such as diazepam, may produce muscle weakness. The therapeutic context in which the patient is willing to accept reduction in spasticity and reduction in strength is frequently a compromise. Side effects, such as drowsiness or blunting of affect, from benzodiazopines are a frequent reason to reduce or discontinue them. Concerns about habituation or abuse have led to fewer prescriptions. Use of implantable Baclofen pumps may lead to steady-state suppression of spasticity. Unfortunately, sudden withdrawal of these medications (as in a pump failure), is an emergency because seizures and vasomotor instability may occur with fatal consequences.

THE NATIONAL MODEL SPINAL CORD INJURY SYSTEM

The Model Spinal Cord System has evolved to optimize patient management. The goal is to assume encompassing care from the onset of the traumatic event, including transport and acute care, to acute rehabilitation, psychosocial and vocational services, and community reintegration together with lifelong follow-up and maintenance (11). The spinal cord injury team becomes involved early in the acute hospitalization. Early specialized intervention results in significantly fewer complications (12), including reduction in the incidence of:

- Pressure ulcers
- Pulmonary atelectasis
- Abnormal renal function
- Contractures, especially in the hand
- Decreased overall mortality (13,14)
- Additional benefits that follow with shorter hospitalization (15) and higher possibility of discharge to the community; reduced medical costs are only one of many arguments in favor of the Model System (16).

RECONSTRUCTION STRATEGIES

Elbow Extension for C5 and C6 Patients

Tetraplegic patients without triceps function are able to benefit from two important substitution maneuvers to achieve elbow extension. External

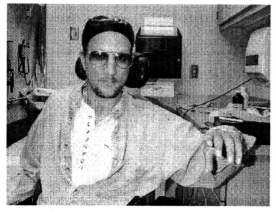
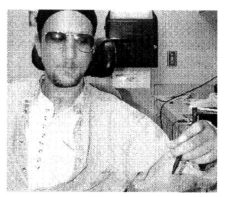

FIGURE 17-1   In high tetraplegia, the patient uses the arm in a fixed abducted position, like a crane, with hand pronated and fingers in palmar pinch orientation. Shoulder pain from this posture, with scapular instability, winging, and trapezius muscle overuse is common. This posture must be considered in surgical planning, especially to avoid excessive pronation or reduced supination. This patient requires additional supination by osteotomy to bring a fork to the mouth.

shoulder rotation followed by forward shoulder flexion results in gravity-assisted elbow extension. A second maneuver involves a closed kinetic chain, with the hand fixed to a point while the patient activates the pectoralis major and the anterior deltoid. However, there are severe functional limitations for patients who lack active extension. The workspace is reduced and activities occur predominantly around the chest and lap. Objects are frequently beyond reach and items on the chest or face, like a blanket, cannot be removed. The hands are frequently in front of the face and the lack of coordinated hand movement is awkward for gesturing or pointing.

Restoration of active elbow extension is often the most satisfying procedure in the tetraplegic patient, and elbow extension is the most important function to be added, providing an eight-fold increase in the functional workspace of the patient (17). Active elbow extension is necessary for trunk control, transfers, and independent self-care. A patient with active elbow extension is able to prevent pressure sores by performing "pressure releases" or "weight shifts" while in bed or in a wheelchair. In many countries where electric wheelchairs are not commonly available, patients depend on their forward humeral flexion and elbow extension to propel their chairs. Providing mobility correlates with life satisfaction, social integration, and occupation (18,19). Active elbow extension provides a stabilizing antagonist to otherwise unopposed elbow flexion, thus permitting simple tasks such as drinking from a glass, pouring, writing, and so forth (20). Active elbow extension also stabilizes the activity of the brachioradialis, leading to better function of the muscle when used as a transfer. In short, active elbow extension is a significant determinant for independence and self-care (21,22).

PROCEDURES FOR RESTORING ELBOW EXTENSION

Experienced surgeons have each modified their techniques to improve their results. Hentz and Ladd recommended the technique of Castro-

Sierra and Lopez-Pita (23) with the modification described by Mennen and Boonzar when there is a long triceps tendon that begins proximal to the midpoint of the humerus. On the other hand, he now favors the original description by Hentz: "entubulating" the detached deltoid insertion with a cone of fascia lata graft and lacing the distal end of the graft through the olecranon (24,25).

We have used various interposition grafts, including the tibialis anterior. Stretching of the graft is now minimized using a modification of the technique by Castro-Sierra augmented with four core sutures of 5mm Dacron tape. Elbow flexion contractures should be corrected to improve reach. Small contractures may respond to serial cast correction. Contractures beyond 20 degrees are released prior to transfer of the posterior deltoid (PD) to the triceps. Grover et al. (26) studied the effects of elbow contractures in C6 tetraplegic patients. The six patients in the study had similar baseline function with ability to transfer assisted with a sliding board and to lift their bodies on their extended extremities to relieve pressure on their ischia. Extension blocking braces were used to limit the patients' range of motion. Patients with weaker extension, MRC grades 2 and 3, were not able to transfer or lift themselves when the simulated flexion contracture was greater than 25 degrees. Patients with elbow extension strength of 4 were disabled, with simulated contractions beyond 45 degrees. Zancolli (27) advocates a biceps-to-triceps transfer for patients with significant elbow contractures combined with anterior elbow release.

Intraoperative Electrical Stimulation

In our center, we have adopted intraoperative electrical stimulation to adjust the resting tension of our tendon transfers. The stimulator produces a balanced charge square step of 0 to 20 milliamperes at 0 to 200 microseconds pulse width with a frequency of 12 Hz. A reference electrode is placed in contact proximally, and the stimulating electrode is then placed near the nerve entry point into the muscle on the epimysial surface. Full force contractions test the suture and recruited contractions measure the force peak over varied tensions.

Biceps-to-Triceps Transfer

This procedure was first performed by Leo Meyer (28) in 1951 to restore elbow extension in a polio patient. The patient had bilateral elbow contractures of 50 degrees and wished to ambulate with crutches. Meyer divided the lacertus fibrosus and the biceps tendon as far distally as possible. As part of the elbow release, he divided the brachialis at the level of the coronoid. He then tunneled the biceps tendon-lacertus fibrosus around the arm subcutaneously and sutured them into the triceps. He did not specify whether the subcutaneous tunnel was medial or lateral. His patient lacked the final 30 degrees of elbow extension and was not able to use crutches in the end but was very satisfied with his ability to hold objects in front of him and to use a typewriter, and he became independent for self-care.

Freidenberg (28) published his experience with a polio patient who had a full range of elbow motion. He divided the biceps tendon from the lacertus fibrosus and transferred the tendon around the lateral subcutaneous border of the arm. A distally based flap of triceps tendon of 2.5 cm was needed to suture to the biceps tendon. The patient retained full elbow range of motion and was able to hold 7- and 8-pound weights with the elbow extended against gravity. He became independent for transfers and his ability to ambulate with crutches increased.

Zancolli reported his first five cases of lateral subcutaneous biceps-to-triceps transfer in 1979 (5) and his updated series of 13 cases in 1987 (27). His larger series had an average follow-up of 37 months, with 80 percent good to excellent results. Clinical evaluation is important to distinguish biceps function from supinator function and brachioradialis function. Typically, strong brachioradialis and wrist extension predict active supinator and brachialis function (Figure 17-1). However, with spotty recovery, the supinator or brachialis may not be strong enough, and transfer of the biceps would seriously compromise the ability of the patient to flex and supinate. Supinator strength is isolated with the elbow in extension, eliminating the pull of the biceps. Brachioradialis strength, although difficult to assess independently, is evaluated with resisted flexion of the elbow from a position of flexion and pronation. If the clinical exam is equivocal, Zancolli recommends nerve blocks to the musculocutaneous nerve or electromyography to differentiate biceps and supinator function. At follow-up, all of his patients had preservation of supination. Functional active elbow flexion was also preserved, although there was a 25 percent loss of flexion strength (29). One patient had radial nerve palsy that resolved in 4 months. Zancolli also concluded that although a flexion contracture greater than 20 degrees was a contraindication to PD transfer, one could readily transfer the biceps at the time of elbow release.

Ejeskar (30) reported two failures and one case of radial nerve palsy with recovery after five months in his series of five patients with lateral subcutaneous transfer. He concluded that this is the procedure of choice, with results exceeding those of the posterior deltoid (PD) transfer, especially for patients with elbow contractures and those who do not require a very strong active elbow flexor.

We have limited experience with successful biceps-to-triceps transfer, although we have attempted the procedure. In one case, we had to abandon the procedure in an ASIA C5 patient who preoperatively had strong elbow flexion and supination. Intraoperatively we observed biceps atrophy with healthy brachialis and supinator muscles. A second patient with C5 level demonstrated spastic contracture of the elbow and forearm with 80 degrees of flexion contracture and 80 to 100 degrees of supination to pronation. Following elbow release, anterior capsulotomy and fractional lengthening of the brachialis muscle, the biceps tendon and its bicipital aponeurosis were sutured into the intact distal brachialis tendon. Elbow flexion was regained. Later, this patient received a posterior deltoid transfer, radius pronation osteotomy, and brachioradialis-to-extensor carpi radialis brevis transfer. One further patient had the procedure reversed due to inability to extend the elbow. We analyze that the patient had developed adhesions to the flexor attachments or inability to train the transfer.

Kuz (31) reports excellent results in three tetraplegic patients (four extremities) who underwent a biceps-to-triceps transfer. Patient selection is very important; none of the patients had contractures greater than 15 degrees preoperatively. They recommend examination for active supinator and brachialis function independent from biceps prior to the biceps transfer. After the procedure, no patient had a flexion contracture greater than 8 degrees, none had lost supination or flexion strength, and all had an extension strength of 4 or better. Casting is in place for 3 weeks in 30 degrees of flexion, followed by 6 weeks of flexion block splinting, advancing 15 degrees per week. Active elbow extension is performed with the arm supported over a "power board," thus eliminating the gravitational pull. The authors conclude the procedure is beneficial to those patients with dynamic flexion–supination deformities attributable to the biceps, and although not supported by their data, they claim that the procedure is advantageous for patients with flexion supination contractures greater than 30 degrees from an unopposed biceps pull.

Biceps-to-Triceps Transfer: Technique. A curvilinear incision is made in the antecubital fossa (Figure 17-2). The lacertus fibrosus is identified and harvested together with a long slip of forearm fascia. The median nerve and brachial artery are identified medially and laterally, the lateral cutaneous nerve to the forearm. The recurrent radial artery and vena commitantes are ligated. The forearm is stressed into maximal supination, which protects the posterior interosseous nerve (PIN), and the biceps tendon is detached from the radial tuberosity. Damage to the radial nerve and PIN is avoided. A separate incision is made on the posterior distal arm,

and the broad triceps tendon is clearly exposed. The freed biceps tendon and the lacertus fibrosus are delivered into the posterior wound via a generous subcutaneous tunnel around the medial distal arm. Any fibrous septa interfering with an optimal line of pull for the transfer are eliminated. Via a stab incision in the triceps insertion, a 4-mm drill hole is made in the olecranon. The distal cortex is not drilled, but instead, two smaller holes are made with .045-inch k-wires for later intra-osseous anchoring of the biceps. With the arm in full extension, the biceps tendon is woven into the central strongest portion of the triceps. The tension is readjusted so that functional flexion is not limited. Nonabsorbable sutures into the tendon are mounted on straight free needles and passed into the olecranon drill whole and tied. Interweaving the lacertus fibrosus reinforces the repair. The arm is immobilized in a cast for 3 weeks in 30 degrees of flexion, followed by 6 weeks of flexion block splinting, advancing 15 degrees per week. Active elbow extension is performed with the arm supported over a "power board," eliminating the gravitational pull.

Preliminary prospective studies by Kozin (personal communication) indicate that this procedure should not be performed if subsequent tendon transfers or functional electric stimulation (FES) produce strong finger flexion and pronation of the forearm. The remaining supinator strength, without the supination provided by the biceps, may be insufficient for hand positioning at the face.

Reinforced Posterior Deltoid Transfer: Technique

The posterior half of the deltoid is approached via a proximal incision that follows the inferior, lateral border of the deltoid muscle from the deltoid tuberosity to a point approximately 5 cm distal to the acromion. The deltoid muscle is dissected from the overlying subcutaneous fat so that its lateral surface is visualized and the point at which fibers converge on the tuberosities from the anterior and posterior halves is easily seen.

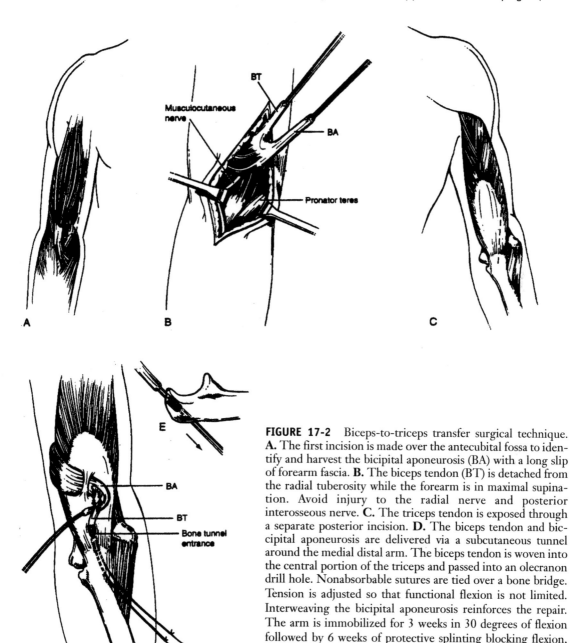

FIGURE 17-2 Biceps-to-triceps transfer surgical technique. **A.** The first incision is made over the antecubital fossa to identify and harvest the bicipital aponeurosis (BA) with a long slip of forearm fascia. **B.** The biceps tendon (BT) is detached from the radial tuberosity while the forearm is in maximal supination. Avoid injury to the radial nerve and posterior interosseous nerve. **C.** The triceps tendon is exposed through a separate posterior incision. **D.** The biceps tendon and bicipital aponeurosis are delivered via a subcutaneous tunnel around the medial distal arm. The biceps tendon is woven into the central portion of the triceps and passed into an olecranon drill hole. Nonabsorbable sutures are tied over a bone bridge. Tension is adjusted so that functional flexion is not limited. Interweaving the bicipital aponeurosis reinforces the repair. The arm is immobilized for 3 weeks in 30 degrees of flexion followed by 6 weeks of protective splinting blocking flexion, advancing 15 degrees/week. (Adapted from Kuz, et al. [Kuz, 1999 #447].)

Elevating the deltoid muscle, the under surface is visualized, and the attachment of the deltoid, including the arcuate fibers and periosteum of the humerus, are elevated to create a strong tendon of insertion for the donor muscle. The triceps insertion is approached through a posterior incision that deviates to the lateral side of the olecranon at the elbow. The distal triceps is dissect-ed until the entire expansion of the tendon is appreciated and so that the central third, composed of heavy tendinous tissue, can be differentiated from the muscular attachments. This center third is elevated, including the strip of periosteum distally, and reflected proximally. Underlying muscle is left in place and attached to the remaining two-thirds of the triceps tendon as described by Castro-Sierra (23). A 4.5-mm drill hole is made from medial to lateral, carefully protecting the ulnar nerve at the level of the olecranon process of the ulna. A subcutaneous tunnel is made between the posterior incision and the deltoid incision beneath the remaining intact bridge of skin and subcutaneous tissue. Sutures of #2 Tevdec are placed in the deltoid tendon and the triceps tendon, and the triceps are sutured through the distal deltoid. This repair is reinforced by 5-mm Dacron tapes placed from the deltoid and attaching to the distal triceps remaining insertion and a second tape from the olecranon process to the deltoid tendon, as depicted in Figure 17-3. The Dacron tape at the olecranon is crossed to prevent its subluxation along the sides of the humerus, and the remaining triceps tendon is oversewn using interrupted sutures of #1 Tevdec to encapsulate this Dacron reinforcement graft. Tension is set with the elbow in full extension to 30 degrees of flexion, with the arm abducted to 90 degrees. To prevent stripping of the tendon graft from the triceps, it is further reinforced at its departure from the triceps. These wounds are closed with 3/0 and 4/0 Vicryl and a long cast applied in full extension to 30 degrees of flexion. Tendon is tested by intraoperative electrical stimulation of the deltoid muscle in a position of 90 degrees of forward humeral flexion and tension adjusted so that full elbow extension can be obtained. Because the excursion of the deltoid is limited, flexion is usually tight at 30 degrees of flexion of the elbow.

Release of Elbow Contractures

Concomitant mild to moderate elbow flexion contractures and forearm supination deformities in tetraplegia often respond to conservative measures with serial casting in extension and pronation at weekly intervals. Freehafer (32) has attributed the combined deformity to a contracted biceps, such that pronation of the forearm accentuates the flexion deformity. He proposed serial casting, followed by tenotomy of the biceps tendon, once casting alone had reached full benefit. After surgery, the arm again undergoes further serial casting to maximize the effectiveness of the procedure. In 1977, he published his experience with eight patients (12 arms) with a C5 level. These patients had paralysis below the elbow that eventually improved, with recovery of strong brachioradialis and radial wrist extensors. Flexion strength about the elbow was maintained, and recurrence observed in two patients who continued to posture their extremities in elbow flexion without splinting.

Our current management algorithm (Figure 17-4), for mild to moderate flexion supination contractures includes serial casting to reduce the flexion contracture to less than 20 or 30 degrees, followed by a transfer of the biceps or posterior deltoid to the triceps for elbow extension. Biceps pronatorplasty may be an option; however, in those patients with severe elbow and forearm contractures we have not found it possible to perform a satisfactory anterior elbow release and still be able to reattach the biceps, despite a carefully devised z-plasty lengthening of the tendon without an intercalary graft. Severe deformities require more aggressive intervention, including elbow capsular release, biceps tendon lengthening, brachialis fractional lengthening, and forearm pronation osteotomy.

Restoration of Pronation and Supination

In Group 0 patients, supination is the only voluntary motion about the forearm. Pronation may be accomplished by a substitution maneuver involving shoulder abduction, elbow flexion, internal rotation, and the force of gravity on the limb. Supination contracture of the forearm severely limits the patient's ability to pronate.

In Group 1—patients without elbow flexion or forearm supination or internal rotation contracture—pronation is possible by a combination of activities of the brachioradialis, shoulder abduction, wrist extension, and gravity (33). Pronation is initiated from a position of forearm supination by the action of the brachioradialis that is a forearm neutralizer. The center of gravity of the forearm is further shifted in favor of pronation by slight shoulder abduction. Based

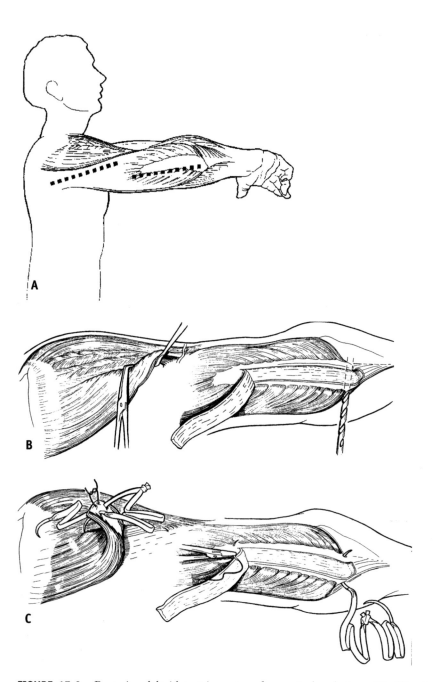

FIGURE 17-3 Posterior deltoid-to-triceps transfer surgical technique. Modification of the Castro-Sierra and Lopez-Pita triceps turn-down requires four strands of 5 mm Dacron as reinforcement. **A.** The distal incision curves laterally around the olecranon, while the proximal incision runs along the posterior border of the deltoid. The patient is positioned supine. Dissection of the triceps and harvest of the tendinous central-third is done under (sterile) tourniquet. Proximal dissection is done after the tourniquet is removed. **B.** The central-third of the tendinous portion is turned down. A 4.5-mm drill hole of the olecranon is made from medial to lateral. Harvesting of the posterior one-half of deltoid requires subperiosteal elevation, starting with the posterior distal border. Neighboring septal perforating vessels are cauterized. A right-angle clamp helps delineate the tendinous raphe and the extent of the muscle to be detached. The muscle is mobilized until the desired excursion is obtained. The muscle can be stimulated intra-operatively to best determine its useful excursion. **C.** The distance to the tendinous portion of the posterior deltoid is measured and the length of the turn-down tongue determined. Locking sutures in the proximal portion of turn-down are applied to prevent tear propagation. Two strands of 5–0 Dacron tape are tied together and passed into the olecranon drill hole, anchoring the large knot into the bone tunnel. Two other strands of Dacron tape are tied and sutured to the tendinous undersurface of the deltoid. A locking suture with 0-ethibond prevents cutting-out of the Dacron tape.

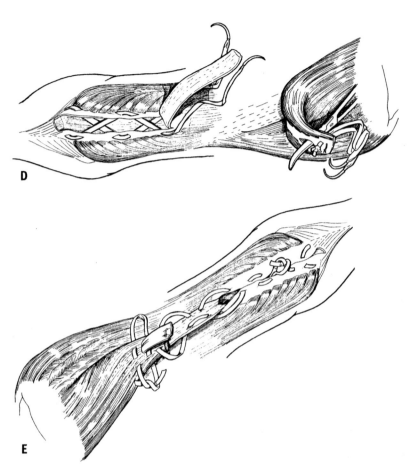

FIGURE 17-3 (continued)   **D.** The interval between the distal medial and lateral tendinous portions is closed by shoe-lacing the Dacron strands. The triceps turn-down is delivered into the proximal wound via a generous subcutaneous tunnel. A large Kelly clamp is used to make a hole in the deltoid tendon. **E.** The free end of the triceps turn-down, together with the distally anchored Dacron tapes, is passed from the undersurface of the distal deltoid. The triceps turn down is sutured to itself in maximum tension while assistant holds the elbow extended and in slight abduction. The distally anchored Dacron tapes are woven to the tendinous distal deltoid in a nonconstricting fashion. The proximally anchored Dacron strands are woven into the triceps turn-down and into the intact medial and lateral tendinous triceps and tied to each other.

on mathematical modeling, a small shoulder abduction of 10 degrees is sufficient to tip the forearm into pronation (33). On the other hand, the inability to adduct the shoulder eliminates the ability of the brachioradialis to accomplish pronation. Brachioradialis (BR) transfer to extensor carpi radialis brevis (ECRB) for wrist extension could improve pronation (33).

Schottstaedt et al (34) are credited with the original description of a biceps pronator-plasty. "The biceps brachii can be transferred to the side of the radial tuberosity opposite its normal insertion. . . ." To restore lost supination in polio

patients, they also transferred the insertion of the pronation teres to the opposite surface of the radial shaft, thus alternating the function of these muscles. Pronation can be restored with a biceps rerouting procedure (Figure 17-5) (35). Adequate z-lengthening of the biceps tendon is an essential component of the procedure. Release of the interosseous membrane and distal radio-ulnar joint posterior capsule may be needed in cases of severe supination contracture. In his report, Zancolli included two patients with tetraplegia managed successfully. Both patients had supple forearms; one underwent rerouting

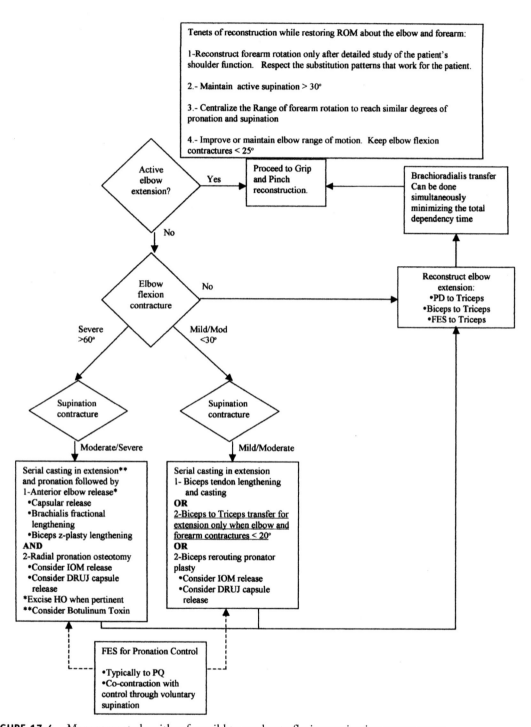

Tenets of reconstruction while restoring ROM about the elbow and forearm:

1-Reconstruct forearm rotation only after detailed study of the patient's shoulder function. Respect the substitution patterns that work for the patient.

2.- Maintain active supination > 30°

3.- Centralize the Range of forearm rotation to reach similar degrees of pronation and supination

4.- Improve or maintain elbow range of motion. Keep elbow flexion contractures < 25°

Active elbow extension? — Yes → Proceed to Grip and Pinch reconstruction.

Brachioradialis transfer Can be done simultaneously minimizing the total dependency time

No

Elbow flexion contracture — No → Reconstruct elbow extension:
• PD to Triceps
• Biceps to Triceps
• FES to Triceps

Severe >60°   Mild/Mod <30°

Supination contracture   Supination contracture

Moderate/Severe   Mild/Moderate

Serial casting in extension** and pronation followed by
1-Anterior elbow release*
• Capsular release
• Brachialis fractional lengthening
• Biceps z-plasty lengthening
AND
2-Radial pronation osteotomy
• Consider IOM release
• Consider DRUJ capsule release
*Excise HO when pertinent
**Consider Botulinum Toxin

Serial casting in extension
1- Biceps tendon lengthening and casting
OR
2-Biceps to Triceps transfer for extension only when elbow and forearm contractures < 20°
OR
2-Biceps rerouting pronator plasty
• Consider IOM release
• Consider DRUJ capsule release

FES for Pronation Control

• Typically to PQ
• Co-contraction with control through voluntary supination

FIGURE 17-4 Management algorithm for mild to moderate flexion supination contractures.

of the biceps tendon, and a second patient had transfer of the biceps to the brachialis to remove unopposed bicipital supination.

Pronation Osteotomy of the Radius: Technique

Osteotomy is indicated when limited passive pronation prevents positioning the arm and reaching in the workspace. Surgery is performed when conservative management, such as serial casting, passive stretching, and exercise with therapy, has failed to produce a useful range of passive forearm pronation. The procedure is useful when the supination contracture of the forearm is combined with flexion contracture of the elbow. When the elbow flexion contracture exceeds 30 degrees, it is difficult to elongate the biceps tendon enough by z-plasty to reinsert it into the radius as a pronator (Figure 17-5) (35). Biceps z-plasty and fractional lengthening of the brachialis and capsulectomy are often required to correct this flexion contracture.

Radial pronation osteotomy is done at the time of other tendon transfers with postoperative immobilization dictated by the specific tendon transfer performed, without additional immobilization time for the radial osteotomy itself. A standard Henry approach to the middle third of the radius is ideal, allowing access to the pronator teres, brachioradialis, flexor digitorum profundus, and flexor pollicis longus. Tendon transfers can be performed through the same incision. A longitudinal incision is made along the ulnar border of the brachioradialis. The insertion of the pronator teres into the radius is identified, and its distal third elevated to make room for a plate. We recommend conventional dynamic compression plating with 3.5 mm AO/ASIF implants (Chur, Switzerland) but have found that such rigid fixation is not always necessary in these patients. A 4- or 6-hole, 1/3 tubular plate is now our implant of choice because of its low profile. The implant is placed directly on the convex surface of the radius. Application of the plate onto the volar flat surface of the radius can result in an undesirable longitudinal angular deformity (bowing) if the plate is not perfectly contoured. Occasionally, such longitudinal angular deformity leads to abnormal motion about the DRUJ, including subluxation, or undue restriction of forearm rotation. A proxi-

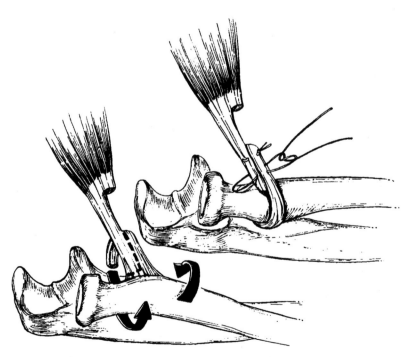

FIGURE 17-5 Biceps rerouting procedure restores pronation.

mal screw hole is made to hold the plate temporarily to the radius. The site of transverse osteotomy can be marked. The plate is removed and longitudinal reference marks across the planned osteotomy site are made to assist in controlling the amount of rotation. After the transverse osteotomy is completed, the plate is reapplied to the proximal fragment. Release of 3 to 4 cm of the interosseous membrane on the radial border is usually sufficient. The distal fragment is then reduced to the proximal fragment-plate and held with a reduction clamp. Forearm rotation is evaluated and final adjustments are made based on the ability to grasp and bring the hand to the mouth in supination. Full pronation can be augmented by humeral internal rotation. The position recommended is neutral position with 40 degrees of pronation and 40 degrees of supination. Release of the dorsal DRUJ capsule has not been required with this procedure, but it may be necessary in some patients.

Gellman et al. (36) reported their results with the biceps rerouting procedure in six tetraplegic patients (eight limbs) with supination deformity. They caution against the procedure when there is a co-existing elbow contracture greater than 90 degrees. In one case, they used an intercalary free graft to connect the distal and proximal stumps of the rerouted biceps tendon. This patient, with elbow flexion contracture of 90 degrees preoperatively, had an unsatisfactory result. They concluded that:

- Supination decreased an average of 41 degrees, with unsatisfactory results in patients who had no active supination after the surgery.
- In addition to lack of active supination, unsatisfactory results were seen in patients with limited elbow ROM. Satisfied patients had flexion from 22 to 145 degrees and unsatisfied patients, 55 to 113 degrees.
- Sixty degrees of active pronation was possible without having to release the interosseous membrane. Additional gains in active pronation were documented over the passive pronation obtained intraoperatively.

- More predictable results follow when the dominant extremity is operated.

Based on our experience, following anterior elbow release for flexion contracture greater than 90 degrees, including fractional lengthening of the brachialis, we prefer to simply z-lengthen the biceps tendon without rerouting it as a pronator. The supination deformity is managed with an osteotomy about the mid-shaft of the radius. The surgical procedure is simple and has the added advantage of avoiding any damage to the posterior interosseous nerve, a risk inherent in procedures on the radial proximal forearm. Further, the high risk of developing a radio-ulnar synostosis, as in the more proximal radial osteotomy procedure, is also avoided.

Radial Osteotomy: Outcomes. Hentz (17) briefly discusses his experience with osteotomy of the radius at its mid-shaft with compression plating for supination deformity. His results were "beneficial" in four patients.

Peljovich has reviewed our experience with pronation osteotomies in five tetraplegic patients (six arms) from the first 58 patients managed in the Cleveland FES Center. Five arms were classified as C5 ASIA level and one as C6. According to the international classification, five arms were Ocu:1 and one Cu:3. Two patients with elbow contractures underwent simultaneous biceps-to-triceps transfer and biceps lengthening. Passive range of motion (PROM) improved from 84 degrees to 131 degrees (from 0 ± 13 degrees of pronation to 84 ± 9 degrees of supination preoperatively to 79 ± 20 degrees of pronation to 52 ± 36 degrees of supination postoperatively). Average active supination after the procedure was 13 ± 31 degrees, and the resting pronation position was 50 ± 22 degrees, for a functional range of 62.4 degrees. Four patients sensed their forearms were overpronated and one underpronated. Functional evaluation included testing seven representative tasks from a list of ADLs: writing, dialing a phone number, drinking from a glass, eating with a fork, using a telephone receiver, brushing hair, and inserting a diskette into a computer. The first two tasks required 9 degrees of supination to 42 degrees of pronation; the second two tasks required 30 degrees of supination to 55 degrees of pronation; and the last two tasks required 60 and 70 degrees of supination. Task completion was related to remaining active supination and the newly acquired pronation. Only two arms, with active supination to 34 and 50 degrees, were able to complete all the tasks. One arm with active supination to 28 degrees completed six tasks, and three other arms with inability to actively supinate completed only three tasks (Fig. 17-6).

SURGICAL PROCEDURES THAT IMPROVE HAND FUNCTION

Procedures that increase the force of grasp and release, add new movements, or improve alignment of the hand improve function and independence.

Brachioradialis Transfer

The brachioradialis (BR) is a most readily available muscle and is versatile for reconstructive transfers in tetraplegia. Several tendon transfers have been described. The specific transfer to be performed will depend on the patient's remaining function as well as on his or her individual needs and requirements:

- BR to ECRB for wrist extension (37)
- BR to FDP for grip (7)
- BR to FPL for pinch (39,39)
- BR for adduction opponensplasty (7,40)
- BR to EDC, EPL for finger and thumb extension (41)

Anatomy. The BR has a broad origin along the lateral epicondylar ridge measuring about 7 to 7.5 cm from 10 cm to 2.5 cm proximal to the elbow joint (42). The distal tendinous portion is bound to the distal radius and forearm fascia and does not glide over the distal third of the forearm. Its final insertion on the lateral surface of the radius is located beneath the tendons of the APL and

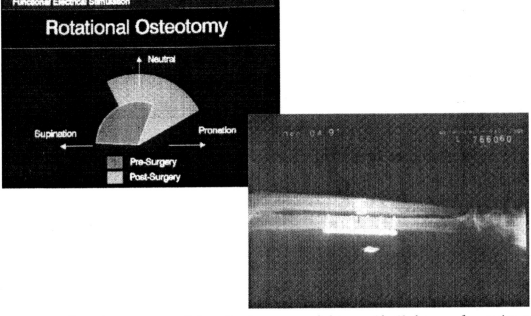

FIGURE 17-6 Pronation osteotomy of the radius is recommended to provide 40 degrees of pronation and supination.

EBP. Its proximal muscle belly has significant fibrofascial tethers that limit its passive ROM. Innervation from the radial nerve usually originates above the elbow. The radial sensory nerve travels beneath the flattened muscle belly and exits dorsally along the distal tendinous portion.

Physiology. We have studied the muscle characteristics of the brachioradialis while performing tendon transfers in tetraplegic patients (42). The total excursion of the muscle was calculated in 70 patients from the sum of the passive lengthening from the resting length plus active unloaded contraction following electrical stimulation. Measurements were made with the elbow in 90 degrees of flexion. The average total excursion was 41.7 mm and increased to 77.9 mm following dissection from the perimuscular soft tissue. The muscle is freed as far back as its proximal third without compromising its innervation from the radial nerve. Brand (43) found that the BR has a mass fraction of 7.7 percent, which is larger than any other muscle in the forearm. The excursion of muscles that may be available for transfer in some patients—the extensor carpi radialis longus (ECRL) averages 59 mm; the pronator teres (PT), 36 mm; and the ECU, 65 mm—and fall short of the "freed" BR muscle excursion, and shorter yet of the excursion needed for full digital flexion of 85 mm. The length–tension characteristics of the BR were studied with intraoperative measurements in 27 patients (42). Isometric force measurements at different muscle lengths were measured using electrical stimulation while the free tendinous end was connected to a strain gauge. The active force produced by the BR was quite flat over a range of 1.5 to 2 cm; it was found to be above 90 percent or greater of the maximal force developed over a range from -0.5 cm to 1.5 cm relative to the resting undisturbed length.

Some surgeons and therapists believe that the brachioradialis is difficult to train, especially in the absence of elbow stabilization. Studies have shown that when the elbow is stabilized either by a brace, the mass of a held object, or by provision of an elbow extensor such as a posterior

deltoid transfer, the brachioradialis becomes a more effective distal transfer (22,39,42). The antagonist action to the BR at the elbow is active elbow extension affected by an intact triceps, a posterior deltoid-to-triceps transfer, a biceps-to-triceps transfer, or electric stimulation to the triceps. Others have performed similar studies demonstrating the strength developed in grip, when the BR was transferred to the FDP, and pinch, when the FPL increases.

We advocate that elbow extensor plasty be performed as a first stage or combined with the brachioradialis transfer. Combining these two procedures reduces overall operative time and, because of the long, flat, length–tension curve of the brachioradialis, adequate function results from the co-immobilization of the elbow in extension and the wrist extension in the postoperative period. The transfer is especially effective because as the patient reaches, the elbow extension tensions the brachioradialis, providing some tenodesis wrist extension; when recruited with the wrist extensors or alone, additional wrist extension occurs.

In people in Group 1, ASIA C5, the brachioradialis is the only potential strong donor muscle for reconstruction. We believe that the vast majority of patients would benefit from transfer of the voluntary brachioradialis to augment wrist extension. The International Classification of Group 1 includes some patients who have grade 3 wrist extension; that is, antigravity for the mass of the hand. Many of these patients do not have sufficient strength to handle objects associated with activities of daily living, and they should be tested with these familiar objects before a determination is made that they have sufficient wrist strength. Patients in this group are always better with very strong wrist extension that allows the tenodesis of distal muscles to provide simple lateral prehension.

Brachioradialis transfer for thumb adduction opponensplasty can be accomplished by extending the BR tendon with the ring finger superficialis and suturing it into the tendinous insertion of the abductor pollicis brevis. Pronator teres is usually used in this transfer currently.

Wrist Arthrodesis

Wrist arthrodesis is indicated to replace an external splint, or if insufficient motors are available, for wrist extension. Some patients select the procedure for cosmetic qualities and to be brace-free. The radiocarpal joint is approached through a dorsal midline incision, and the extensor retinaculum is reflected along the third extensor compartment. By subperiosteal dissection, the attachments of the third and fourth compartments are elevated from the radius, and the extensor pollicis longus is transposed to a subcutaneous position. An AO/ASIF (Synthes, Chur, Switzerland) wrist arthrodesis plate is used to span the third metacarpal to the radius with either neutral or 30 degrees of wrist extension, depending upon patient preference and the requirements from balance and posture of other tendon transfers across the fingers and thumb. The wrist is decorticated on the dorsal 75 percent of the joint surfaces. A bone graft, if required, is taken from the radius. The plate is positioned to avoid fraying of adjacent extensor tendons and can be covered using the nonfunctional wrist extensor tendons. The extensor retinaculum is re-opposed to protect the fourth compartment and beneath the extensor pollicis longus. Immobilization, protection from weight-bearing, and radiographic examinations are repeated from 3 months or until trabecular bone traverses the wrist joint.

Proximal Row Carpectomy (PRC)

Proximal row carpectomy is a rarely performed procedure in the setting of spinal cord injury; rather it is usually done for severe wrist contracture release. Schroer et al. (44) demonstrated a higher incidence of mid-carpal instability of the volar-intercalated segment variety in paraplegics. These patients utilize their upper extremities in a variety of weight bearing activities, including transfers, wheelchair propulsion, sports, and weight shifts throughout their lives. High tetraplegics impose similar demands on their upper extremities. Static instability pattern

was documented in 6 percent of all paraplegics and in as much as 18 percent in those whose injuries occurred 20 years prior. The patterns of degenerative arthritis that accompany the long-standing nondissociative mid-carpal instability pattern in these patients have not been clearly documented. As lifespan increases, so does the possibility of such findings, and PRC may become a useful salvage procedure.

We use intraoperative fluoroscopy during the procedure. The carpus is approached from a dorsal longitudinal incision over the third and fourth extensor compartments. The EPL is freed from its tunnel, and the floor of the fourth compartment is elevated at the subperiosteal level. A longitudinal capsulotomy exposes the radiocarpal joint. The scaphoid and lunate bones are excised first. The soft tissues are freed sharply. With adequate exposure, we prefer to use a microsagittal saw or small osteotomes to fracture the bones into two or three smaller pieces. Often, pins are driven into the pieces to act as joysticks for manipulation. The soft tissues are then divided systematically from the fragments. Ulnar deviation delivers the triquetrum into the field for excision. Transection of the volar radioscaphocapitate ligament, the median nerve, or the flexor carpi radialis (FCR) should be avoided. These structures are at risk while excising the scaphoid. The capitate should articulate within the lunate fossa. If there is excessive laxity of the carpus with respect to the radius, even after soft capsule repair, it is advisable to hold the capitate in the lunate fossa with Kirschner wires. The wrist is immobilized in neutral position. Immobilization and wires, when used, are discontinued at 4 weeks and ROM started.

Carpometacarpal Arthrodesis

Carpometacarpal (CMC) arthrodesis to position the thumb for lateral pinch has been incorporated into modifications of Moberg's key pinch by numerous authors. The pre-positioning of the thumb in the high spinal cord injured patient is critical because of the paucity of muscle forces available and the necessity of using a single move-ment, wrist extension and flexion, as a single ten-don transfer to move the thumb and fingers for strong pinch. Carpometacarpal arthrodesis elimi-nates the need for abduction and adduction forces, and it improves the extensor pollicis longus tenodesis by adjusting CMC extension. We favor a position of 25 degrees of extension and 45 degrees of abduction. Pronation of 10 to 20 degrees is adjusted so that the desired pinch is as shown in Figure 17-7. The degree of pronation of the CMC joint is important because in some persons with adduction contracture, the degree of thumb extension, and therefore, the opening of key pinch can be increased by overpronating an additional 20 degrees. This additional positioning can be useful when the patient wants to grasp larger objects than is normally possible with key grip. The CMC joint is approached through a dorsal incision between the extensor pollicis bre-vis and abductor pollicis longus. The dorsal cap-sule of the joint is divided and a subperiosteal dis-section exposes the joint. A 0.62 Kirschner wire is used to temporarily transfix the joint while the position, angle, and alignment of the pinch are established.

The CMC joint can then be decorticated around the wire and an additional wire placed across the joint or to the adjacent index metacarpal to stabilize the arthrodesis. A bone graft is seldom required. The pins are cut off below the level of the skin and the pins across the CMC joint itself are often left in place. Postoperative immobilization should be contin-ued for a minimum of 6 weeks without weight bearing or forceful movement to prevent a CMC nonunion. The Kirschner wires can be removed if prominent.

Reconstruction According to Level of Voluntary Function

Moberg was instrumental in renewing interest on the surgical reconstruction of the tetraplegic hand when he proposed his method of elbow extension and simple pinch in 1975 (4). That same year, Zancolli (6) published his experience

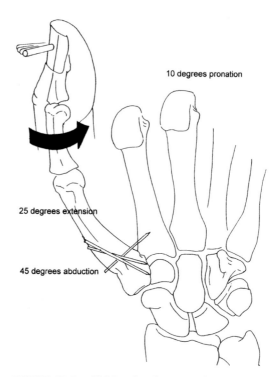

FIGURE 17-7 CMC arthrodesis. **A.** The position for CMC arthrodesis is 45 degrees of abduction, 25 degrees of extension, and 15 degrees of pronation. The precise position for arthrodesis is ultimately determined intra-operatively. Excessive abduction places the thumb too anterior to the flexed digits, missing them altogether attempting pinch. **B.** Adding pronation at the fusion site, has two important advan-tages: 1) better thumb pulp opposition; and 2) better toleration of abduction because the plane of thumb IP joint flexion is made to coincide on the platform made by the flexed digits. Abduction at the thumb metacarpal improves first web space opening during the release phase, which translates into ability to grasp larger objects. In addition, with a more abducted thumb, the plane for lateral key pinch is shifted into pronation such that it is easier for patients with limit-ed forearm pronation to grab objects from a horizon-tal table top. Patients are able to substitute for the lack of pronation with shoulder abduction and internal rotation. Those with weaker triceps function will have difficulty with this substitution maneuver when trying to reach an object, because the extending the elbow with the arm abducted and internally rotated requires an active elbow extensor working against gravity. **C.** Typical lateral key pinch and release pattern after reconstruction in high tetraplegia C5 patient with a Moberg reconstruction or a motor transfer to FPL and IP stabilization without metacarpal abduction or pronation. **D.** Lateral key pinch and release after reconstruction in C5 tetraplegia with a Cleveland modification of Moberg reconstruction. CMC arthrodesis of the thumb significantly improves the posture of the thumb for pinch and release.

with 97 cases of patients with mid-cervical tetraplegia. He performed complex staged reconstructions starting with an "extensor" phase, and later, after a healing period, a "flexor" phase. His combination of muscle, tendon, and joint procedures produced grasp and key grip in an entirely synergistic neuromuscular reconstruction. This elegant combination of procedures influenced surgeons to perform staged procedures and combined tendon transfers. House sustained the enthusiasm for staged reconstruction and enhanced the technique by adding intrinsic transfers. Optimism for restoration of hand grasp in these patients continues to grow.

Group 0 (ASIA C4)

These patients have no motor function remaining below the level of the elbow. Current tendon transfer techniques offer little hope of achieving hand function. The posterior deltoid may be too weak for transfer. Elbow flexors and shoulder muscles are partially denervated. They may achieve simple substitution using a brace. Functional electric stimulation (FES) is the predominant method of reconstruction, with eight functioning muscles or tendon transfers, permitting hand grasp, pinch, and release, often without a brace, and elbow extension. Some selected patients request a wrist arthrodesis to simplify the reconstruction and ensure that they are brace-free. (See the FES section that follows.)

Group 1 (ASIA C5)

This group is among the most common of patients. Brachioradialis function in this patient population is of sufficient strength, above a grade 4 BMRC, to offer reliable transfers. The reconstruction effort includes restoration of active elbow extension. An elbow stabilizer improves the function of the BR transfer (22,39,42). The distal reconstruction consists of restoring key pinch and is typically done at the same time as the transfers for wrist extension.

Moberg described the original "simple grip" procedure. The BR is transferred to ECRB, for wrist extension, while wrist flexion is assisted by gravity. Thumb ray control includes interphalangeal (IP) stabilization with a large threaded Kirschner wire. Hyperflexion of the thumb metacarpo phalangeal (MP) joint is observed in some individuals and could be prevented by tenodesis of the extensor hood to the metacarpal. Release of the thumb A1 pulley and the second extensor compartment containing the ECRL and ECRB are performed to provide better mechanical advantage at the expense of range of motion; it contributes to the MP flexion posture. Brand (64) suggested alternative routing of the FPL, the procedure avoiding release of the A1 pulley, via Guyon's canal, effectively producing a flexion adduction moment. Brand also tenodesed the EPL to the radius to reduce the tendency for MP hyperflexion. Thumb abduction is improved when the site of the EPL tenodesis was more radial than its third extensor compartment. McDowell (45,46) applied these modifications in six patients, with disappointing results.

In 1992, House reported on his one-stage key pinch release technique (47). He advocates elbow extension reconstruction before BR-to-ECRB transfer and pinch reconstruction. Thumb control begins with carpometacarpal joint fusion as recommended by Zancolli. The position of the thumb metacarpal, with respect to the index metacarpal, is in 40 degrees of abduction and 25 degrees of extension. Ten degrees of pronation are added for improved pulp pinch. The EPL and FPL are tenodesed to the distal radius. The New Zealand split FPL transfer is recommended in place of arthrodesis of the IP joint.

This split transfer is a simple technique to prevent hyperflexion of the IP joint and has been used for patients with other paralytic conditions. Alternatively, House advises against performing the FPL split tenodesis on patients who are satisfied with their grip function despite having a hyperflexed IP joint. These patients have grown accustomed to and value their pinch pattern and a more normal appearance of the pinch does not equate to better function for them.

Authors' Approach

The preferred procedure for elbow extension at our center is the posterior deltoid-to-triceps transfer described in Figure 17-3. The BR transfer to the ECRB can be performed safely as a simultaneous procedure (48). The combined

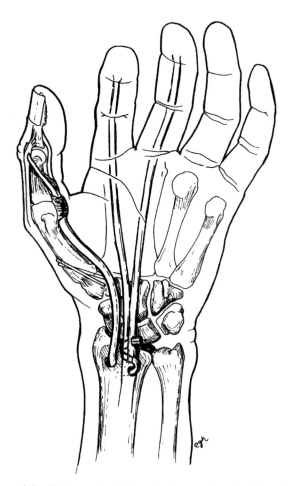

FIGURE 17-8   Modification of the Moberg simple key pinch procedure. **A.** Transfer of the brachioradialis BR into the ECRB for wrist extension; BR is mobilized proximally and its detached distal tendon interwoven into the ECRB. Tension of the transfer is set later while adjusting other transfers. The elbow is held in 90 degrees of flexion and the BR is electrically stimulated. **B.** Thumb CMC arthrodesis in 20–30 of extension, 30–40 of abduction, and 10–15 of pronation. **C.** FPL split tenodesis through a single radial mid-axial incision. **D.** FPL is tenodesed to the distal radius; the proximal free end is woven in and out of the volar distal radius through 4.5 mm drill holes, 1.5 cm apart. **E.** As the FPL emerges from the radius, it is interwoven to the index and long finger flexor profundi. The tension of the tenodesis is adjusted to create a reverse cascade with slightly more flexion in the index finger. **F.** The EPL is tenodesed to the distal radius by weaving it through the retinaculum over its fibro-osseous tunnel. **G.** EDC synchronization and tenodesis.

The seven surgical steps are part of a single-stage reconstruction. The flexor pulleys of the thumb are left undisturbed. Arthrodesis of the CMC joint of the thumb is an important early step. Tension of tenodeses around the thumb and wrist can be adjusted properly until the desired 'release' is accomplished with the wrist in 20 degrees of flexion. With the wrist in 20 to 30 degrees of extension, lateral key pinch should be restored. The extremity is immobilized with the elbow in 90 degrees of flexion, and the wrist and fingers in a position of 'function.'

Biceps rerouting pronatorplasty.   The biceps tendon is z-lengthened and rerouted around the lateral aspect of the proximal radius to restore pronation (Zancolli, 1967 #472). Release of the interosseous membrane and occasionally distal radio-ulnar joint posterior capsule is necessary in cases of severe supination contracture.

procedure effectively reduces the hospitalization time and the period of complete dependence of the patient. This might be a critical factor in some individuals, where the family or support structure is unable to tolerate the demands of repeat, prolonged hospitalizations.

Modified Moberg Lateral Pinch Procedure: Technique

We have modified Moberg's original procedure based on subsequent clinical experience over two decades. We emphasize assuring that the thumb pulp contacts the index finger at the flexed PIP joint, that the thumb IP joint is stabilized by tenodesis, that volar thumb flexor tendon pulleys are preserved, and that EPL tenodesis permits extension.

Through a volar midline incision, the distal radius, flexor pollicis longus, flexor digitorum profundus, and sublimis muscles are identified. A drill hole is placed within the radius at two locations, approximately 1 cm apart, as depicted in Figure 17-8. The tendon of the flexor pollicis longus is dissected from the muscle at the musculotendinous junction and passed through the drill holes. The tendon is interwoven into the tendon of the flexor digitorum profundus and/or sublimis to stabilize the index finger and/or the long finger, as a stable platform for pinch against the thumb IP joint. This creation of a loop of tendon simplifies the alignment of the thumb in key grip. If the patient requires a carpometacarpal arthrodesis to position the thumb in the adduction–abduction plane, this is performed prior to the tensioning of the tenodesis. We do not advocate release of the A1 or oblique pulley or arthrodesis of the thumb IP joint as originally described by Moberg. The long-term appearance of the thumb with FPL tenodesis done by the original procedure is that of excessive metacarpophalangeal flexion. Although Moberg advocated reversible IP joint pinning and later surgeons performed arthrodeses, it is more common today to create a split transfer or tenodesis of the FPL to EPL (49), as in Figure 17-9. IP arthrodesis is seldom performed due to excessive rigidity. When CMC and IP arthrodeses are combined, all subsequent mobility is located at the metacarpophalangeal joint.

The extensor pollicis longus is tenodesed into the extensor retinaculum and the thumb balanced for full extension in wrist flexion. The degree of CMC extension is balanced to achieve this posture. FPL tension is adjusted so that the thumb contacts the index finger at neutral wrist position and increases pinch with wrist extension (Fig. 17-10). The EPL may need to be re-routed to the second extensor compartment to reduce the adduction moment. Patient outcome is illustrated in Figure 17-11.

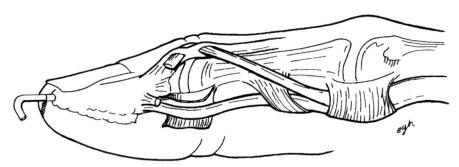

FIGURE 17-9 Modified Split Transfer, FPL to EPL. **A.** A single mid-lateral, radial incision, expose the A2 pulley, which is volar to the IP joint. **B.** The A2 pulley is released, leaving the volar plate of the IP joint intact. The more radial fascicle of the FPL is divided at its insertion on the distal phalanx and dissected proximally, preserving the oblique pulley of the thumb. **C.** The detached FPL slip is rerouted, in a direct line of pull, to the extensor pollicis longus tendon EPL, and woven into it. Tension is adjusted by tensioning the FPL at the wrist level, stabilizing the IP joint in neutral. The Pulvertaft weave is sutured with 4/0 nonabsorbable braided suture. A .062 k-wire is placed across the IP joint and removed at 4 to 6 weeks.

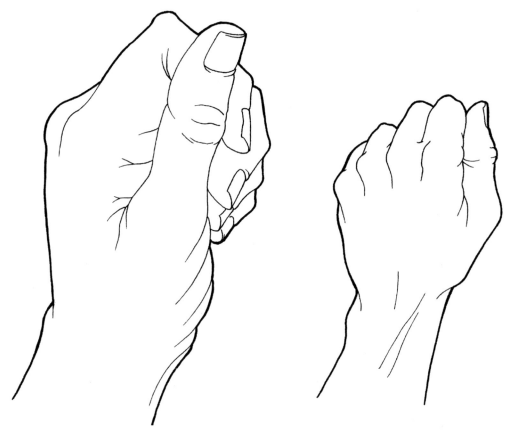

FIGURE 17-10   In lateral pinch, the thumb should contact the index finger at the proximal interphalangeal joint.

Extensor Tenodesis

The EPL is approached through a dorsal incision at the third compartment and divided at the musculotendinous junction. Several techniques are possible for interweaving the tendon through the retinaculum or around Lister's tubercle or re-routing it through the adjacent second compartment, should more extension and less adduction moment be required (Figs. 17-12, 17-13). The transfer cannot be routed through the first extensor compartment because it loses its moment for extension. Tension is set so that maximum MCP extension is created in conjunction with approximately 30 degrees of carpometacarpal extension. The combination of these procedures, FPL tenodesis, CMC arthrodesis, and EPL tenodesis provides a well-balanced thumb with optimum contact and pinch.

FPL Split Transfer

The concept of a stabilizing transfer of the radial half of the flexor pollicis longus to extensor pollicis longus is credited to Mohammed (49). Further studies have demonstrated that this simple procedure has a broad latitude of tension and alignment, which makes it both easy to perform and faster-healing than IP arthrodesis, and is an excellent method of stabilizing the thumb during pinch. The original technique requires two incisions, volar and dorsal. At our center, we accomplish this procedure through a single midlateral, radial incision and by the use of a curved tendon braiding forceps. The exposure of the flexor pollicis longus is achieved by flexing the thumb and noting the two fascicles of FPL. The A2 pulley is entered radially, leaving the volar plate of the IP joint intact, as in Figure 17-9. The more radial fascicle is divided at the level of

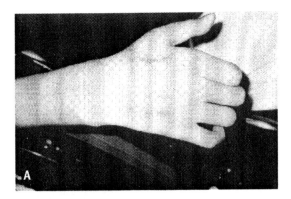

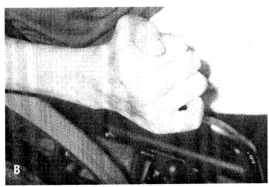

FIGURE 17-11 **A.** Demonstration of contemporary one stage lateral prehension reconstruction in C6/OCu:3 patient. Finger flexion demonstrates the "reversed cascade" with greater finger flexion in the radial digits. **B.** The extensor reconstruction included: EDC tenodesis, EPL tenodesis, and FPL split transfer. Flexion reconstruction included: BR to FPL transfer, ECRB to FDP via IOM transfer and CMC arthrodesis for thumb control.

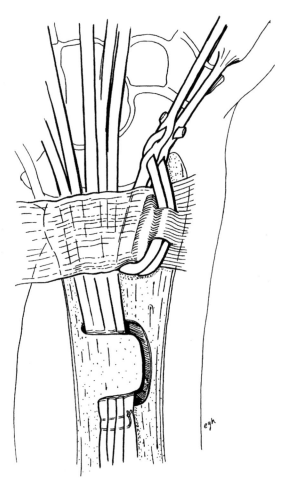

FIGURE 17-12 EPL and APL are sutured to the extensor retinaculum. The EDC tendons are, tenodesed through bone.

the distal phalanx and dissected proximally, preserving the oblique pulley of the thumb and routing this detached slip from a point proximal to it in a direct line of pull to the extensor pollicis longus tendon. A Pulvertaft interweave is performed and repaired with 4–0, nonabsorbable braided suture. Tension is adjusted by tensioning the flexor pollicis longus at the wrist level or by moving the wrist to adjust the thumb flexion and extension tightness. The advantages of this transfer over IP arthrodesis are the softness of the hand and the ability of the thumb to conform to the wheelchair rim during manual wheelchair propulsion or transfers.

ECRB-to-FDP Transfer

Our group recognized an improvement for restoring grip strength in C6 patients. The ECRB can be transferred into the FDP via a window in the interosseous membrane (IOM). This new procedure has the following advantages:

- It is useful even in the face of a weak ECRB of grade 2 or 3. Extension strength evaluation is not always reliable. Occasionally one has to rely on intraoperative assessment under local anesthesia.
- The ECRL is left undisturbed. This muscle is extremely important when there is uncertain

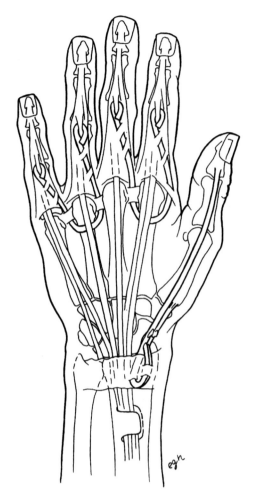

FIGURE 17-13 Extensor phase reconstruction; modified surgical technique. Stage one, extensor phase, reconstruction for Group 4 and 5 patients (Method I). House has proposed two methods for staged reconstructions that can be applied to Group 4 and 5 patients. Active release can be accomplished with a BR transfer into the EPL and EDC as in Method II. Alternatively, in Method I, the EPL, APL, and EDC are tenodesed into the distal radius. The APL is rerouted through the third extensor compartment and together with the EPL, is tenodesed into a bony window in the distal radius or into the extensor retinaculum. The floor of the fourth extensor compartment is exposed, and a 2 by 2 cm ulnar-sided periosteal flap is developed. A high-speed burr is used to create a cortical groove in the shape of a "U." The EDC tendons are sutured together to synchronize finger extension and then are tucked under the "U" bone clip without dividing them proximally.

weakness of the ECRB as the residual wrist extensor.

- The line of pull is straighter for the transfer.

- It avoids the creation of a supination moment as in the ECRL-to-FDP subcutaneous transfer.

The operation was originally performed to act as a superior passive tenodesis in those patients with weak ECRB. Haque reviewed our series of seven patients with spinal cord injury, five with an ASIA level at C6 and two at C7. The total active finger flexion averaged 122 degrees per digit. Key lateral pinch and grip strengths were 4 and 12 pounds, respectively. The patients experienced a variable loss of wrist extension but not of wrist extension strength. It is speculated that the transfer generated a wrist flexion moment that limits the patient's ability to extend. Adhesion formation may also limit range of motion.

Surgical Technique. The procedure requires separate volar and dorsal incisions. The insertion of ECRB into the third metacarpal base is identified and released. The tendon is retrieved proximal to the extensor retinaculum. A volar Henry approach is ideal. One readily identifies the profundus flexor tendons of the digits. The IOM is exposed proximal to the pronator quadratus. The anterior interosseous nerve is protected while a window in the membrane is developed. The tendon of the ECRB is delivered volarly. The FDP tendons are "synchronized" in a reversed cascade with more tension on the radial digits. It is advisable to leave the ulnar one or two digits free, especially for patients with weak ECRB motors. The ECRB is sutured end-to-side into the FDP using a Pulvertaft weave. The tension is adjusted using intraoperative stimulation of the ECRB. Excessive tension limits wrist extension and finger extension. It is imperative that finger extension, for the release phase, is not compromised with excessive tightening of the transfer. A splint is applied with the wrist in slight flexion and the digits in a gentle flexion posture. Immobilization is continued for 4 weeks, followed by active exercises.

A FES neuroprosthesis can provide thumb flexion and extension, adduction, abduction, finger flexion and extension, wrist flexion, pronation, and triceps extension.

Groups 2 and 3 (ASIA C6)

These patients have good BR and ECRL function, while ECRB is present in varying strength. The brachioradialis is available for transfer. Reconstruction can include restoration of active thumb flexion or finger flexion. Moberg proposed a two-stage reconstruction: stage 1 is a simple key pinch procedure where the FPL is tenodesed to the distal radius for thumb flexion. His personal experience with the BR-to-FPL transfer was not favorable. Stage 2 is a BR transfer into the EPL, EPB, or APL to restore abduction of the thumb and thus improve the release phase. Intraoperative evaluation of the EPL, APB, and APL is performed by looking for the best thumb abductor for the individual patient. Once identified, the BR is transferred into it. House performs the same operation on Group 1 patients, except for the transfer of the BR into the FPL for active thumb flexion.

For patients with weak wrist extensors, Group 2, Zancolli (5) prefers to utilize the available BR to actively flex the digits. In stage 1, the extensor phase, the EDC, EPL, and APL are tenodesed to the distal radius. The thumb MP joint is arthrodesed, and the "lasso" procedure is performed for intrinsic reconstruction. In these patients, the lasso operation is done with denervated FDS muscles, and Zancolli refers to it as the "indirect lasso" to distinguish it from the "direct lasso," which involves functioning non-denervated FDS muscles in patients with more remaining function.

In the second stage, the flexor phase, the BR is transferred to the FDP for finger flexion, and the FPL is tenodesed to the distal radius for thumb flexion.

Distinguishing Group 2 from Group 3. Clinical assessment is important to distinguish patients in Group 2 with only BR and ECRL function from those in Group 3, who have an additional wrist extensor, the ECRB. Bean has pointed out that a groove between the ECRL and ECRB is appreciable on examination of the lateral forearm while the patient extends the wrist against resistance (49).

It is still possible to make an error in the clinical assessment, and some researchers advocate intraoperative evaluation. Patients who are dependent on wrist tenodesis mechanics for pinch or sports do not want to lose wrist extension. The tendon of the ECRB can be identified just proximal to the extensor retinaculum via a small incision after infiltration with local anesthetic. The tourniquet is not inflated for this part of the procedure to minimize ischemia. The patient is asked to voluntarily extend the wrist while the tension in the tendon of the ECRB is measured. The ECRL tendon can be transected and the residual ECRB strength determined. If ECRB wrist extension is to be preserved and ECRL transferred to FDP for finger flexion, the moment for wrist flexion attributable to the finger flexors will be increased. If ECRB seems too weak to extend the wrist under these conditions, we transfer it to the finger flexors via the interosseous membrane route and preserve the strong ECRL for wrist extension. These assessments can also be done with intraoperative electrical stimulation of the wrist extensors.

Transfer of a wrist extensor to the finger flexors without an antagonist often leads to a tight fist without finger movement. In many cases, we are adding a finger extensor tenodesis or transferring brachioradialis to the finger extensors to better balance the fingers and prevent this tight hand posture. Although it still functions for key grip, the ECRL transfer becomes a deforming force. Functional electric stimulation (FES) is recommended for persons who want better range of motion and strength without sacrificing wrist extension strength and reliability of BR-to-FPL for pinch.

A FES neuroprosthesis can provide thumb flexion and extension, adduction, abduction, finger flexion and extension, wrist flexion, pronation, and triceps extension.

Groups 4 and 5

Group 4 patients gain control of pronator teres (PT), while Group 5 patients have a strong flexor carpi radialis (FCR). Because of the advantage of FCR as a wrist flexor and finger tenodesis extensor, it is seldom transferred. Staged procedures, as described by Zancolli and House, are recommended. Some investigators avoid manipulating the PT for fear that pronation will be compromised. Loss of pronation is a high price to pay because it is necessary to position the hand in space for useful grip and pinch and for gravity-assisted wrist flexion, which is key for hand opening, the release phase. Zancolli has reported no such loss of pronation and transfers the PT to the FCR or to the FPL during stage 2, the flexor phase of the reconstruction.

Mid-Cervical Reconstruction (Zancolli)

Zancolli describes a complex two-stage reconstruction for mid-cervical tetraplegia. In the first surgical, or extensor phase, a CMC arthrodesis is performed in 30 to 40 degrees of abduction and 20 degrees of extension. Voluntary tendon transfer of brachioradialis to extensor digitorum communis and extensor pollicis longus tendons is performed with the lasso intrinsic procedure to provide more effective finger extension. He advocates tendon transfer to the triceps to improve elbow stability and finger extension. The lasso procedure is adjusted with sutured tension with the finger in complete extension of the IP joints and 20 degrees of flexion of the MP joint. Zancolli believes that the lasso procedure improves the brachioradialis effect and synchronizes finger flexion by applying a uniform tension. The carpometacarpal arthrodesis is immobilized for 8 weeks and then a second surgical stage is performed, as depicted in Figure 17-14 and 17-15. Tendon transfer of extensor carpi radialis to flexor digitorum profundus and the attachment of flexor pollicis longus to extensor carpi radialis brevis at the musculotendinous junction permits finger and thumb flexion. Careful attention should be paid to avoid damaging the tendon of FPL or its adhesion to the radius by preserving the periosteum along its pathway. Alternatively, pronator teres may be transferred to flexor pollicis longus as an inde-

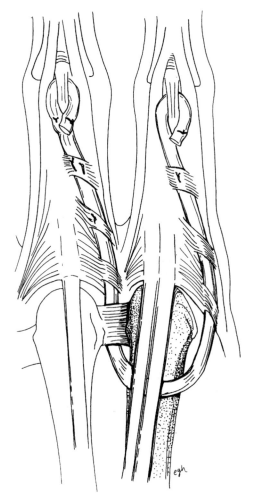

FIGURE 17-14 Intrinsic reconstruction-surgical technique. A free tendon graft, such as the EDQ, is harvested. One free end of the graft is woven and sutured into the radial lateral band about the index finger MP joint. The other free end is passed under the extrinsic extensors of the index and into the lumbrical canal of the long finger, passing deep to the transverse intermetacarpal ligament. It is woven into the radial lateral band of the long finger. A second graft is used around the dorsum of the forth metacarpal neck for intrinsic tenodesis of the ring and small digits.

pendent thumb flexor, or pronator teres may be transferred to flexor carpi radialis to further augment wrist flexion and therefore stabilize finger extension. This combination of muscle, tendon, and joint procedures produces grasp and key grip and an entirely synergistic neuromuscular reconstruction.

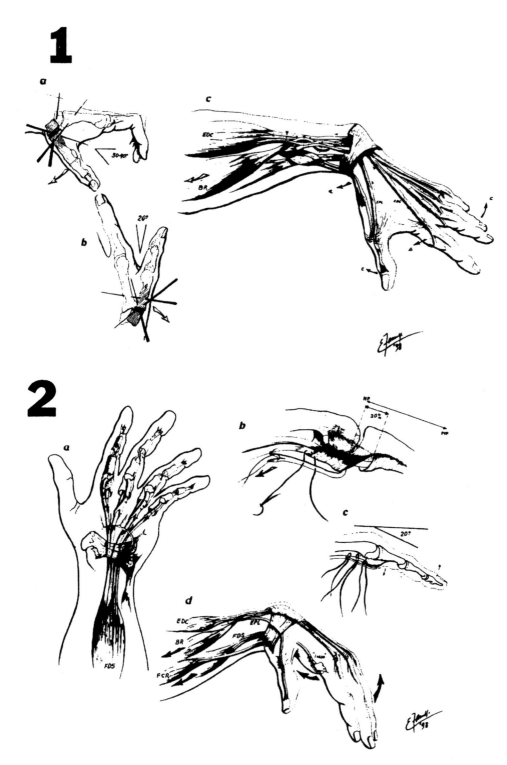

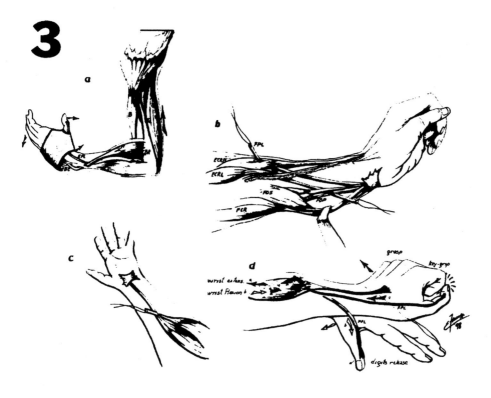

FIGURE 17-15 Mid-cervical synergistic reconstruction (Zancolli, 1999).

Two-stage reconstruction for patients with strong wrist extension.

1. First surgical stage, the extensor phase. *a.* Reconstruction begins with CMC fusion; 30 to 40 degrees of abduction and 20 degrees of extension. *b.* Brachioradialis BR transfer to the extensor digitorum communis EDC, extensor pollicis longus EPL.

2. Stabilization of the MP joints is accomplished with FDS lasso procedure during first surgical stage of the reconstruction. *a.* Expose flexor digitorum sublimis FDS through a transverse incision at the distal metacarpophalangeal flexion crease where the chiasm of Camper is visualized by flexing the fingers and tensioning the FDS. *b.* The FDS is detached between A1 and A2 pulleys and sutured to itself proximally over the A1 pulley. Zancolli has shown that the A1 pulley spans to the proximal fifth, or 20 percent, of the proximal phalanx. *c.* Zancolli adjusts the tension of the with the MP joins in 20 degrees of flexion, the IP joints in full extension, and the wrist in neutral. *d.* By preventing hyperextension of the proximal phalanx, the lasso procedure improves finger IP extension by the transferred BR and synchronizes finger flexion.

3. Postoperative management after extensor phase reconstruction and second stage reconstruction (flexor stage). *a.* The extremity is immobilized in a long arm cast across the wrist and elbow. At 4 weeks the cast is removed, and a small wrist-based cast is used to protect the CMC fusion for 4 additional weeks. The elbow may be immobilized separately in 90 degrees of flexion for the same time. With the elbow stabilized, re-education of the BR transfer is easier. Restoring active elbow extension potentiates the function of the BR transfer. *b.* Four to 6 months after the first stage, the patient undergoes second stage reconstruction (flexor phase). The ECRL is transferred to the FDP for active finger flexion. The FPL tendon is freed proximally and sutured into the ECRB. *c.* When the pronator teres PT is available, it is transferred into the paralyzed FCR to restore wrist flexion. Active wrist flexion stabilizes the wrist and further improve finger extension. *d.* The flexor phase reconstruction is based on synergistic muscles that are readily re-educated for automatic grasp and key pinch.

Staged Reconstruction (House)

House reports favorable experience with the transfer of the PT into the FPL since the early 1970s. His approach for Group 4 patients is outlined:

Stage 1, the extensor phase, encompasses five procedures: 1) thumb CMC fusion; 2) APL and EPL tenodesis; 3) EDC tenodesis or BR to EDC–EPL transfer; 4) intrinsic balancing, with an intrinsic tenodesis or later with a Zancolli indirect lasso during the flexor phase; and 5) FPL split transfer.

Tenodesis of the extensor digitorum communis and extensor pollicis longus is performed, as depicted in Figure 17-13. Tunneling the tendons beneath the flapped radius (as modified by Hamlin), and setting the tension between tendons using an additional Kirschner wire provides a reliable and strong tenodesis. The CMC joint is approached along the radial border of the APL. A pin is advanced to hold the thumb metacarpal in the desired position with respect to the index metacarpal—40 to 45 degrees of abduction, 25 degrees of extension, and 10 degrees of pronation. The pin is temporarily backed out of the index metacarpal while the CMC joint is debrided. The pin is advanced into the index, and the CMC joint is cross-pinned.

House discovered that intrinsic passive tenodesis, using a tendon graft from extensor digiti quinti between the index and long fingers, alleviates intrinsic minus posturing and strengthens the tension that could be applied in the second flexor phase. A lasso in the flexor phase is recommended for patients with PIP flexion contracture associated with spastic FDS and central slip deficits. The intrinsic tenodesis is performed with a free-tendon graft, as in Figure 17-15. In bilateral reconstructions, different methods for grip and pinch are recommended for each hand, based on patient preference.

Postoperatively, the hand is supported in wrist neutral and in finger extension position for 4 weeks, and weight-bearing or passive flexion against the fingers is prevented for a total of 8 weeks.

Stage 2, the flexor phase, includes motor transfers to the FDP and FPL and, when necessary, a Zancolli indirect lasso. Extensor carpi radialis longus is transferred around the radial side of the forearm and interwoven into flexor digitorum profundus. Either the brachioradialis or pronator teres may be used to power flexor pollicis longus (Fig. 17-16).

All tendon repairs are done by a Pulvertaft interweave of at least three passes and sutured with interrupted sutures of 3/0 or 4/0 nonabsorbable braided suture. Because this is a single muscle to a four-tailed graft, tension in the finger flexors must be adjusted so that there is not excessive fifth finger flexion. We prefer a reversed cascade in which the index is tighter than the long, tighter than the ring, and tighter than the fifth finger. In some cases, this requires that the tendon transfer not be passed to the FDP at the fourth and fifth fingers or that it should be done in a lengthened position. Creation of an excessively tight grasp overcomes the extensor tenodesis and provides a clenched fist, which is less functional in this group of patients, who have the potential for large and small object grasp. Because these are voluntary transfers, tension is best suggested by intraoperative electrical stimulation that demonstrates sufficient range of motion and force. The adjustment can be made by changing the degree of interweave until the appropriate tension is established. Establishing tension by tenodesis alone will overemphasize the need for extensive tension and place the finger flexors in too tight a tension.

After the second stage, tenodesis movements are begun at 4 weeks to emphasize the automatic control, and these transfers augment the synergistic balance inherent in the hand. Force is then applied with wrist extension to provide additional thumb and finger flexion. Practice with objects of increasing weight and smoother texture in different orientations of shoulder, elbow, and wrist position will eventually train the patient to use the tenodesis aided by gravity and the rotational movement of the forearm. Maximum power grip is permitted after an additional 6 weeks.

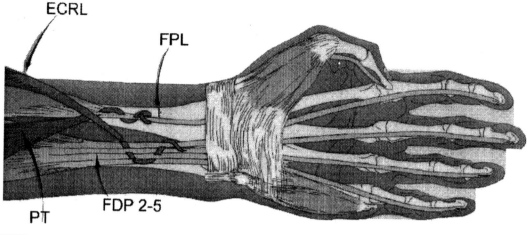

FIGURE 17-16   Flexor phase reconstruction in Groups 4 and 5. House has proposed two methods of reconstruction, one restoring strong lateral key pinch for smaller objects and the other restoring palmar grasp for larger objects. Key pinch reconstruction is based around fusion of the CMC joint of the thumb, while palmar grasp reconstruction utilizes an adduction opponensplasty for thumb control. Both methods, however, prescribe the same flexor phase transfers, including ECRL-to-FDP 2–5 for grip and PT-to-FPL for thumb flexion.

For the same group of patients, Zancolli recommends EDRL-to-FDP 2–5 transfer and transfer of the FPL tendon into the ECRB, which is left in situ, as illustrated in Figure 17-15.

Flexor phase-surgical technique.   The ECRL is first transferred to the FDP to facilitate later positioning of the thumb. It is important to avoid over-tightening the transfer. The proper tension is adjusted such that with the elbow in 90 degrees of flexion, finger MP and IP extension is possible when the wrist is brought into slight flexion. Next the PT is transferred into the FPL. Raising the PT with a periosteal sleeve facilitates the transfer. Finally, if intrinsic balance is necessary, the FDS lasso is used at this stage. Active rehabilitation with finger and thumb flexion is begun in three weeks. Early active ROM is thought to minimize scar formation.

Group 6

These patients have strong finger extension but lack thumb extension. The two-phase reconstruction can be performed in the same operation or as separate procedures. The EPL is sutured to the EDC either side-to-side or incised proximally and woven through the EDC tendon. One can then proceed immediately with the flexion phase or postpone it.

Group 7

These patients may require only finger flexion reconstruction. We recommend an adduction opponensplasty for strong thumb control and an indirect lasso procedure for MP flexion.

Group 8

These patients have remaining extrinsic finger flexors that are usually stronger on the ulnar side. In addition to the thumb adductor opponensplasty and the indirect lasso, the FDP tendons are sutured together to synchronize flexion. The FPL is motored with an ECRL or a BR transfer. McDowell prefers a two-stage reconstruction according to Zancolli for Groups 7 and 8. In stage 1, all the flexors are sutured together to synchronize flexion and the BR is transferred to the FPL for thumb flexion. In stage 2, thumb control is through a modified adductor opponensplasty. A free-tendon graft is sutured into the APB tendon and looped around a pulley, based on the pisiform, and woven into the FCU tendon. Intrinsic balance is accomplished with a direct lasso, where the FDS is motorized by the ECRL in Group 7 patients.

Group 9

These patients' only deficit is intrinsic musculature. Thumb intrinsic reconstruction is done according to Zancolli or an adductor opponensplasty. Intrinsic balance is best accomplished with a direct lasso.

Intrinsic Reconstruction

In the tetraplegic patient with flaccid paralysis of both extrinsic and intrinsic muscles of the hand, no deformity should develop given proper splinting and a ROM program to maintain a supple hand. It is the presence of hypertonicity, spasticity, unbalanced extrinsic force, external forces (such as gravity and conformation of the hand to objects), and, often, neglect or intentional splinting that produces fixed contractures and tight finger posturing. The surgical transfer of an available voluntary motor unit for extrinsic finger flexion without restoration of intrinsic balance can produce a worsening of the imbalance. Intrinsic reconstruction should be undertaken when the surgeon identifies an established or potential intrinsic imbalance.

Intrinsic function is necessary for the coordinated motion of the fingers for grasp. Without intrinsic function, an asynchronous, nonintegrated grasp with early digital roll-up is produced by the action of the extrinsic flexors or a transfer. Such a pattern of distal to proximal sequence of joint flexion beginning at the DIP, PIP, and finally, flexion of the hyperextended MP, is functional only for hook grasp. Grasping large objects requires digital flexion to be initiated at the MP joint with simultaneous IP flexion following closely, as in palmar prehension. Grip strength is compromised with intrinsic weakness or imbalance. Kozin et al. (50) demonstrated a loss of strength of up to 49 percent after ulnar nerve block at the wrist level in 20 volunteers. Pinch strength loss is even more severe, from 75 to 80 percent (51) or 85 percent (50). Brand states that "the combined tension of the two interossei is of the same order as that of an extrinsic finger flexor" (52).

In a recent study in our center (53), the moments generated by the interossei were characterized following electrical stimulation. The flexion–extension and adduction–abduction moments generated were measured with a three-dimensional force transducer in five able-bodied volunteers and two tetraplegic patients. Isometric measurements were made in three different finger positions with various degrees of MP and IP flexion. Moments generated by the lumbricals were approximately 70 percent of other interossei. The muscles tested in the tetraplegic patients generated 80 to 90 percent of the force measured in the able-bodied subjects. The dorsal interossei-generated moments are finger abduction, MP flexion, and IP extension, and the volar interossei for finger adduction, MP flexion, and IP extension.

House and colleagues have studied intrinsic balance in tetraplegic reconstruction. Their treatment algorithm (54,55) is reproduced in Figure 17-17 (55). In Groups 1, 2, and 3, they advocate simple extrinsic, one-stage key pinch reconstruction plus an FDS lasso if the MP joint is hyperextended, or a Stiles-Bunnell tenodesis if the PIP joint is too flexed.

In Groups 4 and 5, a thumb adductor-opponensplasty is performed in method one. An intrinsic tenodesis in the extensor phase is preferred. In method two, the CMC joint of the thumb is fused and an FDS lasso in the flexor phase is favored. For patients in Groups 4 and 5, they recommend either a lasso procedure or an intrinsic tenodesis.

In Groups 6 and 7, one-stage grasp–pinch release reconstruction is done. A lasso is performed when there is intrinsic balance. In Group 6, patients' thumb position and control is by CMC fusion, EPL tenodesis, and tendon transfer to FPL. In Group 7 patients, an adductor-opponensplasty is performed with an intervening graft from FDS IV powered by FCU. The lasso for the third and fourth digits is performed, splitting the FDS of III. Group 6 and 7 patients requiring intrinsic balance for MP extension or clawing after motor transfer into FDP are best managed with a lasso procedure.

For patients with hyperlax joints or a hyperextensible PIP joint, we advise against tenodesis into the lateral bands to avoid the development of a swan-neck deformity. When we have encountered an established swan-neck deformi-

Intrinsic Balance: Two-stage Grasp Pinch and Release.

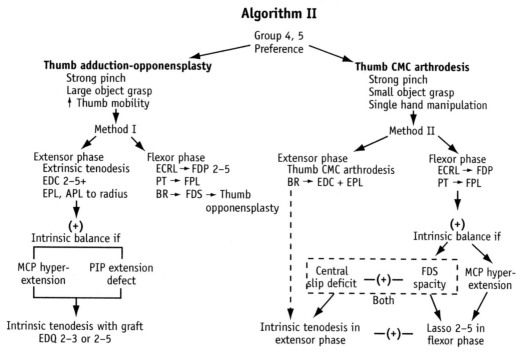

Algorithm II

Group 4, 5
Preference

Thumb adduction-opponensplasty
Strong pinch
Large object grasp
↑ Thumb mobility

Method I

Extensor phase
Extrinsic tenodesis
EDC 2–5+
EPL, APL to radius

Flexor phase
ECRL → FDP 2–5
PT → FPL
BR → FDS → Thumb
opponensplasty

(+)
Intrinsic balance if

MCP hyper-
extension

PIP extension
defect

Intrinsic tenodesis with graft
EDQ 2–3 or 2–5

Thumb CMC arthrodesis
Strong pinch
Small object grasp
Single hand manipulation

Method II

Extensor phase
Thumb CMC arthrodesis
BR → EDC + EPL

Flexor phase
ECRL → FDP
PT → FPL

(+)
Intrinsic balance if

Central
slip deficit

—(+)—

FDS
spacity

MCP hyper-
extension

Both

Intrinsic tenodesis in
extensor phase

—(+)—

Lasso 2–5 in
flexor phase

Courtesty of James House MD, JHS 22A, 1997

FIGURE 17-17 Intrinsic reconstruction algorithm (after House Instructional Course Lecture 1999, ASSH). Intrinsic reconstruction by groups: For Group 4 and 5 patients, House performs a two-stage key pinch release reconstruction. He recommends two different methods according to thumb reconstruction. In Method I, a thumb adductor-opponensplasty is performed, and an intrinsic tenodesis in the extensor phase is preferred. In Method II, the CMC joint of the thumb is fused and an FDS lasso in the flexor phase is favored.

His approach to Group 1, 2, and 3 reconstructions includes an extrinsic, one-stage key pinch reconstruction plus either an FDS lasso (if MP joint is hyperextended) or a Stiles–Bunnell tenodesis (if PIP joint is too flexed).

Group 6 and 7 patients undergo a one-stage grasp/pinch release reconstruction. Intrinsic balance, whenever necessary, is accomplished with a Zancolli lasso regardless of the method for thumb reconstruction. In Group 6, patients' thumb position and control is by CMC fusion, EPL tenodesis, and tendon transfer to FPL. In Group 7 patients, an adductor-opponensplasty is performed with an intervening graft from FDS IV motorized by FCU. The lasso for the third and fourth digits is performed by splitting the FDS of III.

ty in a tetraplegic hand, we perform a tenodesis procedure with a slip of FDS detached proximally and sutured to the A2 pulley (Fig. 17-18). In our experience, clawing or chronic flexor posturing of the fifth finger is often best treated by PIP arthrodesis in 40 degrees of flexion, and we seldom perform a tenodesis on the fourth and fifth fingers. Some patients experience a stretching out of the extensor tendon tenodesis, so we advocate suture of the extensor tendons to the retinaculum as well to avoid this laxity.

Metacarpophalangeal (MP) hyperextension deformity with PIP flexion deformity (with or without EDC central slip attenuation) results in the inability to create a functional grip and is indications for intrinsic balance procedures. The FDS lasso procedure, shown in Figure 17-18, is useful for patients who have MP joint hyperextension or clawing. Flexion deformity of the PIP joint without central slip defects can be managed with an intrinsic tenodesis. Both of these procedures are passive methods that depend on

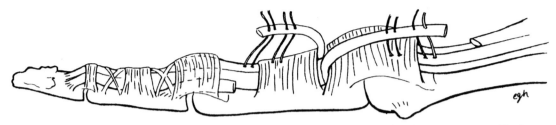

FIGURE 17-18 FDS lasso procedure-surgical technique. It is important to either interweave or scarify the tendon of FDS; we recommend a tendon interweave to minimize the likelihood of stretching out of the transfer. In addition, the tension of each tendon can be adjusted independently by the tightness of the weave. Suture is with 3/0 or 4/0 nonabsorbable braided suture.

motion about the wrist and are referred to as a "dynamic tenodesis." We use the lasso procedure and intrinsic tenodesis in those patients who have a combination of PIP flexion contracture secondary to FDS spasticity or excessive adhesions and an extensor lag due to attenuation of the extensor central slip. Intrinsic tenodesis is performed in the extensor phase and the lasso procedure added in the flexor phase.

The reconstruction can only be successful when the PIP shows passive range of motion. PIP flexion deformities must be treated aggressively, including tightening of the extensor tendons or transfer of the lateral bands dorsally. Failure to achieve sufficient PIP extension will result in deficient palmar prehension and large object grasp. For the late reconstruction with poor extensor tendon structure, a PIP arthrodesis is preferred.

Lasso Intrinsicplasty: Technique

The lasso procedure was described by Zancolli to balance metacarpophalangeal flexion and intrinsic balance where claw hand, (intrinsic minus), posturing had developed in an otherwise supple hand. Finger flexion contractures are often the result of excessive tightness within flexor digitorum sublimis or adhesions posterior to the tendon and to the adjacent flexor digitorum profundus. Release of the hypertonic FDS removes the deforming force from the PIP joint and creates an MP joint flexion tenodesis. Balancing the tension allows extensor digitorum communis, either as a tenodesis or motored by

an active transfer, to be a more effective PIP joint extensor. Expose the flexor digitorum sublimis through a transverse incision at the distal metacarpophalangeal flexion crease. If the hand is flexible and PIP hyperextension is expected, then a volar Bruner incision is needed to allow transfer of a slip of the FDS to the A2 pulley as a restraint. The chiasm of Camper can be visualized by flexing the fingers and tensioning the FDS while performing the lasso procedure. The FDS is detached between A1 and A2, and if the PIP joint is tight or contracted, both limbs are cut at equal lengths and interwoven over the A1 pulley to the proximal tendon of the flexor digitorum sublimis as originally described.

Zancolli has modified the procedure to address stretching of the reconstruction with time. He loops the superficialis tendon through the A2 pulley so that the amount of pulley captured in the tendon loop spans the proximal fifth, or 20 percent, of the proximal phalanx, as shown in Figure 17-18. He then sutures the tendon to itself proximal to the A1 pulley. If the PIP joint is hyperextensible or lax, one slip can be cut long and interwoven to the A2 pulley to provide a tenodesis at the PIP joint that prevents hyperextension. It is important to either interweave or scarify the tendon of FDS. We prefer a tendon interweave because there is less likelihood of stretching out of the transfer. In addition, the tension of each of the tendons can be adjusted independently by the tightness of the weave. Suture is with 3/0 or 4/0 nonabsorbable braided suture. Gauging the tension of the lasso is somewhat imprecise if the patient was given paralytic agents during anesthesia or if the muscle is in fact denervated. If the FDS is innervated and under voluntary control, the intraoperative stimulation of the FDS will demonstrate the appropriate balance that the patient will have when awake. If the tension is being set in a paralyzed muscle, the transfer should not be set too tight; that is, the metacarpophalangeal joints should still extend during wrist flexion. Excessive tightness limits the size of objects that can be grasped in the hand and may lead to swan-neck deformities if a tight lasso is combined with a strong extensor digitorum communis. The lasso procedure, like other soft tissue realignments, is protected in a relaxed posture, depending upon the balance of additional transfers. Usual healing time is 4 weeks or longer.

Adductor-Opponensplasty: Technique

Adductor-opponensplasty was described by Thompson and modified by Royle. For patients with sufficient motors to allow transfer of the pronator teres (International Group 4), strong pinch can be created. The pronator teres is detached from the radius through an anterior exposure. The tendon is extended with a strip of periosteum and sutured end-to-end to the tendon of the flexor digitorum sublimis of the ring finger in the forearm. The distal end of the tendon is detached from the middle phalanx and rerouted across the palm, using the distal edge of the transverse carpal ligament as a pulley. It is sutured to the extensor mechanism at the abductor pollicis brevis attachment. Tension is adjusted to produce greater abduction as the wrist passes through neutral to extension. Care should be taken to avoid excessive tension or the thumb becomes fixed in anteversion and flexion. An antagonistic thumb extensor is needed by tenodesis or transfer (Fig. 17-19).

FUNCTIONAL ELECTRICAL STIMULATION (FES) NEUROPROSTHESIS

The Functional Electrical Stimulation (FES) neuroprosthesis plays an important role in per-

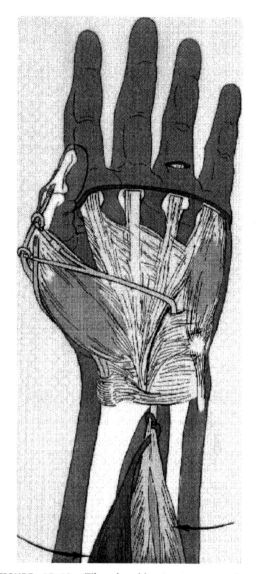

FIGURE 17-19 Thumb adduction-opponensplasty. Transfer is accomplished by elongating the BR or the PT, whenever available, with a suitable free tendon graft, usually the ring finger superficialis insitu, proximally. The FDS is detached at its distal insertion and rerouted subcutaneously around the ulnar edge of the palmar fascia, according to Royle–Thompson. The tendon is sutured into the tendinous insertion of the abductor pollicis brevis APB. The Riordan–Brand modification to the distal insertion is a further refinement of the technique; the FDS is split and one slip is sutured to the adductor pollicis ADD aponeurosis around the dorsum of the MP joint; the other slip is woven into the APB and around the EPL. We continue to perform this useful operation at our center, especially when a non-FES reconstruction is planned. It is advisable to perform different type of pinch/grip reconstruction in bilateral cases. Patients appreciate their different abilities.

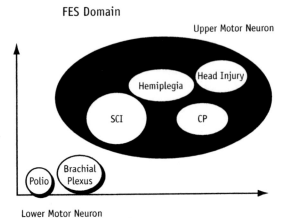

FES Domain

FIGURE 17-20 FES domain. Functional electric stimulation can be a useful therapeutic and management modality in conditions of neuromuscular paralysis with intact lower motor neuron innervation to target muscles. In stroke, traumatic brain injury, and cerebral palsy, FES may be useful in combination with spasmolytic agents and botulinum toxin to regain control of spastic motor units.

sons with upper motor neuron disorders such as spinal cord injury, cerebral palsy, stroke, and head injury (Fig. 17-20). By applying a natural stimulus to the intact peripheral axon, the FES neuroprosthesis is able to elicit and recruit muscle movements and provide functional patterning familiar to the user (Fig. 17-21).

High-level spinal cord injury leaves few opportunities for reconstruction of the hand. At levels ASIA C5 and C6, among the most common injuries, only key pinch can be created using traditional tendon transfer and rehabilitation tools. With the FDA approval in 1997 of the NeuroControl Freehand Functional Electrical Stimulation (FES) Neuroprostheses, additional muscles become available for control (56–61). This section describes the indications, surgical techniques, and results of treatment with this new standard of care for high spinal cord injury.

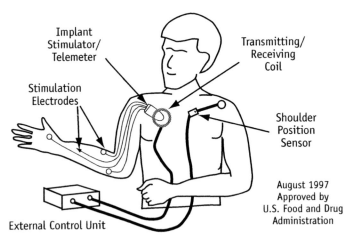

FIGURE 17-21 The implantable FES hand grasp neuroprosthesis (FreeHand System®) was approved for use by the U.S. Food and Drug Administration in August 1997. An external shoulder position sensor translates patient's voluntary motion into input signals for a program within an external control unit housing a microprocessor and memory. The external control unit delivers a radio frequency (RF) signal to a transmitting coil taped to the skin over the implanted stimulator receiver. The radio frequency signal is transmitted to the implanted receiver stimulator below the skin. RF current powers the stimulator and codes specific instructions, which the stimulator processes into appropriate electric pulses to be delivered by implanted epimyseal electrodes. Target muscles have been selected to restore missing function.

The therapist and patient, selecting those muscle groups and forces that provide the best adaptation of the paralyzed hand to activities of daily living, determine program parameters within the external controller. Typically, two grasp patterns are created: lateral pinch for small object grasp in a horizontal plane and palmar prehension for large object grasp in a more vertical plane.

Neurophysiology

Following traumatic spinal cord injury, three types of motor units are identifiable. Above the level of injury, lower motor neurons (LMNs) are spared and remain connected to upper motor neurons (UMNs) in the motor cortex. The corresponding motor continues under volitional control. At the injury segment, the corresponding motor units become totally denervated from combined UMN tract and spinal cord LMN cell body damage. Muscle undergoes irreversible atrophy as a result of disuse and loss of neurogenic trophic transmitters such as acetylcholine. Below the level of injury, LMNs are intact but disconnected from the motor cortex. The corresponding motor units are not under voluntary control, yet remain electrically excitable. The muscle may undergo atrophy and develop type II glycolytic metabolism because of the higher discharge rate of anterior horn cells. These changes can be reversed by electrical stimulation of the intact peripheral nerve branch in a conditioning

and exercise program. A suprathreshold stimulus applied directly to the muscle at a frequency of 10 hertz for 8 hours a day has been effective in changing the contractile properties of the muscle to a slow oxidative metabolic state, rendering them more fatigue resistant (62). Over time, consistent exercise will yield a softening of joint capsular contracture and a reduction in spasticity during the stimulation. Through FES, these innervated muscles can be excited and called upon to perform their primary activity or transferred surgically to perform a more functionally useful activity (Fig. 17-22).

Indications for Treatment

The selection criteria for upper extremity FES neuroprosthesis has not changed significantly since it was outlined in 1988 by Peckham, Keith, and Freehafer (63). The FES neuroprosthesis is indicated for C5 and C6 spinal cord injured persons who have good general health, are free of major infections, and have pharmacologically

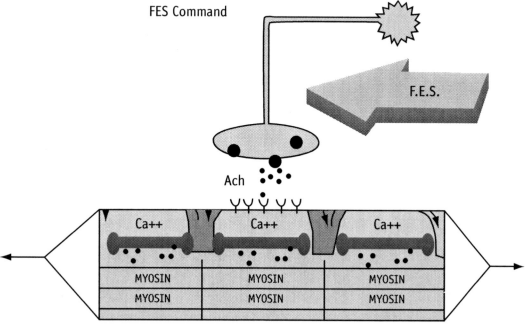

FIGURE 17-22 FES electrical command replaces the discharge from the anterior horn cell. The application of the electrical current causes the usual release of acetylcholine from the motor end plate and subsequent muscle membrane depolarization and contraction. The frequency of the stimulus conditions the muscle to slow oxidative metabolism.

Surgical Treatment for Cervical SCI

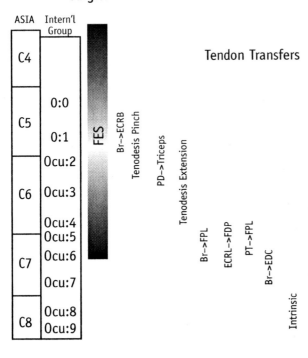

FIGURE 17-23 Application of commonly performed tendon transfer and FES techniques ranked according to neurologic classification (ASIA, International Classification, Surgical Reconstruction for Tetraplegia). The extent of FES application is not yet delimited.

controlled spasticity. To use the hands at this level, good sitting posture and proximal shoulder control is required. ASIA C5 patients typically have an intact, innervated deltoid and brachioradialis with at least Grade 3 strength. C6 patients have one or more wrist extensors, providing a minimum of Grade 3 wrist extension strength. Figure 17-23 shows the relationship of the indications of functional electrical stimulation to other common upper extremity reconstructive procedures. The system consists of an external shoulder position controller or manual switch that activates a program within an external control unit housing a microprocessor and memory. It delivers a radio frequency signal to an implanted stimulator receiver that applies pulses to peripheral nerve branches within selected target muscles. The parameters in the program are determined by the therapist and the patient to select those muscle groups and forces that provide the best adaptation of the paralyzed hand to the activities of daily living. Typically, two grasp patterns are developed—lateral pinch for small object grasp in a horizontal plane and

palmar prehension for large object grasp in a more vertical plane. Patients are selected, and initially their forearm muscles are conditioned using surface stimulation. Over a period of 3 to 6 weeks, muscle strength, fatigue resistance, and controllability increases.

FES Tendon Transfers

Tendon transfers powered by FES-stimulated muscles play in important role in filling deficits where lower motor neuron muscles are inexcitable. To achieve balanced torque of the wrist under the influence of strong stimulated flexor digitorum profundus, strong wrist extension is needed. Typically a voluntary transfer, brachioradialis to extensor carpi radialis brevis, can provide some wrist extension of Grade 3. In addition, a stimulated transfer of extensor carpi ulnaris to extensor carpi radialis brevis increases the force sufficiently to balance the wrist flexion torque provided by strong stimulation of finger flexors. This relationship is illustrated in Figure 17-24. Tendon transfers of this type expand the

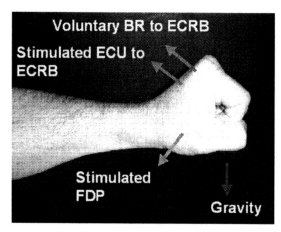

FIGURE 17-24 Balance of torques about the wrist. FES grasp system usually recruits FDS and FDP, FPL, and a wrist flexor. Consequently, strong wrist extension is necessary for proper torque balance about the wrist. Traditional transfer of a voluntary brachioradialis (BR) does not generate sufficient extension moment, especially when the FDP is recruited by a FES system. We recommend transfer of the extensor carpi ulnaris ECU, stimulated by FES, to the ECRB with excellent results.

usefulness of paralyzed muscles and overcome the deficit of denervated functional groups. This transfer allows many patients to be brace free and to use FES-controlled grasp, thus further augmenting the natural tenodesis effects.

FES Neuroprosthesis: Technique

The surgical procedure for implanting the neuroprosthesis requires a general anesthetic without depolarizing blockers, temperature control of the operating room, administration of preoperative antibiotics, and careful anatomic study of the muscles to be stimulated. Surgical incisions are made on the volar and dorsal aspect of the forearm, and the flexor and extensor muscles are identified. Figure 17-25 shows the muscles in the grasp patterns typically used. Intraoperative electrical stimulation and mapping to an optimum force is achieved using a portable stimulator. Epimysial electrodes are sutured in place using a nonabsorbable braided 4/0 suture. The electrode leads are conveyed to an upper arm connector site, and from there, the connections are made to the implantable telemeter stimulator on the pectoralis fascia level. After a brief period of electrode encapsulation and stabilization of other tendon transfers (performed simultaneously), the neuromuscular stimulator is activated, and exercises are resumed. Typically, at about the 12th week, the patient has recovered control of grasp and release in eight muscles of the forearm and wrist. See Figure 17-26 for the implementation timeline.

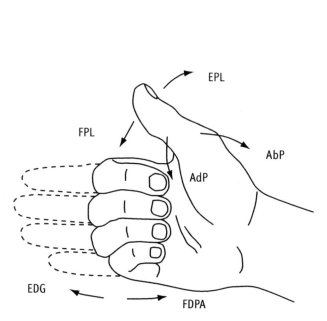

FIGURE 17-25 FES-based reconstruction of upper extremity in C5–C6 tetraplegia is built by targeting muscles for grasp and release function. The current implantable stimulator has eight channels. In 1986, one channel was committed for sensory feedback. A standard epimyseal electrode was implanted in the subcutaneous supraclavicular region with its metal surface facing 'up.' This 'sensory' electrode functions as a primitive proprioceptor to inform the patient of the status of a grip/pinch stimulated pattern. The patient and therapist agree on the signal output of the 'sensory' electrode and how to best accomplish its function as an 'informant.' Overpowering flexion torque about the wrist frequently requires bracing the wrist. Patients themselves have found no significant benefit to the 'sensory' electrode and have asked for brace-free function and more motor channels to be added to the system. A standard FES-based reconstruction provides strong reliable wrist extension with an ECU to ECRB.

Implementation Timeline

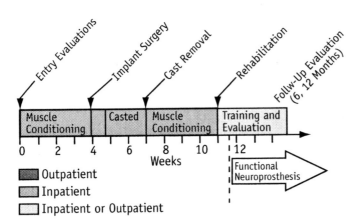

Entry Evaluations

Implant Surgery

Cast Removal

Rehabilitation

Follw-Up Evaluation (6, 12 Months)

| Muscle Conditioning | Casted | Muscle Conditioning | Training and Evaluation |

0   2   4   6   8   10   12
              Weeks

▨ Outpatient
▨ Inpatient
☐ Inpatient or Outpatient

Functional Neuroprosthesis

FIGURE 17-26 Timeline for FES implantation. Following proper patient selection at the entry evaluation, the patient undergoes a period of surface stimulation for muscle conditioning. Stimulation is applied to the radial, ulnar, and median nerves to exercise the fore-arm musculature for 6 hours a day for 4 weeks preceding surgery. The patient undergoes surgical implantation of the FES system and remains hospitalized for 1 day. Cast immobilization continues for 4 weeks to permit electrode encapsulation and tendon transfer healing. When FES exercise resumes, the patient works closely with the therapist to adjust the stimulus parameters for coordinated function. The patient has a functional neuroprosthesis at 12 weeks.

Reachable Workspace

Crago et al. (64) have substantiated the intuitive notion of increased "reachable workspace" in patients with C6 level tetraplegia who had restoration of active elbow extension with a FES neuroprosthesis (Fig. 17-27). Objective evaluation was performed with a book-like object weighing 300 g and instrumented with strain gauges and accelerometers. Grasp force, object orientation, and speed of task performance were recorded. The patient is able to position his arm within the reachable workspace but is only able to perform a specified task within the subset called the *controllable workspace*. Object orientation is also a primary determinant for task performance inside the controllable workspace. The simple task of moving the book was divided into four phases: reach, acquisition, move, and release. The acquisition phase began with detectable grasp force of 0.2 N on the book and ended when the instrumented shelf recorded lift-off. The move phase ended when the book made contact with the new location. Thus, the investigators could evaluate task completion together with quality of the motion. Far and near locations were subdivided into low, medium, and high, as defined. The largest difference was with task completion in the high locations, with greater than 95 percent with the neuroprosthesis "on" and less than 50 percent, and even as low as 2 percent, with the neu-roprosthesis "off." Acquisition time, when averaged over all locations, decreased roughly by half with the neuroprosthesis "on."

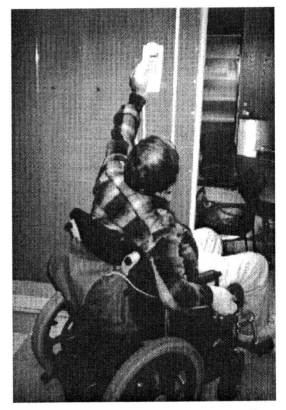

FIGURE 17-27 FES0stimulated triceps allows increased reachable workspace when a tendon transfer is not strong enough, usually in the C5 patient.

FES for Forearm Rotation

Current technology with an implantable Freehand System can be used to achieve rotational forearm control (33). The requirements include strong wrist extension (Groups 2 and 3), supple forearm rotation, and intact lower motor neuron to a forearm pronator. We have found pronator quadratus (PQ) more consistently excitable. Pronator teres (PT) has not been a good candidate for stimulation for patients with strong wrist extensor who could benefit from restoration of pronation because often the patient will have damage to the LMN innervating it. When PQ is stimulated, it can produce pronation moments greater than 30 N/cm. The torque developed by stimulated pronation compares favorably with that developed by mechanical pronation splints (65). Control of forearm rotation is achieved by voluntary supination against the constant activity of the stimulated pronator. This method of control based on co-contraction of agonist and antagonist has also been applied to elbow extension FNS and intrinsic control FNS, as discussed in the corresponding sections.

FES, Grasp, Thumb Control

A voluntary control movement can trigger hand movement. A suitable proportional proximal voluntary control is used to modulate the execution of the programmed functional pattern—for instance, the pinch force developed in a grasp pattern. In C5/C6 patients, contralateral shoulder motion provides such ideal proximal proportional voluntary control. A miniature joystick is adhered to the skin over the shoulder. An extension rod to the clavicle provides the input into the joystick. Two orthogonal motion axes are available: shoulder elevation–depression and shoulder protraction–retraction. One axis of motion is necessary for graded grip control. Most patients find the horizontal axis more natural for the graded or proportional control. A second axis, usually the vertical axis, provides the locking/unlocking com-

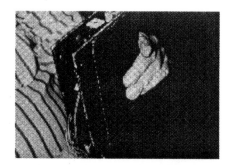
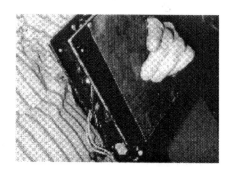
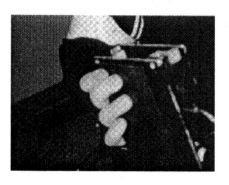
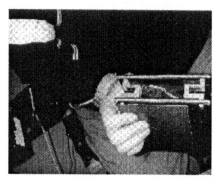

FIGURE 17-28 Intrinsic muscles add better contact of the pulp of the fingers in flat object acquisition. The patient is handling a smart object, which senses the force applied to it. The intrinsic muscles prevent excessive DIP flexion.

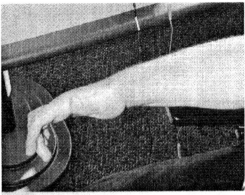
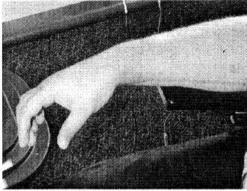
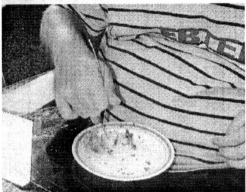
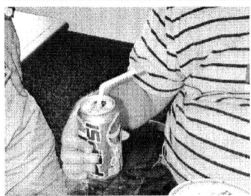

FIGURE 17-29 Lateral pinch and palmar prehension using a neuroprosthesis and reconstruction based on the FES system. Only this technology permits the patient to switch from a lateral key pinch mode to a palmar grasp. Lateral key pinch permits the patient to hold smaller objects with significant strength. Palmar grasp allows the patient to hold larger objects. The therapist, according to patient recruitment pattern, programs the coordinated muscle contraction. Traditional non-FES reconstruction commits the patient to single mode pinch/grasp pattern.

mand and is independent of movement in the graded control axis. A small rapid movement is translated into a lock or unlock command. There are significant limitations to restoring function in tetraplegia that should be recognized before embarking on any reconstructive effort.

Intrinsic Reconstruction

Our center has studied subjects in whom electrodes have been implanted into intrinsic muscles (53). Placement of electrodes into the intermetacarpal spaces was intended to activate more than one interossei en masse. The desired stimulation response was achieved in three or four procedures. Electrodes are placed through dorsal incisions over the second and third interspaces. The dorsal interossei have independent-

ly innervated superficial and deep bellies with insertions into the base of the proximal phalanx and into the lateral band of the dorsal extensor apparatus, respectively. The third dorsal interossei is an exception, with only a deep belly inserting into the lateral band (66). The fascia of the dorsal interossei is incised longitudinally and the fibers spread in an atraumatic fashion with blunt-tipped fine hemostats. The intramuscular electrodes (Memberg design) are placed into the volar (deep muscle belly) of the dorsal interossei and into the volar interossei to maximize the moment generated for MP flexion and IP extension, while minimizing moments in the coronal plane. The highly mobile lumbricals are not stimulated, partly because of the mechanical demands on the electrodes. Stimulation of the second and third interspaces generated function-

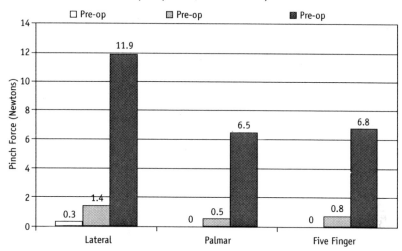

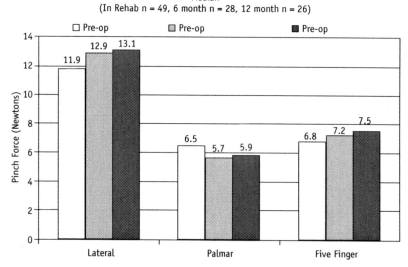

FIGURE 17-30 **A.** Pinch force increases for lateral, palmar, and five-finger grasp patterns. All forces are significantly stronger than required for ADL for tetraplegic patients, compared to pre-operative values. **B.** Pinch force was noted to be stable or increase in the follow-up period for all grasp patterns.

al moments for MP flexion and IP extension (Fig. 17-28).

Outcomes

Typically, pinch force and range of motion increase with time to a plateau over 3 to 6 months (Fig. 17-29). Pinch force is depicted in Figure 17-

30, and stimulated range of motion is shown in Figure 17-31. Antagonist stiffness, contractures of joints, and the number of muscles that can be incorporated into the grasp pattern limit the degree of range of motion. Greater finger extension can be achieved using intrinsic muscles, and greater finger flexion can be achieved by combining flexor digitorum sublimis and profundus.

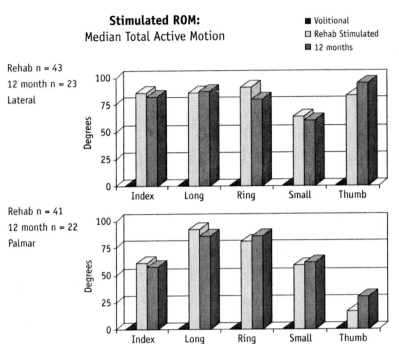

Stimulated ROM:
Median Total Active Motion

■ Volitional
☐ Rehab Stimulated
▨ 12 months

Rehab n = 43
12 month n = 23
Lateral

Rehab n = 41
12 month n = 22
Palmar

FIGURE 17-31 Stimulated range of motion reflects the passive range of the finger joints, often contracted, as well as the limitations of movement without intrinsic extension of the PIP joints. Intrinsic plus posture is common and only improved if tendon transfers or activation of intrinsics are done.

We studied patients in a grasp–release test designed to assess the ability to handle common objects (Fig. 17-32). Patients in our study have shown improvement in independence in activities of daily living, as depicted in Figure 17-33. Improvements in activities in daily living, as depicted in Figure 17-34, show both preference and improvement in skill level across common activities of daily living. We feel that the FES neuroprosthesis is a preferential treatment for patients with high-level spinal cord injury where eight additional muscles primarily (or as tendon transfers) can be provided, exceed improvement in impairments that might be

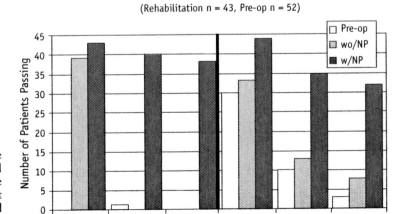

Grasp-Release Test
Pretest
(Rehabilitation n = 43, Pre-op n = 52)

☐ Pre-op
▨ wo/NP
▨ w/NP

FIGURE 17-32 A grasp-release test demonstrates substantial improvement over pre-operative values for heavy or large object manipulation in both lateral and palmar grasp. Small, light objects may be handled without grasp force.

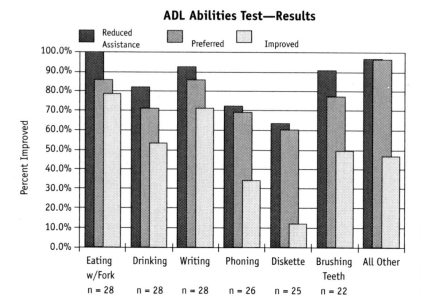

FIGURE 17-33 ADL abilities test shows that patients have reduced assistance, improved performance, and preferred the neuroprosthesis hand grasp to alternative methods for most tasks.

achieved by traditional tendon transfers and tenodesis alone.

Evolving Technologies

The selection criteria remains valid for most of our patients with C5/C6 tetraplegia, yet evolving technologies will soon allow the inclusion of patients with more proximal lesions. Absolute requirements that are not likely to change include proximal control alone. It is hoped that soon we can provide neurotrophic factors necessary to maintain skeletal muscle without atrophy. Another option includes surgical transfer of LMNs to the muscles of interest, either by nerve transfer or direct nerve cell body implantation into the muscle of interest.

Promising research in our center shows that proximal control could be provided by an EEG signal measured from the skin surface. The patient learns to control the cortical beta signal amplitude, conditioned with biofeedback and translated into a reproducible recognizable EEG pattern, and thus a FES command.

The implantable joint angle transducer (IJAT) was developed at our center. The signal from the transducer can function as a sensor. Technology can help us, but we are reminded that the subjec-

tive human element plays a most important role in the perceived well-being of these patients (18).

CONCLUSION

The modern approach to rehabilitation of the upper limbs of spinal cord injured individuals includes surgical and nonsurgical methods. Continually evolving surgical techniques are based on the need for life-long productivity and self-sufficiency. New technologies permit the extension of traditional surgical methods to a larger number of tetraplegics and allow them progress toward a rewarding life.

REFERENCES

1. Ditunno J, Formal C. Chronic spinal cord injury. *N Engl J Med*, 1995; 330(8):550.
2. Medical Research Council. Aids to investigation of peripheral nerve injuries, 2nd ed. *War Memorandum*, Vol. 7. London: His Majesty's Stationery Office, 1943.
3. Blackwood W, Holmes W. Histopathology of nerve injury. In *Peripheral Nerve Injuries*. London: Her Majesty's Stationery Office, 1954. Pp. 88–132.
4. Moberg E. Surgical treatment for absent single-hand grip and elbow extension in quadriplegia: principles and preliminary experience. *J Bone Joint Surg [Am]* 1975; 57(2):196–206.

TABLE 17-3 Procedures Described for Restoration of Elbow Extension.

Procedure	Graft Material	Author
Posterior Deltoid-to-Triceps Transfer	Toe extensors.	Moberg [Moberg, 1975 #187] DeBenedetti [DeBenedetti, 1979 #417] Rackza et. al. [Raczka, 1984 #429] Vastamaki et. al. [Vastamaki, 1995 #454] Lamb [Lamb, 1987 #455] Lamb, Landry [Lamb, 1971 #385] [Lamb, 1972 #192] Lamb, Chan [Lanb, 1983 #67]
	Fascia lata; tubed around deltoid, inserted distally into olecranon drill holes.	Hentz, Keoshian [Hentz, 1979 #180] Hentz, Ladd [Hentz, #433] Now preferred by McDowell and House [McDowell, 1998 #434]
	Fascia lata; two stages—stage one for proximal attachment into deltoid and state two.	Ejeskar [Ejeskar, 1988 #43] [Ejeskar, 1988 #139]
	Tibialis anterior.	Lacey et. al.[Lacey, 1986 #435] Keith, Lacey [Keith, 1991 #458] Gellman [LeClercq, 1991 #452] [Paul, 1994 #17]
	Fascia lata wrapped around a Dacron graft.	Allieu et. al. [Allieu, 1985 #347] [Allieu, 1986 #55] [Allieu, 1993 #309] Rabischong et. al. [Rabischong, 1993 #460]
	Triceps central-third turn- down.	Castro-Sierra, Lopez-Pita [Castro-Sierra, 1983 #413] Mennen, Bonzar[Mennen, 1991 #462]
	Central-third turn-down with olecranon bony block.	Method now preferred by Hentz and Ladd [Hentz, #433]
	Central-third-turn-down reinforced with synthetic graft into olecranon drill holes.	Method preferred by Keith
Biceps-to-Triceps Transfer	Lateral subcutaneous route.	Leo Meyer [Friedenberg, 1954 #445] Friedenberg [Friedenberg, 1954 #445] Zancolli [Zancolli, 1979 #448] Moberg ([Moberg, 1989 #494]) Ejeskar[Ejeskar, 1988 #139]
	Medial subcutaneous route.	Ejeskar [Moberg, 1989 #494] McDowell, House[McDowell, 1998 #434] Kuz, Van Heest, House[Kuz, 1999 #447] Hentz [Hentz, #433]
Brachialis-to-Triceps Transfer		Ober, Barr [Ober, 1938 #486]
Latissimus Dorsi-to-Triceps Transfer		Harmon Crago et. al. [Crago, 1998 #195]
Functional Electrical		Grill, Peckham [Grill, 1998 #206] Miller, Peckham, Keith [Miller, 1989 #450] Carroll et. al. [Carroll, 1997 #456]

5. Zancolli E. Functional Restoration of the Upper Limb in Traumatic Quadriplegia, in *Structural and Dynamic Bases of Hand Surgery*. JB Lippincott, 1979. Pp. 229–262.

6. Zancolli E. Surgery for the quadriplegic hand with active, strong wrist extension preserved: a study of 97 cases. *Clin Orthop* 1975; (112):101–113.

7. Freehafer A, Vonhaam V. Tendon transfer to improve grasp after injuries of the cervical spinal cord. *J Bone Joint Surg* 1974; 56A: 951–959.

8. Freehafer A. Tendon transfers in patients with cervical spinal cord injury. *J Hand Surg [Am]* 1991; 16(5):804–809.

9. Lamb DW, Landry RM. The hand in quadriplegia. *Paraplegia* 1972; 9(4):204–212.

10. Moberg E. Two-point discrimination test: a valuable part of hand surgical rehabilitation, e.g. in tetraplegia. *Scand J Rehabil Med* 1990; 22(3): 127–134.

11. Thomas J. Definition of the model system of spinal cord injury care. In *Proceedings of the National Consensus Conference on Catastrophic Illness and Injury*, Atlanta, Georgia, 1990.

12. Maynard F, Weingarden S. Secondary complications of spinal cord injury. In *Proceedings of the National Consensus Conference on Catastrophic Illness and Injury*, Atlanta, Georgia, 1990.

13. DeVivo M, Kartus P, Stover SEA. Seven-year survival following spinal cord injury. *Arch Neurol* 1967; 44:872–875.

14. DeVivo M. Life expectancy and causes of death for persons with spinal cord injuries. In *Proceedings of the National Consensus Conference on Catastrophic Illness and Injury*, Atlanta, Georgia, 1990.

15. Gibson C. Criteria for evaluating performance of the system. In *Proceedings of the National Consensus Conference on Catastrophic Illness and Injury*, Atlanta, Georgia, 1990.

16. DeVivo M. The cost of spinal cord injury: a growing national dilemma. In *Proceedings of the National Consensus Conference on Catastrophic Illness and Injury*, Atlanta, Georgia, 1990.

17. Hentz V, Ladd A. Functional restoration of the upper extremity in tetraplegia. In Peimer C, ed. *Surgery of the Hand and Upper Extremity*. Pp. 1499–1516.

18. Fuhrer M., et al. Relationship of life satisfaction to impairment, disability and handicap among persons with spinal cord injury living in the community. *Arch Phys Med Rehabil* 1992; 73:552–557.

19. Carroll SG, Bird SF, Brown DJ. Electrical stimulation of the lumbrical muscles in an incomplete quadriplegic patient: case report. *Paraplegia* 1992; 30(3):223–226.

20. Carroll S, et al. Electrical activation of triceps brachii using the Freehand system: a case report. In *Proceedings of the 2nd Annual IFESS Conference*, Vancouver, Canada: IFESS, 1997.

21. Welch R, et al. Functional independence in quadriplegia: critical levels. *Arch Phys Med Rehab* 1986; 67:235–240.

22. Brys D, Waters RL. Effect of triceps function on the brachioradialis transfer in quadriplegia. *J Hand Surg [Am]* 1987; 12(2):237–239.

23. Castro-Sierra A, Lopez-Pita A. A new surgical technique to correct triceps paralysis. *Hand* 1983; 15(1):42–46.

24. Hentz VR, Keoshian LA. Changing perspectives in surgical hand rehabilitation in quadriplegic patients. *Plast Reconstr Surg* 1979; 64(4):509–515.

25. McDowell C, House J. Tetraplegia. In Green D, Hochkiss R, WC P, eds., *Green's Operative Hand Surgery*. Churchill Livingstone, 1988. Pp. 1588–1606.

26. Grover J, Gellman H, Waters R. The effect of a flexion contracture of the elbow on the ability to transfer in patients who have quadriplegia at the sixth cervical level. *J Bone Joint Surg* 1996; 78(A):1397–1400.

27. Zancolli E. Tetraplegia. In McFarlane R. ed., *Unsatisfactory Results in Hand Surgery the Hand and Upper Limb*. New York: Churchill Livingstone, 1987. Pp. 274–280.

28. Friedenberg Z. Transposition of the biceps brachii for triceps weakness. *J Bone Joint Surg* 1954; 36(A): 656–658.

29. McDowell C, Mobert E, House J. The second international conference on surgical rehabilitation of the upper limb in tetraplegia (quadriplegia). *J Hand Surg* 1986; 11(A): 604–608.

30. Ejeskar A. Upper limb surgical rehabilitation in high-level tetraplegia. *Hand Clin* 1988; 4(4): 585–599.

31. Kuz J, Van Heest A, House J. Biceps-to-triceps transfer in tetraplegic patients: report of the medial routing technique and follow-up of three cases. *J Hand Surg* 1999; 24(A):161–172.

32. Freehafer A. Flexion and supination deformities of the elbow in tetraplegics. *Paraplegia* 1977; 15:221–225.

33. Lemay M, Crago P, MW K. Restoration of pronosupination control by FNS in tetraplegia: experimental and biomechanical evaluation of feasibility. Submitted to *J Biomechanics*.

34. Schottstaedt E, Larsen L, Bost F. The surgical reconstruction of the upper extremity paralyzed by poliomyelitis. *J Bone Joint Surg* 1958; 40A: 633–643.

35. Zancolli E. Paralytic supination contracture of the forearm. *J Bone Joint Surg* 1967; 49(A): 1275–1284.

36. Gellman H, et al. Rerouting of the biceps brachii for paralytic supination contracture of the forearm in tetraplegia due to trauma. *J Bone Joint Surg [Am]* 1994; 76(3): 398–402.

37. Freehafer A, Mast W. Transfer of the brachioradialis to improve wrist extension in high spinal cord injury. *J Bone Joint Surg* 1967; 44(A):648–652.

38. Lipscomb P, Elkins EC, Henderson ED. Tendon transfers to restore function of hands in tetraplegia, especially after fracture-dislocation of the sixth cervical vertebra on the seventh. *J Bone Joint Surg* 1958; 40(A): 1071–1080.

39. Waters R, et al. Brachioradialis to flexor pollicis longus tendon transfer for active lateral pinch in the tetraplegic. *J Hand Surg [Am]* 1985; 10(3):385–391.

40. House JH, Gwathmey FW, Lundsgaard DK. Restoration of strong grasp and lateral pinch in tetraplegia due to cervical spinal cord injury. *J Hand Surg [Am]* 1976; 1(2):152–159.

41. Zancolli E. *Structural and Dynamic Basis of Hand Surgery*, 2nd ed. Philadelphia: JB Lippincott, 1979.

42. Freehafer AA, et al. The brachioradialis: anatomy, properties, and value for tendon transfer in the tetraplegic. *J Hand Surg [Am]* 1988; 13(1): 99–104.

43. Brand P. Clinical Mechanics of the Hand. Mosby, 1985.

44. Schroer W, et al. Carpal instability in the weight-bearing upper extremity. *J Bone Joint Surg Am* 1996; 78(12):1838–1843.

45. Hentz V, et al. Rehabilitation and surgical reconstruction of the upper limb in tetraplegia: an update. *J Hand Surg* 1992; 17(A):964–967.

46. LeClercq C, McDowell C. Fourth International Conference on Surgical Rehabilitation of the Upper Limb in *Tetraplegia*. Ann Chir Main Membre Superievr 1991; 10:258–260.

47. House JH, Comadoll J, Dahl AL. One-stage key pinch and release with thumb carpalmetacarpal fusion in tetraplegia. *J Hand Surg [Am]* 1992; 17(3):530–538.

48. Paul SD, et al. Single-stage reconstruction of key pinch and extension of the elbow in tetraplegic patients [see comments]. *J Bone Joint Surg [Am]* 1994; 76(10):1451–1456.

49. Mohammed K, Rothwell AG, Sinclair SW, Willems SM, Bean AR. Upper limb surgery for tetraplegia. *J Bone Joint Surg* 1992; 74(B):873–879.

50. Kozin S, et al. The contribution of the intrinsic muscles to grip and pinch strength. *J Hand Surg* 1999; 24(A):64–72.

51. Smith R. *Tendon transfers of the hand and forearm*. Boston: Little, Brown, 1987. Pp. 103–133.

52. Brand P, Beach R, Thompson D. Relative tension and potential excursion of the muscles in the forearm and the hand. *J Hand Surg* 1981; 6(A): 209–219.

53. Lauer R, et al. The function of finger intrinsic muscles in the response to electrical stimulation. *IEEE Trans Rehab Eng* 1999; 7(1):19–26.

54. House J, et al. Intrinsic balancing in reconstruction of the tetraplegic hand. In Vaastamaki M. ed., *Current Trends in Hand Surgery*. Elsevier Siene, 1995. Pp. 373–378.

55. McCarthy CK, et al. Intrinsic balancing in reconstruction of the tetraplegic hand. *J Hand Surg [Am]* 1997; 22(4):596–604.

56. Keith MW, et al. Functional neuromuscular stimulation neuroprostheses for the tetraplegic hand. *Clin Orthop* 1988; 233:25–33.

57. Peckham PH, Creasey GH. Neural prostheses: clinical applications of functional electrical stimulation in spinal cord injury. *Paraplegia* 1992; 30(2):96–101.

58. Crago PE, Peckham PH, Thrope GB. Modulation of muscle force by recruitment during intramuscular stimulation. *IEEE Trans Biomed Eng* 1980; 27(12):679–684.

59. Kilgore KL, et al. An implanted upper-extremity neuroprosthesis: follow-up of five patients. *J Bone Joint Surg Am* 1997; 79(4):533–541.

60. Keith MW, et al. Tendon transfers and functional electrical stimulation for restoration of hand function in spinal cord injury. *J Hand Surg [Am]* 1996; 21(1):89–99.

61. Keith MW, et al. Implantable functional neuromuscular stimulation in the tetraplegic hand. *J Hand Surg [Am]* 1989; 14(3):524–530.

62. Peckham PH, Mortimer JT, Marsolais EB. Upper and lower motor neuron lesions in the upper extremity muscles of tetraplegics. *Paraplegia* 1976; 14(2):115–121.

63. Peckham P, Keith M, Freehafer A. Restoration of functional control by electrical stimulation in the upper extremity of the quadriplegic patient. *J Bone Joint Surg* 1988; 70(A):144–148.

64. Crago PE, et al. An elbow extension neuroprosthesis for individuals with tetraplegia. *IEEE Trans Rehabil Eng* 1998; 6(1):1–6.

65. Hokken W, et al. A dynamic pronation orthosis for the C6 tetraplegic arm. *Arch Phys Med Rehabil* 1993; 74:104–105.

66. Smith R. Intrinsic muscles of the finger: function, dysfunction and surgical reconstruction. In *AAOS Instructional Course Lectures*. St. Louis: CV Mosby, 1975. Pp. 200–220.

18 Pressure Ulcers: Overview

BOK Y. LEE, MD
MARCELO C. DASILVA, MD
LEE E. OSTRANDER, PhD

PRESSURE ULCERS ARE A SERIOUS PROBLEM in patients with spinal cord injury (SCI). Pressure ulcers have a tremendous impact on the well-being of these patients and on their morbidity and mortality as well. They increase the overall cost of patient care by prolonging hospital stays and escalating nursing costs and time. Additional losses may incur from consequent liquidation. Miller and Delozier reviewed the costs of pressure ulcers as a primary and a secondary diagnosis in patients in which the primary diagnosis was fractured hip (1). The mean hospital charges for the former was $21,675, and $10,986 in additional hospital charges for the latter. They conservatively estimated that in 1992, the costs of pressure ulcer care in hospitals, nursing homes, and home-care settings were $1.335 billion (1). Although the estimated costs of healing a single pressure ulcer range from $2,000 to $40,000, up to 95 percent of pressure ulcers are preventable (2). Judicious and prudent resource allocation is best directed toward this goal.

The agency for Health Care Policy and Research (AHCPR) (3) has identified pressure ulcers as one of the seven conditions affecting a large number of patients involving relatively expensive treatment and urgently needing strategies for prevention and cost containment. This reflects concerns about the aging of the population and the use of life support technologies to prolong the life of these and SCI patients.

INCIDENCE

Improvements in the medical care and antibiotic therapy available to SCI patients have effectively decreased their mortality. Paradoxically, their increase in survival has put them at high risk for the development of pressure sores. Indeed, the most common setting for pressure ulcer formation is in SCI patients. El-Toraei and Chung (4) state that 50 percent of spinal cord admissions were for management and treatment of pressure ulcers. Pressure ulcers occur in 25 to 85 percent of SCI patients. They have a mortality rate of 7 to 8 percent. Surveys conducted by Manley (5) and Peterson and Bitman (6) have shown that 3 to 4.5 percent of SCI patients develop pressure ulcers during hospitalization. Furthermore, in a retrospective study of pressure ulcers in SCI patients, 60% of the patients with complete cervical cord injury developed pressure ulcers; the majority had multiple ulcers, and 50 percent of all paraplegics developed at least one pressure ulcer (7).

PATHOPHYISOLOGY

Pressure ulcers develop as a result of an active metabolic and inflammatory process that begins when sufficient pressure is applied to the skin to overcome the normal capillary pressure—32 mmHg at the arterial end (8). This results in tissue anoxia and cellular death (9–11). The removal of the pressure can reverse the process. Hinsdale (12) reported that a constant pressure of 70 mmHg for 2 hours caused irreversible damage to the tissues but that pressure up to 240 mmHg could be sustained if the pressure was relieved intermittently. Kosiak (10,11) also showed that application of 70 mmHg pressure for 2 hours produced pressure sores, but if the pressure was relieved every 5 minutes, tissue effects were minimal. The discomfort associated with prolonged application of pressure usually causes the person to move to relieve the pressure. Unfortunately, the SCI patient is unaware of the associated discomfort from prolonged pressure application and is unable to move to relieve the pressure.

Although the first clinical sign of impending necrosis is inflammation, it is very likely that by that time necrosis of the subcutaneous tissue and fat and the underlying muscle has already begun. The affected area is usually larger in deep tissue than is apparent from the areas of skin loss (13). Muscle is much more susceptible than skin to pressure injury (14). Indeed, in normal human weight-bearing positions over bony prominence, muscle is seldom interposed between bone and skin (15). The distribution of pressure points in humans lying prone and supine and in the seated position has been documented (Figs. 18-1 and 18-2) (16). The areas of highest pressure in the

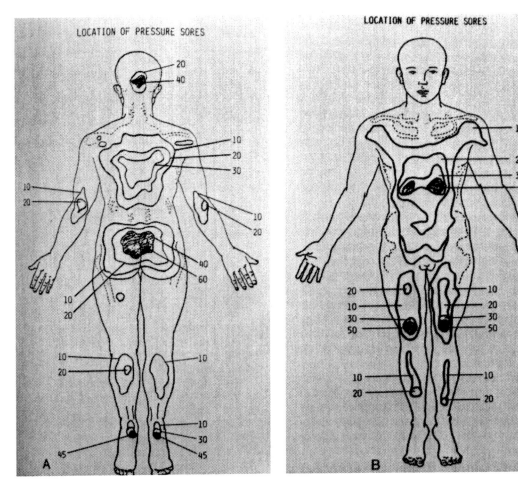

FIGURE 18-1 **A.** The regions of highest pressure for the supine patient. **B.** The regions of highest pressure for the prone patient.

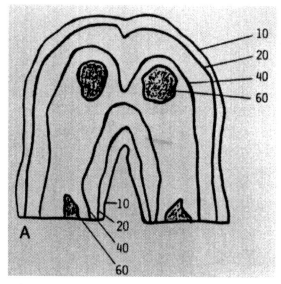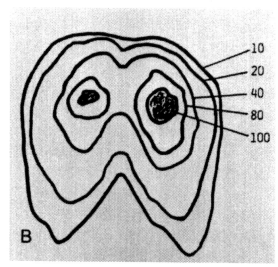

FIGURE 18-2 Examples of pressure distribution in the seated position.

supine position include the sacrum, buttocks, heel, and occiput (40 to 60 mmHg of pressure). The knees and chest receive the most pressure in a prone position (approximately 50 mmHg). In the seated position, a hard surface provides for less distribution of pressure and thus produces higher pressures. Seated, pressures of 40 to 60 mmHg are seen at the ischial tuberosities and the thighs when the feet are dangling free; pressures at the ischial tuberosities rise to about 100 mmHg when the feet are supported.

Normal capillary hydrostatic pressures vary from 15 to 30 mmHg and, in areas over bony prominence, from 40 to 75 mmHg (8). The pressure is transmitted from the skin to the underlying bone and compresses all the underlying tissue; the greatest pressure is over the bone and gradually decreases toward the surface. Thus, because of the greater pressure over the bony prominence and the greater susceptibility of muscle to pressure injury, the greatest extent of necrosis is at the bony interface and not at the surface. It has been shown that relieving pressure for as little as 5 minutes allows tissues to withstand greater pressures (10,11). Husain (9) has confirmed the relationship between intensity of pressure and duration of application: low pressures for long periods produce more damage

than high pressures for short periods.

Shear pressure is also an important contributing factor (16–18). Hinsdale (12) concluded that friction was additive to pressure, producing ulceration of the skin. He showed that shear did not stretch and compress muscle-perforating vessels to lead to ischemia but that it contributed to skin ulceration by a direct application of mechanical forces to the epidermis (12). Shear pressure is manifested whenever the patient is pulled up in the bed or when the head of the bed is elevated.

Other factors contributing to the formation of pressure ulcers include heat in the form of stress and fever, thus increasing the already compromised demand of oxygen caused by tissue compression; and moisture in the form of sweat, urine, and feces that reduces the skin's resistance and predisposes it to maceration. A negative nitrogen balance, along with hypoproteinemia, anemia, and weight loss, predispose the patient to infection in the pressure ulcer (19).

INCIDENCE AND SITES OF FORMATION OF PRESSURE ULCERS

The incidence of pressure ulcer formation increases as the life span of the spinal cord injured patient is prolonged with improved medical care and antibiotics. This longer life span increases the patient's risk time for pressure ulcer development. Prior to 1940, spinal cord injury was associated with a 61 percent mortality rate within the first two months of injury and 81 percent within two years of injury; after World War II, the mortality rate decreased to 3.8 percent and 7.8 percent, respectively (20).

Most pressure ulcers occur in the lower part of the body (96 percent), followed by the hip and buttocks (67 percent) and the lower limbs (29 percent) (6); however, any part of the body is at risk (Fig. 18-3). Some areas are easier to protect. For example, heel pads can prevent ulceration of the foot, and a patient in the prone position also limits the areas at risk to those that are easy to care for: anterosuperior iliac spine, knees, and elbows (21). In SCI patients, the incidence of

pressures at the ischial tuberosity has been shown to range from 5 to 8 percent annually (22), with 25 to 85 percent having an ulcer at some time (4). An increase in the incidence of ischial ulceration is evidence of the patient being moved in a wheelchair (29). Between 3 and 4.5 percent of SCI patients develop sores while hospitalized (5,6), and 7 to 8 percent of deaths in paraplegics are due to pressure sores (12).

PREVENTION

The key to prevention of pressure ulcers is patient and physician awareness of developing signs and symptoms. A clinically useful outline for assessing the stages of development and appropriate care is shown in Table 18-1 (23). Pressure ulcers can also be graded using the system from the National Spinal Cord Injury Data Collection Center (Table 18-2) (24).

Basic skin care has been reviewed by Ungar (25). It includes elimination of particulate matter from the bed, reduction of excess moisture, alternation of position, and limitation of skin

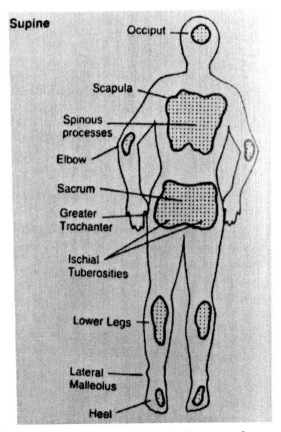

FIGURE 18-3 Areas at risk for development of pressure sores.

TABLE 18-1 Assessment of Stage of Pressure Sore Development

Hyperemia	Stage 1	Seen within 30 minutes of application of pressure as a redness of the skin that disappears within one hour after removal of pressure
Ischemia	Stage II	Observed with continuous pressure of 2 to 6 hours duration; redness of ischemia requires 36 or more hours to disappear after removal of pressure
Necrosis	Stage III	Characterized clinically by a blueness of the skin or a hard lump after more than 6 hours of pressure; does not disappear after pressure removal
Ulceration	Stage IV	Observed within 2 weeks as ulceration and infection; may progress to involve bony prominences

TABLE 18-2 Grading of Pressure Sore Development from the National Spinal Cord Injury Data Collection Center

Grade I	Pressure sore limited to superficial epidermal and dermal layers
Grade II	Pressure sore extends into adipose tissue
Grade III	Pressure sore involves all superficial structures as well as underlying muscle
Grade IV	Pressure sore has destroyed all soft tissues down to and including bone and/or joint structure

soilage through the combination of good nursing care and an indwelling catheter or even urinary or fecal diversion procedures, if necessary (22).

Proper position of the patient is essential for uniform pressure distribution and relief of spasticity (26). Additionally, numerous devices for weight distribution have been developed, including pads for chairs and beds and specifically designed beds. Houle (27) has found, however, that such padding for seats and beds does not reduce ischial pressure below capillary pressure and is therefore not a substitute for alternating pressure. A number of beds have been developed that reduce pressure to 15 to 30 mmHg. They include air-fluidized beds, mud beds, and low-air loss beds (Figs. 18-4 and 18-5).

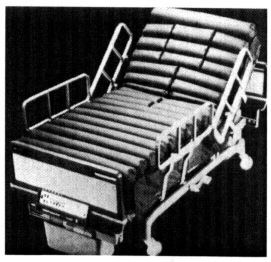

FIGURE 18-5 A low-air loss bed.

If used properly, these beds can maintain pressure below capillary arterial pressure (22). Other methods include the Stryker frame, circle electric bed, ripple mattresses, and rocking beds, all based on Kosiak's theory that tissue tolerates higher pressure if there are intermittent periods of relief (10,11).

NONSURGICAL TREATMENT

Local therapy of the pressure sore is the same, whether for definitive treatment or to prepare for surgery. Local treatment involves 1) debridement of necrotic tissues; 2) wound cleansing; 3) application of dressings; 4) control of sepsis; and 5) possibly, adjunct therapy. The basic principle is to monitor the healing of the ulcer at least once a week. If the current plan of care is not promoting improvement, it should be reassessed and implemented.

Debridement

Experienced health care personnel should be involved with the removal of necrotic or moist tissues. This is necessary for wound healing, because these devitalized tissues are a perfect medium for bacterial and fungal growth. They are avascular, thus inaccessible for antimicrobial action. They initiate an initially acute inflammatory response—

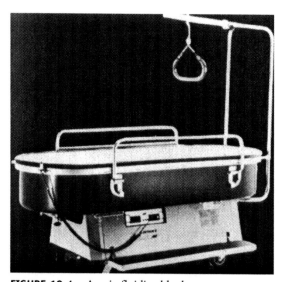

FIGURE 18-4 An air-fluidized bed.

developing into chronic—which usually further delays wound healing. Mechanical, sharp, enzymatic, and/or autolytic debridement techniques may be used. Mechanical debridement includes wet-to-dry dressings, hydrotherapy, wound irrigation, and dextranomers. Enzymatic debridement is usually reserved for patients in nursing homes or those who cannot tolerate surgery. The area must be infection-free. Applying topical enzymatic agents, such as collagenase, a biologic licensed by the Food and Drug Administration (FDA) promotes debridement (28).

The enzyme, collagenase, plays an important role in all stages of cutaneous repair, guiding the continuous breakdown and reshaping of collagen to restructure and promote healing. Collagenase is selective in removing nonviable tissue, leaving intact the viable granulation tissue. Collagenase may be used alone or in conjunction with a topical microbial agent, such as Polysporin powder. Research findings indicate that collagenase promotes debridement and growth of granulation tissue within 3 to 30 days (29–32).

Wound Cleansing

Removing necrotic, devitalized tissue depends on the nature of the solution used and the amount of pressure applied to the area. Normal saline is the preferred cleansing solution because it is physiologic and adequately cleanses most wounds. Antiseptic agents are reactive chemicals that are cytotoxic to wound tissue, delay wound healing, and should not be used as wound cleansers. Foresman et al. (33) studied the required amounts of dilution needed for various skin and wound-cleanser agents to maintain white cell viability and phagocytic function (Table 18-3). They developed a skin and wound toxicity index, which indicates the dilution required by a specific chemical agent to maintain white cell viability and phagocytic efficiency. Pressurized irrigation of 8 to 15 psi effectively cleanses the wound and reduces the risk of trauma and wound infection. Irrigation pressure less than 4 psi will not cleanse the wound. In con-

TABLE 18-3 Toxicity Index for Wound and Skin Cleansers

Test Agent	Toxicity Index
Shur Clens®	1:10
Biolex™	1:100
Saf Clens™	1:100
Cara Klenz™	1:100
Ultra Klenz™	1:1,000
Clinical Care™	1:1,000
Uni Wash®™	1:1,000
Ivory Soap® (0.5%)™	1:1,000
Constant Clens™	1:10,000
Dermal Wound Cleanser™	1:10,000
Puri-Cleans™	1:10,000
Hibiclens™	1:10,000
Betadine® Surgical Scrub	1:10,000
Techni-Care™ Scrub	1:100,000
Bard™ Skin Cleanser™	1:100,000
Hollister™	1:100,000

Adapted from *Clinical Practice Guidelines*, No. 15. Treatment of Pressure Ulcers. U.S. Department of Health and Human Services. Public Health Service Agency for Health Care Policy and Research. Rockville, Maryland: AHCPR Publication No. 95-0652, December 1994. Pp. 51.

trast, an irrigation delivery system capable of delivering more than 15 psi to the wound may cause trauma and drive bacteria into the tissue (34). In some instances when the ulcer is too large or difficult to access at bedside, or the area to be cleansed has thick exudate, slough, or necrotic tissue, whirlpool therapy should be considered.

Application of Dressings

A wound dressing should be biocompatible, keep the wound surface moist, and protect the wound while keeping the surrounding skin (periulcer) intact. Studies have shown that wet-to-dry dressings should be used only for wound debridement. Several investigators found that the rate of healing is better with moist wound-healing dressings than with wet-to-dry ones (35–37). Furthermore, in five controlled trials, there were no significant differences between moist saline gauze and other types of moist wound dressing in pressure ulcer healing (38–42).

Adjunct Therapy

These therapies include electrotherapy; hyperbaric oxygen; infrared, ultraviolet, and low-energy laser irradiation; ultrasonography; miscellaneous topical agents; and systemic drugs other than antibiotics. So far, the only therapy with supporting evidence to warrant recommendation is electrical stimulation (28). Its use is recommended for Stage III and IV pressure ulcers that fail to respond to conventional therapy (28,43–47). Topical agents, such as sugar, honey, zinc, magnesium, gold, aluminum, phenytoin, aloe vera gel, yeast extract, and insulin have been used, but only zinc acetate and aluminum hydroxide ointment (48) and phenytoin (49) were evaluated in a controlled and blinded fashion. Recently, pharmacologically active therapies such as basic fibroblast growth factor (bFGF) (50) and recombinant platelet-derived growth factor-BB (rPDGF-BB—Becaplermin) (51,52) have been studied in clinical trials for use as wound healing enhancers. Only Becaplermin has shown enough significant effectiveness to be approved by the FDA for use in chronic wounds. Its current approval is for diabetic lower extremity ulcers, with ongoing studies of its effectiveness in pressure ulcers. Becaplermin is produced by recombinant DNA technology. Insertion of the gene for the B chain of PDGF into the yeast *Saccharomyces cerevisiae* produces a biological molecule similar to that of naturally occurring PDGF (53,54). In a prospective, multicenter, double-blind, parallel group, placebo-controlled trial of 124 patients with chronic, full-thickness pressure ulcers, 100 µg/g of Becaplermin gel once a day significantly increased the incidence of complete healing and >90 percent healing when compared to placebo (p <0.05) (54). Nonetheless, when 100 µg/g of Becaplermin gel twice a day was compared with placebo, it did not show a significant statistic difference. Furthermore, there was neither clinical benefit nor significant statistical difference between treatments with Becaplermin gel at 300 µg/g or 100 µg/g once a day. The authors concluded that Becaplermin gel at 100 µg/g once a day increased the incidence of complete healing and >90 percent healing in patients with stage III and IV pressure ulcers (54).

Recent research in utilizing the body's own energy is being carried out. This treatment uses a machine producing currents in the nanoampere range. It is thought that these currents, which produce specific waveforms, are able to stimulate mitochondrial DNA to produce the necessary energy to regenerate tissue and thus lead to rapid healing of these more intractable ulcers. A positive energy balance seems to be achieved in the body as a whole, and many patients treated by this method develop a feeling of well-being. Preliminary studies show a rapid subsiding of edema, clearing of infection, ingrowth of epithelium, and healing of the wound. Concomitant pain seems to subside simultaneously. Results are obtained rapidly, and improvements are often noted within hours of the commencement of treatment. Early results in the research of this noninvasive therapy appear extremely promising.

Control of Sepsis

Wound healing is generally impaired when bacteria levels are $>10^5$ organisms per gram of tissue. By definition, all Stage II, III, and IV pressure ulcers are colonized with bacteria and

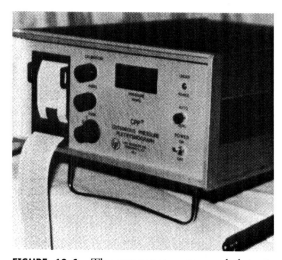

FIGURE 18-6 The cutaneous pressure plethysmograph.

should, therefore, be treated with effective wound cleansing and debridement. Swab cultures are usually inadequate, because they only reveal the superficial microflora. Instead, the Center for Disease Control (CDC) recommends either needle aspiration of the fluid or tissue ulcer biopsy when a culture is required. Whenever a clean ulcer fails to heal or continues to produce exudate for 2 to 4 weeks, one should consider a 2-week trial of topical antibiotics (silver sulfadiazine or triple antibiotic ointment). Topical antiseptics should not be used. Systemic antibiotics should be given to patients with bacteremia, sepsis, advancing cellulitis, or osteomyelitis. If purulent or foul odor develops, sharp debridement and/or surgery should be performed.

SURGICAL MANAGEMENT

The management of pressure ulcers is difficult. The traditional approaches of conventional rotation flap and primary closure yield less than optimal results. In a series of 374 surgically managed pressure ulcers, multiple procedures were required to achieve successful healing in 148 ulcers (55). Nevertheless, a surgical approach should be considered for those individuals with clean Stage II or IV pressure ulcers that do not respond to optimal care (28). Candidates should be medically stable, adequately nourished (albumin $\geqslant 3.5$ mg/dl, TLC $\geqslant 1,800$ mm^3, body weight >80 percent of ideal), and able to tolerate operative blood loss and postoperative immobility. Factors that have a negative effect on wound healing are smoking, spasticity, levels of bacterial colonization ($\geqslant 10^5$), incontinence, and urinary tract infection. A number of techniques are available to the surgeon managing a patient with pressure ulcers: primary closure, skin grafting and flaps, and free flaps.

Much morbidity can be avoided through the use of a technique for assessing the healing potential of pressure ulcers. The cutaneous pressure plethysmograph (Fig. 18-6) is a vascular diagnostic instrument that senses the flow of blood in the skin to various skin-bearing pres-

sures using a hand-held probe. With the application of incremental pressures, the blood flow waveform is gradually reduced and obliterated at a critical pressure. The technician gradually reduces the pressure until the waveform reappears (Fig. 18-7). The probe can be applied to any skin surface area (Fig. 18-8) and provide a systematic quantitative analysis of cutaneous pressure (Fig. 18-9).

Surgical techniques may be inappropriate for some patients. For example, split-thickness skin grafts are not for definitive treatment, but are of value in patients unable to undergo immediate flap repair. Excision and closure are only functional in temporarily closing the skin defect because increased tension at the suture line often leads to a recurrence of the lesion. These flaps require a lengthy procedure with numerous stages. Perhaps the best approach is the use of a myocutaneous flap.

The myocutaneous rotation flap is a single unit of skin and underlying muscle that is transferred to cover a defect. The use of a myocutaneous rotation flap is advantageous because it brings a new vascular supply to an avascular area while providing bulk for filling defects or covering bone grafts. It also supplies a mass of tissue to cushion a pressure-bearing area.

We have recently reviewed our experience with a total of 142 surgical repairs of pressure ulcers in 70 patients (56). The ischium was most frequently involved (47 percent), followed by the sacrum (27 percent), trochanter (23 percent), and calcaneous, hips, ribs, thorax, and thigh (each 1 percent). Short-term success (i.e., no need for additional surgery during the first subsequent month) was similar for all procedures; long-term success was greatest for myocutaneous rotation flap.

CONCLUSION

Pressure ulcers remain a difficult problem. Pressure shear forces, friction, and moisture contribute to the formation of a pressure ulcer. Operative management is difficult because no single procedure is appropriate for all patients.

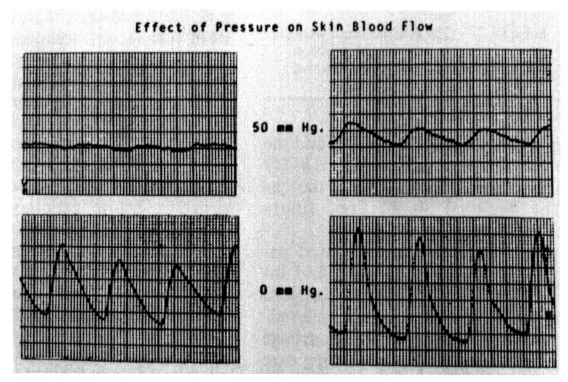

FIGURE 18-7 Effect of pressure on skin blood flow.

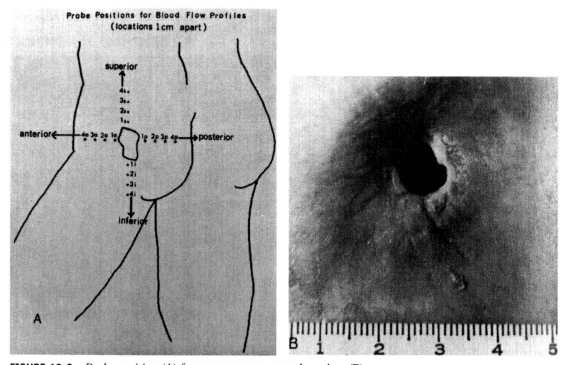

FIGURE 18-8 Probe position (**A**) for measurement around an ulcer (**B**).

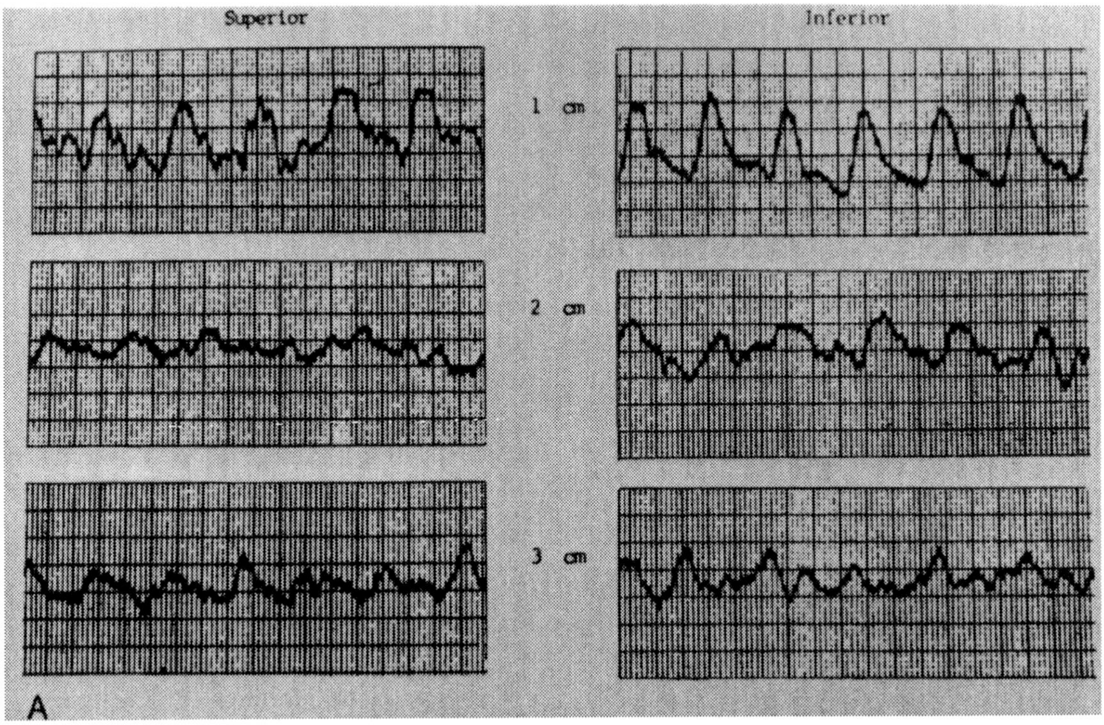

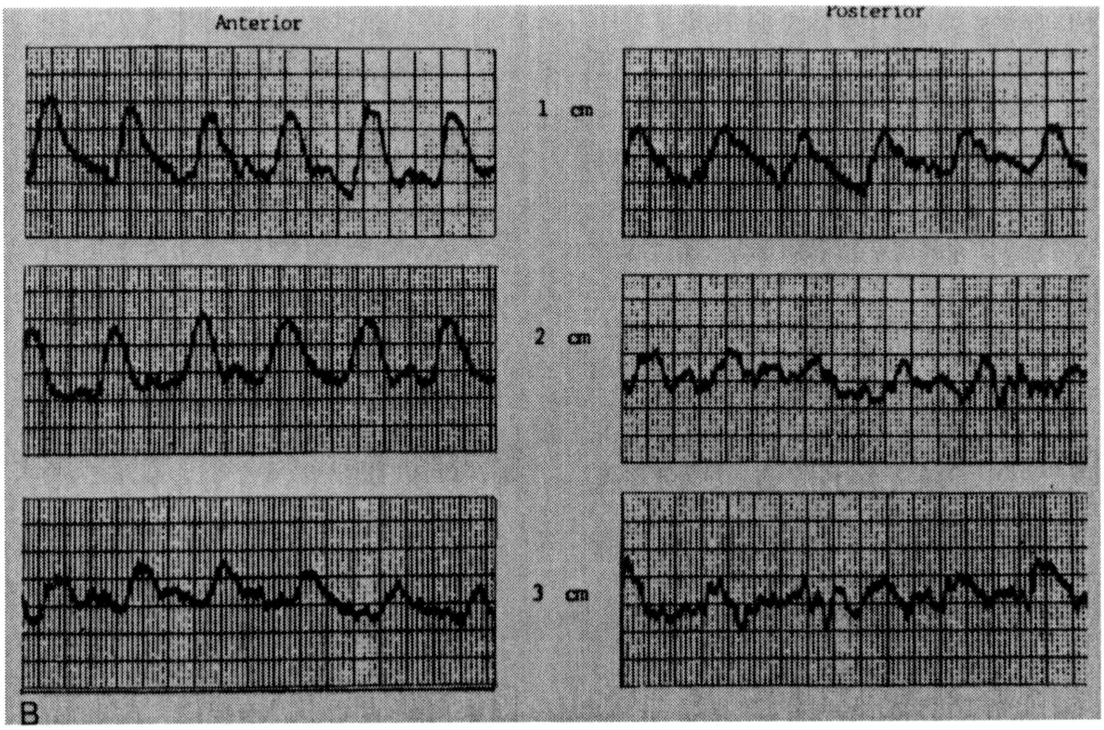

FIGURE 18-9 **A** and **B**. Systematic quantitative analysis at selected measurement sites.

The use of the cutaneous pressure photoplethysmograph is of value in noninvasive assessment of the healing potential of a pressure ulcer and in assisting the surgeon in a proper patient selection. The myocutaneous rotation flap is advantageous in providing a healthy vascular supply and cushioning over the pressure-bearing area.

REFERENCES

1. Miller H, Delozier J. Cost implications of the pressure ulcer treatment guideline. Columbia, Maryland: Center for Health Policy Studies, 1994. Contract No. 282-91-0070. Sponsored by the Agency for Health Care Policy and Research.
2. Fowler E. Chronic wounds: an overview. In D. Krasner, ed., *Chronic Wound Care*. King of Prussia, Pennsylvania: Health Management Publications, 1990. Pp. 212–218.
3. Pressure Ulcers in Adults: Prediction and Prevention. In *Clinical Practice Guideline Number 3*, U.S. Department of Health and Human Services, Public Health Service, Agency for Health Care Policy and Research, Publication No. 92-0047, May 1992; 3:1–63.
4. El-Toraei I, Chung B. The management of pressure sores. *J Dermatol Surg Oncol* 1977; 3:507.
5. Manley MT. Incidence, contributory factors and costs of pressure sores. *S Afr Med J* 1978; 53:217.
6. Peterson NC, Bittman S. The epidemiology of pressure sores. *Scand J Plast Reconstr Surg* 1971; 5:62.
7. Nola GT, Vistnes LM. Differential response of skin and muscle in the experimental production of pressures sores. *Plast Reconstr Surg* 1980; 66:728.
8. Landis E. Studies of capillary blood pressure in human skin. *Heart* 1930; 15:209.
9. Husain T. An experimental study of some pressure effects on tissues with reference to the bedsore problem. *J Pathol Bacteriol* 1953; 66:347.
10. Kosiak M. Etiology and pathology of decubitus ulcers. *Arch Phys Med* 1959; 40:62.
11. Kosiak M. Etiology of decubitus ulcers. *Arch Phys Med* 1961; 42:19.
12. Hinsdale SM. Decubitus ulcers: role of pressure and friction in causation. *Arch Phys Med Rehabil* 1974; 55:147.
13. Shea JD. Pressure sores. *Clin Orthop* 1975; 112:89.
14. Keane FX. The function of the rump in relation to sitting and the Keane reciprocating wheelchair seat. *Paraplegia* 1978–1979; 16:390.
15. Daniel RK. Muscle coverage of pressure points: the role of myocutaneous flaps. *Ann Plast Surg* 1982; 8:446.
16. Lindan O, Greenway RM, Piazza JM. Pressure distribution on the surface of the human body: evaluation in lying and sitting positions using a "bed springs and nails." *Arch Phys Med Rehabil* 1965; 46:378.
17. Reichel S. Shearing forces as a factor in decubitus ulcers in paraplegics. *JAMA* 1958; 166:762.
18. Bennett L, Kavner D, Lee BY, Trainor FS. Shear versus pressure as causative factors in skin blood flow occlusion. *Arch Phys Med Rehabil* 1979; 60:307.
19. Mulholland JH, Tui C, Wright AM, et al. Protein metabolism and bedsores. *Ann Surg* 1943; 118:1015.
20. Taylor RG. Spinal cord injury: its many complications. *Am Fam Physician* 1973; 8:138.
21. Vasconez LO, Schneider WJ, Jurkiewicz MJ. Pressure sores. *Curr Probl Surg* 1977; 14;1.
22. Snively SL, Tebbetts JB. Pressure sores (overview). *Selected Readings in Plastic Surgery* 1986; 3:1.
23. Edberg EL, Cerny K, Stauffer ES. Prevention and treatment of pressure sores. *Phys Ther* 1973; 53:246.
24. Staas WE, LaMantia JG. Decubitus ulcers and rehabilitation medicine. *Int J Dermatol* 1982; 21:437.
25. Ungar GH. The care of the skin in paraplegics. *Practitioner* 1971; 206:507.
26. Reuler JB, Cooney TG. The pressure sore: pathophysiology and principles of management. *Ann Inter Med* 1981; 94:661.
27. Houle RJ. Evaluation of seat devices designed to prevent ischemic ulcers in paraplegic patients. *Arch Phys Med Rehabil* 1969; 50:587.
28. Clinical Practice Guidelines, No. 15. Treatment of Pressure Ulcers. U.S. Department of Health and Human Services. Public Health Service Agency for Health Care Policy and Research. Rockville, Maryland: AHCPR Publication No. 95-0652. December 1994.
29. Boxer AM, Gottesman N, Bernstein H, Mandl I. Debridement of dermal ulcers and decubiti with collagenase. *Geriatrics* 1969; 24(7):75–86.
30. Lee L. K, Ambrus J. L. Collagenase therapy for decubitus ulcers. *Geriatrics* 1975; 30(5):91–93, 97–98.
31. Rao D. B, Sane P. G, Georgiev E. L. Collagenase in the treatment of dermal and decubitus ulcers. *J Am Geriatric Soc* 1975; 23(1):22–30.
32. Varma AO, Bugatch E, German EM. Debridement of dermal ulcers with collagenase. *Surg Gynecol Obstet* 1973; 136(2):281–282.

33. Foresman PA, Payne DS, Becker D, Lewis D, Rodeheaver GT. A relative toxicity index for wound cleansers. *Wounds* 1993; 5(5):226–231.

34. Bhaskar SN, Cutright DE, Gross A. Effect of water lavage on infected wounds in the rat. *J Periodontol* 1969; 40(11):671–672.

35. Fowler E, Goupil DL. Comparison of the wet-to-dry dressing and a copolymer starch in the management of debrided pressure sores. *J Enterostomal Ther* 1984; 11(1):22–25.

36. Gorse GJ, Messner RL. Improved pressure sore healing with hydrocolloid dressings. *Arch Dermatol* 1987; 123(6):766–771.

37. Sebern MD. Pressure ulcer management in home health care: efficacy and cost effectiveness of moisture vapor permeable dressing. *Arch Phys Med Rehabil* 1986; 67(10):726–729.

38. Alm A, Hornmark AM, Fall PA, Linder L, Bergstrand B, Ehrnebo M, Madsen SM, Setterberg G. Care of pressure sores: a controlled study of the use of a hydrocolloid dressing compared with wet saline gauze compresses. *Acta Derm Venereol* (Stockholm) 1989; 149 Suppl:1–10.

39. Colwell JC, Foreman MD, Trotter JP. A comparison of the efficacy and cost-effectiveness of two methods of managing pressure ulcers. *Decubitus* 1992; 6(4):28–36.

40. Neil KM, Conforti C, Kedas A, Burris JF. Pressure sore response to a new hydrocolloid dressing. *Wounds* 1989; 1(3):173–185.

41. Oleske DM, Smith XP, White P, Pottage J, Donovan MI. A randomized clinical trial of two dressing methods for the treatment of low-grade pressure ulcers. *J Enterostomal Ther* 1986; 13(3):90–98.

42. Xakellis GC, Chrischilles EA. Hydrocolloid versus saline gauze dressing in treating pressure ulcers: a cost-effectiveness analysis. *Arch Phys Med Rehabil* 1992; 73:463–469.

43. Carley PJ, Wainapel SF. Electrotherapy for acceleration of wound healing: low intensity direct current. *Arch Phys Med Rehabil* 1985; 66(7):443–446.

44. Kloth LC, Feedar JA. Acceleration of wound healing with high voltage, monophasic, pulsed current. *Phys Ther* 1988; 68(4):503–508. [See Erratum in: *Phys Ther* 1989; 69(8):702.]

45. Feedar JA, Kloth LC, Gentzkow GD. Chronic dermal ulcer healing enhanced with monophasic pulsed electrical stimulation. *Phys Ther* 1991; 71(9):639–649.

46. Gentzkow GD, Pollack SV, Kloth LC, Stubbs HA. Improved healing of pressure ulcers using dermapulse, a new electrical stimulation device. *Wound* 1991; 3(5):158–170.

47. Griffin JW, Tooms RE, Mendius RA, Clifft JK, Vander Zwaag R, El-Zeky F. Efficacy of high voltage pulsed current for healing of pressure ulcers in patients with spinal cord injury. *Phys Ther* 1991; 71(6):433–432.

48. Motta GJ. The effectiveness of Dermagram topical therapy for treating chronic wounds in nursing facility residents. *Ostomy Wound Manage* 1991; 36:35–38.

49. El Zayat SG. Preliminary experience with topical phenytoin in wound healing in a war zone. *Mil Med* 1989; 154(4):178–180.

50. Robson MC, Phillips LG, Lawrence WT, Bishop JB, Youngerman JS, Hayward PG, Broemeling LD, Heggers JP. The safety and effect of topically applied recombinant basic fibroblast growth factor on the healing of chronic pressure sores. *Ann Surg* 1992; 216(4):401–408.

51. Robson M, Phillips LG, Thomason A, Robson LF, Pierce GF. Recombinant human growth factor-bb for the treatment of chronic pressure ulcers. *Ann Plast Surg* 1992; 29:193–201.

52. Robson M, Phillips LG, Thomason A, Robson LF, Pierce GF. Platelet-derived factors BB for treatment of chronic pressure ulcers. *Lancet* 1992; 339:23–25.

53. Robson MC, Maggi SP, Smith PD, Wassermann RJ, Mosiello GC, Hill DP, Cooper DM. Ease of wound closure as an endpoint of treatment efficacy. *Wound Rep Reg* 1999; 7:90–96.

54. Rees RS, Robson MC, Smiell JM, Perry BH, et al. Becaplermin gel in the treatment of pressure ulcers: a phase II randomized, double-blinded, placebo-controlled study. *Wound Rep Reg* 1999; 7:141–147.

55. Conway H, Griffith BH. Plastic surgery for closure of decubitus ulcers in patients with paraplegia. *Am J Surg* 1956; 91:9.

56. Lee BY, Shaw WW, Madden JL, et al. Surgical management of pressure sores. *Contemp Orthop* 1982; 5:49.

19

Prevention and Management of Pressure Ulcers in the Spinal Cord Injured Patient: Responsibilities of the Nurse

MARY L. SHANNON, EdD, RN

THE ESTIMATES OF SPINAL CORD INJURY (SCI) prevalence are highly variable. Kurtzke (1) estimated prevalence to be 500 to 600 injuries per million. However, De Vivo, Fine, Maetz, and Stover (2) estimated prevalence to be more than 30 percent higher: 906 spinal cord injuries per million. Based on 1998 figures, 227,000 people in the U.S. have a spinal cord injury, and roughly 50,000 of those are military veterans (3,4). Pressure ulcers are a special concern in the SCI patient because they are the fourth leading cause of death in this population (5). In a questionnaire study done by Salzberg, Byrne, Cayten, Kabir, et al. (4) of 800 SCI members of the Eastern Paralyzed Veterans Association (EPVA), 17 percent had a pressure ulcer at the time of the study, and 70.3 percent gave a history of one or more pressure ulcers. The authors estimated that this 17 percent prevalence translated to

38,000 people with SCIs suffering from a pressure ulcer at any given time (4). Studies from two other countries show much higher prevalence rates among SCI patients: Brazil, 54 percent (6) and Iceland, 58 percent (7). Regardless of the actual prevalence of pressure ulcers in SCI patients in the U.S., pressure sores are a major and very expensive problem. It is estimated that the annual treatment cost of all pressure ulcers in all types of patients in the U.S. is more than $1.3 billion dollars (4).

Spinal cord injury is clearly a condition whose onset occurs in a young and overwhelmingly male population. Most peacetime injuries occur in the 16- to 30-year age group, with the modal age at injury being 19 years. The National Spinal Cord Injury Statistical Center, whose figures derive from 17 federally funded SCI Care Systems, categorizes 38 separate causes of injury into five major categories: motor vehicle accidents (MVA), falls, acts of violence, recreational sporting injuries, and other. Of these, MVAs account for nearly half. Falls are the second leading cause of SCI (5).

Much of the medical research and management of the SCI patient was necessitated by the volume and severity of injuries suffered by military personnel in times of active warfare. However, not until 1944 was a focused effort made to manage spinal cord injured patients in units designed specifically for that purpose. The British Medical Research Council implemented planning for large potential numbers of military and civilian casualties resulting from World War II. The Council agreed to send all SCI patients to special SCI units, which were established throughout Great Britain. One of these units was at Stoke Mandeville Hospital in Aylesbury, England, where Dr. Ludwig Guttmann established a comprehensive treatment and rehabilitation program (5). Guttmann stated that "the cardinal prophylaxis [in the prevention of pressure ulcers] is frequent change of posture, at least every 2 hours *day and night*, to redistribute pressure" (8). Guttmann is generally acknowledged to be responsible for establishing the 2-hour turning schedule for prevention of pressure ulcers in patients unable to turn themselves. It is possible that he was also the first to recognize the effect of shearing on the skin and its supporting tissues:

> The degree and extent of the disastrous effects of local pressure in paraplegia, causing ischaemia of skin and deeper tissues, are determined by its intensity, duration, and direction. With regard to direction, I consider the effect of sheering (sic) stress to be much more disastrous than the more vertical pressure, as the former cuts off larger areas from their vascular supply (8).

Not until 1970 was there a federally sponsored system of SCI care in the U.S. with the founding of the Southwest Regional System for Treatment of Spinal Injury (5).

The demographics of the United States SCI population today is very different from that during WWII, the Korean War, and Vietnam. Overwhelmingly, those military SCI patients were young, physically fit men with no other major health problems. Their SCIs were treated and they underwent rehabilitation programs in the Veterans Administration Medical Centers (VAMC) throughout the country. Many of them made maximum physiologic and psychologic recoveries from their injuries and were able to make places in society for themselves. For these men, the health problems associated with their SCIs required regular self-monitoring with infrequent need for medical assistance and hospitalization. However, for other ex-servicemen recovery was less satisfactory. Often, the psychologic adjustment of these men to SCI was poor. Their failure to adjust to the permanence of their injuries affected their management of physical health as well.

Much has been written about the nature of the psychologic problems encountered by veterans with SCI. Many studies have shown depression, anger, inability to cope, suicidal thoughts, etc. These findings continue to be observed among many veterans as well as in non-military SCI patients (9–12) . Since WWII, the VAMCs continue to furnish physical and psychological care to these ex-military personnel, who now range in age from 50 to 80-plus years. The medical and nursing care for this segment of the SCI population is demanding, both from the problems associated with the cord damage and those associated with aging.

Following the war in Vietnam, the U.S. has had limited, short-term military operations. These engagements have resulted in fewer casualties of all types. Therefore, the major SCI population seen at present is largely the result of civilian accidents. Many SCIs occur in young males engaging in high-risk behaviors such as high-speed MVAs, violence, drug use, and sports, especially diving. SCIs occur in the 16- to 30-year age group more often than in all other age groups combined (5). These young men probably have a post-injury life expectancy of 30 to 40 years (13). The medical and nursing care for this segment of the SCI population requires physical and psychologic counseling that differs in several major respects from that of the first group. In service-connected injuries, both a formal and informal support system exists because:

- Among servicemen the injury is usually a result of fighting in defense of one's country; there is generally widespread public sympathy and support for these men.
- Large numbers of other servicemen suffered the same or similar injuries at about the same time. Therefore, injured individuals are not alone in having to adjust to a very traumatic, permanent condition.
- The military and VAMC hospitals provide excellent rehabilitation and long-term care without cost, as needed, to those who served during periods of active warfare.

In civilians suffering catastrophic SCIs as a result of accidents or high-risk behaviors, such support systems are seldom found, and the individual may suffer from guilt about the injury. They differ from the military SCI patient in several significant respects, such as:

- The person may blame himself for his injury if it results from driving too fast, drinking too much, diving into shallow water, etc.; there is little or no public sympathy and financial support available to him.
- The person may feel guilt if others were injured as a result of his behavior.
- Civilian SCIs usually involve only one person. Therefore, there are few others experiencing the same problems at the same time. The support system of similarly injured individuals available to VAMC patients is not available to nonmilitary SCI patients.
- There are fewer SCI centers available to civilian patients, and care outside these centers is seldom comprehensive.
- These SCI patients may not have adequate insurance to defray the cost of care. Many times they have no insurance.

- The SCI patient may perceive himself as a drain on his family's resources.

There is a third group of civilian SCI patients comprised of older individuals. Falls are the predominant etiology for their SCIs. Falls are the primary reason for spinal cord injury from the age of 46. By age 75, it is the overwhelming reason for injury, accounting for 59.6 percent of SCIs, while MVAs account for only 32.3 percent (5). These patients differ from the previous two categories in certain respects such as:

- They are often physically frail and have other major health problems.
- They may have changes in their mental acuity ranging from forgetfulness to Alzheimer's disease.
- These patients often have limited or no support systems from family and/or friends.
- Their rehabilitation is more difficult because of age, physical condition, mental condition, financial resources, etc.
- There is a dramatic increase in the proportion of neurologically incomplete quadriplegics among this age group as compared with other groups. Generally, this level of injury in the elderly makes complete rehabilitation to independent living status an impossibility.

The psychologic difficulties experienced by SCI patients may include emotions such as anger, denial, dependence, fear, frustration, unreasonable demands, neglect of self, refusal to cooperate, and others. These behaviors are most common within the first few months post-injury, but may persist or appear at anytime. All health care providers should be aware of the patient's psychologic state, so that referral to appropriate professional help can be made in a timely manner.

In planning nursing care for the SCI patient, many things must be taken into consideration, particularly the neurologic level of injury and its extent. For example, the patient with C-5 motor and sensory function has the ability to feed and groom himself; with C-6 motor and sensory function, he can be independent in grooming, bathing, driving, and preparing a simple meal. With T-1 through T-6 injuries the patient should be able to live independently in a wheelchair-accessible environment. With lower levels of spinal cord function, the person's motor and sensory functions improve, with the possible exception of spinal reflex activity that regulates bladder and bowel function. Above T-12 that activity is preserved, below L-1, it is usually absent (5). If the SCI lesion is *complete*, there is loss of sensation and voluntary muscle control below the level of the lesion. If the injury is *incomplete* there may be preservation of sensation or of some degree of motor function below the injury (5).

Both neurologic level of injury and its extent are basic to the patient's needs and subsequent plan of care. SCI patients often suffer from one or more complications that result from their cord injury. Their primary causes of death in order of frequency are: respiratory deaths, predominantly from pneumonia; heart disease; accidents, poisonings, and violence; and infective and parasitic disease, which is virtually always septicemia usually associated with pressure ulcers (5).

The remainder of the chapter focuses on pressure ulcer prevention and management in the SCI with particular reference to nursing care. Without question, prevention of skin breakdown is the most effective treatment. Daily assessment using one of several scales developed for the purpose of pressure ulcer prevention helps to raise personnel awareness. The difficulties in choosing the proper assessment instrument have been pointed out by various authors (14–17); none of those in common use are specifically designed for assessing the SCI patient. Salzberg, Byrne, Cayton, et al. (18) published a proposed scale in 1996 for use with the SCI population and later refined it (4). However, no statistics on validity or reliability are given. Whatever assessment instrument is used, personnel should be trained to use it properly and often, but not to rely on it completely. Such scales raise personnel awareness but do not substitute for the nurse's own eyes and judgment.

SCI patients are at very high risk for skin breakdown for all of the same reasons as other patients, but they also have some intrinsic changes that relate to the nature of their spinal cord injuries. In the initial stage of SCI, spinal shock lowers tissue resistance to pressure because of the loss of vasomotor control and flaccid paraplegia. The loss of vasomotor control causes a decrease of tone in the vascular bed of the paralyzed parts of the body, resulting in vasodilatation in these areas. A loss of vascular tone means that capillary closing pressure in these patients is probably considerably less than that of the 32 mm Hg commonly cited in the professional literature. Later there is spasticity of the paralyzed limbs, with adductor and flexor spasms being predominate. If not carefully managed, these spasms cause the development of pressure ulcers in certain areas of the body, such as the inner aspect of the knees and ankles, and produce shearing stress on the covering skin because of continuous rubbing. After the spasms subside, there is decreased muscle tone and wasting with time. If the patient is in a spinal cord treatment center, these alterations can be controlled or minimized. However, if the patient is not in a comprehensive spinal cord center, then management is often less satisfactory and can result in serious skin problems.

The concept of prevention of skin damage is one that must be embraced by the patient and the entire health care team, particularly the nurse. The patient may not practice prevention for a variety of reasons: self-neglect or self-destructive behaviors, depression or other psychologic causes, poor social adjustment, cognitive impairment, lack of information about cause and prevention of the problem, desire to be readmitted to the hospital where he can benefit from a stay in a therapeutic environment and enjoy the company of others with injuries similar to his own, and others (9–11,19–21). Whatever the reason(s) for the individual's failure to practice prevention, attempts must be made by health professionals to understand those reasons and plan approaches so that an acceptable solution can be found. These plans must include the patient's participation in their formulation if they are to succeed. There are a number of ways that this can be done. The following example is an approach used by one agency for SCI patients who have failed to practice preventive skin care.

Shepherd Center, Crawford Research Institute, Atlanta, Georgia, is a 100-bed neurology hospital that treats SCI injuries. They report success with a pilot program designed to decrease readmission of SCI patients who failed to practice preventive skin care. These were SCI patients with high rates of recidivism admitted for surgical revision of pressure ulcer wounds. Personnel instituted a "contingency management" program designed to show that individual behavior responds to its consequences. The program was designed to pay SCI patients who agreed to participate (via a contract) a small fee for maintaining skin integrity. Many of the agency's patients are indigent and regard the hospital stay as a respite from the constant and stressful responsibility of self-care. In this exploratory study, patient compensation was more successful in fostering prevention of pressure ulcers in several SCI patients "who possess the capacity but little or no motivation for avoiding pressure ulcers" (19). The authors point out that even with patient compensation for maintaining intact skin there is potential for tremendous cost savings by possibly preventing the need for pressure ulcer surgery at a cost of approximately $24,575 per patient versus an actual cost of $846 (including compensation and nursing management) in one of their subjects (19).

The Shepherd Center Contingency Management approach is not necessary for most SCI patients, but it might prove useful in unmotivated patients. One of the main strengths of such an approach is that it emphasizes that a partnership between patient and care-givers can sometimes achieve results that directive care from the health professional cannot. (This is a point worth remembering for all who believe that they know what is best for the patient.)

Teaching the SCI individual about skin care begins when the patient's condition is stabilized.

Prior to that time it is the responsibility of the health care providers to act in the best interests of the patient to prevent skin breakdown. That responsibility begins with transport of the injured person to a hospital for definitive treatment. When transporting a spinal cord injured patient, the method chosen should meet two criteria: it should provide stability of the spine and pressure reduction on soft tissues. The initial concerns are to maintain airway, deliver oxygen to all tissues, treat neurogenic shock, effectively immobilize the spine, and manage any other life-threatening conditions. In the immediate post-injury period, prevention of pressure ulcer development is of secondary importance. The use of rigid backboards with head restraints by emergency personnel is common. Usually the time of transport is of sufficient brevity to prevent any real risk of pressure ulcer development as a result of the high interface pressures that result, especially over bony prominences. However, there are times when transport time is lengthy. If that is the case, then one type of transport surface presently available has the capability of reducing the likelihood of skin injury: the vacuum pack. Consisting of polystyrene beads contained in a sealed bag on which the injured person is placed, the bag is emptied of air within 30 seconds by using a manual pump. The beads conform to the person's body configuration. The vacuum pack possesses stabilization and pressure reduction characteristics. It does not lower pressures below capillary closing pressure, but one study showed that pressures over the lower sacrum and the mid-lumbar area decreased to 36.7 mmHg, a value considerably less than the 115.5 mmHg found with padded backboards and the 147.3 mmHg found with non-padded backboards (22). A second study confirmed that vacuum packs provide lower interface pressures than do backboards and other conventional stretchers (23).

Following transport of the newly injured SCI patient to a hospital, he is transported to the intensive care unit (ICU) for stabilization of his condition. ICU staff are primarily concerned with the life-threatening condition changes manifested by patients, rather than skin care. However, every ICU should be equipped with beds that have pressure-reducing capabilities. These usually include foam, static air, alternating air, gel, or water mattresses, although these products are not of equal effectiveness in reducing pressure. The choice of ICU bed should be made based upon an assessment of the needs of the patient, and every ICU patient should be placed on the type of support surface that his condition warrants.

ICU staff often believe that mattresses that are advertised as being "pressure-relieving" can prevent pressure ulcer development in all patients. However, no support surface presently in use can do this. All must be supplemented with a regular turning schedule. With selection of an appropriate bed support surface and frequent turning, skin integrity in the SCI patient can usually be preserved. The caveat is that SCI patients must be on a bed that furnishes firm support while providing the ability to move the patient's body as a unit, to prevent any further damage to the spinal cord. Two beds used with SCI patients can accomplish these objectives: RotoRest (Kinetic Concepts) and the Stryker Frame (Stryker). The RotoRest provides continuous lateral rotation through an arc of 60 degrees. This movement changes maximum pressure points and aids in the control of such respiratory conditions as atelectasis and pneumonia by preventing the pooling of respiratory secretions. Whether shearing forces, both internal and external, are possible factors of concern with lateral rotation beds has not been established. The Stryker Frame provides for turning from supine to prone positions and movement on the frame is not continuous.

Failure to place a SCI patient on a safe bed that can provide safe support and turn the body as a unit is to place him at unacceptable risk for skin breakdown and possible additional cord injury. Consultation with the physician, the skin care nurse, and bioengineers may be necessary to make a proper decision about a safe support surface for the SCI patient. All ICUs should have an established policy about the type of support surface that is acceptable for SCI management. This allows a decision to be made before the patient reaches the ICU and avoids the need to move him from one support surface to another unnecessarily. Each move increases the risk to the patient and places an avoidable demand on staff (up to eight people can be required to move a critically ill patient from one bed to another). It is particularly important that nurses know that foam or foam combination mattresses: 1) do not provide sufficient support to stabilize a spinal injury; 2) are usually not of sufficient thickness and deformation capability to reduce interface pressures to safe levels in any patient: and 3) deform and deteriorate over time. Krouskop, Randall, Davis et al. (24) have shown that interface pressures on foam mattresses begin to increase within 24 months of use because of increasing stiffness of the foam. This is especially problematic in the heaviest load-bearing areas under the sacrum and heels.

Skin breakdown is not only a function of unrelieved supracapillary closing pressure, although this is a necessary piece of the equation. Three other factors figure in the etiology as well: friction, shear, and significantly impaired nutrition.

The SCI patient in the ICU falls prey to friction and shear from reasons that differ from those of the non-SCI patient. In the non-SCI patient, friction and shear are most often associated with elevation of the head of the bed to allow eating, watching TV, conversing with visitors, and/or for comfort. Gravity pulls the patient down in the bed while friction attempts to hold the skin in its original position on the mattress. Shear, which only occurs in the presence of friction and pressure, causes severe angulation of the circulatory vessels to the skin and subcutaneous tissues and deprives them of blood supply. The SCI patient, on the other hand, is not subjected to elevation of the head of the bed while in the immediate post-injury phase. The friction and shear encountered comes as a result of turning the patient on either a lateral turning bed or a Stryker Frame. Friction and shear are both lateral movements, as opposed to the up and down and lateral movements that the non-SCI patient experiences. It is not possible to eliminate any of the three primary causes of skin breakdown: pressure, friction, or shear; they can only be minimized. The fourth factor, significant nutritional compromise or previously existent nutritional deficiencies, can be corrected in most patients.

Significant nutritional depletion has a direct impact on the intact skin's ability to withstand pressure injury. The major changes associated with it are: 1) weakened immune response and phagocytosis; 2) interstitial edema due to hypoproteinemia; total protein levels of less than 5.4 g/dl result in a failure to maintain normal colloid osmotic pressure; 3) decreased angiogenesis, fibroblast production, and collagen synthesis; 4) decreased muscle mass because muscle protein is used as an energy source that is reflected in a creatinine height index below 40 percent of standard; 40 to 60 percent is regarded as marginal depletion; and 5) intestinal absorption problems due to hypoproteinemia. This decreases protein oncotic pressure to less than that of capillary hydrostatic pressure. The result is that water is not absorbed from the intestines.

Regaining lost weight and re-establishing nitrogen balance in the nutritionally compromised individual who has recently suffered a SCI is very difficult. Albumin, a major body protein, is essential to transport amino acids for creation of protein; it also binds zinc, which is needed for collagen cross-linking, and transports free fatty acids, which provide energy, and albumin serves as one of the components of the cell membrane (25,26) Clinically significant malnutrition is diagnosed if 1) serum albumin is less than 3.5 mg/dL, 2) total lymphocyte count is less than 1800 mm, or 3) body weight has decreased more than 15 percent (14).

If the intact skin is breached by a stage III or IV pressure ulcer, then protein loss is accelerated and the ability to improve protein and other nutrient levels is much harder to achieve. Baseline nutritional measurements must be obtained so that deficiencies can be corrected. These include weight, height, body-mass index,

serum albumin, and total lymphocyte count. Monitoring should continue at periodic intervals as determined by the physician so that treatment may be altered as needed. The nurse should be aware that serum albumin level is not reflective of recent change in protein status; its half-life is 20 days. Total lymphocyte count is the more commonly accepted measure of recent body protein change. Total lymphocyte count is reflective of malnutrition if below 1500 cells/mm, and this also serves as a measure of impaired immunity (27). Proteins that have shorter half-lives than albumin are pre-albumin, retinol-binding protein, and fibronectin; level checks of these may be ordered at times (27–30).

In patients with severe protein losses with albumin levels below 2.5 g/dL, treatment attempts are made to rapidly improve the patient's protein stores because mortality rises six-fold in these patients (26). Obviously, any nutritional plan requires the input of a trained nutritionist who can advise on the types of products that are available and can best meet the patient's nutritional needs. The physician may attempt rapid improvement in protein status by giving intravenous solutions of amino acids and supplementing the IV with 12.5 grams of albumin per liter for a limited time. This approach is effective, but must be closely monitored. Fluid shift occurs as the patient's protein oncotic pressure rises and exceeds hydrostatic pressure (31). The shift causes symptoms of acute respiratory distress and other fluid overload problems. Only careful, frequent observation and fluid therapy management prevents this. Once the intestinal absorption problems have been stabilized, tube or oral feedings are begun as tolerated. In patients with severe protein depletion, it may take 2.0 grams of protein/kg/day to replace that loss (14). If the patient has renal problems, then nutritional consultation is necessary to achieve positive nitrogen balance safely.

The SCI patient is incontinent of bowel and bladder in the initial period of injury. The normal skin pH is slightly acidic. However, when urine and stool mix, bacteria normally present in the stool convert urea to ammonia, which changes the skin pH to alkaline. The loss of this "acid mantle" renders skin more subject to irritation, which can influence permeability and make infection a possibility. Ammonia also converts the stool pH into an alkaline range. This reactivates stool enzymes that help to break down intact skin. The bar soaps used by most hospitals to bathe patients are also alkaline. The additive factors of bowel and bladder incontinence plus the use of alkaline bar soaps or other inappropriate skin and wound cleansers makes the intact skin more prone to bacterial, yeast, and fungal infections.

The skin of the incontinent patient should be kept clean and dry to discourage skin breakdown. For intact skin, a mild soap with warm water is usually satisfactory. In patients with sensitive or fragile skin there are commercial skin care products that provide less irritation and drying than soap. One example of a skin cleansing product line is represented by Aloe Vesta, Sensi-Care, and Septi-Soft (ConvaTec). Other similar products are available from several companies.

The best cleansing agent for an open wound is one that does not damage normal tissue. All commercial skin and wound cleansers are ionically charged. These agents interact with the cell membrane and interfere with its ability to withstand invasion by bacteria. Isotonic saline (0.9 percent) is the only nonionic cleanser, but it lacks surfactant properties. Surfactants include wetting agents, surface tension depressants, detergents, dispersing agents, emulsifiers, quaternary ammonium antiseptics, and more. If a surfactant is needed to rid the wound of exudate, residual topical agents, or metabolic wastes, then mild commercial cleansers such as Dermagran (Derma Sciences, Inc.) or Shur-Clens (ConvaTec) have the lowest toxicity index—10—as measured in a study by Hellewell, Major, Foresman, and Rodeheaver (32). The study found that nonantimicrobial and antimicrobial wound cleansers varied in their toxicities to normal cells from a toxicity index of 10 to 10,000. Some cleansers are particularly toxic to white blood cells and phagocytes (33).

There may be times when cleansing agents with greater surfactant strength will be needed in a wound. However, these stronger preparations are much more toxic to normal cells in the wound bed. Their use should be discontinued as soon as the wound is clean enough to allow the use of a less toxic cleanser. Hellewell, Major, Foresman, and Rodeheaver (32) found that the addition of an antiseptic to the cleansing solution raised the toxicity index to 10,000. Rodeheaver points out that "the benefit of antiseptics in cleansing solutions has not been documented" (34).

If there is a need to irrigate the wound, excessive mechanical force must be avoided to avoid disruption of the wound bed. The AHCPR Guideline on Treatment of Pressure Ulcers (14) states that safe irrigation pressures range between 4 to 15 psi. If the pressure is too low, it will not clean the wound bed sufficiently, and if it is too high it will disrupt normal cellular growth and may drive bacteria deeper into the wound. Since the guidelines were published, several wound irrigation systems have been marketed, generally of three types: syringes, squeezable bottles with special tips, and battery-powered irrigation devices.

Rodeheaver (34) states that the battery-powered irrigation devices illustrate the most dramatic new development in wound irrigation. These are disposable, pulsatile, irrigation devices. Their ability to both deliver and remove the irrigation fluid and all of the loosened wound debris make them an alternative to whirlpool therapy, especially useful for the patient who is not a candidate for whirlpool treatment. These devices have been found to decrease the possibility of wound cross-contamination, which is always a possibility with whirlpool treatments. Additionally, they increase wound healing and decrease hospital length of stay because of their efficacy. Davol, Inc., Stryker Instruments, and Zimmer, Inc. currently make these products.

In an agency where budgetary concerns dictate the use of nondisposables whenever possible, wound irrigation can be performed with a 35 ml syringe with a 19–gauge blunt-tipped needle or an angiocath held 1 to 2 inches above the wound surface. Such a device will deliver irrigating fluid at 8 psi, a level that can remove bacteria without damaging normal cellular components of the wound bed. Wounds with adherent material may require the use of commercial cleansers with minimal toxicity (14).

Moisture-barrier products are essential components of skin management in the incontinent patient. Applied to clean, dry, intact skin after each incontinence episode, these products prevent subsequent stool and urine evacuations from coming into direct contact with the skin. They can be applied over fungal powders if a fungal infection is present (35). Examples of moisture barriers are Aloe Vesta (Calgon Vestal Laboratories), Baza Pro (Sween), and Barri-Care (Care-Tech Laboratories).

Indwelling urinary catheters may be used in the initial management of SCI patients. Such devices decrease the risk of skin breakdown from the action of urine on the skin surface and its pH but at the expense of placing the patient at increased risk for the development of infection (36). The incidence of urinary tract infections in spinal cord injured patients is high, ranging from 10 to 66 percent (37). Infections in pressure ulcers originate from endogenous as well as exogenous sources, a fact often overlooked by clinicians. Urinary catheters should be removed as quickly as possible and a bladder retraining program instituted if possible.

Stool incontinence is harder to manage effectively than urinary incontinence for several reasons: stool contains autolytic enzymes and bacteria; stool cannot be totally prevented from coming in contact with skin and/or wounds in the perineal area; and care-givers may regard stool clean-up as repellent and avoid cleaning patients as frequently and thoroughly as needed.

There are some products advertised as being helpful in stool management. Some are safer and more useful than others, but none are entirely satisfactory. Rectal Foley catheters can be inserted into the rectum. However, they may cause rectal necrosis and bowel perforation if not used properly. Perianal pouches that are properly applied and frequently observed by the nurse are less likely to cause damage. They can, however, cause skin irritation, possibly leading to breakdown.

Adult diapers should be avoided whenever possible. These products encourage skin maceration by holding moisture next to the skin. If their use is unavoidable, then polymer-based chux and diapers should be used (38), and they should be changed upon soiling. In the patient who suffers from diarrhea, the etiology must be sought and treated; otherwise the skin care regimen will not be able to prevent skin breakdown.

The presence of an infection in any patient, but particularly in the SCI patient, is always a cause for concern. Never has that concern been more significant than at present. Handwashing was carefully practiced until the advent of antibiotics seemed to make it less important. Health care personnel became more complacent about the need to "wash your hands and drown the germs." For the past few years, the scientific press has contained articles documenting the rise of resistant bacteria that place patients at significant risk for infection and death once more, thus making careful handwashing and attention to asepsis essential. The bacterial strains that have been most commonly associated with pressure ulcer infections have varied somewhat over time. Guttmann (8) stated that *Staphylococcus aureus, B. strep. Haemolyticus, Proteus, B. coli,* and *Ps. Pyocyanea* were those commonly found in the 1950s. In 1999, the most commonly found organisms infecting pressure ulcers are *Proteus mirabilis, Group D streptococci, Escherichia coli, Staphylococcus aureus, Pseudomonas aeruginosa, Bacteroides fragilis,* and *Peptostreptococcus* sp., plus other antibiotic-resistant strains such as *Methicillin-resistant Staphylococcus aureus* (MRSA) and Enterococcus (once a relatively nonpathogenic organism). *Enterococcus* has become one of the top three nosocomial bacterial pathogens in the U.S. (39,40). Strains of MRSA have recently been isolated from patients in the U.S. and Japan that show intermediate resistance to Vancomycin. Enterococci have become resistant to both β-lactams and aminoglycosides. As Devlin (41) points out, these resistant strains are especially difficult to treat because they have the ability to escape antimicrobials control almost as rapidly as the drugs are developed. In patients at high risk, such as the SCI patient, infection control measures must be assiduously practiced by all care-givers.

All pressure ulcers are colonized bacterially. The bacteria become problematic only when their concentrations increase above 100,000 organisms per gram of tissue, as determined by tissue biopsy or needle aspiration. The signs and symptoms of infection are recognizable by the experienced nurse: increasing fever, cellulitis and/or induration in the peri-wound area, and presence of purulent drainage with foul odor. However, in the older patient with spinal cord injury, these symptoms may be altered. A mild temperature elevation (less than 100 degrees Fahrenheit), lethargy, confusion, and loss of appetite may be the initial symptoms. Cellulitis may be mild or not apparent, but wound drainage is usually present. If there is failure to recognize the signs of infection, sepsis results. It is essential that signs and symptoms of infection be quickly reported so that systemic antibiotic coverage can be started as soon as infection is identified and cultures are obtained.

Galpin (42) found in a study of 21 patients that all who were septic and older than age 60 died in spite of appropriate antibiotic therapy. Systemic antibiotics that are effective in the treatment of pressure ulcer infections include cefoxitin, piperacillin, imipenem, clindamycin, metronidazole, and ciprofloxacin. These potent drugs must be monitored carefully by the nurse, particularly in the older SCI patient. In these patients renal function may be decreased and imipenem, cephalosporins, and aminoglycosides may build to toxic levels (43,44).

Each year the number of products available for the prevention and treatment of chronic wounds grows. They include antimicrobial/anti-fungal preparations; cleansers; moisture barriers; moisturizers; sealants and protectants; tapes; bed systems; mattress overlays; replacement mattress systems; chair cushions; foot, ankle, heel, and elbow protectors; and a multitude of wound care dressings and topical agents. This latter category seems to grow exponentially each year. In part, the growth is fueled by the development of new approaches to wound care, but it also may reflect the realization by various manufacturers that wound care products comprise a market that continues to have enormous growth potential as the U.S. population ages, chronic wounds become more numerous, and patients become more physically compromised.

Some dressings and topical products exhibit remarkable effects on wound healing while others are less effective. The health care provider must be able to sort fact from fiction to determine which of these products is best for the patient with a pressure ulcer. Major dressing and topical categories used in the prevention and/or treatment of pressure ulcers are listed below (45).

- **Absorptive products.** This category includes calcium alginates; hypertonic saline dressings; and absorptive powders, pastes, beads, and granules. The most commonly used product in this category is calcium alginate dressing. Derived from brown seaweed, these dressings are designed for use in moderate to heavily draining wounds. They have the capability to help reduce wound odor and activate macrophages in the wound. They are not indicated in wounds that are dry or covered with eschar. DMERC Medical Policy for Surgical Dressings covers alginates for moderately to highly exudative full-thickness wounds, such as Stage III and IV pressure ulcers, and as fillers for wound cavities with moderate and high exudates. The product comes in a variety of forms: pads, ribbons for wounds of narrow dimension, and ropes for packing cavities. Common brands are KALTOSTAT (ConvaTec) and SORBSAN (Dow Hickam).

- **Antimicrobial dressings.** This category includes dressings that have been impregnated with antibacterial or bactericidal substances designed to reduce the bioburden of the wound. Examples of these dressings are Thermazene (Silver Sulfadiazine), Kendall, and Arglaes (Medline Industries). Such medicated dressings are not without a negative side. In addition to helping control bacteria in the wound, they may also exert cytotoxic effects on healing cells. Fibroblasts are especially vulnerable to their chemical reactivity.

- **Biosynthetic dressings and skin substitutes.** These dressings are designed to provide temporary covering for wounds such as burns, skin tears, donor sites, and the like. The skin substitutes are bioengineered products created from a bioabsorbable matrix containing human dermal and epidermal cells often obtained from neonatal foreskin. These products are capable of secreting certain growth factors that may improve the healing process, usually from the wound edges. Examples of biosynthetic dressings are BIO-BRANE (Dow Hickam), E-Z DERM, and MEDISKIN (Brennan Medical). A synthetic skin product is Apligraf (Novartis).
- **Collagen dressings.** These products come as pads, powders, gels, and packing strips/ribbons. Collagenous protein in the products helps to promote the development of new tissue and debridement. An example is FIBRA-COL (Johnson & Johnson).
- **Composite dressings.** These dressings contain a combination of components. DMERC Policy states that these dressings must have at least the following capabilities: 1) a bacterial barrier, 2) an absorptive layer other than an alginate, foam, hydrocolloid, or hydrogel, 3) either a semi-adherent or nonadherent property over the wound site, and 4) an adhesive border. Examples are Tegaderm with Absorbent Pad (3M HealthCare), COVA-DERM PLUS (DeRoyal), BAND-AID Surgical Dressing (Johnson & Johnson), TELFA XTRA (Kendall), and OpSite Plus (Smith & Nephew).
- **Creams, ointments, and solutions.** This category consists of topicals used for the prevention or treatment of skin breakdown. Their active ingredients are not categorized as drugs. Examples are GRANULEX (Dow Hickam) and Dermagran (Derma Sciences).

- **Polyurethane foam.** These dressings may be either hydrophilic (absorb fluids) or hydrophobic (repel fluids). Most are moderately fluid absorptive. They create a moist wound environment and provide thermal insulation for the wound. They are designed for use with pressure ulcers, stasis ulcers, certain types of small burns, donor graft sites, postoperative incisions, and moderately exudative wounds. DMERC Medical Policy for Surgical Dressings covers foam dressings when used on full-thickness wounds with moderate to heavy exudate. Some brands contain activated charcoal to help control wound odor. Examples are HYDRASORB, Lyofoam (ConvaTec), and Allevyn (Smith & Nephew).
- **Gauze dressings.** This is the oldest dressing category in continuous wound use. These dressings come in many sizes and shapes. They may be woven or nonwoven sponges, pads, ropes, ribbons, strips, rolls, or tubes. Woven gauze is manufactured from 100 percent cotton that is woven like a fabric. Nonwoven gauze is usually manufactured from a blend of materials. Both types of gauze may be impregnated with a variety of substances. The DMERC Medical Policy for Surgical Dressings divides gauzes into three sections: nonimpregnated, impregnated with water or normal saline, and impregnated with something other than water or normal saline. Examples are Topper, Kling, ABD pads, Kerlix, Mesalt, Adaptic, Telfa, and more.
- **Growth factors.** These specific proteins found normally in the body play a number of roles in wound healing. Secreted by platelets, keratinocytes, macrophages, and fibroblasts, growth factors bind to target cell receptors and stimulate that cell's growth, proliferation, movement, or differentiation. They may be isolated from the person's own cells and concentrated to be readministered to stimulate wound healing, or they may be made by recombinant DNA processes. In both cases, when topically applied to a wound, their purpose is to accelerate healing. An example is

REGRANEX (Ortho-McNeil). To date, there is little data specific to their effectiveness in pressure ulcers.

- **Hydrocolloids.** These dressings are composed of an outer polyurethane layer that covers an inner layer composed of gumlike materials such as guar, karaya, gelatin, pectin, or carboxymethylcellulose. They protect the wound from injury, prevent bacteria from entering the wound externally, and maintain a moist wound environment. They are occlusive and should not be used on infected wounds because they encourage anaerobic bacterial growth. These dressings may be used for a variety of wounds, both acute and chronic, such as partial-thickness wounds, wounds with necrosis or slough, and wounds with light to moderate exudate. They encourage autolysis of the wound and therefore, debridement. The DMERC Medical Policy for Surgical Dressings covers their use on wounds with light to moderate exudate. Examples include Tegasorb (3M), Cutinova (Beiersdorf-Jobst), DuoDerm (ConvaTec), and Restore (Hollister).

- **Hydrogels.** These water- or glycerin-based amorphous gels can be used in clean and infected wounds. They do not have the ability to adhere when placed on a wound and require the use of an appropriate secondary dressing to hold the hydrogel in place. Primarily composed of water (80 to 99 percent), they cool and soothe the wound surface by reducing the temperature as much as 5 degrees. They are transparent, so that the wound can be observed. They are minimally absorptive and cannot be used on wounds with much exudate. If used alone, they cannot protect the wound from bacteria. The DMERC Medical Policy for Surgical Dressings covers hydrogels when used on full-thickness wounds with minimal or no exudate, such as Stage III and IV clean wounds. They are not covered for Stage II pressure ulcers without substantial documentation. Examples are Vigilon (Bard), NuGel (Johnson & Johnson), and Restore (Hollister).

- **Transparent film dressings.** Adhesive, semipermeable, and transparent, these dressings allow passage of oxygen from the atmosphere to the wound surface and water vapor from the wound surface to the atmosphere. The pores of the dressing are small enough to prevent bacteria or atmospheric particles from penetrating to the wound. They maintain a moist environment that promotes granulation tissue formation and the body's autolysis of necrotic tissue. The DMERC Medical Policy for Surgical Dressings covers their use on open partial-thickness wounds with minimal exudate or on closed wounds such as Stage I and II pressure ulcers. Examples are OpSite (Smith & Nephew), Tegaderm (3M), and Bioocclusive (Johnson & Johnson).

- **Wound fillers.** These gels, pads, or powders are designed to pharmacologically debride devitalized tissue in the wound, absorb exudate, and clean the wound. The DMERC Medical Policy for Surgical Dressings recommends once daily dressing change but does not specify wound type or stage for reimbursement.

- **Debriding agents.** Enzymatic debriding agents are papain-urea-, or collagenase-based. Designed to pharmacologically debride devitalized tissue in the wound, these agents are slower and less effective than sharp debridement. Examples include Accuzyme (Healthpoint), Collagenase, and SANTYL (Knoll).

The AHCPR14 recommends the following wound dressing guidelines:

- Use a dressing that will keep the ulcer bed continuously moist. Wet-to-dry dressings should be used only for debridement and are not considered continuously moist saline dressings.
- Use clinical judgment when selecting a type of moist wound dressing suitable for the ulcer. Studies of different types of moist wound dressings show no differences in pressure ulcer healing outcomes.

- Choose a dressing that keeps the surrounding intact (periulcer) skin dry while keeping the ulcer bed moist.
- Choose a dressing that controls exudate but does not desiccate the ulcer bed.
- Consider care-giver time when selecting a dressing.
- Eliminate wound dead space by loosely filling all cavities with dressing material.
- Avoid overpacking the wound.
- Monitor dressings applied near the anus, because they are difficult to keep intact.

Many other products exist that do not fall clearly into one of the categories listed previously. They generally have more specific applications and are not included here. There are yearly compendia of wound care products published by Springhouse Corporation entitled *Resources in Wound Care, 1999 Directory* (46) and *The 1999 O/WM Buyers Guide* (45) by the publisher of *Ostomy/Wound Management* magazine. These publications list all products currently available for wound care and the indications for their use. They are excellent resources and are recommended to any reader who is responsible for wound care.

The SCI patient is a prime example of the person who needs to learn about and accept responsibility for self-care. He will live with his injury for a lifetime. Once rehabilitation begins he must master new ways of performing activities of daily living. Depending upon the level and completeness of the cord injury, the patient may be able to perform self-care unassisted, with minimal assistance, or may require maximal assistance.

The nurse plays a key role in the education of patients and their care-givers. Whether the SCI patient suffers preventable complications of his injury is a function of many factors, which include understanding how the complications are produced, his or his caregiver's responsibility in prevention, his feelings about his injury and its aftermath, self-esteem, satisfaction with life, relationships with health care professionals, and others.

LaMantia, Hirschwald, Goodman, et al. (47) report the results of a Pressure Sore Readmission Program designed for the SCI patient. Forty-two patients were enrolled and 28 completed the program. Of those completing, 24 remained healed at three months. Of 23 patients who reached 1 year post-discharge from the program, 15 remained healed, four had skin breakdowns, and four were not evaluated. The findings were unexpected in that "there was a lack of significance between healed skin and the program components of psychosocial intervention (attendance and quality of participation in groups and individual sessions)." The authors note that several studies suggest that the individual's ability to develop personal goals will not necessarily bring about a high degree of behavior change. They postulate that patients who were unable to define their own life goals were able to follow those of the program, and therefore, maintain skin integrity. The study did show "a positive association between teaching, reinforcement of specific behaviors, and healed skin."

There are no clear stimuli to always motivate a SCI person to practice good preventive skin care. However, the nurse should try to understand patients and their concerns, strengths, and limitations. There is an art to determining "teachable moments" and the same approach cannot be used with all. For some, conveyance of factual information is sufficient. For others, interest in them as individuals is primary to their learning and practicing good skin care habits.

It is important that the teaching plan cover essential information such as regular position changes while in the bed or chair, the frequency with which these position changes should be done, the importance of keeping the skin clean and moisturized, the importance of daily skin examination, good nutrition, and other aspects of skin hygiene. Bandura (48,49) found the process of changing an individual's health behavior to be extremely complex and the process to require varied approaches at regular intervals. The fact that roughly 30 percent of all SCI patients develop a pressure ulcer each year following initial discharge says that we still have much to learn about how to teach the SCI person effectively and motivate him to assume responsibility for his own health and well-being.

REFERENCES

1. Kurtzke JF. Epidemiology of spinal cord injury. *Exp Neurol* 1975; 48:163–236.
2. DeVivo MJ, Fine PR, Maetz HM, Stover SL. Prevalence of spinal cord injury: a re-estimation employing life table techniques. *Arch Neurol* 1980; 37: 707–708.
3. Lasfargues JE, Custis D, Morrone F, Carswell J, Nguyen T. (1995) A model for estimating spinal cord injury prevalence in the United States. *Paraplegia.* 33, 62 – 68.
4. Salzberg CA, Byrne DW, Cayten CG, Kabir R, van Niewerburgh MA, Viehbeck M, Long H, Jones EC. Predicting and preventing pressure ulcers in adults with paralysis. *Advances in Wound Care* 1998; 11(5):237–246.
5. Stover SL, Fine PR. *Spinal Cord Injury: The Facts and Figures.* Birmingham, Alabama: The University of Alabama at Birmingham, 1986.
6. daPaz AC, Beraldo PS, Almeida MC, Neves EG, Alves CM, Khan P. Traumatic injury to the spinal cord: prevalence in Brazilian hospitals. *Paraplegia* 1992; 30(9):636–640.
7. Knutsdottir S. Spinal cord injuries in Iceland 1973–1989: a follow-up study. *Paraplegia* 1993; 31:68–72.
8. Guttmann L. The problem of treatment of pressure sores in spinal paraplegics. *British J of Plastic Surgery* 1955; 8:196–213.
9. Anderson TP, Andber MM. Psychosocial factors associated with pressure sores. *Arch Phys Med Rehabil* 1979; 60:341–346.
10. Gordon WA, Bellile S, Harasymiew S, Hehman L, Sherman B. The relationship between pressure sores and psychosocial adjustment in person with spinal cord injury. *Rehabilitation Psychologist* 1982; 3:185–191.
11. Heilporn A. Psychological factors in the causation of pressure sores: case reports. *Paraplegia* 1991; 29:137–139.
12. Krause JS. Skin sores after spinal cord injury: relationship to life adjustment. Spinal Cord 1998; 36:51–56. Nehemkis AM, Groot, H. Indirect self-destructive behavior in spinal cord injury. In N. Faberow, ed. *The Many Faces of Suicide.* New York: McGraw-Hill, 1980. Pp. 99–115.
13. Geisler WO, Jousse AT, Wynne-Jones M. Survival in traumatic transverse myelitis. *Paraplegia* 1977; 14:262–275.
14. Bergstrom N, Bennett MA, Carlson CE, et al. *Treatment of Pressure Ulcers. Clinical Practice Guideline,* No. 15. Rockville, Maryland: U.S. Department of Health and Human Services. Public Health Service, Agency for Health Care Policy and Research. AHCPR Publication No. 95-0652. December, 1994.
15. Cooper DM. Wound assessment and evaluation of healing. In R. Bryant, ed., *Acute and Chronic Wounds: Nursing Management.* St. Louis: Mosby Yearbook,1992. Pp. 69–90.
16. Woodbury MG, Houghton PE, Campbell KE, Keast DH. Pressure ulcer assessment instruments: a critical appraisal. *Ostomy/Wound Management* 1999; 45(5):42–55.
17. Haalboom JRE, den Boer J, Buskens E. Risk assessment tools in the prevention of pressure ulcers. *Ostomy/Wound Management* 1999; 45(2): 20–34.
18. Salzberg CA, Byrne DW, Cayten CG, van Niewerburgh P, Murphy JG, Viehbeck M. A new pressure ulcer risk assessment scale for individuals with spinal cord injury. *Am J Phys Med Rehabil* 1996; 75:96–104.
19. Adkins VK, Mathewseon C, Ayllon T, Jones ML. The ethics of using contingency management to reduce pressure ulcers: Data from an exploratory study. *Ostomy/Wound Management* 1999; 45(3): 56–61.
20. Gosnell D. Pressure sore risk assessment, part II: analysis of risk factors. *Decubitus* 1989; 2(3):40–43.
21. Shannon ML, Skorga P. Pressure ulcer prevalence in two general hospitals. *Decubitus* 1989; 2(4):38–43.
22. Lovell ME, Evans JH. A comparison of the spinal board and the vacuum stretcher, spinal stability and interface pressure. *Injury* 1994; 25(3):179–180.
23. Main PW, Lovell ME. A review of seven support surfaces with emphasis on their protection of the spinally injured. *J Accid Emerg Med* 1996; 13(1): 34–37.
24. Krouskop TA, Randall C, Davis J, et al. Evaluating the long-term performance of a foam-core hospital replacement mattress. *J of Wound, Ostomy & Continence Nursing* 1994; 21:241–246.
25. Himes D. Protein-calorie malnutrition and involvuntary weight loss: the role of aggressive nutritional intervention in wound healing. *Ostomy/Wound Management* 1999; 45(3):46–55.
26. Pinchcofsky-Devin G. Why won't this wound heal? *Ostomy/Wound Management* 1998; 24:42–51.
27. Shelty PS, Jungs RT, Watragewies KE, et al. Rapid turnover transport proteins: An indicator of subclinical protein energy malnutrition. *Lancet* 1979; 2:23–232.

28. Wallach J. *Intrepretation of Diagnostic Tests* 6th ed. Boston: Little, Brown & Co., 1996. Pp. 464.

29. Vaziri ND, Eltorai I, Gonzales E, et al. Pressure ulcer, fibronectin, and related proteins in spinal cord injured patients. *Arch Phys Med Rehabil* 1992; 73:803–806.

30. Fuoco U, Scivoletto G, Pace A, Vona VU, Castellano V. Anemia and serum protein alteration in patients with pressure ulcers. *Spinal Cord* 1997; 35(1):58–60.

31. Kaminsky MV Jr, Pinchcofsky-Devin G, Williams SD. Nutritional management of decubitus ulcers in the elderly. *Decubitus* 1989; 2:20–30.

32. Hellewell TB, Major DA, Foresman PA, Rodeheaver GT. A cytotoxic evaluation of antimicrobial and nonantimicrobial wound cleansers. *Wounds* 1997; 9(1):15–20.

33. Foresman PA, Payne DS, Becker D, Lewis D, Rodeheaver GT. A relative toxicity index for wound cleansers. *Wounds* 1993; 5(5):226–231.

34. Rodeheaver GT. Pressure ulcer debridement and cleansing: a review of current literature. *Ostomy/Wound Management* 1999; 45 (1A suppl):S80–85.

35. Jeter KF. The special skin care needs of incontinent patients: An ET clinician's view. *Wound and Skin Care* 1992; 3–5:11.

36. Mertz PM, Marshall DA, Davis SC, et al. The wound environment: implications from research studies for healing and infection. In D. Krasner, ed.,*Chronic Wound Care: A Clinical Source Book* for Healthcare Professionals. King of Prussia, Pennsylvania: Health Management Publications, 1990. Pp. 66–73.

37. Fletcher DJ, Taddonio RF, Byrne DW, Wexler LM, Cayten CG, Nealon SM, Carson W. Incidence of acute care complications on vertebral column fracture patients with and without spinal cord injury. *Spine* 1995; 20(10):1136–1146.

38. Brown DS. Diapers and underpads, part 2: cost outcomes. *Ostomy/Wound Management* 1994; 40:34–44.

39. Davis JM, Huycke MM, Wells CL, et al. Surgical Infection Society Position on Vancomycin-resistant enterococcus. *Arch Surg* 1996; 131:1061–1068.

40. Brown DL, Smith DJ. Bacterial colonization/infection and the surgical management of pressure ulcers. *Ostomy/Wound Management* 1999; 45(1A suppl):S109–118.

41. Devlin HR. Bacteria for the nineties. *Ostomy/Wound Management* 1998; 44(8):32–40.

42. Galpin JE, Chow AW, Bayer AS. Sepsis associated with decubitus ulcers. *Am J Med* 1976; 61:346–350.

43. Calandra GB, Wang C, Aziz M, et al. The safety profile of imipenem/cilastatin: world-wide clinical experience based on 3470 patients. *J Antimicrob Chemother* 1986; 18 (Suppl E):193–202.

44. Kertesz D, Chow AW. Infected pressure and diabetic ulcers. Clin Geriatr Med 1992; 8:835–852.

45. The 1999 O/WM Buyers Guide. *Ostomy/Wound Management* 1999; 45(7).

46. Resources in Wound Care: 1999 Directory. *Advances in Wound Care.* 12(4).

47. LaMantia JG, Hirschwald JF, Goodman CL, Wooden VM, Delisser O, Staas WE Jr. A program design to reduce chronic readmissions for pressure sores. *Rehabil Nurs* 1987; 12(1):22–25.

48. Bandura A. *Principles of Behavior Modification.* New York: Holt, Rinehart, Winston 1969.

49. Bandura A. Psychotherapy based upon modeling principles. In AE Bergin & SL Garfield, eds., *An Empirical Analysis.* New York: John Wiley & Sons, 1971. Pp. 653–672.

20 Operative Reconstruction in the Spinal Cord Injured · Patient

ZAHID B.M. NIAZI, MD
C. ANDREW SALZBERG, MD

THE MANAGEMENT OF A SPINAL CORD injured patient with pressure ulcers starts with prevention, and if general principles of good care are followed, a large number of initial and recurrent pressure ulcers can be prevented. Initial surgical treatment must be planned so that the flap design does not violate other vascular territories or pedicles that would make future flaps impossible. Pressure ulcers can recur whether treated surgically or by conservative measures in up to 91 percent of spinal cord injured (SCI) individuals. Such high incidence rates may be due to associated factors rather than the surgical technique used or the standard conservative management provided. Recurrent, extensive or multiple truncal pressure ulcers are difficult to manage and are a challenge for even the most experienced reconstructive surgeon. In centers of excellence, utilizing individual patient-focused treatment and the standard workhorse flaps, or with the occasional use of the most difficult and involved surgical reconstruction in a reconstructive surgeon's armamentarium, an appropriate long-term stable outcome is possible.

For most individuals, normal sensation and the ability to move protects them from the contact forces of pressure, friction, or shear, but these become a problem for persons lacking mobility or those with impaired sensibility, and thus leads to the development of pressure ulcers. Pressure ulcers remain a common problem with a significant financial impact on health care budgets, whether in the acute care, nursing home, or home care populations. The incidence and prevalence varies, but several populations are at significantly higher risk and these include spinal cord injured (SCI) individuals. Spinal cord injuries are usually the result of automobile accidents in individuals injured younger than 50 years of age and of falls in individuals injured when older than 50 years of age. Patients surviving late life injury are much more likely to have incomplete injuries predominantly affecting the cervical spine (1).

Most spinal cord injured patients will develop a pressure ulcer at some point in their lives. Spinal cord injuries affect nearly 200,000 people in the United States with a quarter of these patients going on to develop a pressure ulcer during their first admission (2,3). With the high cost (nearly \$60,000) of treating a patient with an initial pressure ulcer, the increase in the total number of spinal cord injured patients, and the shrinking size and budgets of hospitals, management of these ulcers is a major economic and logistic problem. The estimated annual cost of treating patients with pressure ulcers in the United States is between $1 billion and $5 billion (4–6).

Pressure ulcers remain a major health risk for persons with SCI, despite enormous published research describing their risk factors. With more than 200 risk factors identified in the published literature, pressure ulcers still occur in more than 30 percent of the patients who enter an emergency room setting with a spinal cord injury (6). Of these initial ulcerations, nearly a quarter will be stage III or IV and will become candidates for operative repair.

Spinal cord injuries account for a large number of admissions into specialized treatment and rehabilitation units. As many as 80 to 85 percent of individuals with SCI develop a pressure ulcer (7) at some point during their lifetimes, at the rate of 23 to 30 percent per year. It has been the experience of dedicated teams caring for SCI patients that early admission and treatment in an organized multidisciplinary care system is beneficial. Results demonstrate statistically significant reductions in acute care and total lengths of stay coupled with a highly significant reduction in the incidence of pressure ulcers for patients admitted within 1 day of injury to these units. Moreover, for patients admitted within 1 day of injury, mortality rates were lower than reported previously for patients not admitted to an organized SCI care system (8).

Each year, 60,000 people die of pressure ulcer-related complications (2,3). More than 70 percent of spinal cord injured patients with a pressure ulcer have multiple ulcers. With thousands of new admissions and the high cost of treating an individual with a pressure ulcer, management of these ulcers is not only a logistic problem but also a huge economic burden. Pressure ulcers may account for one-fourth of the cost of caring for SCI patients and the cost of pressure ulcer prevention is one-tenth of pressure ulcer treatment (6).

The U.S. Department Public Health Service has recommended guidelines that make specific recommendations to identify at-risk adults and define early interventions for prevention of pressure ulcers (9). Prevention and early intervention programs can help in reducing the prevalence of pressure ulcers. A person's risk for developing a pressure ulcer can be predicted by using the Braden scale or SCIPUS scale. In a study carried out by Hunter et al. (10) using the Braden scale, there was a 60 percent decrease in prevalence from the 25 percent baseline to the 10 percent found at the audits carried out up to 16 months from implementation of protocols consistent with the National Pressure Ulcer Advisory Panel (NPUAP) consensus statement. Salzberg et al. compared the different scales and found that the SCIPUS was more accurate than the Braden, and identified a new acute version, referred to as SCIPUS-A in their study, to be an accurate predictor of pressure ulcers during the first hospitalization after a spinal cord injury (11,12).

A study by Maklebust et al. (13) from data obtained through five hospital-wide pressure ulcer audits were pooled for exploratory analysis. This secondary data analysis suggested that the odds of having a pressure ulcer were 22 times greater for hospitalized adult patients with fecal incontinence compared to hospitalized adult patients without fecal incontinence.

Clinicians involved in conservative care of these chronic wounds have many treatment interventions from which to choose, including debridement/irrigation, dressings, pressure-relieving devices, hyberbaric or topically applied oxygen, whirlpool/pulsed lavage, ultrasonography, topical antibiotics, and cytokine growth factors. Unfortunately, many wounds heal very slowly, do not heal, or worsen despite the best efforts to promote tissue repair. In such instances, another modality that has shown promise is the use of electrical stimulation (14).

SURGICAL PLAN FOR SCI PRESSURE ULCERS

Patients with Stage II, III, or IV ulcerations will have their ulcers treated by conservative methods, whereas others will undergo surgical reconstruction (15) of the defects following debridement of the bursal sac. The spinal cord patient who becomes a surgical candidate for repair presents a unique situation for the reconstructive surgeon. The decreased or lack of sensation, poor mobility, and medical conditions (including autonomic dysreflexia) complicate the pre-operative, the intra-operative, and the postoperative care needed for these individuals. The decision to undergo surgical repair of the pressure ulcer should be made with the full knowledge of the risks and benefits, surgical and nonsurgical alternatives, and the complications associated with each procedure. Such inherent risks and complications include loss of flap viability, recurrence of ulceration, bleeding (hematoma), infection, and the need for future surgery. The relative weight given to each of these complications must be balanced with the advantage of a closed or a healed wound. No patient would prefer an open ulceration with its associated problems if given the choice for closure with a low-risk, simple procedure and a healed wound (16).

The medical management of the patient lays the groundwork for the success of any surgical procedure. Patients suffering from cardiopulmonary or metabolic disorders must be treated and stabilized prior to surgery. Anemia must be corrected by diet, nutritional supplements, and medication. Correction by blood transfusions may be reserved for patients needing surgery urgently or if conservative management fails to correct the anemia. Inadequate nutrition and local wound care must be improved preoperatively to ensure a better chance for the definitive surgery to be effective. If necessary, hyperalimentation by enteral or parenteral routes should be instituted.

It is imperative at the time of surgery for these pressure ulcers that the bursal sac is removed completely and that partial resection of any bony prominences is performed to reduce the likelihood of recurrence. Similarly, the importance of proper postoperative rehabilitation must be emphasized. Relief of pressure is mandatory, and the patients are nursed initially on low air loss or zero-pressure inlays and then gradually switched when appropriate. Flexion contractures, if left untreated prior to definitive surgery, can result in undue tension on the flaps and result in other unnecessary complications. Similarly, appropriate medication is given to treat spasmodic episodes. All patients are given perioperative, culture specific intravenous antibiotics before surgery and for 1 week postoperatively. All patients have a mechanical bowel prep as a part of their preoperative preparation. In most cases, debridement of nonviable tissue is performed by sharp technique, with enzymatic or autolytic debridement. Serial minor debridements can be performed at the bedside to prepare the wound for definitive surgery, but in some patients extensive debridement may be required, which is best performed in the operating room as these procedures may induce pain and anxiety for the patient. Blood loss during extensive pressure ulcer debridement is usually underestimated, and blood should be replaced intraoperatively or in the immediate postoperative period (16). If possible, autogenous blood should be considered; if required, however, most surgery can be accomplished without significant blood loss and possible risk of transfusion.

Soft tissue coverage for closure of pressure ulcers was initiated by John Staige Davies, who recommended that the scar epithelium should be replaced and extra padding provided over bony prominences by use of skin flaps, thus reducing the chances of recurrence (17). Even this breakthrough surgical option of the 1930s and its variations has not completely prevented recurrence of pressure ulcers. In treating pressure ulcers, certain surgical options such as split-thickness skin grafts on a granulating bed, simple excision of ulcer edges and closure under tension, stellate closure or closure with thin (less than 1 cm thick) flaps over bony prominences, or flaps that fail to fill up the dead space, are not recommended because they produce high failure and recurrence rates, result in additional scars that may lie over pressure areas, and may compromise the future use of more reliable flaps (16).

Dependable closure can be obtained by reserving primary advancement closure to patients with small defects, following excision of the bursal sac and closure without tension for patients who have very lax skin. The coverage of all other wounds is based on the aforementioned protocol of excising the bursal sac, contouring bony prominences, and insetting large, well-vascularized myocutaneous flaps. SCI patients always require the surgical consideration for possible recurrence, and these flaps should be designed in such a way that they can be re-rotated if an ulcer recurs in the future. In ambulatory patients, muscle flaps must be used prudently not to affect gait (16).

The surgical reconstructive options vary with the site of the pressure ulcer, the previous operations performed, and the vascularity and sensibility of the area. As a general rule, patients with small pressure ulcers or ulcers less than 10 cm2 and who have adequate quantity and quality of local tissue available can be managed easily with local tissue rearrangement. Those patients who have adequate quality but inadequate quantity of local tissue may need to undergo a two-stage, definitive procedure with tissue expansion as a first stage. In the most extreme group of patients with both inadequate quality and quantity of local tissue, tissue from a distant site must be transferred. This procedure can be in the form of a microvascular free-tissue transfer or as a fillet flap in patients with life-threatening sepsis

secondary to multiple or extensive truncal or other complex ulcers. Table 20-1 summarizes this treatment algorithm.

SITE-SPECIFIC CHARACTERISTIC FINDINGS AND MANAGEMENT OF PRESSURE ULCERS

The trunk is the most common site for pressure ulcers. The anatomic distribution of ulceration, however, is related directly to patient positioning, mobilization, periods of pressure, and periods of pressure relief. The injury in pressure ulcers begins from within and progresses outwards, with the underlying muscle being most sensitive to pressure. Therefore the skin wound usually represents a small area of damage to the tissues and may truly be the "tip of the iceberg." Pressure ulcers develop in SCI patients who have unrelieved pressure on bony prominences and are unable to transfer by themselves, who have suffered a stroke or are comatose, or who have undergone prolonged surgery under general anesthesia.

Ischial Ulcers

An ischial ulcer is characterized by a small area of skin ulceration and a large undermined cavity. These occur from prolonged sitting in a wheelchair or seat and almost always involve bony exposure. The ischium forms the base of the ulcer and requires surgical excision and contour in almost all

---

TABLE 20-1 SCI Surgical Plan

Presence of Pressure Ulcer, New or Recurrent	
Tissue of adequate quality, sensate/insensate, but inadequate quantity (i.e. local tissue available but pressure ulcer > 10cm²)	Tissue of inadequate quality and inadequate quantity (i.e. no local tissue available and large pressure ulcer > 10cm²)
↓	↓
Rx–Tissue expansion If too much scarring then ↓	Rx–Tissue transfers: Pedicled or free flaps
Rx–Tissue transfers: Pedicled or free flaps	

If tissue transfers are required, then local or distant muscle flaps can be mobilized and transferred as muscle alone or as a myocutaneous transfer (18–23) or one can proceed to free-tissue transfer (24–27).

cases. A partial rather than radical ischiectomy should be carried out because the latter may lead to unnecessary complications (28,29).

A superiorly based gluteus maximus myocutaneous flap is the primary choice for flap reconstruction of ischial ulcer, because of its large size, reliable blood supply, and ability to be re-rotated if required for treatment of recurrences. Alternatively, if the skin defect is large, the hamstring may be advanced as a V-Y advancement myocutaneous flap. This provides a large surface that can also be re-rotated for future breakdowns. This large, muscle-based flap is reliable and will cover larger defects when needed. On rarer occasions, the tensor fascia lata (TFL) may prove useful in covering the ischium and can be utilized to cover both trochanteric and ischial ulcers at the same operative time.

Sacral Ulcers

A sacral ulcer is centered over the sacral prominence and is usually characterized by a large skin defect with overhanging edges. These ulcers originate by unrelieved pressure on the sacrum in the lying position. In the acute spinal cord injured patient, the time initially spent recumbent may be correlated with development of ulceration. The ulcer is usually shallow, with the sacrum in its base. An inferiorly based, large gluteus maximus myocutaneous flap is the primary reconstructive choice for these typically broad, yet shallow, ulcers. Random cutaneous flaps have been used in the past, however, these do not provide the reliability, the soft tissue volume, and the increased blood supply which is inherent in a myocutaneous flap. The gluteus maximus myocutaneous flap may be designed as a V-Y advancement flap, and for larger defects a bilateral advancement can prove extremely useful. In patients with low-level spinal cord injuries, the potential for reconstruction with a sensate intercostal or tensor fascia lata flap can also be considered. As always, flap design and vascular territories are taken into consideration preoperatively so as to plan for subsequent surgery that may be required in the future.

Greater Trochanteric Ulcers

A trochanteric ulcer occurs over the lateral-most aspect of the femur just distal to the femoral neck. These ulcers may have a modest skin defect overlying a similar, deeper defect. The tensor fascia lata flap is the treatment of choice. This flap can be used as a transposition, an island, or a V-Y rotation advancement flap. The large amount of skin and fascia available for rotation makes this "workhorse" flap the most utilized and dependable choice. The vastas lateralis muscle flap is an excellent choice to fill large defects in the hip because it can be turned back into a large femoral cavity or after a girdlestone procedure. It is both reliable and bulky, but requires additional skin coverage. The rectus femoris myocutaneous flap can also be used as an island flap for treatment of trochanteric ulcers. Keeping future reconstructions in mind, random skin rotations or transposition flaps (rhomboid flaps) and even bipedicle fasciocutaneous flaps can be designed easily for smaller defects, but should be reserved for special situations where the surgeon believes that recurrence is not probable.

Quadriplegics and paraplegics may develop ulcers at other sites (i.e., heel, ankles, knee, iliac crests, elbows, scapula, thoracic spine, and occipital scalp). These patients can be treated on the same principles of pressure ulcer management and the defects covered with local cutaneous, muscle, or fasciocutaneous flaps; however, if no local tissue is available, then a pedicled flap or free-tissue transfer reconstruction has to be considered.

Multiple Pressure Ulcers

Extensive ulcerations may be associated with complications like osteomyelitis, perineal, and urethral fistulas. Some persons may have recurrent ulcers or ulcers that have been present for a long time. In cases of long-standing ulceration, one must be aware of malignant degeneration occurring, and a biopsy may be considered to rule out squamous cell carcinoma. Berkwits et al. (30) reported on a case of a squamous cell carcinoma that was found on biopsy during surgical reconstruction of a pressure ulcer in a paraplegic patient 15 years after spinal cord injury and 14 years after development of a sacral pressure ulcer. They also state that occurrence of a Marjolin's ulcer in chronic pressure ulcers and other chronic skin ulcerations may become more widespread as the life span of spinal cord injured patients increases.

POSTOPERATIVE MANAGEMENT

Surgical treatment of pressure ulcers is only a small part in the management of the ulcer. Postoperative care and rehabilitation includes an absolute pressure-free environment for a period of 3 weeks. All reconstructive patients are placed on either low air loss or air fluidized mattresses in the immediate postoperative period. Gradual transfer to other mattresses and cushions to prevent pressure and shearing can be initiated according to individual surgical preference. Adequate control of urinary and fecal output helps to minimize surgical site contamination. Diversion of fecal stream with colostomy is not routinely required for most persons, even in the face of a recurrence or lack of tissue for closure. It is reserved for only the most difficult situation where control is the only mechanism.

Nutritional support and chest and general physical therapy are maintained until mobilization out of bed is initiated and the patient can be transferred to a low-pressure mattress system.

RECURRENT PRESSURE ULCERS IN SPINAL CORD INJURED PATIENTS

The recurrent pressure ulcer is a failure in which not all contributing factors may be recognized. Rehabilitation centers struggle with a certain number of ulcer recurrences, which become an enormous logistic and economic problem as the SCI patient population increases annually. The surgical options for this group of patients are usually limited because of a shortage of available useful tissue and vary with the site of the pressure ulcer, the previous operations performed, and the vascularity and sensibility of the area. Recurrent pressure ulcers are a difficult surgical problem and those patients who develop them because of a failure, albeit uncontrollable in some instances, of the previous surgical procedure, are physically and psychologically impaired to some extent. These patients may have extensive or multiple ulcers, and surgical repair in patients who have paucity of viable tissue, or chronic, extensive, or recurrent postsurgical ulcers, necessitates the consideration of additional reconstructive options. Surgeons, therefore, must consider the surgical options of tissue expansion, comprised of expanded cutaneous or myocutaneous flaps; sensate flaps; filleted leg/thigh flaps; or free fasciocutaneous, free muscle, or myocutaneous flaps, any of which may be used as necessary to close these wounds in patients who may be chronically ill.

In a retrospective study of 176-SCI patients, all who had a history of one or more pressure ulcers had an equal rate of recurrence of approximately 35 percent for both surgically and medically treated patients. The recurrence rate was higher in smokers, diabetics, and patients with cardiovascular disease. Current smokers and patients who had a long history of smoking had a higher risk than former smokers. Patients who smoked had a higher recurrence rate (42.2 percent) while nonsmokers had a recurrence rate of 26.2 percent (P = 0.057) (4).

A review of the literature reveals an extremely wide range of recurrence rates ranging from as low as 0 percent to as high as 91 percent (31–41). The highest recurrence rate was reported by Evans et al. (34) in the 85- to 90-year age group in their series. They also reported an 82 percent recurrence of ulcer at site of surgical correction and 64 percent at a different site in 22 paraplegic patients. Disa et al. (33), in their series of 40, reported a 76 percent recurrence in traumatic paraplegic patients and no recurrence in nontraumatic paraplegics, while the nontraumatic, nonparaplegics had a recurrence of 69 percent. Relander and Palmer (39) reported a 48 percent recurrence in 66 operated ulcers in a 39-patient series with a two- to 12-year follow-up.

Two-thirds of their patients had a neurologic deficit. Goodman et al. (42) reported ulcer recurrence or new ulcer development in postsurgical patients to be 79.2 percent.

Even major rehabilitation centers dealing with spinal cord injured patients struggle with a certain number of recurrences. In 1964, Dansereau and Conway (32) reported the surgical treatment of 2,000 pressure ulcers. Recurrences developed in 5 percent of ischial ulcers, 14 percent of trochanteric ulcers, and 15 percent of sacral ulcers. Conservative treatment of truncal pressure ulcers also does not give long-term healed results in a great majority of patients. In those spinal cord injured individuals who develop pressure ulcers, it appears that associated medical factors may be responsible for the higher incidence rather than the surgical technique used or the standard conservative management provided.

Level of activity is one of the most significant risk factors (43–45) associated with pressure ulcer development, and results show that the bedfast and motorized chairfast patients have a higher incidence of recurrence than the patients with nonpowered chairs. An altered level of consciousness, history of cerebrovascular accident, and dementia can also result in long periods of immobility and thus predispose to ulcer development. Malnutrition, hypoalbuminemia, and anemia are predisposing factors (46) and must be corrected to improve chances of healing whether treating the patient surgically or nonsurgically. Other factors like urinary incontinence and moist clothes and sheets have been consistently associated with pressure ulcers (47). In the SCI population there is a bimodal curve (7) for an increase in pressure ulcer development after age 35 and again after age 65.

Some authors (37,48–51) maintain that tobacco use plays a crucial role in the development of pressure ulcers while others (52,53) believe that it does not contribute to pressure ulcer development, let alone its recurrence. The proponents of an association between smoking and pressure ulcer development state that current smokers are at a significantly increased risk

for pressure ulcers (37,48–51). Pressure ulcers of the heel are four times as common in smokers (51), probably related to the decreased vascularity of ischemic limbs. In a study of 38 SCI patients (37), cigarette smoking was positively correlated with higher incidence and more severe ulcers. Individuals who cease smoking may significantly reduce their risk of developing pressure ulcers, and the effects of smoking may be partially reversible (7). Recurrence of pressure ulcers statistically showed that smoking was an independent risk factor and that patients who had been smoking for a longer time had a higher risk of developing a recurrence (7).

Arteriosclerotic heart disease has been linked to pressure ulcers (54). Patients who suffer from cardiovascular disease have nearly double the incidence of recurrent pressure ulcers (7). The same is true for diabetics in this series, as compared to nondiabetics, and confirms other workers' reports (55).

TREATMENT OF THE DIFFICULT OR RECURRENT PRESSURE ULCER

The recurrent pressure ulcer requires new insights into tissue availability and its sensibilty and remains a challenge for the plastic and reconstructive surgeon (56). These ulcers are a difficult surgical problem because the traditional methods of reconstruction have either already been used or cannot give the appropriate outcome.

It has been our experience over the last four years that in a nonsurgical approach some refractory ulcers may be temporized or managed to full healing with the vacuum-assisted closure device (VAC™, KCI Corporation). A recent publication (57) echoes the beneficial effect of negative pressure therapy in treating stage IV pressure ulcers.

The surgical repair of the pressure ulcer in a patient who has paucity of viable tissue or chronic, extensive, or recurrent postsurgical ulcers, necessitates the consideration of additional reconstructive options. We therefore must consider tissue expansion, uncommonly used muscle flaps, sensate flaps, free-tissue transfers, or flaps harvested from amputated legs or limbs to reconstruct these difficult recurrent pressure ulcers. The operative procedures are more extensive, time-consuming, may require blood transfusions, and are associated with a higher patient morbidity.

The authors Rubayi and Bernett (58), discuss their experience with one-stage reconstruction of multiple pressure ulcers over a 10-year period (between 1986 and 1996) in 120 spinal cord injured patients and present certain advantages of this comprehensive method of surgical management. They state that although cumulative operating time and intra-operative blood loss were somewhat increased, the number of anesthetic episodes and the hospital stay were less than that seen in patients managed in multiple stages. Accordingly, rehabilitation and societal reintegration could be initiated earlier, and overall hospital cost may be better contained.

Expanded Cutaneous or Myocutaneous Flaps

We have utilized the concept of tissue expansion to increase the reconstructive options to meet the needs of some of these patients (59–61). Tissue expansion has been shown to give more tissue of good quality, good vascularity, and even has the ability to bring sensate flaps to the area. This is well documented in the literature, as exemplified by the work of Cherry et al. (60), who demonstrated an increase in blood flow in expanded tissue caused by an increased vascularity appearing at the interface between the host and capsule tissue. In expanded tissue there is an increase in the number and size of vessels. Studies have shown not only an increase in the microvascularity of expanded flaps (61) but also a demonstrably increased pedicle flow. Furthermore, expanded flaps exhibit an increased survival length of 117 percent over nonexpanded control flaps (60).

The patients selected for tissue expansion can be both the high spinal cord (quadriplegic) and low spinal cord (paraplegic) injured patients with recurrent pressure ulcers, patients with a large

ulcer, or those having a limited amount of remaining viable tissue available for reconstructive purposes. In some of these patients an expanded sensate flap can be transposed to provide cover. The tissue expanders need to be defect specific and can either be round, rectangular, crescentic, or tubular shaped. Incisions for insertion of the expanders should be made away from the ulcer, usually on the lateral margin of the planned incision of the future flap. Newer techniques now allow for endoscopic placement using remote sites. For removal of wrinkles, approximately 60 to 75 cc of sterile saline must injected into the expander at the time of expander insertion. Following 1 to 2 weeks of postoperative healing time, they are then injected with amounts varying from 20-50 cc of sterile saline every 4 to 5 days, depending on the degree of skin tension and capillary refill of the overlying skin. The paraplegic patient presents a unique situation to the use of tissue expansion because symptoms of discomfort or pain from overexpansion (ordinarily one of the criteria used as a clinical gauge) cannot be used in these neuropathic individuals. Expansion is continued until enough tissue is created to close the defect. Usually a 550 to 600 cc expander may require a 6- to 8-week period for inflation to its maximum, after which the expander is removed, the ulcer is excised, and the expanded tissue incorporated into a standard myocutaneus flap (i.e., gluteus maximus, tensor fascia lata, or any other local myocutaneus flap available) to close the wound. Suction drains are inserted and left in situ for 2 to 3 weeks postoperatively. All patients are given perioperative, culture-specific intravenous antibiotics, on call to the operating room, and then 1 week postoperatively. All patients have a mechanical bowel prep as part of their preoperative preparation.

The concept of using local myocutaneous tissue that is of adequate quality but inadequate quantity, expanding it, and creating a larger surface area has been well documented to heal wounds and improve cosmesis in other areas of the body. This principle of tissue expansion was used in recurrent or difficult pressure ulcers in a prospective series of 10 consecutive patients seen over a 24-month period (59). Tissue expansion in this situation resulted in good cover of the defect with a complication rate of 10 to 15 percent. In this series, nine out of 10 patients had the gluteus myocutaneous flap expanded, and in only one patient was the tensor fascia lata flap expanded. Since reporting this consecutive series of patients, we have continued to use this concept of the expanded myocutaneous flap in many different reconstructive situations in the pressure ulcer patient with excellent results and low complication rates. A similar concept has been utilized by expanding adequate quality sensate skin in an adjacent area to provide soft tissue coverage for pressure ulcers and reduce the recurrence rate. Neves et al. (62) reported using tissue expansion of the sensate skin of the back for treatment of pressure ulcers with good results.

Muscle Flaps

SCI patients with an ischial pressure ulcer may develop perineal complications with the development of urethral fistulas and ulcerations. Kauer et al. (18) reported a 19-case series using the gracilis musculocutaneous flap to prevent such complications and emphasized that this flap has many advantages. The flap is thick, it protects the urethra from injury, it can be raised as a myocutaneous flap with a large amount of good quality skin for cutaneous defects, it has an ample arc of rotation especially as an island flap, the donor site can be closed easily, and the posterior musculocutaneous region of the thigh remains uncompromised for use in treating other ulcers. Alternatively we and others (19,20) have utilized the inferiorly based rectus abdominis myocutaneous flap with good results. Pena et al. (19) utilized an inferiorly based rectus abdominis myocutaneous flap in a series of eight recurrent or chronic perineal and ischial pressure ulcers in neurologically impaired patients, and reported distinct advantages of using this flap in such patients and a low complication rate. Bunkis et al. (21) used this inferiorly based pedicled myocutaneous flap to cover perineal and

ischial wounds, especially in previously amputated pelvises.

In refractory pressure ulcers with hip joint involvement, Evans et al. (22) reported carrying out a girdlestone arthroplasty in a 15-patient series, with no femoral stabilization, and reconstructed the soft tissue with a vastas lateralis muscle flap with good results. Paletta et al. (20) in 1993 reported use of 22 posterior thigh flaps in 21 patients for soft tissue coverage of trochanteric, ischial, and some sacral wounds. They also state that the posterior thigh flap can be used as a pedicled flap in the management of heel and foot wounds.

Sensate Flaps and Re-innervation

The concept of re-innervation of the gluteal region in paraplegics by mobilizing intercostal nerves and extending their reach by sural nerve grafts and neurotization of the required area without involving other skin areas is interesting because it is purpoted to achieve: 1) re-innervation of skin to gain protective sensibility in the pressure bearing area; and 2) re-innervation of the gluteus maximus muscle to gain voluntary muscle contraction to improve blood flow and diminish ischaemia (63).

Mackinnon et al. (64) reported a technique of re-innervating the territory of the lateral femoral cutaneous nerve (the tensor fascia lata musculocutaneous flap) using the medial antebrachial cutaneous nerve of the forearm. This neurotization procedure restored sensibilty to the area of the healed pressure ulcer. We have found that these flaps are technically demanding and usually do not serve to give enough sensation to these patients to warrant their routine use.

Another sensate flap that has been used for preventing pressure ulcer recurrence is the upper-quadrant (intercostal flap) based on the ninth, tenth, or eleventh intercostal bundles. This was reported by Spear et al. (65), who stated that the flap-covered area, with transferred sensibility, appears to be protected by referred sensation; they recommend its use in certain specific conditions where the benefit of a sensory flap outweighs the price of a more extensive procedure.

Luscher et al. (31) reported a 0 percent incidence of local recurrence in 19 consecutive neurosensory tensor fascia lata flaps and state that if the neurological pattern permits a neurosensory flap, then such flaps should be the primary choice of reconstruction to minimize long-term morbidity. This series is commendable for achieving a perfect result in their patients. Neves et al. (62) used tissue expansion of sensate skin of the back for providing adequate tissue coverage of debrided pressure ulcers without a donor site deficit, however these patients required a two-stage procedure.

Salvage Flaps (Filleted Leg/Thigh) from Amputations

The concept of using tissue that is to be discarded allows the reconstructive surgeon to treat even the most extensive, difficult, recurrent, or multiple pressure ulcers. The total thigh flap provides a large bulk of tissue for use when all other options have failed or the tissue available is inadequate for coverage of a large ulcer. This procedure is sometimes performed to save life rather than limb in severely ill patients with uncontrollable infection involving the underlying bone and in whom the ulcer is extensive. The amount of soft tissue required determines the type and length of the flap that is needed; the surgeon can use flaps of varying lengths from the knee down to the mid-lower leg region. Georgiade et al. (66) suggested making the lower incision at the knee level in carrying out a total thigh flap. For covering large sacral defects, Spira et al. (67) suggested a longer length of flap and making the lower incision approximately 9 inches below the knee joint level to allow the flap to reach; whereas Weeks et al. (68) used the entire length of soft tissue of the leg down to the level of the malleoli as an island flap for covering extensive ulcers.

In the treatment of extensive or recurrent ulceration, Berger et al. (69) describe a modification in the total thigh flap procedure by splitting the flap according to its vascularity to achieve closure of multiple pressure ulcers in a one-stage procedure.

Microvascular Free-tissue Transfer

In 1992, Yamamoto et al. (24) reported two successful reconstructions of recurrent pressure ulcers with free microvascular fasciocutaneous flaps. In the first case, a free lateral thigh pedicled on the first and third direct cutaneous branches of the deep femoral vessels was used to cover a large recurrent sacral pressure ulcer. The vascular pedicle was dissected to the deep femoral trunk proximally and anastamosed to the inferior gluteal vessels. In the second case, a free medial plantar flap was transferred to a recurrent ischial pressure ulcer. The vascular pedicle was dissected to the posterior tibial vessels proximally. The long vascular pedicle of the flap was passed through the femoral subcutaneous tunnel, and end-to-side microvascular anastomoses were performed to the superficial femoral trunk without any vein grafts. The authors advocate the use of free-tissue transfer for recurrent pressure ulcer reconstruction.

Daniel et al. (25) reported using a myocutaneous intercostal neurovascular flap that failed on day 10 post-op. Morrison et al. (26) reported using a free medial plantar flap of one side to reconstruct the heel defect of the other foot. Chen et al. (27) reported using a single, filleted lower leg myocutaneous free flap to cover multiple extensive pressure ulcers. One could utilize free-muscle flaps and fasciocutaneous flaps for pressure ulcers in insensate areas on the ankle and foot. Free-tissue transfers for pressure ulcers are long operative procedures, technically challenging, and require postoperative monitoring with specialized units to obtain consistent flap survival and healing. Even with these limitations, free flaps should be considered as an option in all reconstructive plans. Our experience demonstrates that although the use of microvascular transfer appears to be a good option, the use of other reconstructive procedures usually provides stable, long-term coverage without significant recurrence.

CONCLUSION

In conclusion, spinal cord injury is a sudden, traumatic event that not only is complicated by sensory and motor function loss but also contributes to the development of secondary conditions such as pressure ulcers. Pressure ulcers can lead to significant morbidity, prolonged or recurrent hospitalization, and diminished quality of life. Using the general principles of good medical management of the spinal cord injured patient allows the surgeon to carry out the most simple or even the most extensive surgery in this patient population to expedite healing. Initial surgical treatment must be planned so that the flap design does not violate other vascular territories or pedicles that would make future flaps impossible. Recurrent, extensive, or multiple truncal pressure ulcers are difficult to manage but become a challenge in spinal cord injured patients. A long-term stable outcome is possible in most rehabilitation centers, with dedicated reconstructive surgeons and teams.

REFERENCES

1. McGlinchey-Beroth R, Morrow L, Ahlquist M, Sarkarati M, Minaker KL. Late-life spinal cord injury and aging with a long term injury: characteristics of two emerging populations. *J Spinal Cord Med* 1995; 18(3):183–193.
2. Stover SL, Fine PR, eds., *Spinal Cord Injury: The Facts and Figures*. Birmingham, Alabama: University of Alabama at Birmingham, 1986.
3. Kynes PM. A new perspective on pressure sores prevention. *J Enterost Ther* 1986; 13(2):42–3.
4. Niazi ZBM, Salzberg CA, Byrne DW, Viehbeck M. Recurrence of initial pressure ulcer in persons with spinal cord injured injuries. *Advances in Wound Care* 1997; 10(3):38–42.
5. Trott A. Chronic skin ulcers. *Emerg Med Clin North Am* 1992; 10:823–845.
6. Byrne DW, Salzberg CA. Major risk factors for pressure ulcers in the spinal cord disabled: a literature review. *Spinal Cord* 1996; 34:255–263.
7. Salzberg CA, Byrne DW, Cayten CG, Niewerburgh PV, Murphy JG, Viehbeck M. A new pressure ulcer risk assessment scale for individuals with spinal cord injury. *Am J Phys Med Rehabil* 1996; 75(2):96–104.
8. DeVivo MJ, Kartus PL, Stover SL, Fine PR. Benefits of early admission to an organized spinal cord injury care system. *Paraplegia* 1990; 28(9):545–555.
9. Pressure ulcers in adults: prediction and prevention. Clinical practice guideline. U.S. Dept Hhs Publ Public Health Serv 1992; No. AHCPR 92-0047.
10. Hunter SM, Langemo DK, Olson B, Hanson D, Cathcart-Silberberg T, Burd C, Sauvage TR. The effectiveness of skin care protocols for pressure ulcers. *Rehabil Nurs* 1995; 20(5):250–255.
11. Salzberg CA, Byrne DW, Kabir R, van-Niewerburg P; Cayten CG. Predicting pressure ulcers during initial hospitalization for acute spinal cord injury. *Wounds* 1999; 11(2):45–57.
12. Salzberg CA, Byrne DW, Cayten CG, Kabir R, van-Niewerburgh P, Viehbeck M, Long H, Jones EC. Predicting and preventing pressure ulcers in adults with paralysis. *Advances in Wound Care* 1998; 11(5):237–246.
13. Maklebust J, Magnan MA. Risk factors associated with having a pressure ulcer: a secondary data analysis. *Adv Wound Care* 1994; 7(6):25–34.
14. Kloth LC, McCulloch JM. Promotion of wound healing and electrical stimulation. *Advances in Wound Care* 1996; 9(5):42–45.
15. Niazi ZBM, Salzberg CA. Surgical management of pressure ulcers. *Wounds* 1997; 9(3):87–93.
16. Niazi ZBM, Salzberg CA. Operative repair of pressure ulcers. In Thomas DR, Altman RM, (eds.), *Clinics in Geriatric Medicine*. Philadelphia: W.B. Saunders, Publishers 1997 August; 13(3):587–597.
17. Davies JS. Operative treatment of scars following bed sores. *Surgery* 1938; 3:1–7.
18. Kauer C, Andourah A. Perineal complications and gracilis musculocutaneous flap in patients with paraplegia: apropos of 19 cases. *Ann Chir Plast Esthet* 1991; 36(4):347–352.
19. Pena MM, Drew GS, Smith SJ, Given KS. The inferiorly based rectus abdominis myocutaneous flap for reconstruction of recurrent pressure sores. *Plast Reconstr Surg* 1992; 89(1):90–95.
20. Paletta C, Bartell T, Shehadi S. Applications of the posterior thigh flap. *Ann Plast Surg* 1993; 30(1):41–47.
21. Bunkis J, Fudem GM. Rectus abdominis flap closure of ischiosacral pressure sore. *Ann Plast Surg* 1989; 23:447.
22. Evans GR, Lewis VL Jr, Manson PN, Loomis M, Vander-kolk CA. Hip joint communication with pressure sore: the refractory wound and the role of Girdlestone arthroplasty. *Plast Reconstr Surg* 1993; 91(2):288–294.
23. Daniel RK, Faibisoff B. Muscle coverage of pressure points: the role of myocutaneous flaps. *Ann Plast Surg* 1982; 8:446.

24. Yamamoto Y, Nohira K, Shintomi Y, Igawa H, Ohura T. Reconstruction of recurrent pressure sores using free flaps. *J Reconstr Microsurg* 1992; 8(6):433–436.

25. Daniel RK, Terzis JK, Cunningham DM. Sensory skin flaps for coverage of pressure sores in paraplegic patients. *Plast Reconstr Surg* 1976; 58:317.

26. Morrison WA, Crabb DM, O'Brien BM, Jenkins A. The instep of the foot as a fasciocutaneous island and as a free flap for heel defects. *Plast Reconstr Surg* 1983; 72:56–63.

27. Chen H, Weng C, Noordhoff MS. Coverage of multiple extensive pressure sores with a single filleted lower leg myocutaneous free flap. *Plast Reconstr Surg* 1986; 78:396.

28. Karaca A, Binns J, and Blumenthal F. Complications of total ischiectomy for the treatment of ischial pressure sores. *Plast Reconstr Surg* 1974; 62:96.

29. Berlemont M, Keromest R. The dangers of removal of the ischium in the treatment of paraplegic ulcers: a review of 236 case records (Translated from French). *Revue de Chirurge Orthopedique* 1987; 73:656–664.

30. Berkwits L, Yarkony GM, Lewis V. Marjolin's ulcer complicating a pressure ulcer: case report and literature review. *Arch Phys Med Rehabil* 1986; 67(11):831–833.

31. Luscher NJ, De Roche R, Krupp S, Kuhn W, Zach GA. The sensory tensor fascia latae flap: a 9-year follow-up. *Ann Plast Surg* 1991; 26(4):306–310. Discussion 311.

32. Dansereau JG, Conway H. Closure of decubitus in paraplegics: report on 2000 cases. *PRS* 1964; 33:474.

33. Disa JJ, Curlton JM, Goldberg NH. Efficacy of operative cure in pressure sore patients. *PRS* 1992; 89:272–278.

34. Evans GRD, Dufresne CR, Manson PN. Surgical correction of pressure ulcers in an urban center: is it efficacious? *Advances in Wound Care* 1994; 7(1):40–46.

35. Griffith BH and Schultz RC. The prevention and surgical tratment of recurrent decubitus ulcer. *Acta Chirurgica Scandinavia* 1942; 87(76S):207.

36. Harding RL. An analysis of 100 rehabilitated paraplegics. *PRS* 1961; 27:235.

37. Lamid S, El Ghatit AZ. Smoking, spasticity, and pressure sores in spinal cord injured patients. *Am J Phys Med* 1983; 62(6):300–306.

38. Mathes SJ, Feng LJ, Hunt TK. Coverage of the infected wound. Ann Surg 1983; 198(4):420–429.

39. Relander M, Palmer B. Recurrence or surgically treated pressure sores. *Scand J Plast Reconstr Surg* 1988; 22:89–92.

40. Rubayi S, Cousins S, Valentine WA. Myocutaneous flaps: surgical treatment of severe pressure ulcers. *AORN J* 1990; 52(1):40–55.

41. Salzberg CA. Recurrence of pressure ulcers in 219 spinal cord injured patients. 40th Annual Conference of the American Paraplegic Society. September 1994, Las Vegas.

42. Goodman CM, Cohen V, Armenta A, Thornby J, Netscher DT. Evaluation of results and treatment variables for pressure ulcers in 48 veteran spinal cord injured patients. *Annals of Plastic Surgery* 1999; 42(6):665–672.

43. Manley MT. Incidence, contributory factors, and cost of pressure sores. *South African Medical Journal* 1978; 53:217–222.

44. Gosnell DJ. An assessment tool to identify pressure sores. *Nurs Res* 1973; 22:55–59.

45. Oot-Giromini BA. Pressure ulcer prevalence, incidence and associated risk factors in the community. *Decubitus* 1993; 6:24–32.

46. Bogie KM, Nusibeh I, Bader DL. New concepts in the prevention of pressure sores. In Frankel HL ed., *Handbook of Clinical Neurology—Spinal Cord Trauma* 1992; 17:347–366.

47. Reuler JB, Cooney TG. The pressure sore: pathophysiology and principles of management. *Ann Intern Med* 1981; 94:661–666.

48. Guralnik JM, Harris TB, White LR, Coroini-Huntley JC. Occurrence and predictors of pressure sores in National Health and Nutrition Examination survey follow-up. *J Am Geriatr Soc* 1988; 36:807–812.

49. Langemo DK, Catheart-Silberberg T. Incidence and prediction of pressure ulcers in five patient care settings. *Decubitus* 1991; 4:25–36.

50. Salzberg CA. Smoking and pressure sores in spinal cord injured patients. 40th Annual Conference of the American Paraplegia Society, September 1994, Las Vegas.

51. Barton AA. Prevention of pressure sores. *Nurs Times* 1977; 73:1593–1595.

52. Copeland-Fields LD, Hoshiko BR. Clinical validation of Braden and Bergstrom's conceptual schema of pressure sore risk factors. *Rehabil Nurs* 1989; 14(5):257–260.

53. Jensen TT, Juncker Y. Pressure sores common after hip operations. *Acta Orthop Scand* 1987; 58(3):209–211.

54. Petersen NC, Bittmann S. The epidemiology of pressure sores. *Scand J Plast Reconstr Surg* 1971; 5:62–66.

55. Berlowitz DR, Wilking SVB. Risk factors for pressure sores: a comparison of cross-sectional and cohort-derived data. *J Am Geriatr Soc* 1988; 36:1043–1050.

56. Niazi ZBM, Salzberg CA. Surgical management of the difficult recurrent pressure sore. In Lee BY, ed., *Cutaneous Ulcers and Pressure Ulcers.* Chapman and Hall Publishers, New York 1998. Pp. 246–252.

57. Baynham SA, Kohlman P, Katner HP. Treating Stage IV pressure ulcers with negative pressure therapy: a case report. *Ostomy Wound Management* 1999; 45(4):28–35.

58. Rubayi S, Burnett CC. The efficacy of single-stage surgical management of multiple pressure sores in spinal cord-injured patients. *Ann Plast Surg* 1999; 42(5):533–539.

59. Gray CG, Salzberg CA, Petro JA, Salisbury RE. The expanded flap for reconstruction of the difficult pressure sore. *Decubitus* 1990; 3(2):17–20.

60. Cherry GW, Austed ED, Pasyk K, et al. Increased survival and vascularity of random-pattern skin flaps elevated in controlled expanded skin. *Plast Reconstr Surg* 1983; 72:680.

61. Forte V, Middleton WG, Briant TD. Expansion of myocutaneous flaps. *Arch Otolaryngology* 1983; 11:371.

62. Neves RI, Kahler SH, Banducci DR, Manders EK. Tissue expansion of sensate skin for pressure sores. *Ann Plast Surg* 1992; 29(5):433–437.

63. Hauge EN. The anatomical basis of a new method for re-innervation of the gluteal region in paraplegics. *Acta Physiol Scand Suppl* 1991:603:19–21.

64. Mackinnon SE, Dellon AL, Patterson GA, Gruss JS. Medial antebrachial cutaneous–lateral femoral cutaneous neurotization to provide sensation to pressure-bearing areas in the paraplegic patient. *Ann Plast Surg* 1985; 14:541–544.

65. Spear SL, Kroll SS, Little JW. Bilateral upper-quadrant (intercostal) flaps: the value of protective sensation in preventing pressure sore recurrence. *Plast Reconstr Surg* 1987; 80:734–736.

66. Georgiade N, Pickrell K, Maguire C. Total thigh flaps for extensive decubitus ulcer. *Plast Reconstr Surg* 1956; 17:220.

67. Spira M, Hardy SB. Our experience with high thigh amputations in paraplegics. *Plast Reconstr Surg* 1963; 31:344.

68. Weeks PM, Brower TD. Island flap coverage of extensive decubitus ulcers. *Plast Reconstr Surg* 1968; 42:433.

69. Berger SR, Rubayi S, Griffin AC. Closure of multiple pressure sores with split total thigh flap. *Ann Plast Surg* 1994; 33(5):548–551.

21

Nutrition in Spinal Cord Injured Patients

NANAKRAM AGARWAL, MD, MPH, FRCS, FACS

APPROXIMATELY 10,000 PERSONS sustain spinal cord injuries in the United States each year. Through technologic advances, these patients can live out near-normal life spans (30 to 40 years post-injury). The leading causes of death in spinal cord injured patients are pneumonia (20.5 percent), heart disease (15 percent), accidents (9.7 percent), infections (8.8 percent), and pulmonary complications (8.5 percent) (1). One of the major problems, however, continues to be infection, leading to repeated hospitalizations.

Malnutrition is a significant covariable in the occurrence of infection and prognosis of the spinal cord injured patient. Studies on hospitalized patients show that malnutrition contributes to an increased incidence of morbidity and mortality (2) and is a significant factor in the development of acquired immune deficiencies (3), defective wound healing (4), pressure sore formation (5), cardiac (6) and respiratory insufficiency (7), and infectious complications (8). The preservation of nutritional status would, therefore, appear to be a major factor in improving the prognosis in these patients. Fortunately, most patients are healthy and well-nourished before their injuries. A better understanding of the physiology of trauma, the prevention of malnutrition and appropriate treatment when present, and the provision of adequate amounts of nitrogen and fuel, based on the patient's nutri-

tional requirements are essential in achieving this goal.

METABOLIC RESPONSE TO SPINAL CORD INJURY

Many of the metabolic changes seen in spinal cord injury (SCI) are nonspecific and are subsequent to the trauma. O'Connell and Gardner (9) have divided the clinical course of spinal cord injury into two major periods: the stage of flaccidity, or *spinal shock*, and the return of reflex activity. The stage of flaccidity averages 6 weeks after the initial transaction of the spinal cord and is characterized by an acute vasodepression and fall in basal metabolic rate roughly proportional to the degree of shock. Nitrogen balance becomes negative from day 1 (10) and can reach a peak of up to 25 grams per day 2 to 4 weeks after injury (11). This negative nitrogen balance after SCI is obligatory and correlates with the extent of SCI or degree of motor dysfunction (12). There is also a negative fluid balance in the initial 3 to 4 weeks, orthostatic hypertension is severe, and gastrointestinal function can be either hypoactive or hyperactive (13).

The return of reflex activity is associated with abnormal loss of nitrogen, progressive weight loss, increased proportion of body fat, decreased lean body mass, and a reduction in energy expenditure (14–17). Despite more than adequate protein and calorie administration, nitrogen losses are not minimized (18). There is a drastic loss of total body potassium that is more pronounced in quadriplegia than in paraplegia. Although the decrease in total body water parallels the loss in body weight, sodium is retained, resulting in a relative increase in extracellular water (19). There is a decrease in muscle blood flow, and atrophied muscle cells are eventually replaced by connective tissue (14). Hypercalciuria and hyperphosphaturia induced by immobilization and inactivity occur in the early stages of the disease and remain until mobilization occurs (9, 19).

NUTRITIONAL ASSESSMENT

Controversy still exists over methods of identifying or classifying malnutrition (20). Currently available methods range from simple clinical judgment to highly sophisticated and expensive tests for estimating body composition. Some form of objective data is generally required to document the type and degree of nutritional depletion. Objective information also provides a means of monitoring the efficacy of therapeutic interventions. Most importantly, serial objective measurements enable early identification of the high-risk patient and early institution of aggressive nutritional support to reduce morbidity and mortality (21).

Body Weight

Body weight, a simple and valuable gross measurement of body composition, is measured inexactly and infrequently. In the trauma setting, Kinney and associates (22) have demonstrated that there is a high risk of death with a 25 percent weight loss. The percentage of ideal body weight is determined with reference to weights for age, sex, and height using Metropolitan Life Insurance tables. Mild protein-calorie malnutrition is defined as a body weight of 80 to 90 percent of ideal body weight, moderate malnutrition as 70 to 80 percent of ideal body weight,

and severe malnutrition as less than 70 percent of ideal body weight (23). It is far more valuable, however, to assess the percentage of usual body weight or percent weight change over a given period of time. A loss of 1 to 2 percent of body weight in 1 week, 5 percent in 1 month, or 10 percent in 6 months is considered clinically significant (24).

The interpretation of changes in body weight requires careful consideration of various factors. A gain or loss of greater than 0.2 kg/day is uncommon. Rapid changes in body weight (10 percent of body weight in 2 weeks or less) most likely reflect changes in total body water as seen with overhydration, dehydration, ascites, pleural effusion, or edema (24).

From a practical standpoint, daily measurements of body weight provide valuable diagnostic and therapeutic information.

After the initial weight loss over the first 3 to 4 months after injury, there should be very little change in the patient's body weight. However, chronic spinal cord injured patients have a tendency toward weight gain, with weight changes seen in individual patients related to changes in fat content (25). Peiffer suggests that the ideal body weight of spinal cord injured patients should be maintained at 4.5 kg and 9.0 kg below calculated ideal body weight for paraplegics and quadriplegics, respectively (26).

Body Fat

In clinical practice, body fat mass is most commonly assessed by measuring the triceps skinfold thickness with Lange skinfold calipers. A mean of three readings taken from the back of the nondominant arm, midway between the acromial process and the olecranon process of the ulna, is usually expressed as a percentage of the standard (50th percentile) value. Severe depletion is indicated by a value less than 60 to 80 percent of the standard value (24). Certain precautions are needed in interpreting body fat measurements: individual observer variation, position of patient, duration and amount of pressure, presence of edema or subcutaneous emphysema, or change of site by more than 1 cm can result in a significant variation (27).

Muscle Mass or Somatic Protein Mass

The size of the skeletal muscle mass varies considerably according to the physical condition of the body, presence or absence of disease, and disuse (28). Skeletal muscle mass represents 4 to 6 kg of the body's total 10 to 12 kg of protein and serves as the major source of protein during periods of starvation and stress. Alterations in work capacity are also related to muscle mass. Of the various methods described in the literature for assessing muscle mass, anthropometry and 24-hour urinary creatinine levels are commonly used (24).

Midarm Circumference and Midarm Muscle Circumference. The midarm circumference is measured at the same site as the triceps skinfold thickness. The midarm muscle circumference (MAMC) is derived from the midarm circumference (MAC) and the triceps skinfold (TSF): MAMC = MAC − (0.314 × TSF). Both values are also expressed as a percentage of standard. Severe protein-caloric malnutrition is indicated by a value less than 60 percent of standard (24). Anthropometric measurements, although simple, quick, noninvasive, and inexpensive, have limited accuracy because they measure individual muscle groups rather than total muscle mass and are subject to all the errors mentioned for triceps skinfold measurements.

24-Hour Urinary Creatinine. The 24-hour urinary excretion of creatinine is a simple, inexpensive, and noninvasive index of muscle mass (29). A significant relationship has been demonstrated between muscle mass and urinary creatinine excretion in both adults and children. As compared with a mean creatinine excretion of 23 mg/kg/day in healthy men, 24-hour urinary creatinine excretion in chronic spinal cord injured patients is decreased. There is a greater decrease in quadriplegics (11.81 + 3.53 mg/kg) than in paraplegics (17.06 ± 5.21 mg/kg), and the decrease correlates with the level of spinal cord

injury (30). In this manner, 24-hour urinary creatinine excretion has the potential for use in monitoring muscle mass in spinal cord injured patients.

Visceral Protein Mass

Visceral protein mass, the second component of body cell mass, accounts for approximately 2 kg of the total protein in a healthy adult man. It is generally measured by albumin, transferrin, retinol-binding protein, and thyroxine-binding prealbumin. The levels of these plasma proteins are more sensitive measuring criteria for protein-caloric malnutrition than anthropometric measurements. In the presence of stress secondary to surgery, trauma, or sepsis, profound deficiencies in visceral proteins occur before any significant decrease in anthropometric measurements is seen (24). Their fall represents decreased liver biosynthesis and turnover, and their rise parallels nutritional recovery. Besides malnutrition, other factors known to influence the levels of visceral proteins include the rate of metabolic utilization, excretion, intravascular–extravascular transfer, hydration, and type of resuscitation fluid (31).

Albumin. Serum albumin is still the most widely studied objective measurement and is considered by some to be the most useful indicator of malnutrition (32). An albumin level of 3.0 to 3.5 gm/dL is suggestive of mild malnutrition; a level between 2.1 and 2.9 gm/dL suggests moderate malnutrition; and a level of 2.0 gm/dL or less suggests severe malnutrition (24).

Transferrin. Serum transferrin, a more sensitive visceral protein, has a shorter half-life (8.8 days) and a smaller plasma pool (5.29 gm) than albumin (33). Thus, serum transferrin levels more rapidly reflect changes in visceral protein. Actual serum transferrin values are measured by radioimmunodiffusion. However, because this technique is not readily available, transferrin values are generally calculated from the total iron-binding capacity (TIBC) (24): transferrin (mg/dL) = (0.8 × TIBC) − 43. A value between

151 and 175 mg/dL suggests mild malnutrition; a value between 100 and 150 mg/dL suggests moderate depletion; and a value less than 100 mg/dL suggests severe malnutrition.

Immunologic Assessment

The importance of immunocompetence to the survival of patients who have had surgery or sepsis has been recognized for the past decade. In many patients, the competence of the immune system is clearly related to nutritional status (3,8), but in others this relationship may not be as direct. An immunologic assessment includes a total lymphocyte count, a delayed cutaneous hypersensitivity test, serum complement levels, and tests for other cellular immune functions.

Total Lymphocyte Count. Total lymphocyte count, readily available in most patients within hours of admission, has been described as a "poor man's" assessment of immunocompetency (34) and predictor of postoperative sepsis (35). The count, derived by multiplying the percentage of lymphocytes in peripheral smear by the white blood cell count, is considered abnormal if it is less than 1,500/ mm^3 and is suggestive of severe malnutrition if less than 800/mm^3.

Delayed Cutaneous Hypersensitivity. Delayed hypersensitivity is determined by intradermal injections of 0.1 mL of four recall antigens: mumps, *Candida albicans*, purified protein derivative of tuberculin, and trichophytin. The skin test is considered positive if there is an induration with a diameter of 5 mm or greater at either 24 or 48 hours. Persons are classified as normal if they have test results with two or more positive readings, relatively anergic if only one test is positive, and anergic if all tests are negative.

Besides malnutrition, a large number of non-nutritional factors can influence the results of these tests. These factors include infections, uremia, cirrhosis, hepatitis, trauma, burns, hemorrhage, steroids, immunosuppressants, general anesthesia, and surgery (36); these tests, therefore, may have limited applicability in the SCI patient.

Nutritional Status of Spinal Cord Injured Patients

An unexpectedly large percentage of patients with spinal cord injury show characteristics of malnutrition. In the acute phase, nutrient deficiencies such as albumin (100 percent of patients), carotene (62 percent), transferrin (37 percent), ascorbate (25 percent), thiamine (24 percent), folate (20 percent), and copper (11 percent) were documented most frequently at 2 weeks post-injury. There was an average of 2.0, 1.6, and 1.2 nutrient abnormalities per patient at 2, 4, and 8 weeks post-injury, respectively, and dependent plasma proteins such as albumin and transferrin remained low throughout the entire 8 week post-injury study period (37). Similarly, a nutritional assessment of 17 otherwise healthy chronic paraplegic men revealed that none of the patients had normal values for all four objective measurements (albumin, transferrin, total lymphocyte count, and cutaneous hypersensitivity). Mild malnutrition was evident in 47 percent of patients, 53 percent demonstrated some index of moderate malnutrition, and a large majority (82 percent) were immunodeficient (38).

ENERGY EXPENDITURE

The spinal cord injured, when compared with sex-and-age matched control subjects, have lower 24-hour energy expenditures. This lower energy expenditure in SCI persons can be explained by lower values of spontaneous physical activity, resting metabolic rate, fat free mass, and thermic effect of food (39). The basal metabolic rate and total energy expenditure correlates with the level of lesion and is significantly less than that predicted by standard formulas based on the normal population (40, 41). This decrease in energy expenditure is, however, most marked in quadriplegics, with individual paraplegics exhibiting significant variations in their measured resting energy expenditure, ranging from 82 to 125 percent of predicted values.

The energy costs of ambulation and even simple activities are higher in spinal cord injured patients than those of a normal person. In their extensive literature review, Fisher and Gullickson (42) found that a normal person walks at a rate of about 83 meters/min with an energy expenditure of 0.063 Kcal/min/kg. The disabled person walks more slowly to avoid incurring an increase in energy expenditure per minute. The more disabled the person, the more slowly he walks and the less efficient he becomes in terms of energy expenditure/Kcal/unit distance. Clinkingbeard et al. (43) have shown that paraplegics consume nine times the energy per meter expended by a normal person walking at his comfortable walking speed. Furthermore, patients with a lumbar lesion walked five times faster than those with a thoracic lesion and used 320 percent less energy expenditure per unit distance. Proper prescription braces in paraplegics reduce energy consumption, but no matter how well prescribed and fitted the braces are, a severe loss of function still exists that causes a very large energy expenditure of ambulation. Energy expenditure for propelling a wheelchair is not significantly less than that used in walking at corresponding speeds but requires 9 percent more Kcal/min than normal ambulation. Energy expenditure during wheelchair locomotion is directly related to speed and is also greater with use of upper extremities than with use of lower extremities (42).

The activity level of quadriplegics with high-level lesions is profoundly decreased by their motor deficits. The activity level of quadriplegics with low-level lesions and paraplegics varies widely on the basis of physical abilities, individual personality, motivation, and interest. Not surprisingly, total energy expenditure and caloric needs in quadriplegics with high-level lesions are significantly less than in quadriplegics with lower lesions and in paraplegics. In contrast, total energy expenditure in many paraplegics may exceed the energy expenditure of normal patients (40).

NUTRITIONAL REQUIREMENTS

SCI patients, in general, should be given a low caloric diet. Cox et al. (41) have demonstrated

that stable, rehabilitating patients require 23.4 Kcal/kg/day, with quadriplegics requiring 22.7 Kcal/kg/day and paraplegics requiring 27.9 Kcal/kg/day. Rodriguez et al. (12) recommend that elimination of the activity factor of 1.2 (due to the diminished activity arising from paralysis) and a diminution of the stress factor from initial predicted energy expenditure calculation will provide more appropriate caloric needs.

Spinal cord injured patients have a tendency toward weight gain and are at increased risk for developing obesity-related disorders such as diabetes (44) and cardiovascular disease (45). Obesity and loss of weight are the result of an imbalance between caloric intake and energy output. In a study of 17 paraplegics, significant differences in energy expenditure were observed: only 29.4 percent were normometabolic with a measured resting energy expenditure (MREE) of 90 to 110 percent of predicted resting energy expenditure (PREE); 35.3 percent were hypermetabolic with an MREE more than 110 percent PREE; and 35.3 percent were hypometabolic with an MREE less than 90 percent PREE. Although caloric intake of the three metabolic groups was identical, none of the patients in the hypermetabolic group were overweight, because caloric intake was identical to measured energy expenditure. In contrast, the hypometabolic patients were consuming significantly more calories than were expended, and obesity (weight >110 percent ideal body weight) was maximum in hypometabolic patients (83.3 percent) (38). Optimal calorie intake should be established according to the patient's previous state of nutrition and metabolic status. A large majority may benefit from weight loss, while a few may require higher levels of caloric intake.

Spinal cord injured patients require more protein because they experience increased nitrogen loss. Albumin elimination rates are increased in paraplegics (46), protein loss through pressure sores is directly related to the size of the sore (5), and the negative nitrogen balance is accentuated by the presence of infection or stress of surgery. All the aforementioned factors should be taken into account when calculating the amount of protein required to keep the patient in a positive nitrogen balance. The recommended intake of protein is 1.5 to 2.0 gm/kg/day with a ratio of nonprotein calories to nitrogen of approximately 100 calories per gram of nitrogen (47). Sources of protein that contain the highest percentage of essential amino acids (fish, egg, milk) are more efficiently utilized than plant proteins.

Both carbohydrates and fat should be used as nonprotein sources of energy following injury. The maximal rate of glucose oxidation is around 6 to 7 mg/kg/min, and higher infusion rates stimulate lipogenesis. As such, glucose infusion should not exceed 4 to 5 mg/kg/min, equivalent to 400 to 500 g/day of glucose in a 70-kg person, and providing approximately 50 percent to 60 percent of the total caloric requirement. Excess carbohydrate has been associated with hyperglycemia, hypercarbia, increased ventilatory drive, inability to wean from the ventilator, and a fatty liver. Blood glucose levels greater than 220 mg/dI have been shown to be associated with a significantly greater incidence of severe infection, bacteremia, or pneumonia. Insulin should be administered to maintain blood glucose levels below 200 mg/dl, as far as possible (48).

The balance of the 40 to 50 percent of the total caloric requirement should be 20 to 30 percent from lipids (not to exceed 2.5 g/kg/day) and 20 to 30 percent from protein. At least 3 percent of the total calories should be provided as fat to prevent essential fatty acid deficiency. Increasing fat calories up to 50 percent of total calories may be helpful in weaning patients off ventilators and achieving a better blood glucose control in diabetics and patients receiving high doses of steroids (47). However, increased fat administration has been associated with hyperlipidemia, hypoxia, cholestasis, and an increased rate of infection (48).

Overfeeding is deleterious and should be avoided. Overfeeding cannot reverse tissue catabolism (49). In effect, overfeeding increases the risk of mortality. Postoperative patients receiving calories equal to 150 percent of measured energy expenditure (MEE), when compared to patients given calories equal to MEE,

had a significantly greater mortality (40 versus 28 percent) (50). Therefore, it is suggested that during the acute stress period, the best goal is "moderation." Caloric intake should be reduced to 80 percent of caloric needs with adequate protein supplements provided (47). In addition, daily requirements of electrolytes, vitamins, and trace elements should be provided. It is generally agreed that there is an increased need for vitamins (especially A, C, and E) and minerals (zinc, selenium, and magnesium) (47). It has been recommended that 25,000 IU of vitamin A per day be given to patients receiving steroids (51).

TIMING AND ROUTE OF NUTRITIONAL SUPPORT

Several studies have shown that malnutrition develop within the first several days following admission. The critical times for nutritional assessment are at admission and whenever patient condition or mobility is compromised. If a deficit in dietary intake or nutritional status is identified, nutrient intake must be increased by dietary modification, supplementation, or spoon feeding.

Tube feeding should be considered if oral intake is compromised. Current evidence suggests that besides the advantages of safety, convenience, and cost, enteral feeding preserves gut mucosal mass and normal gut flora, prevents increased gut permeability to bacteria and other toxins, maintains mucosal immunity and gut-associated lymphoid tissue, and attenuates the hypermetabolic response to injury (52). When compared to total parenteral nutrition, institution of early enteral nutrition significantly lowers the incidence of septic morbidity. Parenteral nutrition should be administered only when enteral access cannot be obtained, when enteral nutrition support fails to meet nutritional requirements, or when feeding into the gastrointestinal tract is contraindicated. Subsequent transition to oral feeding should be implemented as soon as enteral access is obtained or gastrointestinal function improves. Either gastric or small bowel feeding is acceptable. Small bowel feedings via nasoenteric tubes placed under flwith fluroscopic or endoscopic guidance does increase tolerance to feeds but does not effectively reduce the risk of aspiration and pneumonia. As such, enteral feeding should not be delayed in order to establish small bowel access. A majority of patients tolerate some amount of intragastric feedings, and small bowel feedings may be reserved for those patients who do not tolerate gastric feeds (53).

Although provision of nutrients by tube feeding is beneficial, there are also inherent disadvantages. In the individual more prone to development of pressure sores, fecal incontinence, diarrhea, and moisture can increase the likelihood of the sores occurring or worsen their conditions. Second, the use of restraints after the insertion of tubes can possibly limit mobility. Third, enteral nutrition promotes gastric colonization with potentially pathogenic microorganisms, and there is a significant risk of aspiration (54). Fourth, although they are difficult to estimate, adverse effects can result from loss of mealtime socialization and interaction with staff, including loss of self-esteem (55).

PHYSICAL ACTIVITY AND NUTRITIONAL SUPPORT

A positive nitrogen balance is often not achieved in patients despite the provision of sufficient amounts of both calories and amino acids. An important factor contributing to this may be immobility. In their classic studies, Deitrick et al. (56) have shown that immobilization of normal men with adequate nutrient intake resulted in a net loss of nitrogen, potassium, phosphorous, calcium, and sulfur. These deleterious effects were significantly reduced by the use of an oscillating bed (57).

As early as 1932, Cutbertson (58), in a study of patients recuperating from lower extremity fractures or osteotomy of long bones, demonstrated that massage, "an ancient therapeutic adjunct," supplemented by passive movement of the affected extremity, resulted in increased retention of nitrogen, sulfur, and phosphorus.

Recently, Gibson et al. (59), in their study of patients with long leg casts for fracture of the tibia, observed that short periods of low-voltage percutaneous electrical stimulation of muscles improved muscle-protein synthesis and prevented disuse muscle atrophy.

CONCLUSION

A multidisciplinary approach is required for optimal care of spinal cord injured patients. They are at significant risk nutritionally, and successful management requires close attention to their nutritional status, tailoring of nutritional therapy to their needs, early intensive treatment, aggressive physical therapy, and early ambulation.

REFERENCES

1. Stover SL, File PR. *Spinal Cord Injury: The Facts and Figures.* Birmingham, Alabama: University of Alabama, 1986.
2. Mullen J, Buzby GP, Matthews DC, et al. Reduction of operative morbidity and mortality by combined preoperative and postoperative nutritional support. *Ann Surg* 1980; 192:604.
3. Law DK, Durdrick SJ, Abdou NI. The effects of protein caloric malnutrition on immune competence of the surgical patient. *Sur & Gynecol Obstet* 1974; 139:257.
4. Greenhaigh DG, Gamelli RL. Is impaired wound healing caused by infection or nutritional depletion? *Surgery* 1987; 102:306.
5. Mulholland JH, Tui C, Wright AM, et al. Protein metabolism and bed sores. *Ann Surg* 1943; 118:1015.
6. Viart P. Hemodynamic findings during treatment of protein-caloric malnutrition. *Am J Clin Nutr* 1978; 31:911.
7. Askanazi J, Weissman C, Rosenbaum SH, et al. Nutrition and the respiratory system. *Crit Care Med* 1982; 10:163.
8. Newmann CG. Interaction of malnutrition and infection—a neglected clinical concept. *Arch Intern Med* 1977; 137:1364.
9. O'Connell FB Jr., Gardner WJ. Metabolism in paraplegia. *JAMA* 1953; 153:706.
10. Kaufman HH, Rowlands BJ, Stein DK, et al. General metabolism in patients with acute paraplegia and quadriplegia. *Neurosurgery* 1985; 16:309.

11. Cooper IS, Hoen TI. Metabolic disorders in paraplegia. *Neurology* 1952; 2:332.

12. Rodriguez DJ, Benzel EC, Clevenger FW. The metabolic response to spinal cord injury. *Spinal Cord* 1997; 35:599–604.

13. Claus-Walker J, Halstead LS. Metabolic and endocrine changes in spinal cord injury. II: Partial decentralization of the autonomic nervous system. *Arch Phys Med Rehabil* 1982; 63:576.

14. Claus-Walker J, Halstead LS. Metabolic and endocrine changes in spinal cord injury: the nervous system before and after transaction of the spinal cord. *Arch Phys Med Rehabil* 1981; 62:595.

15. Nuhlicek DN, Spurr GB, Barboriak JJ, et al. Body composition of patients with spinal cord injury. *Eur J Clin Nutr* 1988; 42:765–773.

16. Shizgal HM, Rosa A, Leduc B, et al. Body composition in quadriplegic patient. *J Parenteral Enteral Nutr* 1986; 10:364.

17. Sedlock DA, Laventure SJ. Body composition and resting energy expenditure in long term spinal cord injury. *Paraplegia* 1990; 28:448–454.

18. Rodriguez DJ, Clevenger FW, Osler TM, et al. Obligatory negative nitrogen balance following spinal cord injury. *JPEN* 1991; 35:319–322.

19. Cardus D, McTaggart WG. Body sodium and potassium in men with spinal cord injury. *Arch Phys Med Rehabil* 1985; 66:156.

20. Laren DS, Meguid MM. Nutritional assessment at the crossroad. *J Parenteral Enteral Nutr* 1983; 7:575.

21. Agarwal N. Nutritional and metabolic assessment and monitoring in trauma. *Trauma Q* 1987; 3(3):64.

22. Kinney JH, Duke JH Jr, Long CL. Tissue fuel and weight loss after injury. *J Clin Pathol* (Suppl) 1978; 4:65.

23. Grant JP, Custer PB, Tliurlow J. Current techniques of nutritional assessment. *Surg Clin North Am* 1981; 61:437.

24. Blackburn GL, Bistrain BR, Maini BS, et al. Nutritional and metabolic assessment of the hospitalized patient. *J Parenteral Enteral Nutr* 1977; 1:11.

25. Greenway RM, Houser HB, Lindan O, Weir DR. Long-term changes in gross body composition of paraplegic and quadriplegic patients. *Paraplegia* 1969; 7:301.

26. Peiffer SC, Blust P, Leyson JF. Nutritional assessment of the spinal cord injured patient. *J Am Diet Assoc* 1981; 78:501.

27. Hull JC, O'Quigley J, Giles GR, et al. Upper limb anthropometry: the value of measurement variance studies. *Am J Clin Nutr* 1980; 33:1846.

28. Moore FD, Oleson KH, McMurphy JD, et al. The body cell mass and its supporting environment. In Body Composition in Health and Disease. Philadelphia: W.B. Saunders, 1963. Pp. 485.

29. Heymsfield SB, Arleaga C, McManus C, et al. Measurement of muscle mass in humans: validity of the 24 urinary creatinine method. *Am J Clin Nutr* 1983; 37:478.

30. Agarwal N, Lee BY, DelGuercio LRM. Urinary creatinine excretion in spinal cord injured patients. *Nutrition* 1987; 3:192.

31. Godan MHN, Wateriow JC, Picun D. Protein turn-over, synthesis and breakdown before and after recovery from protein-energy malnutrition. *Clin Sci Mol Med* 1977; 53:473.

32. Agarwal N, Acevedo F, Leighton LS, et al. Predictive ability of various nutritional variables for mortality in elderly people. *Am J Clin Nutr* 1988; 48:1173.

33. Awai M, Brown EB. Studies of the metabolism of I-131 labeled human transferrin. *J Lab Clin Med* 1963; 61:363.

34. Seltzer MH, Bastidas JA, Cooper DM, et al. Instant nutritional assessment. *J Parenteral Enteral Nutr* 1979; 3:157.

35. Lewis RT, Klein H. Risk factors in postoperative sepsis: significance of preoperative lymphocytopenia. *J Surg Res* 1975; 26:365.

36. Blackburn, GL, Harvey, KB. Nutritional assessment as a routine in clinical medicine. *Postgrad Med* 1982; 71:46–63.

37. Laven GT, Huang CT, De Vivo MJ, et al. Nutritional status during the acute stage of spinal cord injury. *Arch Phys Med Rehabil* 1989; 70:277–282.

38. Lee BY, Agarwal N, Corcoran L, et al. Assessment of nutritional and metabolic status of paraplegics. *J Rehabil Res* 1985; 22:11.

39. Monroe MB, Tataranni PA, Pratley R, et al. Lower daily energy expenditure as measured by a respiratory chamber in subjects with spinal cord injury compared with control subjects. *Am J Clin Nutr* 1998; 68:1223–1227.

40. Mollinger LS, Spurr GB, El Ghatit AZ, et al. Daily energy expenditure and basal metabolic rates of patients with spinal cord injury. *Arch Phys Med Rehabil* 1985; 66:420.

41. Cox SAR, Weiss SM, Posuniak EA, et al. Energy expenditure after spinal cord injury: an evaluation of stable rehabilitating patients. *J Trauma* 1985; 25:419.

42. Fisher SV, Gullickson G Jr. Energy cost of ambulation in health and disability: a literature review. *Arch Phys Med Rehabil* 1978; 59:124.

43. Clinkingbeard JR, Gersten JW, Hoehn D. Energy cost of ambulation in the traumatic paraplegic. Am J Phys Med 1964; 43:157.

44. Bauman WA, Spungen AM. Disorders of carbohydrate and lipid metabolism in veterans with paraplegia or quadriplegia: a model of premature aging *J Clin Invest* 1990; 85:893–898.

45. Krum H, Howes LG, Brown DJ, et al. Risk factors for cardiovascular disease in chronic spinal cord injury patients. *Paraplegia* 1992; 30:381–388.

46. Ring J, Seirert J, Lob G, et al. Elimination rate of human albumin in paraplegic patients. *Paraplegia* 1974; 12:139.

47. DeBiasse MA, Whilmore DW. What is optimal nutritional support? *New Horizons* 1994; 2:122–130.

48. Frankel WL, Evans NJ, Rombeau JL. Scientific rational and clinical application of parenteral nutrition in critically ill patients. In Rombeau JL, Caldwell MD, eds., *Clinical Nutrition, Parenteral Nutrition*, 2nd ed., Philadelphia: W.B. Saunders, 1993. Pp. 597–616.

49. Chwals WJ. Overfeeding the critically ill child: fact or fantasy? New Horizon 1994; 2:147–155.

50. Vo NM, Wayscaster M, Acuff RV, et al. Effect of postoperative carbohydrate overfeeding. *Am Surg* 1987; 53:632–635.

51. Levenson SM, Demetriou AA. Metabolic factors. In Cohen IK, Diegelmann RF, Lindblad WJ, eds., *Wound Healing: Biochemical and Chemical Aspects*. Philadelphia: W.B. Saunders, 1992. Pp. 248–273.

52. Minard G, Kudsk KA. Is early feeding beneficial? How early is early? *New Horizons* 1994; 2:156–163.

53. Heyland DK. Nutritional support in the critically ill patient: a critical review of the evidence. *Critical Care Clinics* 1998; 14:423–439.

54. Pingleton S, Hinthorn D, Liu C. Enteral nutrition in patients receiving mechanical ventilation. *Am J Med* 1986; 80:827–832.

55. Finucane T E. Malnutrition, tube feeding and pressure sores: data are incomplete. *J Am Geriatr Soc* 1995; 43:447–451.

56. Deitrick JE, Wheldon GD, Shorr E. The effects of immobilization upon various metabolic and physiologic functions of normal men. *Am J Med* 1948; 4:3–36.

57. Wheldon GD, Deitrick JE, Shorr E. Modifications of the effects of immobilization upon metabolic and physiologic functions of normal men by the use of an oscillating bed. *Am J Med* 1949; 6:684–711.

58. Cutbertson DP. Certain effects of massage on the metabolism of convalescing fracture cases. *O J Med* 1932; 25:401–408.

59. Gibson JNA, Smith K, Rennie MJ. Prevention of disuse muscle atrophy by means of electrical stimulation: maintenance of protein synthesis. *Lancet* 1988; 2:767–771.

22 Psychosocial Aspects of Spinal Cord Injury

NEIL R. BOCKIAN, PhD
CLAUDIA S. FIDANQUE, PsyD
ANGELA LEE, MA, CSW

SPINAL CORD INJURY (SCI) has a profound impact on the life of the affected individual. In this review, the authors highlight some of the psychological difficulties the individual is more likely to encounter, as well as the strengths and resilience seen in this population. Key topics include Axis I conditions (especially depression, substance abuse, and PTSD), Axis II conditions (i.e. personality disorders), and quality of life issues (including sexuality, vocational rehabilitation, and the impact of chronic pain). Selected case material is used to illustrate some of the major issues encountered by our clients.

AXIS I CONDITIONS

Although individuals with spinal cord injury may have any of the DSM-IV Axis I conditions, three will be explored in some depth. Depression is a common response to loss, and, for most, SCI represents a dramatic loss of both physical functioning and self-image. Substance abuse, in many cases of traumatic SCI, has an etiological connection: alcohol- and drug-related motor vehicle accidents are a leading cause of traumatic SCI. Finally, posttraumatic stress disorder, although given inadequate attention in the literature for quite some time, has recently been brought to the forefront. Many situations that lead to SCI are emotionally traumatic and carry the risk of death; as such, individuals with traumatic SCI are often at risk for PTSD.

Depression

Depression following spinal cord injury (SCI) is a common problem. In a comprehensive review of the literature, Boekamp et al. (1) found that recent studies using structured diagnostic interviews have reported prevalence estimates between 20 to 45 percent for clinical depression within the first year after spinal cord injury. In comparison, the 1-year prevalence of major depression in the general population was approximately 6 percent. Risk factors for depression include prior episodes of depression, family history of depressive or bipolar disorder, family history of suicide attempts, current suicidal ideation, age of onset under 40, chronic pain, female gender, lack of social support, postpartum, life stressors, concurrent medical illness, and concurrent substance abuse. Specific risk factors for individuals with spinal cord injury were complete neurologic injury and medical comorbidity, including traumatic brain injury (2,3), as well as greater physical impairment (4). Among those who became depressed, one study found that the average time until onset was 21 days (3). Although most depression studies have been done with adults, one study done with a sample of 86 children and a control group of adults (matched on time since injury and level of injury) found similar results in both groups. There were no significant differences between the groups on overall measures of depression, self-esteem, and self-perception. Further, there was no significant difference in psychological adjustment between those with paraplegia or tetraplegia (5).

Care should be taken when using standard screening measures (e.g. self-report inventories). Most self-report measures could not distinguish between the hallmark somatic symptoms of depression and the somatic problems secondary to physical disability. Confounding factors include constipation, impotence, and sleep and appetite disturbance (6,7).

There is no evidence that depressive symptoms are part of a process that will lead to a more thorough "working through" of the grief associated with loss of function; rather, depression has been linked to poorer rehabilitation outcomes (8,9). Therefore, clinicians should actively and quickly address depressive symptoms. In the clinical experience of the authors, early treatment of depressive symptoms is much more efficacious than treating a full-blown depressive episode that has unfolded over time. Problem-solving training (10), psychotherapy, and medications all can be helpful in the prevention and/or treatment of depression.

Substance-Related Disorders

Substance use problems are relatively common in the population at large and tend to be more common in the SCI population. Individuals who became spinally injured as a result of substance-related activities (e.g. driving under the influence or drug-related violence) are relatively likely to have a substance abuse problem. In one study (11), vocational rehabilitation and independent living center clients with SCI had nearly double the rate of moderate and heavy drinking as did the general population (46 vs. 25 percent). Heinemann and his associates (12) found that their SCI rehabilitation sample had a mean

of 5.9 alcoholic beverages per weekday; this was nearly identical to findings by Frisbie and Tun (13), whose sample of individuals with SCI averaged 6 drinks per weekday. Weekend drinking tends to be even higher, with a mean of 17.1 drinks per two-day period (12). Studies of individuals with traumatic injuries have found that approximately 15 to 70 percent were using alcohol or drugs at the time of their injury (13–15,22).

What percentage of individuals with SCI has a substance abuse problem at any given time? No precise answer is known at this time (16) although relevant data is available. In a study using the Michigan Alcohol Screening Test (MAST), a standardized assessment instrument, 49 percent of the sample exceeded the cutoff for an alcohol-use disorder (12). A study by Radnitz and her associates indicates that lifetime prevalence of alcohol dependence in her sample was 33.6 percent (17). O'Donnell et al's sample of 47 individuals with SCI included 41 (87 percent) with a prior history of substance abuse, 32 (68 percent) who were using when injured, and 32 (68 percent) who resumed their drug/alcohol use post-injury (14). In most cases, the pattern of substance abuse predates the injury. Heinemann et al (12) found that 75 percent of their sample reported no change in their drinking pattern following their injury. Sweeney and Foote (23) found that 96 percent of their sample of individuals in an inpatient alcohol dependence/SCI program had alcohol problems that pre-dated their spinal cord injury.

Medications can also be misused, especially medications for pain and spasticity. In a sample of 96 individuals with long-term spinal cord injury, Heinemann et al (18) found that of the 43 percent of their sample who received prescription medications, 24 percent misused them (i.e., took more than prescribed or used medications without a prescription). In other cases, drugs such as marijuana or alcohol may be forms of self-medication for pain and spasticity (19,20).

Treatment of substance-use problems is especially important in SCI, because substance abuse can lead to reduced self-care, and therefore increased problems with pressure sores, infections, and other medical problems (22). Research has found that substance abuse has been found to be associated with the following problems in individuals with SCI: depression, suicide, ruined internal catheterization programs, distended bladder, decreased coordination and mobility, decreased cognitive capacity necessary to learn mobility, poor nutrition (which leads to fatigue and weakness), and lower self esteem (14,21). Despite the obvious importance of treatment, however, there is evidence that substance abuse problems are vastly undertreated in individuals with spinal cord injury. One study showed that problems associated with substance abuse were present in 70 percent of the sample; 52 percent of the sample reported problems post-injury, 16 percent indicated that they would benefit from treatment, *but only 7 percent actually received treatment* (22). These findings suggest the need for increased assessment and referral.

Treatment has been found to be effective. Sweeney and Foote studied a group of 36 individuals with SCI and drug or alcohol addiction who were treated with a multidisciplinary, multimodal inpatient program. The exact length of the program was unspecified, but occurs in three phases, the first of which is a minimum of 14 days. Follow-up data collected 3 to 18 months after discharge revealed that 84 percent of program participants reported using alcohol and drugs significantly less frequently and 56 percent were totally abstinent. These findings were corroborated by reports from significant others. According to the authors, "The best cure for drug abuse is a meaningful life" (23, p. 899), thus the path to success is to help the individual to discover a sense of purpose. Ideally, it is best to have a practitioner who is sensitive to the special issues associated with both substance-related problems and SCI, because a lack of knowledge in either area may impact treatment.

The practitioner should be sensitive not to overgeneralize findings regarding substance abuse in individuals with SCI. Individuals who were not traumatically injured, or whose injury was not sustained during substance use, generally are not at higher risk than others in the population. One study, which investigated substance use in nearly 1,000 members of the Paralyzed Veterans of America (PVA), showed a rate of substance abuse that was substantially lower than that of the general population (24).

Practitioners who are not part of the direct treatment of substance abuse problems can still be vital to effective drug or alcohol rehabilitation of the individual with SCI. There is often a narrow window of opportunity very shortly after the injury when motivation to change peaks (12,21). The person may be experiencing regrets regarding his substance use, and how it led to his injury. However, it may not be long before the individual experiences denial ("the drugs did not lead to the accident") or rationalization ("alcohol is my only pleasure"), and thus becomes far more difficult to treat. The referrer should be familiar with *motivational interviewing* techniques to encourage the individual to enter treatment immediately (25). Motivational interviewing consists of five general principles: 1) express empathy; 2) develop discrepancy (i.e., help the person see how their behavior is discrepant with their life goals); 3) avoid argumentation; 4) roll with resistance; and 5) support self-efficacy. Timely referral, using optimally motivating techniques, can be essential to a successful outcome.

Posttraumatic Stress Disorder (PTSD)

Posttraumatic Stress Disorder (PTSD) is a potentially serious problem for individuals with SCI. Recently, led by Cynthia Radnitz and her associates, scientists have turned their attention to trauma-related symptoms. In a sample of 126 veterans, most of whom have long-term injuries, Radnitz, et al (26) found a relatively high prevalence of PTSD among individuals with SCI. Using structured interviews, Radnitz found that 11.9 to 16.7 percent of the sample had current PTSD, while 28.6 to 34.9 percent of the sample qualified for a PTSD diagnosis at some point during their lives.

Radnitz et al (27) then compared individuals with paraplegia and tetraplegia with control subjects who had traumatic injuries but no spinal cord injury. In a finding that appears counterintuitive, individuals with tetraplegia sustained less severe symptoms and lower prevalence of PTSD (see Table 22-1). Also, measures of symptom intensity produced a significantly lower mean for quadriplegics than paraplegics and controls. These two variables were interpreted to be directly related to impaired peripheral nervous system function. The sympathetic arousal experienced in PTSD is much reduced for those with higher level injures; the psychophysiological element of posttraumatic stress is shut down, blocking what would have been a comprehensive symptom and prognosis course. Binks et al (28) describe similar findings, noting that individuals with injuries above T1–T3 were significantly less likely candidates for current PTSD.

Radnitz (26) also points out that elements of an SCI event itself are traumatizing: consciousness of the injury, losing sensation and motor ability, the demands of rehabilitation and attendant losses of function (i.e., social, sexual, self-image, etc.). She postulates a "double" form of PTSD; it could be that previous traumatic events compound a profound distress reaction to SCI, producing a doubly traumatized patient.

Because PTSD research is in its nascent phase, some researchers have urged caution in interpreting causal connections between paralysis and PTSD. It could be that pre-existing conditions, including personality or other considerations, are more important than paralysis or SCI in determining PTSD symptoms (29,30). Nonetheless, preliminary data strongly suggest that the clinician working with a patient with

spinal cord injury should be keenly aware of the possible presence of trauma related problems.

AXIS II CONDITIONS

Individuals with spinal cord injury (SCI) have long been considered at risk for various kinds of impulsive and acting-out behaviors. In theory, this is because SCI is often sustained during risky activities, such as adventure sports (diving, rock climbing), drug/gang activities (gunshot wounds, stabbings), and high-risk driving (e.g. driving while intoxicated, motorcycle riding). Such behaviors can interfere with a patient's rehabilitation or can disrupt the functioning of the rehabilitation unit as a whole. For example, an individual with borderline personality disorder can undermine his rehabilitation while creating dissension and splitting among staff (31). Further, individuals with a wide array of personality disorders can create challenging countertransference reactions in the rehabilitation specialist (32). Because new treatments are emerging that are successful with personality disorders (33–35), assessment and intervention are increasingly important.

Several research studies demonstrate that traumatically injured individuals with spinal cord injury (SCI) have relatively high degrees of energy, impulsivity, and risk taking. Studies by Fordyce (36) and Taylor (37) used the MMPI, and their results supported the assumption that certain personality characteristics are associated with accidents that involve traumatic disability. Both found SCI patients to have impulse-dominated characteristics based on elevations in scales 4 or 9 or both on the MMPI. These characteristics include impulsivity, acting out, and a subjective sense of high energy and personal drive. Fordyce's analysis revealed that those subjects whose onset of injury was judged to be "imprudent" were more likely to have impulse-dominated behavior than those not judged imprudent. Nonpathological instruments have yielded similar results. A sample of paraplegics evaluated with the Rorschach test revealed characteristics such as impulsiveness, body image

TABLE 22-1 Percentage of Individuals
Diagnosed with PTSD

	Paraplegia*	Quadriplegia**	Control***
Current	22	2	21
Lifetime	44	13	26

*n=45; **n=55; ***n=43
Based on data from Radnitz, et al., 1998.

concerns, and interpersonal distancing (38). Mawson and his associates, using a case control design, found that spinal cord injury was associated with sensation-seeking prior to injury (39). Woodbury (40), in his extensive literature review, also reported similar findings, noting that increased risk taking and impulsivity may have an etiologic role in SCI. These characteristics are in contrast to general medical samples, which often have elevations on scales 1, 2, and 3 (indicating somatic anxiety and depression) and, to a lesser extent, 7 and 8 (indicating anxiety and feelings of alienation) (41–44).

Despite the data available on personality characteristics of individuals with SCI, almost no data is available on the prevalence of diagnosable personality disorders in this population. In one study, 40 SCI subjects and an equal number of matched controls (medical patients) were given a structured diagnostic interview and a self-report personality-disorder instrument. Structured interview data indicated that 27.5 percent of SCI patients, and a similar number of controls, have personality disorders. Unexpectedly, impulsive/externalizing disorders (histrionic, narcissistic, antisocial, and borderline) were not unusually high in SCI patients and were not higher than controls. Avoidant, schizoid, and depressive disorders were unexpectedly frequent. Due to the small sample size and limited geographical and ethnic diversity of the sample, the findings must be considered preliminary; nonetheless, the study does imply that further research on personality disorders in populations with disabilities is warranted (45).

Despite the emphasis on personality pathology, both in the literature and in this review, it should be noted that many of the personality characteristics described for individuals with SCI are positive and adaptive. Malec (46) found that persons with SCI appeared more extroverted than those with nontraumatic injuries or injuries resulting in chronic pain. Kunce and Worley (47), using the Strong Vocational Interest Blank, found that individuals active in receiving their injury were characterized by adventurousness, boldness, and assertiveness.

Preliminary data indicate that personality disorders are present in only a minority of cases (45). Strengths such as a positive attitude and an outgoing personality can facilitate rehabilitation, as well as adjustment to the changes that the acquisition of a disability brings (48). In the senior author's clinical experience, there have been several clients who were difficult to manage within the hospital setting, but who went on to excellent rehabilitation outcomes. The very characteristics that made it hard for them to adapt to the hospital—being assertive, energetic, and demanding, when the conditions of the hospital setting encouraged them to be cooperative and tolerant—helped them to overcome obstacles during the arduous process of comprehensive rehabilitation. In that situation, the team must be far-sighted, supporting the individual's spirit, rather than yielding to institutional convenience.

QUALITY OF LIFE AND THE INDIVIDUAL WITH SCI

Improving quality of life is, in a broad sense, the goal of all SCI rehabilitation. Although there are many definitions of quality of life, elements include life satisfaction, physical integrity, material success/comfort, spiritual satisfaction, a sense of meaning or purpose, and relationship satisfaction. The following sections address overall quality of life, as well as areas that frequently impact the quality of life of individuals with SCI: chronic pain and changes in sexuality.

Studies of Overall Quality of Life

Most individuals with SCI, even those with severe disabilities, have a high quality of life (49). A national study of 1,000 randomly selected individuals found that 69 percent of individuals with disabilities were satisfied or very satisfied with life (50). Whiteneck et al found that approximately three-fourths of their sample of 282 long-term patients with SCI rated their quality of life as good or excellent (51). Several studies have found that, on average, SCI is associated with a somewhat reduced quality of life relative to the general population (52–55). Nonetheless, the overlap between disabled and nondisabled groups in quality of life ratings is generally substantial.

Numerous factors are important in determining the quality of life of an individual following SCI. Life satisfaction has been found to correlate positively with productivity, employment, and mobility, and negatively with dependency (e.g. lack of transportation, low income, and family conflicts), health problems, and emotional distress (53,56–58). Schulz and Decker (55) found that perceived health, income, perceived control, perception of disability, social support, and satisfaction with social contacts were important contributors to life satisfaction. Given the impact of a severe disability such as spinal cord injury, the individual's coping skills are also an important factor (59,60). A 15-year longitudinal study found that, in general, adjustment to SCI continues to improve over time, including gains in life satisfaction, work, sitting tolerance, and decreased need for medical services. Activity level, satisfaction, and (self-rated) adjustment were three of the most stable variables (61). Whiteneck et al (51) found a curvilinear pattern, in which quality of life improved up to age 50 and 30 years post-injury, and then began to decline.

Interestingly, demographic data, such as age and injury severity, were not effective as predictors of life satisfaction in several studies (51,53,58,62,63). Further, although it may seem logical that individuals with paraplegia would have a better overall quality of life than those with quadriplegia, the research has not borne this out. This finding has important ethical implications, as dramatic "right to die" cases are premised on poor quality of life for the severely disabled (64,65).

To place SCI in a long-term perspective, Crewe (66) asked subjects of long-standing injuries (22 years) to narrate life stories which she categorized as comic, romantic, tragic, ironic, and other responses (unclassified). Depending on how positively or negatively one frames not just devastating injury, but attitudes and behaviors before and long afterward determines a rating from an interview. The first of a few telling points from Crewe's work is that traumatic disability is not the pivotal life event. Although one narrator claimed profound change post-injury, his story was analyzed as mirroring the picture of his childhood and youth. More commonly, interviewees recognized the fact that personality continuity was maintained despite catastrophic disability and any other peaks and lows. Crewe briefly considered that respondents may have unintentionally revised their early histories to conform to post-injury attitudes, but she finds such an interpretation a longer reach than the repeated claims to the contrary and story analyses reflecting continuity. She also describes few of the 50 narrators as sustaining hopelessness or negativity about their accidents: nearly half were considered comic, the style evincing the least depressive tone. Crewe also dismisses stereotypical images of the heroic victim who overcomes all obstacles and the embittered anti-hero: supercrip and villains are products of the media.

Spinal Cord Injury and Pain

Chronic pain is common in individuals with SCI and can have a large impact on quality of life. Due to sampling variation and different definitions of what constitutes chronic pain, estimates of the frequency of chronic pain among patients with spinal cord injury vary widely. Summers et al found that the reported incidence of pain in spinal cord injury patients ranged from 14 to 94 percent. Nepomuceno et al (67) surveyed 200 previously hospitalized spinal cord injury patients with intractable pain to characterize and analyze pain reported by patients. Of the 200 respondents, 48 percent reported their abnormal sensation to be painful. The researchers found no apparent relationship between the quality of pain described and the level of the lesions. In order of frequency, spinal cord injury pain was characterized as "burning and/or stinging" (greater than 50 percent); "pulling or pressing" (25 percent); or "cramping, stabbing, and tingling/numbness" (20 percent). Nepomuceno found that 80 percent of the respondents reported abnormal sensation within 6 months to over 4 years after injury. Pain intensity was severe in 25 percent of the respondents and 41 percent reported that their pain increased over time. Medications were used by 38 percent of those experiencing pain, but only 22 percent reported consistent pain relief. In 44 percent of the cases, pain interfered with activities of daily living.

Several studies have investigated factors that predict the impact of pain on the client with SCI. Individuals who reported that pain interfered with activities of daily living were older, scored higher on measures of verbal intelligence, were more depressed, experienced greater levels of distress, and reported a more negative psychosocial situation (67,68). Summers et al (69) found that anger and negative cognitions were associated with greater pain severity. However, anxiety and depression were not significantly correlated with severity of pain. Wade et al (70) found anger and frustration were critical concomitants of chronic nonspinal cord injury pain. They proposed that prolonged anger might exacerbate the emotional unpleasantness associated with pain, making pain less tolerable and intensifying depression over time. Individuals who negatively appraised their pain and were less accepting of their disability experienced more severe pain (69).

Several psychological interventions have been found to be extremely effective for chronic nonmalignant pain. Biofeedback (71) and hypnosis (72,73) often provide excellent relief. A particularly promising approach utilizing a combination of yoga and "mindfulness" meditation has been found to produce a 58 percent reduction in perceived pain (74). Cognitive behavioral approaches to improving clinical pain are well established (75). Skills such as goal setting, self-monitoring, problem solving, relaxation, time management, and positive reappraisal are important in managing pain (76,77). Multidisciplinary assessment and treatment, considering physical and psychosocial aspects of pain, is generally essential to an optimal treatment outcome (78–80).

Unfortunately, many patients with pain problems assume that referral to a psychologist implies that they have a mental health disorder (i.e. they are "crazy") or that the pain is psychogenic (i.e. "all in their head"). Individuals with spinal cord injury, because of the presence of such obvious physical damage, may be very sensitive to any implication that their problem is psychogenic. The manner in which the psychologist is introduced to the client can facilitate the process of implementing treatment. The referring professional should reassure the patient that having a psychologist as part of pain treatment is routine, necessary, and helpful.

Vocational Adjustment

Given the practical and symbolic meaning of work in United States culture, return to work has long been considered a key rehabilitation outcome (81). Although early research investigated only paid employment, more recent researchers have considered a wider variety of roles, such as student or homemaker, to be productive and satisfying.

Obtaining employment following a spinal cord injury can be very difficult. Murphy and Athanasou reviewed 24 studies, representing, 4771 individuals with SCI; the total return-to-work rate was 39.3 percent (82). James et al (83), using a large sample of individuals from the National Spinal Cord Injury Statistical Center database, found that only 18.9 percent of African Americans, and 38.7 percent of whites, had been employed at any time in a 6-year period following their SCI. According to the Spinal Cord Injury Statistics center, employment rates 8 years post-injury for individuals who were between 16 and 59 at injury are 34.4 percent for individuals with paraplegia and 24.3 percent for those with quadriplegia. This compares to a 58.8 percent employment rate prior to injury (84). In one sample of 140 community-based persons with SCI, 27 percent were employed, 35 percent were in unpaid productive activities, while 38 percent were unemployed (85). One survey found that 82 percent of individuals receiving disability benefits would rather be working (86). Individuals with SCI are substantially underemployed.

In categorizing injured individuals into employed, productive-unemployed, and unemployed, Krause (87) found a pattern of differences between the three; employed participants manifested higher motivation, achievement orientation, persistence, and planning. The trade-off they endured was an increase in stress over the other groups. Productive individuals were seen as calmer and lower in achievement needs, who nonetheless evinced stable adjustment post-injury and minimal stress or negative emotions. Those who were categorized as unemployed indicated elevated poor self-control, aggression, alienation, and stress reactivity. They reported lower levels of positive emotions and more intense anger and anxiety. Derived from the same nonpathologically oriented personality questionnaire as the other clusters, this matrix was associated with injury onset. These results led Krause to two claims: the first is that although no direct measure of trait stability is possible, the likelihood is that many traits predating injury were in evidence decades later; the second is that a traumatic disabling condition was not the source of constructive development nor the cause of poor functioning.

Clients identify several factors as interfering with obtaining employment, including health issues, lack of awareness of vocational skills, transportation problems (88), physical limitations imposed by SCI, job environment, and inaccessibility (81). Systemic factors can discourage many individuals from seeking employment. One barrier is fear that one will lose benefits, such as low-cost (Section 8) housing, medical coverage, and prosthetic support (81,89). Changes in the Social Security and Medicare systems have improved this problem, providing ways for individuals to work and to retain part or all of their benefits (86); however, some individuals with SCI may not know about these provisions, and private disability insurance plans may still contain disincentives.

Systematic discrimination against paralyzed individuals has not been scientifically studied, but is likely to exist. An expose by Dateline NBC (John Hockenberry) matched an individual in a wheelchair against an able-bodied individual in a job search. Differences were seen in how potential employers behaved towards the two different applicants. The most striking example occurred at a retail store. The individual in a wheelchair was told by the counter-person that he could not have an interview because the manager was not present, while the able-bodied individual, who entered moments later, *was handed the manager's appointment book* and allowed to select from possible appointment times. Although such media investigations have potential flaws, the findings lend credence to the anecdotes of clients who report feeling disadvantaged when searching for jobs.

There is evidence that people of color are doubly disadvantaged, i.e. being members a minority group and having a disability. Studies have revealed that African American rehabilitation clients have substantially lower rates of employment than white clients. For example, James et al (83) studied 1,042 whites and 196 African-Americans who were drawn from the National Spinal Cord Injury Statistical Center database. One year post-injury, 6.6 percent of African Americans, and 14.9 percent of whites were employed. By 6 years post-injury, a total of 18.9 percent of African Americans, and 38.7 percent of whites, had been employed following their SCI. Feist-Price (90) examined the records of over 70,000 individuals who sought Department of Vocational Rehabilitation services and found a number of differences in the delivery of disability services for African Americans versus European Americans. A significantly higher proportion of European Americans was considered eligible for services. As a proportion, over 10 times as many European Americans (92 percent) received agency purchased services than African Americans (8 percent). African Americans were also less likely to be successfully rehabilitated (e.g. competitively employed), and their cases were more likely to be closed for reasons other than successful rehabilitation (e.g. refusing services or failure to cooperate). The author argues that there are numerous reasons for these findings. Racism, cultural differences between counselors and clients, poor diversity training for counselors, lower education and socioeconomic status in the African American sample, problems with paperwork, and bias in estimating rehabilitation potential of African Americans, all contribute to the observed vocational rehabilitation differences.

Given the difficulties individuals with disabilities may face in obtaining employment, it is extremely important for them to know their rights under the Americans with Disabilities Act (ADA) (91,92), as well as regulations regarding Medicare, Social Security, and Medicaid benefits (86). During acute rehabilitation, with its focus on medical stabilization and functional improvement, vocational rehabilitation can be neglected. Skilled vocational rehabilitation can play a critical role in the comprehensive rehabilitation of the individual with spinal cord injury.

Sexuality

Sexuality has received much attention in the literature, but numerous authorities agree that there has been inadequate attention in clinical practice (93–104). Of the numerous and varied issues covered in a literature review on the subject of SCI and sexuality, this issue is the only one to be so consistently reiterated by contemporary providers and researchers. They offer reports of patient concerns (93,94,96,97,104), what to include in sexuality programs (93,94,97–99,102–104), the positive effect of programs (97,98), and some contrasting elements between men's and women's SCI experience (93–95,104), consistently concluding with a call for sexuality coverage in programs.

The concerns of the spinal cord injured about their significantly altered sexuality are neither surprising nor few. They mourn losses of specific capacities and sexual sensitivity, such as erectile function, orgasm, use of hands or limbs, and arousal thresholds; the power to please a partner may be thought of as diminished or ended (93,97). There is the shocking awareness that their culture considers them asexual (93,97), no longer serious contenders in the competition to attract hetero- or homosexual partners. This attitude may evince initially with a spouse (93) or pre-injury lover and is affirmed at any number of familial or social junctures. A 33-year-old male patient of one of the authors (CF), who had seen himself as successful in attracting women until the time of his accident, was greeted at a friend's wedding with a statement of how "cute" it was for the guy in the wheelchair to move onto the dance floor. Six years post-injury, this man reported that similar comments are made all the time. No wonder fears emerge in injured individuals; abandonment, powerlessness, and no one wanting a cripple, all are common parts of the post-injury period (93,94,96,97). Endangered self-esteem (97,104) that stems from sexuality per se and impacts various realms of interpersonal life is as common as the anxiety that accompanies impaired sexual functioning (97). For some with SCI, pain is a part of one's sex life (97). Many current professionals and patients recognize these psychoemotional burdens.

In response to so many serious stresses surrounding sexuality, those who propose counseling as part of any rehabilitation program have concrete suggestions for what to include in such an effort. Overall, there must be a willingness to be clear and thorough in supplying all information (93,94,97–99). The counselor must address anatomical or physiological facts, commonplace activities, oral sex, or any untried or less traditional modes. Positions and adaptive behaviors (93–95,97,98), anticipated limitations, and frank discussion of the experience of peers is needed. Some SCI patients have requested contact with peers who are farther from time of injury; in that regard, group treatment is often a preferred modality that can help (93,98) to broaden perspectives, share techniques, offer reassurance, and lift spirits. The group counseling session may be one in which the professional gains as well: studies to date are rudimentary, and the physiological idiosyncrasies of lesions and nervous systems can be understood best when described by patients (93). Another priority format is the couple setting when a partner is extant. There can be no progress in reclaiming sexuality for a suddenly disabled person without a supportive, flexible partner (93,97). Learning together and communicating with more depth than a couple may have ever done is the only hope for a realistic retrieval of some of the rewards of sexuality. Clinicians understand that it is only in the context of psycho-emotional life (94,97) that the integrity of sex is protected; intimacy, joy, pride, pleasure, and attachment can all be maintained in the face of major sexual adjustment when feelings and attitudes have been expressed, considered, and respected (95,96).

The proponents of sexuality counseling programs envision similar successes for their graduates; they offer evidence that participants' knowledge, satisfaction, and self-regard have all been rewarded after sexuality programs (97,98). Professionals have revealed their own feelings of being ill equipped (99) to provide such services, again calling attention to the need to focus on the issue in a formal manner. A structured series of individual, couple, or group sessions has resulted in gains for both patients and partners according to current providers, who may be psychologists, social workers, nurses, SCI peers, or others.

Little is written about sexuality for women with SCI (101,102). In contrast to males, females may not sustain the drop in fertility associated with SCI (94,95), so that contraception becomes a consideration (93). Many women whose femininity is affected (93,94) by their injuries sustain some sense of restoration at the news that they can be sexually active and become pregnant and deliver a healthy infant despite severe disability. This may be one reason they exhibit less adjustment problems after injury (93) but to whatever their better coping capacity is attributable, they continue to see themselves as sexual beings, with a host of concerns regarding attractiveness, responsiveness, and the ability to satisfy a partner and themselves.

Section Summary

Despite popular conceptions regarding the quality of life of individuals with disabilities, the majority of individuals with spinal cord injury rate their quality of life as good or excellent. Health, independence, perception of disability, social support, income, and coping skills have an important impact on life satisfaction. In addition, adjustment has been found to be fairly stable, with a general trend toward improvement over time. Proper counseling regarding sexuality, chronic pain, and vocational adjustment can further enhance quality of life. Although the most current research indicates that individuals with SCI rate their quality of life lower than those without disabilities, disability rights advocates would argue that this discrepancy could be eliminated if appropriate social conditions were met (105).

CONCLUSION

Professionals working with clients with spinal cord injury should consider several principles and findings that have been borne out in the research literature. Clients with SCI should be screened for depression, PTSD, substance use disorders, and chronic pain, because the population is clearly at risk for these problems. Because depression has been found to be associated with poorer rehabilitation outcomes, the clinician should treat depression actively, and as early as possible. Psychotherapy, counseling, and medications can all be effective in reducing or eliminating depression. The individual with spinal cord injury, from a personality standpoint, is relatively likely to be energetic and outgoing; these characteristics can be very helpful in a rehabilitation setting. There is also elevated risk for impulsive behavior. Preliminary research suggests that there is a risk for personality disorders that is higher than the general population but approximately the same as other medical populations; routine screening would be a wise precaution.

The quality of life of an individual with SCI is often lower than individuals without SCI, but, contrary to popular belief, the difference between the two populations is generally small. Quality of life can be enhanced in many ways, with sexuality and vocational counseling being emphasized in this review. When issues of chronic pain are involved, integrating a specialist in the behavioral and psychological aspects of chronic pain can make an enormous difference. Several psychological/behavioral approaches have demonstrated pain reductions of 50 percent or more, and substantial reductions in depression and anxiety associated with pain. A team approach, which integrates behavioral and psychological aspects routinely, may be crucial in facilitating the client's openness to these approaches.

REFERENCES

1. Boekamp JR, Overholser JC, Schubert DS. Depression following a spinal cord injury. Intl J Psychiatry in Medicine 1996; 26(3):329–349.
2. Consortium for Spinal Cord Medicine (ed.). *Depression Following Spinal Cord Injury: A Clinical Practice Guideline for Primary Care Physicians.* Washington DC: Paralyzed Veterans of America, August 1998.
3. Fullerton DT, Harvey RF, Klein MH, Howell T. Psychiatric disorders in patients with spinal cord injuries. *Arch Gen Psychiatry* 1981; 38:1369–1371.
4. Kishi Y, Robinson RG, Forrester AW. Comparison between acute and delayed onset major depression after spinal cord injury. *J Nervous and Mental Disease* 1995; 183(5):286–292.
5. Kennedy P, Gotsuch N, Marsh N. Childhood onset of spinal cord injury: self-esteem and self-perception. *British Journal of Clinical Psychology* 1995; 34:581–588.
6. Davidoff G, Roth E, Thomas P, Doljanac R, Dijkers M, Berent S, Wolf L, Morris J, Yarkony G. Depression among acute spinal cord injury patients: a study utilizing the Zung self-rating depression scale. *Rehab Psychology* 1990; 35(3): 171–179.
7. Radnitz CL, Bockian N, Moran AI. (2000). Assessment of psychopathology and personality in persons with physical disabilities. In Frank RG and Elliott TR eds., Handbook of Rehabilitation Psychology. Washington, D.C.: American Psychological Association.
8. Herrick SM, Elliott TR, Crow F. Social support and the prediction of health complications among persons with spinal cord injuries. *Rehabil Psychol,* 1994; 39:231–250.
9. Lawson NC. Significant events in the rehabilitation process: the spinal cord patient's point of view. *Arch Phys Med Rehabil,* 1978; 59:573–579.
10. Elliot TR, Godshall FJ, Herrick SM, Witty TE, Spruell M. Problem-solving appraisal and psychological adjustment following spinal cord injury. *Cognitive Therapy and Research* 1991; 15(5):387–398.
11. Johnson DC. *Alcohol Use by Persons with Disabilities.* Madison, Wisconsin: Wisconsin Department of Health and Social Services, 1985.
12. Heinemann AW, Keen M, Donohue R, Schnoll S. Alcohol use by persons with recent spinal cord injury. *Arch Phys Med Rehabil,* 1988; 69:619–624.
13. Frisbie JH, Tun CG. Drinking and spinal cord injury. *J Am Paraplegia Soc* 1984; 7(4): 71–73.
14. O'Donnell JJ, Cooper JE, Gessner JE, Shehan I, Ashley J. Alcohol, drugs, and spinal cord injury. *Alcohol Health and Research World* 1981; 6(2): 27–29.
15. Heinemann AW, Schnoll S, Brandt MS, Maltz R, Keen M. Toxicology screening in acute spinal cord injury. *Alcoholism: Clinical and Experimental Research* 1988; 12:815–819.
16. Radnitz CL, Tirch D. Substance misuse in individuals with spinal cord injury. *Intl J Addictions* 1995; 30:1117–1140.
17. Radnitz CL, Broderick CP, Perez-Strumolo L, Tirch DD, Festa J, Schlein IS, Walczak S, Willard J, Lillian LB, Binks M. The prevalence of psychiatric disorders in veterans with spinal cord injury: a controlled comparison. *J Nerv Ment Disease* 1996; 184:431–433.
18. Heinemann AW, McGraw TE, Brandt MJ, Roth E, Dell'Oliver C, Schnoll S. Prescription medication misuse among persons with spinal cord injuries. *Intl J Addictions* 1992; 27:301–316.
19. Burke DC. Pain in paraplegia. *Paraplegia* 1973; 10:297–313.
20. Malec J, Harvey R, Cayner J. Cannabis effects on spasticity in spinal cord injury. *Arch Phys Med Rehabil* 1982; 63:116–118.
21. Pollets DF, Glenn MK. Substance abuse and disability: attention and prevention. Presentation at the 8th Annual Conference of the American Association of Spinal Cord Injury Psychologists and Social Workers, Las Vegas, Nevada, September 6, 1994.
22. Heinemann AW, Doll MD, Armstrong KJ, Schnoll S, Yarkony GM. Substance use and receipt of treatment by persons with long-term spinal cord injuries. *Arch Phys Med Rehabil* 1991; 72:482–487.
23. Sweeney TT, Foote JE. Treatment of drug and alcohol abuse in spinal cord injury veterans. *Intl J Addictions* 1982; 17:897–904.

24. Kirubakaran VR, Kumar VN, Powell BJ, Tyler AJ, Armatas PJ. Survey of alcohol and drug misuse in spinal cord injured veterans. *J Studies on Alcohol* 1986; 47(3):223–227.

25. Miller WR, Rollnick S. *Motivational Interviewing*. New York: Guilford, 1991.

26. Radnitz CL, Schlein IS, Walczak S, Broderick CP, Binks M, Tirch DD, Willard J, Perez-Strumolo L, Festa J, Lillian LB, Bockian N, Cytryn A, Green L. The prevalence of post-traumatic stress disorder in veterans with spinal cord injury. *SCI Psychosocial Process* 1995; 8(4):145–49.

27. Radnitz CL, Hsu L, Tirch DD, Willard J, Lillian LB, Walczak S, Festa J, Perz-Strumolo L, Broderick CP, Binks M, Schlein I, Bockian N, Green L, Cytryn A. A comparison of posttraumatic stress disorder in veterans with and without spinal cord injury. *J Abnorm Psychology* 1998; 107:676–680.

28. Binks TM, Radnitz CL, Moran AI, Vinciguerra V. Relationship between level of spinal cord injury and posttraumatic stress disorder symptoms. *Annals of the New York Academy of Sciences* 1997; 821:430–432.

29. McFall ME (1991). Post traumatic stress disorder in spinal cord injury patients. *SCI Psychosocial Process* 1991; 4(3):88–92.

30. Craig AA, Hancock KM, Dickson H, Martin J, Chang E. Psychological consequences of spinal cord injury: a review of the literature. *Australian and New Zealand J of Psychiatry* 1990; 24:418–25.

31. Bockian N. Systemic-behavioral treatment of a personality disorder and abusive behavior on a spinal cord injury unit: a case illustration. *SCI Psychosocial Process* 1994; 7:153–160.

32. Stewart JR. Denial of disabling conditions and specific interventions in the rehabilitation counseling setting. *J Applied Rehab Counseling* 1994; 25(3):7–15.

33. Beck AT, Freeman A. *Cognitive Therapy of Personality Disorders*. New York: Guilford, 1990.

34. Linehan MM. *Cognitive Behavioral Treatment of Borderline Personality Disorder*. New York: Guilford, 1993.

35. Millon T (1999). *Personality Guided Psychotherapy: From Cognitive-Behavioral to Synergistic Treatment of Axis-I and Axis-II*. New York: John Wiley and Sons.

36. Fordyce W. Personality characteristics of men with spinal cord injury as related to manner of onset of disability. *Arch Phys Med and Rehab* 1964; 73:552–557.

37. Taylor GP. Moderator-variable effects on personality-test-item endorsements of physically disabled patients. *J Consulting and Clinical Psychology* 1970; 35:183–188.

38. Mattlar C E, Tarkkanen P, Carlsson A, Aaltonen T, Helenius H. Personality characteristics for 83 paraplegic patients evaluated by the Rorschach method using the comprehensive system. *Brit J Projective Psychology* 1993; 38(2):20–30.

39. Mawson AR, Biundo JJ, Clemmer DI, Jacobs KW, Ktsanes VK, Rice JC. Sensation-seeking, criminality, and spinal cord injury: a case-control study. *Am J Epidemiology* 1996; 144(5):463–472.

40. Woodbury B. Psychological adjustment to spinal cord injury: a literature review, 1950–1977. *Rehab Psychology* 1978; 25(3):119–134.

41. McDaniel JW. *Physical Disability and Human Behavior* 2nd ed. New York: Pergamon Press, 1976.

42. Harper DC, Richman LC. Personality profiles of physically impaired adolescents. *J Clin Psychology* 1978; 34(3):636–642.

43. Spergel P, Erlich GE, Glass D. The rheumatoid arthritic personality: a psychodiagnostic myth. *Psychosomatics* 1978; 19(2):79–86.

44. Wilson H, Olson WH, Gascon GG, Brumback RA. Personality characteristics and multiple sclerosis. *Psychological Reports* 1982; 51:791–806.

45. Bockian N, Lee A, Fidanque C. Personality disorders and spinal cord injury: a controlled study. Paper Presentation at the American Association of Spinal Cord Injury Psychologists and Social Workers, Las Vegas, Nevada, September 3, 1997.

46. Malec J. Personality factors associated with severe traumatic disability. *Rehab Psychology* 1985; 30(3):165–172.

47. Kunce JT, Worley BH.. Interest patterns, accidents, and disability. *J Clin Psychology* 1966; 22: 105–107.

48. Mann K. Winners: characteristics of highly successful rehabilitation clients. *Vocational Evaluation and Work Adjustment Bulletin* 1994; 27(1):15–18.

49. Eisenberg MG, Saltz CC. Quality of life among aging spinal cord injured persons: long-term rehabilitation outcomes. *Paraplegia* 1991; 29: 514–520.

50. International Center for the Disabled. The ICD survey of disabled Americans: bringing the disabled Americans into the mainstream. New York: International Center for the Disabled, 1986.

51. Whiteneck GG, Charlifue SW, Frankel HL, Fraser MH, Garnder BP, Gerhart KA, Krishnan KR, Menter RR, Nuseibeh I, Short DJ, Silver JR. Mortality, morbidity, and psychosocial out-

comes of persons spinal cord injured more than 20 years ago. *Paraplegia* 1992; 30:617–630.

52. Dew MA, Lynch K, Ernst J, Rosentahl R. Reaction and adjustment to spinal cord injury: a descriptive study. *J Applied Rehab Counseling* 1983; 14:32–39.

53. Fuhrer MJ, Rintala DH, Hart KA, Clearman R. Young ME. Relationship of life satisfaction to impairment, disability, and handicap among persons with spinal cord injury living in the community. *Arch Phys Med and Rehab* 1992; 73, 552–557.

54. Menhert T, Krauss HH, Nadler R, Boyd M. Correlates of life satisfaction in those with disabling conditions. *Rehab Psychology* 1990; 35:3–17.

55. Schulz R, Decker S. Long-term adjustment to physical disability: the role of social support, perceived control, and self-blame. *J Pers and Social Psychology* 1985; 48:1162–1172.

56. Krause JS, Crewe NM. Long term prediction of self-reported problems following spinal cord injury. *Paraplegia* 1990; 28:186–202.

57. Krause JS. The relationship of productivity to adjustment following spinal cord injury. *Rehab Counseling Bull* 1990; 33:188–199.

58. Siosteen A, Lundqvist C, Blomstrand C, Sullivan L, Sullivan M. The quality of life of three functional spinal cord injury subgroups in a Swedish community. *Paraplegia* 1990; 28:476–488.

59. De Vivo MJ, Richards JS. Community reintegration and quality of life following spinal cord injury. *Paraplegia* 1992; 30:108–112.

60. Nieves CC, Charter RA, Aspinall MJ. Relationship between effective coping and perceived quality of life in spinal cord injured patients. *Rehab Nursing* 1991; 16(3):129–132.

61. Krause JS. Longitudinal changes in adjustment after spinal cord injury: a 15-year longitudinal study. *Arch Phys Med and Rehab* 1992; 73:564–568.

62. Cushman LA, Hassett J. Spinal cord injury: 10 and 15 years after. *Paraplegia* 1992; 30:690–696.

63. Krause JS, Dawis RV. Prediction of life satisfaction after spinal cord injury: A four-year longitudinal approach. *Rehab Psychology* 1992; 37:49–60.

64. Maynard FM, Muth AS. The choice to end life as a ventilator-dependent quadriplegic. *Arch Phys Med and Rehab* 1987; 68:862–864.

65. Mourer SA. The refusal of treatment: staff reaction and recommendations. *SCI Psychosocial Process* 1991; 3(4):72–76.

66. Crewe NM. Life stories of people with long-term spinal cord injury. *Rehab Counseling Bull* 1997; 41(1):26–42.

67. Nepomuceno C, Fine PR, Richards S, Gowens H, Stover SL, Rantanuabol U, Houston R. Pain in patients with spinal cord injury. *Arch Phys Med Rehabil* 1979; 60:605–609.

68. Richards JS, Meredith RL, Nepomuceno C, Fine PR, Bennett G. Psychosocial aspects of chronic pain in spinal cord injury. *Pain* 1980; 8:355–366.

69. Summers JD, Rapoff MA, Varghese G, Porter K, Palmer RE. Psychosocial factors in chronic spinal cord injury pain. *Pain* 1991; 47:183–189.

70. Wade JB, Price DD, Hamer RM, Schwartz SM, Hart RP. An emotional component analysis of chronic pain. *Pain* 1990; 40:303–310.

71. Keefe FJ, Hoelscher TJ. Biofeedback in the management of chronic pain syndromes. In Hatch JP Fisher JG, Rugh JD eds., *Biofeedback: Studies in Clinical Efficacy*. New York: Plenum, 1987.

72. Brown DP, and Fromm E. *Hypnosis and Behavioral Medicine*. Hillsdale, New Jersey: Lawrence Erlbaum, 1987.

73. Hilgard ER. *Hypnosis in the Relief of Pain*. New York: Bruner/Mazel, 1994.

74. Kabat-Zinn J. *Full Catastrophe Living*. New York: Delta, 1990.

75. Turk DC, Meichenbaum D, Genest M. *Pain and Behavioral Medicine*. New York: Guilford, 1983.

76. Umlauf RL. Psychological interventions for chronic pain following spinal cord injury. *Clin J Pain* 1992; 8:111–118.

77. Hanson RW, Gerber KE. *Coping with chronic Pain: A Guide to Patient Self-management*. New York: Guilford, 1990.

78. Mariano AJ. Chronic pain and spinal cord injury. *The Clin J of Pain* 1992. 8:87–92.

79. Britell CW, Mariano AJ. Chronic pain in spinal cord injury. *Phys Med and Rehab: State of the art reviews* 1991. 5(1):71–82.

80. Wegener ST, Elliott TR. Pain assessment in spinal cord injury. *Clin J Pain* 1992. 8:93–101.

81. Krause JS, Anson CA. Self-perceived reasons for unemployment cited by persons with spinal cord injury: relationship to gender, race, age, and level of injury. *Rehabil Couns Bull* 1996. 39:217–227.

82. Murphy GC, Athanasou JA. Vocational potential and spinal cord injury: a review and evaluation. *J Applied Rehabil Counseling* 1994. 25: 47–52.

83. James M, DeVivo MJ, Richards JS. Postinjury employment outcomes among African-American and White persons with spinal cord injury. *Rehabil Psychol* 1993; 38:151–164.

84. Spinal Cord Injury Statistics Home Page.

http://www.spinalcord.org/resource/Factsheets/factsheet2.html. Information published 5/96.

85. Young ME, Alfred WG, Rintala DH, Hart KA, Fuhrer MJ. Vocational status of persons with spinal cord injury living in the community. *Rehab Couns Bull* 1995; 37:229–243.

86. Working. *Spinal Network Extra* 1990; Summer: 30–44.

87. Krause JS. Personality and traumatic spinal cord injury: relationship to participation in productive activities. *J Applied Rehab Counseling* 1997; 28(2):15–20.

88. Targett PS, Wilson K, Wehman P, McKinley WO. Community needs assessment survey of people with spinal cord injury: an early follow-up study. *J Vocational Rehabil* 1998; 10:169–177.

89. Ernst JL, Day EH. Reducing the penalties of long-term employment: alternatives in vocational rehabilitation and spinal cord injury services. *J Vocational Rehabil* 1998; 10:133–139.

90. Feist-Price S. African Americans with disabilities and equity in vocational rehabilitation services: one state's review. *Rehab Couns Bull* 1995; 39:119–129.

91. Jacobs K. Integrating the Americans with Disabilities Act of 1990 into client intervention. *Am J Occupational Therapy* 1992; 46:445–448.

92. Moakley TJ. Informing spinal cord injured persons about their rights and expectations under the Americans with Disabilities Act. *SCI Psychosocial Process* 1994; 7:8–12.

93. Althof S, Levine S. Clinical approach to the sexuality of patients with spinal cord injury. *Urol Clin North Am* 1993; 20:527–534.

94. Drench M. Impact of altered sexuality and sexual function in spinal cord injury: a review. *Sexuality and Disability* 1992; 10(1):3–13.

95. Grundy D, Russell J. ABC of spinal cord injury: later management and complications—I. *Brit Med J* 1986; 292:677–680.

96. Kreuter M. Sexual adjustment and quality of relationships in spinal paraplegia: A controlled study. *Arch Phys Med and Rehab* 1996; 77:541–547.

97. Lemon M. Sexual counseling and spinal cord injury. *Sexuality and Disability* 1993; 11(1):73–97.

98. Melnyk R, Montgomery R, Over R. Attitude changes following a sexual counseling program for spinal cord injured persons. *Arch Phys Med and Rehab* 1979; 60:601–605.

99. Novak P, Mitchell M. Professional involvement in sexuality counseling for patients with spinal cord injuries. *Am J Occupational Ther* 1988; 42(2):105–111.

100. Richards J, Lloyd L, James J, Brown J. Treatment of erectile dysfunction secondary to spinal cord injury: Sexual and psychosocial impact on couples. *Rehab Psychology* 1992; 37(3):205–213.

101. Sipski M, Alexander C. Sexual activities, response and satisfaction in women pre- and post-spinal cord injury. *Arch Phys Med and Rehab* 1993; 74:1025–1029.

102. Tepper M. Sexual education in spinal cord injury rehabilitation: Current trends and recommendations. *Sexuality and Disability* 1992; 10(1):18–31.

103. White M, Rintala D, Hart K, Young M, Fuhrer M. Sexual activities, concerns and interests of men with spinal cord injury. *Am J Phys Med and Rehab* 1992; 71(4):225–231.

104. Zasler N. Sexuality in neurologic disability: an overview. *Sexuality and Disability* 1991; 9(1):11–27.

105. Connally P, Roberts EV, Gold J. Old attitudes, new attitudes, and disability policy. *SCI Psychosocial Process* 1992; 5(4):124–130.

23

A Changed World: Socioeconomic Problems of Spinal Cord Injured Patients

KRISTIN BALFANZ-VERTIZ, LSW
CARLETON PILSECKER, MSSW

A REVIEW OF THE LITERATURE has shown little change in the social and economic problems that spinal cord injured patients experience. Unfortunately, many of the same barriers still exist, despite the efforts of professionals and the disabled community to educate society about long-term disabilities.

Two changes that have had an impact on socioeconomic problems are an increase in the number of spinal cord injuries and a change in the etiology.

Each year, 20,000 Americans are paralyzed as a result of trauma and disease. Of the more than half-million persons in this country who are paralyzed, a quarter million were injured as a result of trauma (1). From 1973 to 1977, acts of violence were the fourth leading cause of spinal cord injury (13.9 percent). Since 1990, violently acquired spinal cord injuries (VASCI) have nearly doubled as a percentage of all causes of SCI (25.1 percent) and have moved into second place behind motor vehicle crashes (38.1 percent) (2). People who sustain injuries come from various social, ethnic, and economic backgrounds. The only commonality is the inability to be prepared to face a lifelong disability.

A spinal cord injury is not something that can be planned for. Occasionally, a disease process gradually impinges on one's mobility and feeling, and symptoms associated with spinal cord injury increasingly appear. Typical paraplegia or tetraplegia happens in an instant. The life that a person knows and has been accustomed to is altered drastically. The world that was once known—the world one could easily traverse and manipulate and interact with in long-established, sometimes automatic, ways—is instantaneously gone. Even everyday language no longer fits. Family and friends say, "Cross your fingers and hope for the best," or "You'll be fine in no time." But what are these well wishes supposed to mean to a person who is permanently disabled?

Society can be largely indifferent to the fact that the world has changed drastically for spinal cord injured persons, thus leaving most of the responsibility for "adjusting" with the injured person. That complex, challenging, and often frustrating process begins in the unfamiliar environment of a hospital. For a significant period of time immediately post-injury, the hospital constitutes the patient's world. It is here that the newly injured person first learns the meaning of the new label "disabled," fights against some of its premonitions, surrenders to others, and comes to more or less "accept" the fate with which he or she has been presented.

During this time of uncertainty, the hospital staff plays a strong role in assisting the patient with his or her new injury and supporting the patient's progress. This can best be done by providing a multidisciplinary team approach that works with the patient to develop rehabilitation goals. This is often difficult when the patient's primary focus may be on walking, returning to life as it was prior to the injury, or even gaining sympathy from family and friends. The rehabilitation staff focuses primarily on independence. This may be the person's ability to care for himself or to instruct others to care for him when he returns to the community. When there is a difference in rehabilitation goals, the patient and staff quickly become frustrated. Patients may not accept the need for rehabilitation and leave the hospital early, they may challenge the staff or lose interest in the rehabilitation program. The patient is soon labeled as "noncompliant," "unmotivated," and/or "manipulative." When this occurs, the staff also loses interest in treating the challenging needs of this population. This helps neither the patient nor the staff. To avoid this, it is good to recognize that the patient who is seen as noncompliant is often the one who proves most adept at achieving maximum independence in the world.

Independence is both important to and functional for patients. Staff should acknowledge this and support individual goals nonjudgmentally. Patient expectations may change from the acute phase through after discharge. Their early expectations may be unrealistic and extreme. Their first impressions are influenced by the amount and type of education that they receive

about their injury, the reactions of other people, and previous experiences and feelings about people with disabilities. More realistic expectations are found when individual factors become known and as the educational function of rehabilitation takes effect. How staff treats patients also has a large impact on patient success and realistic expectations. Those who are treated as adults and expected to manage their own care will likely have a higher quality of life following rehabilitation.

The expectations and goals will likely change again following discharge from the rehabilitation hospital. This is in part caused by the physical gains that are made. Patients may experience increased stamina and strength, functional return, and learn new techniques to achieve greater independence. Throughout the course of rehabilitation, the goals of the individual must be the priority for the team to achieve a positive outcome.

Society has not been structured to accommodate those with physical disabilities. Restaurants and stores are not always wheelchair accessible, and city sidewalks do not always allow a wheelchair to move easily. Newly injured patients are not aware of everyday barriers until they are faced with them. When the reality of an inaccessible world is put on top of the psychological adjustment to a new injury, it can seem overwhelming and at times impossible. Rehabilitation staff work with persons to prepare for re-entry into the world that they knew before. This includes assisting with day-to-day care, leisure skills, and social relationships; advocating for change for disability needs; managing medical needs, employment, education; and more. Whether it is several weeks or several months, preparation for the real world, in addition to adjustment to a permanent disability, cannot be mastered in this short time frame. The initial rehabilitation process gives patients a basic framework about their injury and how they can provide for their essential personal needs. Unfortunately, many of the following issues of adjustment will not be fully explored until the person is discharged back to the community.

However, it is important that staff be aware of key social and economic barriers that spinal cord injured patients face and how these barriers affect their adjustment to a life-altering disability.

SOCIAL RELATIONSHIPS

Soon after injury, the patient must begin to deal with the impact of the injury on significant social relationships. Anxious family members and friends appear at the bedside, and each party wonders and worries about the future. Obvious changes arise in relationships: spouses seek divorce; parents unable to accept the unhappy new reality discontinue significant contact with their disabled son or daughter; friends no longer find themselves having something in common with the spinal cord injured person; and the patient, on the basis of more-or-less-accurate reality testing, terminates meaningful relationships. But such events, especially when it comes to family members, are the exception rather that the rule. Usually, important people remain important to the injured person, who must assess which aspects of relationships will remain unchanged and which must be different.

This concern cannot be completely resolved while the patient is hospitalized. Time back in society—perhaps considerable time—is necessary before all the strands of significant relationships are once again in place. Nevertheless, the task begins early on, so the rehabilitation program must provide a variety of methods for patients to experience and explore how their relationships are to be defined. Encouraging family members to attend therapy sessions can enable all concerned to understand the patient's possibilities, limitations, and struggles. Patient/family education programs and consumer-oriented books and pamphlets about spinal cord injury also contribute to this goal. Individual counseling sessions between the social worker, the psychologist, and the patient; with family members in family counseling sessions; and group counseling can help clarify options for all parties. When the patient is physically able, day and weekend passes and days of residing with family in the rehabilitation unit's special patient-family living area are crucial experiments whose teaching values must be optimized through individual and group opportunity and discussed afterward with staff.

How one will be accepted into the wider community is also a matter of concern following spinal cord injury. Spinal cord injured patients rehabilitated for a considerable time pass these important words of advice on to their more recently injured compatriots: "The rehabilitation hospital staff is used to you; the world is not." And the reverse is also true: the patient, since injury, has related almost exclusively to hospital personnel within the official and unofficial rules of an institutional setting. Reintegration into the outside world can be made easier with the experience provided by passes and outings.

One of the most valuable relationships that can be formed is interaction with "old injury" people. Peer interaction and development of new relationships with spinal cord injured and other disabled individuals through the rehabilitation hospital and disabled community have proved to be educational and supportive. The feedback given by persons who have been surviving in the "real world" can prevent, as well as provide, a sense of comfort for those with new injuries. They are able to see that it is possible to have productive lives similar to those they knew before their injury.

It is noted in the literature that there has been in increase in the number of younger persons sustaining spinal cord injuries (ages 0–30). Most of these cases are caused by acts of violence. These people are likely to be single; have little, if any, social support; minimal education; have little, if no, work history; and be financially supported by governmental programs. With all of these factors in mind, it is no surprise that the social and life skills of this age group are lacking, if not nonexistent. The rehabilitation program can also assist by providing social skills training. This may be accomplished through educational sessions involving discussions, videotapes, and role-playing focused on the social opportunities and dilemmas an injured person can expect to encounter and positive ways of reacting to them. Unfortunately, this needed type of service is not usually covered by insurance sources and, therefore, is frequently not addressed.

One special area of social interactions that generates much question and concern is the issue of sexual relationships, both in terms of the injured person's ability to be satisfied and to satisfy a partner as well as the ability to produce offspring. Patients, because of their anxiety about their sexuality and in spite of their usual eagerness to re-establish themselves as sexual beings, cannot be rushed into trying out their sexual capabilities.

FINANCES

Financial concerns are considerable for the spinal cord injured and their families, as they begin to wonder about their debts to the hospital and its care providers. If the patient has been the primary wage earner, concerns center on basic living expenses and the adjustments that will be necessary. Many will explore the possibility of whether alternative financial resources are available. Until the time comes when the injured person can return to significant employment—if it comes at all—the means of putting food on the table and paying bills become a central issue. The knowledgeable social worker will give crucial assistance as these concerns surface.

If it were possible to look ahead to their spinal cord injury, perhaps the injured person would do one of the three things: 1) sign up for a comprehensive insurance policy that not only would pay all medical and hospital costs but also provide a considerable ongoing income; 2) plan to be injured in such a manner that someone else— more likely, someone's insurance company— would have to come up with a seven-figure payoff; or 3) enlist in the armed forces and become injured by some means other than their own negligence. In the latter case, the person would have a fairly substantial, tax-exempt lifetime income.

Economic barriers may be the most difficult to overcome and the most important because they can affect solutions to other barriers. Many

people who sustain spinal cord injuries but do not have either adequate medical coverage or plentiful financial resources to fall back on must rely on society's "safety net" programs. These include Medicaid, Social Security Disability, Supplemental Security Income, Aid to Families with Dependent Children, workmen's compensation, or Veterans Administration pension. These programs usually remain in effect unless the person resumes employment. The benefits of these programs are far from generous and, with the added burden of ongoing personal and health care costs, the injured person will likely wind up in difficult financial straits. For people with spinal cord injury, the cost of independence is greater than it is for an able-bodied person. There are costs for home modifications, personal care attendants, and other health-related expenses. Almost regardless of the eventual outcome, it is important for the patient and family to learn early what immediate resources are available and that there are long-term options with which the social worker can assist.

EMPLOYMENT AND EDUCATION

As rehabilitation progresses, the possibility of the injured person returning to former employment will become increasingly clear, although the matter may not be fully resolved until the injured person attempts to return to and function at work following hospital discharge. During the past few years, considerable strides have been made in devising altered work environments and modified tasks for the spinal cord injured employee and, occasionally, some employers have adopted flexible work hours to accommodate the injured person's new capabilities. Computers have created a world of work that can be uniquely adaptable to even severely injured persons. Buildings, sidewalks, and transportation have become significantly more wheelchair accessible, making employment possibilities considerably better than they once were. This is not to state that these issues have been completely corrected, and in retrospect, they should be much farther advanced than they are.

Vocational counselors, both in the rehabilitation setting and in state agencies, have a correspondingly enlarged opportunity to provide a service with a concrete payoff for their clients. However, some previously employed spinal cord injured people will not return to work because the rewards of whatever work is available will not outweigh the difficulties their injuries have created. Others will find themselves sufficiently well compensated for their injury that employment is no longer necessary. Some choose not to work because it would mean losing the financial benefits they receive with uncertain prospects of earning enough additional money to make it worthwhile and being able to sustain substantial employment.

Presently, the Work Incentives Improvement Act is passing through Congress for approval. This bill would send a strong signal that all Americans, including people with disabilities, can and do bring tremendous energy and talent to the American workforce. The unemployment rate for all working-age adults with disabilities is nearly 75 percent. One of the most glaring problems is that people with disabilities frequently become ineligible for Medicaid or Medicare if they go back to work. This puts people with disabilities in the untenable position of choosing between health care coverage and work. The Work Incentives Improvement Act would improve job opportunities for people with disabilities by increasing access to health care and employment services. The foundation for this act was created in response to the alarming unemployment and poverty rate for people with disabilities. This legislation has the ability to effect about 9 million adults who collect federal disability benefits.

Vocational planning may require attention to renew, revise, or generate new educational endeavors. State vocational agencies, federal grant programs, and private funding sources allow people with disabilities to attend school at little or no cost. The reasons for returning to educational programs include furthering vocational goals, developing new career paths, and completing high school. The rehabilitation hospital can assist with this process by stressing the need to finish high school and encouraging higher education as a means of successful community integration. Visits to nearby college campuses during rehabilitation can give clear evidence of their accessibility and, with assistance from the student disabilities department, present the college's interest in making further education a viable and rewarding pursuit. If nothing else, such visits are a useful way of getting young people who are injured into contact with young people who are not.

HOUSING

The prospect of discharge from the rehabilitation setting requires attention to the matter of housing. Only rare individuals whose mobility is scarcely impaired can think of returning to their former home with complete comfort. Most will have to attend to at least the placement of ramps, the widening of doorways, and the altering of the bathroom so it is both accessible and usable. In this, as in many aspects of the newly altered lifestyle, the amount of money available is a key factor. Some patients will be unable to return to their previous homes, and the challenging task of locating affordable, wheelchair-accessible living quarters must begin.

Wheelchair-accessible housing has been increasing in recent years, partly in response to state and local legislation mandating that a certain percentage of new apartments accommodate disabled people. These are not yet easy to find, however, unless a person has more than usual financial assets. The federal government, through the Department of Housing and Urban Development (HUD), has a program that partially subsidizes rents for disabled people. These "Section 8" funds are limited, however, and it is not unusual in some cities for applicants to wait several years before a subsidized apartment becomes available for them.

Many people return to housing that is not accessible. Perhaps a doorway is not wide enough for a wheelchair, the bathroom is not accessible, or there are stairs at the entrance of the home. This requires even an independent person to become dependent on others to enter and exit their home. Many states offer home modification programs with qualifications that are based on income and need for modifications. Some agencies require a person to be working or in school before modifications will be made. Even after the requirements are met, there are extensive waiting lists up to 5 years for basic home modifications.

Unfortunately, many people with spinal cord injuries, because lack of personal assistance and accessible housing, must reside in 24-hour care facilities. Commonly called nursing homes or long-term care facilities, these places are usually not prepared to treat the complex physical, emotional, and psychological needs of this population. Some persons become depressed at the thought of spending the rest of their lives in a nursing home and lose the goal and drive to live independently. Others may use these facilities as a temporary home while securing accessible housing and personal care. The centers for independent living play an instrumental role in assisting the patient to look for and obtain housing and attendant care.

A nursing home bed can usually be found for a cooperative spinal cord injured person. However, if substance abuse, hostile behavior, past social involvement, or psychiatric illness complicates heavy care needs, the prospect of locating a willing nursing home may become quite dim. The ventilator-dependent tetraplegic who has managed to corral the extensive resources necessary to live in the community will probably be particularly disadvantaged should care attendant(s) become unavailable. Nursing homes will not always accommodate these patients and even hospitals may decline to admit. Specialized facilities for ventilator-dependent people are both rare and very expensive.

PERSONAL ATTENDANTS

A crucial question for many patients approaching discharge from the rehabilitation hospital is, who will be providing necessary assistance? For some, this means someone to do household chores, and for others, someone to also provide personal care. Our society tends to assume that the spouse will take on most, if not all, assistance duties. However, even the most dutiful spouse occasionally needs help, and many patients need to hire someone regularly or occasionally as their aide. Some limited state monies are available to partially defray the costs of assistance for low-income disabled persons, and some Veterans Administration funds are available for veterans who meet certain eligibility criteria.

Not all devoted spouses choose to make themselves available for the patient's care—opting, for example, to continue or take up employment to provide a reliable income. Not all spouses are physically capable of providing care, even with all available equipment. Some are willing to take on part, but not all, of the patient's care. Bowel care is an area that is often the most difficult for the spouse to accept. Likewise, some patients refuse to let their spouse provide bowel care, fearing an adverse effect on their overall relationship and, at times, their sexual relations. Others decide that the spouse will be called on for this critical service only in emergencies or when they are traveling and their customary arrangements are not possible.

Both the amount and kind of care needed and the availability of "natural" helpers (spouse, parents, and other family) determine the extent to which community resources must be enlisted. The person with limited personal care needs will likely find the necessary help from a home health agency. In some of these situations, private insurance and state medical programs may assist with or meet these costs. The person who requires a live-in attendant, on the other hand, will probably discover it to be a substantial challenge to meet the care requirements. In recent years, there has been a welcome increase in community training programs for people interested in working as aids for the severely disabled; however, there is still an insufficient supply of well-trained, reliable attendants. The patient needs someone who is knowledgeable and stable; whose personality fits comfortably with that of the patient; and who will perform sometimes arduous, unpleasant tasks at all hours of the day and night for less than substantial wages. It is no small wonder that this challenge is not easily met! For this reason, patients sometimes unwisely agree to be cared for by too-willing family members who are not capable of handling the responsibility, or they sometimes coerce reluctant family members into taking on the work. In both cases, the arrangement seldom persists profitably for either person.

Hiring an attendant is a new experience for almost all recently injured patients. Staff can help the patient think carefully about which care needs must be met, the time intervals during which various kinds of assistance will be necessary, off-duty time that the attendant will have, house rules that should be formulated, and how patient and attendant will interact apart from carrying out care needs (e.g. whether they will eat together, watch TV together, or share social occasions). Some disabled people have found it difficult to be both employer and friend. Being expected to meet the social and emotional needs as well as the physical needs of their employer has overwhelmed some attendants. For some patients it can be helpful to have a chance in advance to "role play" the interview with a prospective attendant. In addition, social skills training can usefully include a segment on how to interact successfully with an attendant.

LEISURE TIME

A spinal cord injury may require a change in some of the patient's leisure activities. What was once comfortable and enjoyable may now be impossible or take more effort than the activity is worth. Some rethinking and experimenting in this area occurs during the patient's free moments during rehabilitation. The matter may not be fully settled until long after rehabilitation is complete. However, evidence of the possibilities available even to the severely disabled must be widely shared during the rehabilitation period. Until fairly recently, even spectator sports were mostly inaccessible to wheelchair-bound people. Not only has that changed for the better, but both individual and competitive sports once thought out of reach for the spinal cord injured person are now commonplace. "Disabled" no longer necessarily equates to "inactive," unless the injured person so chooses.

LIFE IN THE WORLD AFTER REHABILITATION

Once acute rehabilitation is over, full-time life in the "real world" begins; then, the process of testing one's old and new social roles gains momentum. Some will be fortunate enough to be able to pick up—as spouse, parent, employee, friend, church member, student—pretty much where they left off. Others, by virtue of the extent of their injury or the particular choices they make about how to cope, will considerably recast their daily activities. The former breadwinner may become the stay-at-home parent. The former patrolman may become a police dispatcher. The weekend camper and vacation traveler may turn into the housebound invalid. Quickly for some, and more slowly for others, the questions— What do I now expect of myself? And, what do others now expect of me?—will be answered, and then asked again and reanswered.

After living in the community for a while, spinal cord injured people often report an acceleration of the awkward experiences they began encountering early in their disability: "people stare at me," "children ask ridiculous questions about me," " some jerks think I'm totally helpless." They tell of embarrassing moments when their chair tipped over or when they had an involuntary bowel movement. They report surprises: "my neck gets sore from looking up all the time," "people have a hard time understanding what I can and can't do." Nevertheless, their surprise mostly comes from discovering that, in general, other people are both kind and appropriately helpful.

Being back in the world means encountering the full range of socioeconomic problems that beset everyone, plus a variety that are mostly reserved for disabled people. The way these problems play themselves out in the lives of the spinal cord injured illustrates a noteworthy fact concerning this population: there is a continuum, with injured people whose overall behavior can be characterized as prudent on one end and those whose behavior can be called imprudent on the other.

Some people become spinal cord injured essentially by accident. They conduct themselves reasonably, cautiously, and prudently, but fate inflicts an automobile accident or a fall. After a period of adjustment to their injury, they basically return to their former prudent lifestyle, not immune to socioeconomic difficulties. A social security check gets lost in the mail or an attendant becomes ill. They may need temporary assistance with the financial or care emergency that is generated. Sometimes temporary assistance is not easy to locate. If housing is the problem, for example, few shelters can accommodate people in wheelchairs. Thus, the prudent person may be severely frustrated.

On the other end of the continuum are the people who conduct their lives impulsively, recklessly, and imprudently. They drive too fast on their motorcycles; they dive into shallow water; they get behind the wheel of an automobile while under the influence of alcohol or drugs; they attempt to hold up a convenience store. For them, socioeconomic emergencies are just one facet of their emergency-induced way of living. One day a large, lasting result of their lifestyle manifests as a spinal cord injury. Their approach to life will probably not change, so when they return to society from a rehabilitation hospital, they choose friends and housemates who take financial advantage of them. They select aides who cater to their vices, who are co-indulgers with them in their self-destructive habits, and who are impulsive and in need of immediate gratification and therefore provide unreliable, inconsistent, or inadequate care.

The lifestyles of many spinal cord injured people fall in between the two extremes of the prudent–imprudent continuum. Their lives are more or less emergency-induced and impulsively conducted. However, the fact that imprudent people tend more often than prudent people to become spinal cord injured means that emergencies, chaos, and disruptiveness will be more evident in the spinal cord injured population than in the general population. Hospital staff, therefore, must be aware of stereotyping and inaccurately painting all or most spinal cord injured patients with the same unflattering brush.

CONCLUSION

The types of patients that sustain a spinal cord injury have changed dramatically in the last 25 years. The development of comprehensive treatment and rehabilitation programs for spinal cord injured people came from the large number of such injuries in World War II. At that time, the life expectancy was 6 months for a spinal cord injury. Today, things have changed dramatically, and spinal cord injured patients are now experiencing, along with many others in society, the pleasures and problems of aging. Retirement from work and social activities may come earlier than planned or desired. More care may be needed, and long-time caregivers may no longer be able to help. Finances may become tighter, and additional care is needed. The need for nursing home care becomes a larger, possible necessity.

The social and economic burdens of spinal cord injury are often greater for African Americans and Hispanics. This is largely due in part to discrimination, lower educational and socioeconomic status, and lack of social support systems. Rehabilitation hospitals must reshape and develop programs that meet the changing needs of the population. Long-term follow-up must be provided to foster empowerment and enhance community integration.

People who have been injured for several decades continue to talk of adjustment to, rather than acceptance of, the injury. There is grateful approval of the changes that have occurred in society: improved accessibility, better transportation, and overall, more enlightened attitudes in the general public toward disabilities. Life has not been easy since injury, and most would not want to do it again. Even for the most severely disabled, there have been rewards as well as burdens, accomplishments as well as deprivations. They remember clearly the circumstances of their injury: it was the moment the world changed dramatically for them.

REFERENCES

1. *Your World Changes with a Spinal Cord Injury.* National Spinal Cord Injury Association, 1996.
2. Stover S, Richards J, Devivo M. *The Impact of Violence on the Etiology and Outcomes of Spinal Cord Injury.* 1994.

24 Spinal Cord Ischemic Injury: Experimental Model and Prevention

BOK Y. LEE, MD, FACS
MARCELO C. DASILVA, MD

SPINAL CORD ISCHEMIA as a consequence of intra-abdominal arterial reconstruction is a rare complication (1), the outcome of which is partial or complete paraplegia. The occurrence of this complication has been associated with the level and duration of aortic occlusion, intraoperative hypotension, inadequate intraoperative anticoagulation, atheromatous emboli, and occlusive arteriosclerosis of the spinal cord arteries. We present a review of the incidence, clinical factors, and vascular anatomy of the spinal cord. Additionally, we present a report of a patient with spinal cord ischemia with paraplegia secondary to the presence of an abdominal aortic aneurysm (AAA) in the absence of any surgical procedure.

INCIDENCE

Elliott et al. (2) cite 51 published cases of spinal cord ischemia secondary to surgery of the abdominal aorta. Perhaps the largest review of the incidence of this complication at a single institution comes from the Henry Ford Hospital (2–4). In a total of 3,445 surgical procedures involving the abdominal aorta, including 1,861 abdominal aortic aneurysms (259 ruptured and 1,062 elective), aortoiliac occlusive disease in 1,188 procedures, and renal or mesenteric arterial occlusive disease in 396, only eight cases (0.2 percent) were associated with spinal cord ischemia. All instances of complications occurred during surgery for abdominal aortic aneurysms. In a recent report from the University of Rochester (1), seven patients were reported with spinal cord ischemia following 744 abdominal aortic procedures (0.9 percent)—three occurred during surgery for aneurysmal disease and four during surgery for aortoiliac occlusive disease.

CLINICAL FEATURES

Examination of the published cases of spinal cord ischemia following abdominal aortic procedures does not yield any specific clinical features that would indicate why certain patients sustain spinal cord injury. The anatomic features of the blood supply to the spinal cord may be an important precipitating factor.

SPINAL CORD VASCULAR ANATOMY

The vascular anatomy of the spinal cord can be divided into a proximal or extraspinal division, an intermediate division, and a terminal distribution system (2). The proximal or extraspinal division is composed of the vertebral, ascending cervical, deep cervical, intercostal, and lumbar arteries. Collateral interconnections are plentiful in the cervical and sacral regions and less so in the thoracic region. Thus, interruption of the blood supply in the thoracic region cannot be compensated for through collateral pathways as well as in the cervical and sacral regions.

The intermediate division is composed of the spinal radicular arteries connecting the branches of the aorta to the terminal distribution system of blood vessels lying in the spinal cord. In an adult, radicular arteries are few and usually include up to two cervical, three thoracic, two lumbar, and those supplying the sacral spinal cord. The great radicular artery (Adamkiewicz) is usually located at the T-9 to T-12 level and is considered the main feeder of the anterior spinal artery in the distal thoracolumbar spinal cord.

The terminal distribution system is composed of the anterior spinal artery and paired posterolateral spinal arteries. The anterior spinal artery is the largest, extends the full length of the spinal cord, and is fed by branches of the two vertebral arteries. In the region lacking radicular blood vessels, the anterior spinal artery is the sole source of blood.

From the foregoing review of the vascular anatomy of the spinal cord, one can see that the spinal cord, particularly the thoracic segment, is highly vulnerable to any interruption in its blood supply. Elliott et al. (2) point out the relative lack of a collateral circulation between branches of the intercostal arteries in the thoracic segment in contrast to the cervical, lumbar, and sacral segments. They also noted the limited communication among the three spinal arteries, the small number of anterior spinal radicular arteries, and the variability of the level of origin of the great radicular artery.

Case Report. A 63-year-old white man, paraplegic from the level of T-10, was admitted from a community hospital. The patient had a history of stroke, from which he had recovered, generalized arteriosclerosis, myocardial infarction, hypertension, and hypothyroidism. Over the past few years, the patient had developed pro-

gressive spastic paralysis. An extensive neurologic examination was inconclusive; the consensus was the presence of ischemic myelitis secondary to the presence of an abdominal aortic aneurysm.

At the time of admission, physical examination revealed a thin, cachectic man in no obvious distress. The patient's vital signs were within normal limits for his age. His neck had bilateral surgical scar from previous carotid artery endoarterectomies. The lungs and cardiac exam were unremarkable. The abdomen was soft, with a palpable pulsitile mass. A neurologic exam revealed marked wasting of the muscles, particularly evident in the distal muscles of the hands and the muscles of the legs and hips. No fasciculations were visible, and there were marked flexion contractures of the lower extremities with spasticity. Previous computed tomography of the abdomen (Fig. 24-1) revealed a dilated abdominal aorta measuring 5 cm at the largest diameter proximally with a calcified wall. An area of low attenuation within the lumen was thought to be representative of thrombus. A large aneurysm was noted beginning at the level of the renal arteries and extending to the bifurcation. Areas of low attenuation suggested the presence of thrombi within the aneurysm. The aneurysm measured 6 cm × 6.5 cm (anteriorposterior × transverse). An ultrasonographic examination of the abdominal aorta performed 8 months later revealed an aneurysmal sac measuring 11 cm in length and 5 cm anterior-posterior at the level of the umbilicus (Fig. 24-2). The patient's condition remained unchanged since admission.

Comment. This case report demonstrates that the thoracic spinal cord is particularly vulnerable to interruption of its blood supply during surgical intervention, blunt abdominal trauma, or in the presence of a dissecting abdominal aortic aneurysm. As discussed, the thoracic spinal region is relatively poor in collateral circulation, limiting the extent of compensatory blood supply through other routes. Additional complications include the limited intercommunication of the anterior spinal

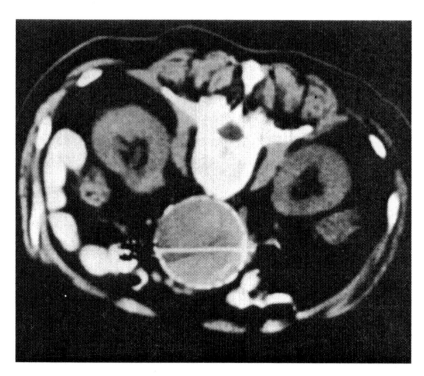

FIGURE 24-1 Computed tomography of the abdomen showing dilated abdominal aorta (5 cm) with a calcified wall and thrombus.

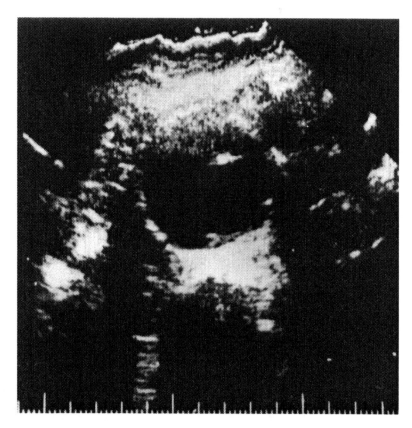

FIGURE 24-2 Ultrasonographic scan showing an aneurysmal sac measuring 11 cm × 5 cm at umbilicus level.

artery and the long length and narrow diameter of the great radicular artery. An additional complicating factor during surgical intervention is the variable origin of the great radicular artery.

In conclusion, steps may be taken to limit the occurrence of spinal cord ischemia following intra-abdominal surgical procedures. As the case report demonstrates, the occurrence of spinal cord ischemia and spontaneous paralysis due to abdominal aortic aneurysm embolization to the great radicular artery in the absence of surgical intervention is unpreventable but is an extremely infrequent source of morbidity.

PREVENTION OF SPINAL CORD ISCHEMIC INJURY BY USE OF A β-AGONIST AGENT

Paraplegia is a complication of thoracoabdominal aortic aneurysm in 4 to 30 percent of patients undergoing repair. This is dependent on the extent of aorta involved, presence of aortic dissection or rupture, hypotension, and aortic cross-clamping time (5–8). This complication has been attributed to temporary or permanent ischemia of the spinal cord caused by the interruption of blood flow during aortic cross-clamping. In most patients who develop paraplegia, neurologic deficits are present at the time they awaken from anesthesia. However, in a subset of patients, paraplegia can develop up to 7 days after surgery (6). This is referred to as *delayed onset paraplegia*.

Recent evidence has indicated that a significant component producing paraplegia is not the result of the ischemia itself. Instead, spinal cord injury occurs after the ischemic interval during the reperfusion period. Reperfusion injury is believed to be partially related to the sudden availability of excess quantities of molecular oxygen in ischemic tissue leading to the production of oxygen-derived free radicals, which in turn causes extensive tissue injury (9). However, the exact mechanism of postoperative paraplegia remains debatable.

We conducted an experimental study to examine the prevention of neuronal degeneration after ischemic injury to the spinal cord using clenbuterol, a selective β-2 adrenergic receptor agonist that has been shown to increase gene expression of nerve growth factor (NGF) and basic fibroblast growth factor (bFGF) in the central nervous system. Nerve growth factor promotes axonal regeneration and synaptic plasticity, while basic fibroblast growth factor antagonizes glutamate-induced increase in intracellular calcium, which causes neurotoxicity. Because glutamate toxicity is believed to occur extensively during and after spinal cord ischemia, clenbuterol may prevent the neuronal cell death and paralysis that occurs within several days of ischemia.

The phenomenon of neuronal preservation after ischemic injury was studied in the New Zealand rabbit model (Fig. 24-3) which, because

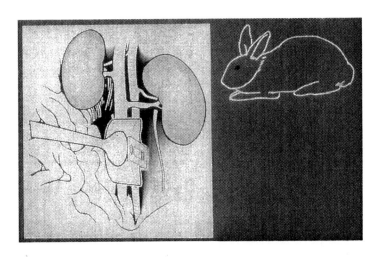

FIGURE 24-3 New Zealand rabbit model.

of its segmental distribution of blood supply to the spinal cord, is an excellent experimental model for reproducing ischemic paraplegia (10). Using the transonic flowmeter (Fig. 24-4A, B), aortic blood flow was measured on the infrarenal aorta. Interestingly, in the rabbits that developed paraplegia, the aortic blood flow measurements were significantly increased following declamping of the aorta, representing a departure from the baseline blood flow measurements. These experimental observations suggest that hyperperfusion following declamping of the aorta may be a significant pathophysiologic event in ischemic spinal cord injury.

Clenbuterol

Clenbuterol is a selective β-2 adrenergic receptor agonist that has been used in patients to increase muscle strength following orthopedic surgery as well as in healthy subjects to enhance rehabilitative muscle growth and prevent atrophy (11,12). Clenbuterol retards denervation atrophy and promotes hypertrophy of skeletal muscle fibers (13,14) via a direction action on the musculature. β-2 agonist treatment promotes long-term recovery of muscle strength following an ischemic injury. Therefore, pharmacologic stimulation of cell membrane β-2 receptors may prevent toxic increases in intracellular calcium concentration, which is triggered by cellular hypoxia-induced glutamate

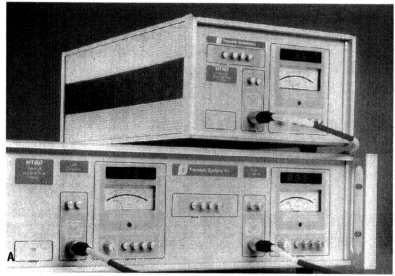

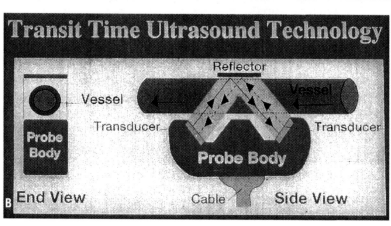

FIGURE 24-4 A. Transonic flowmeter data processor. **B.** Transit time ultrasound technology (The principle of transonic flowmeter). Using wide beam illumination, two transducers pass ultrasound signals back and forth, intersecting the flow in upstream and downstream directions. The flowmeter derives a measure of the "transit time" it takes for the waves to travel from one transducer to the other. The difference between the upstream and downstream transit time is the measure of the volume flow.

release (15,16). In addition, studies of skeletal muscle demonstrate that β-2 adrenergic stimulation can increase the expression of calpastatin, an inhibitor of the protease calpain, which is involved in neurodegeneration (17,18). Studies of the effects of β-2 adrenergic receptor agonists on the central nervous system suggest that these agents have properties that may oppose the neurodegeneration caused by ischemia.

Systemic administration of the β-2 agonist clenbuterol increases central nervous system gene expression of growth factors such as nerve growth factor (NGF) and basic fibroblast growth factor (bFGF) that promote neuronal survival (19,20). Ischemic injury to the central nervous system is thought to result from the toxic effects of excessive release of glutamate, a neurotransmitter released in response to anoxia (16). Glutamate promotes the influx of calcium into neurons, resulting in intracellular calcium overload, which leads to cell death by a variety of mechanisms. In support of this view, calcium chelators have been shown to be at least partially effective in preventing the deleterious effects

of ischemia (21). Interestingly, basic fibroblast growth factor (bFGF) was shown to oppose the ability of glutamate to increase intraneuronal calcium concentration and subsequent cell death (15). Because glutamate toxicity is believed to occur extensively during and after spinal cord ischemia, clenbuterol may prevent the neuronal cell death and paralysis that occurs within several days of ischemia. Together, these studies suggest that clenbuterol may exert a protective effect on the central nervous system during and following periods of ischemia, such as those caused by stroke, trauma, and surgical procedures involving vascular clamping. The phenomenon of neuronal preservation after ischemic injury was studied in a New Zealand rabbit model (10).

In our study, there were 30 evaluable rabbits (15 controls, 15 experimental) weighing 4 to 6 kg. The experimental group was given clenbuterol (9 mg) in drinking water 24 hours prior to surgery. All subjects were premedicated with atropine sulfate (0.005 mg/kg) administered subcutaneously and anesthetized with I.M. keta-

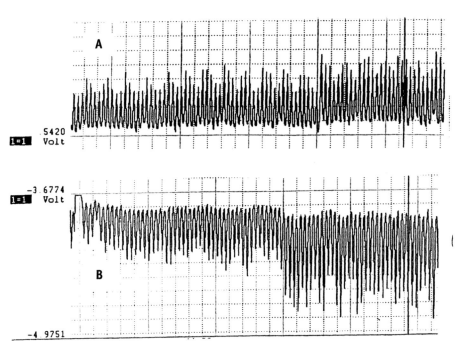

FIGURE 24-5 Transonic flowmeter real-time recording. **A.** Baseline aortic blood flow before clamping. **B.** Aortic blood flow after declamping.

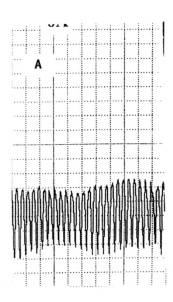
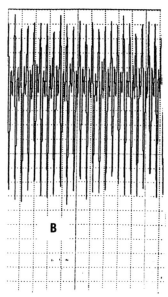

FIGURE 24-6 Transonic flowmeter real-time recording. **A.** Baseline aortic blood flow before clamping. **B.** Aortic blood flow after declamping. Note the marked increase in post-declamping aortic blood flow.

mine hydrochloride (40 mg/kg) and xylazine (3 mg/kg). The fur on the abdomen was clipped with an electric shaver just prior to the surgery, and the skin was prepared with betadine solution. Heparin (70 units/kg) was given intravenously 5 minutes prior to the skin incision. Intermittent IV administration of one-quarter dose of the anesthetic agents maintained an adequate level of anesthesia, and there was no need for endotracheal intubation and mechanical ventilation. Via mask, the rabbits were maintained at 100 percent oxygen during the procedure. The rabbit was placed in the supine position, and a midline incision of approximately 5 cm was made between xiphisternum and pubic symphysis. The abdominal aorta was identified and a transonic flowmeter probe was placed 1 cm below the renal arteries (Fig. 24-3). Direct blood flow measurements were recorded at the infrarenal aorta before and after aortic cross-clamping (Fig. 24-5). The degree of reproducible ischemic injury was established by cross-clamping the infrarenal aorta for a period of either 22 or 30 minutes. Confirmation of aortic occlusion was obtained by a zero reading of the transonic flowmeter. Abdominal aortic blood

flow was recorded at the time of declamping of the aorta until the blood flow readings peaked and returned to baseline (Fig. 24-6A). At the end of the procedure, the abdomen was closed in layers with absorbable fascial and nonabsorbable skin sutures. All rabbits were observed closely postoperatively. Neurologic assessment was recorded according to Tarlov's neurological scale (Table 24-1). The anal and bladder sphincter functions were also assessed daily. The rabbits were euthanized at the end of 30 days.

Assessment of the degree of paralysis of the hind limbs was recorded according to Tarlov's neurologic scale. All of the rabbits with a 30-minute cross-clamping time of the aorta (two control and two experimental, n = 4) developed

TABLE 24-1 Tarlov's Neurologic Scale

Tarlov's Neurologic Scale	
0	Paraplegia, no movement of the lower limb
1	Paraplegia, slight movement of the lower limb
2	Good movement of the lower limbs but unable to stand
3	Able to stand, but not able to walk
4	Complete recovery

Control Group (n=13)

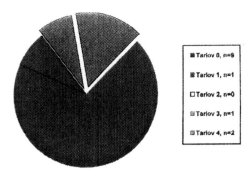

β-Agonist (Clenbuterol) Group (n=13)

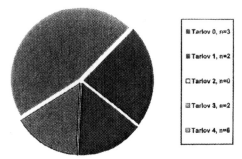

FIGURE 24-7 Neurological outcome of 22-minute infrarenal aortic clamping and declamping. The top pie chart shows the control group (n = 13), in which 77 percent rabbits developed paraplegia (Tarlov 0 and 1, n = 10). The bottom pie chart shows the β-agonist (clenbuterol) group. In contrast to the control group, only half as many rabbits (38 percent) developed paraplegia (Tarlov 0 and 1, n = 5) in this group.

complete paraplegia. Of the 13 control group rabbits with a 22-minute minute cross-clamping time of the aorta, 77 percent developed paraplegia (Tarlov 0, n = 9; Tarlov 1, n = 1), and 23 percent did not develop paraplegia (Tarlov 3, n = 1; Tarlov 4, n = 2). Of the 13 experimental rabbits who were administered clenbuterol 24 hours prior to surgery with 22-minute minute cross-clamping time of the aorta, 38 percent developed paraplegia (Tarlov 0, n = 3; Tarlov 1, n = 2), and 62 percent did not develop paraplegia (Tarlov 3, n = 2; Tarlov 4, n = 6) (Fig. 24-7). An interesting and fairly consistent laboratory observation was that the rabbits who did not develop paraplegia had minimal increases in

post-declamping aortic blood flow, whereas the rabbits who developed paraplegia had a significant marked increase in post-declamping aortic blood flow (Fig. 24-6B). Experimental animals with this kind of post-declamping hyperperfusion showed complete postoperative paraplegia.

Although the exact mechanism of paraplegia following intraoperative aortic clamping and declamping remains unknown, our preliminary laboratory observations in the rabbit ischemic injury model suggest that variations in aortic blood flow following declamping of the aorta may play a role in the development of paraplegia. This may be due to ischemia and/or declamping hyperperfusion; thus, controlling variations in aortic blood pressure following aortic declamping may help to prevent paraplegia. Further aortic blood flow studies will help to clarify the causes of paraplegia following thoracoabdominal aortic aneurysm repair.

REFERENCES

1. Picone AL, Green RM, Ricotta JR, May AG, DeWeese JA. Spinal cord ischemia following operations on the abdominal aorta. *J Vasc Surg* 1986; 3(1):94–103.
2. Elliott JP, Szilagyi DE, Hageman JH, et al. Spinal cord ischemia: secondary to surgery of the abdominal aorta. In Berhard VM, Towne JB, eds.. *Complications in Vascular Surgery*, 2nd ed. Philadelphia: Grune & Stratton, 1985. Pp. 291–310.
3. Szilagyi DE, Hageman JH, Smith RF, Elliott JP. Spinal cord damage in surgery of the abdominal aorta. *Surgery* 1978; 83(1):38–56.
4. Elliott JP, Szilagyi DE, Hageman JH, Smith RF. Spinal cord ischemia: secondary to surgery of the abdominal aorta. In Berhard VM, Towne JB, eds., *Complications in Vascular Surgery*. Philadelphia: Grune & Stratton 1980. Pp. 407–426.
5. Hollier LH. Protecting the brain and spinal cord. *J Vasc Surg* 1987; 5(3):524–528.
6. Crawford ES, Crawford JL, Safi HJ, Coselli JS, Hess KR, Brooks B, Norton HJ, Glaeser DH. Thoracoabdominal aortic aneurysms: preoperative and intraoperative factors determining immediate and long-term results of operations in 605 patients. *J Vasc Surg* 1986; 3(3):389–404.
7. Hollier LH, Money SR, Naslund TC, Proctor CD, Sr, Buhrman WC, Marino RJ, Harmon DE,

Kazmier FJ. Risk of spinal cord dysfunction in patients undergoing thoracoabdominal aortic replacement. *Am J Surg* 1992; 164(3):210–215.

8. Svensson LG, Crawford ES, Hess KR, Coselli JS, Safi HJ. Experience with 1509 patients undergoing thoracoabdominal aortic operations. *J Vasc Surg* 1993; 17(2):357–370.

9. Parks DA, Granger DN. Ischemia-reperfusion injury: a radical view. *Hepatology* 1988; 8(3): 680–682.

10. Moore WM Jr., Hollier LH. The influence of severity of spinal cord ischemia in the etiology of delayed-onset paraplegia. *Ann Surg* 1991; 213(5): 427–432.

11. Maltin CA, Delday MI, Watson JS, Heys SD, Nevison IM, Ritchie IK, Gibson PH. Clenbuterol, a beta-adrenoceptor agonist, increases relative muscle strength in orthopaedic patients. *Clin Sci* 1993; 84(6):651–654.

12. Martineau L, Horan MA, Rothwell NJ, Little RA. Salbutamol, a beta 2-adrenoceptor agonist, increases skeletal muscle strength in young men. *Clin Sci* 1992; 83(5):615–621 [See Erratum in *Clin Sci* 1993;84(6).]

13. Zeman RJ, Hirschman A, Hirschman ML, Guo G, Etlinger JD. Clenbuterol, a beta 2-receptor agonist, reduces net bone loss in denervated hindlimbs. *Am J Physiol* 1991; 261(2 Pt 1): E285–289.

14. Zeman RJ, Ludemann R, Etlinger JD. Clenbuterol, a beta 2-agonist, retards atrophy in denervated muscles. *Am J Physiol* 1987; 252(1 Pt 1):E152–155.

15. Mattson MP, Murrain M, Guthrie PB, Kater SB. Fibroblast growth factor and glutamate: opposing roles in the generation and degeneration of hippocampal neuroarchitecture. *J Neuroscience* 1989; 9(11):3728–3740.

16. Choi DW. Excitotoxic cell death. *J Neurobiology* 1992; 23(9):1261–1276.

17. Bardsley RG, Allcock SM, Dawson JM, Dumelow NW, Higgins JA, Lasslett YV, Lockley AK, Parr T, Buttery PJ. Effect of beta-agonists on expression of calpain and calpastatin activity in skeletal muscle. *Biochimie* 1992; 74(3):267–273.

18. Najm I, Vanderklish P, Etebari A, Lynch G, Baudry M. Complex interactions between polyamines and calpain-mediated proteolysis in rat brain. *J Neuroch* 1991; 57(4):1151–1158.

19. Follesa P, Mocchetti I. Regulation of basic fibroblast growth factor and nerve growth factor mRNA by beta-adrenergic receptor activation and adrenal steroids in rat central nervous system. *Mol Pharm* 1993; 43(2):132–138.

20. Hayes VY, Isackson PJ, Fabrazzo M, Follesa P, Mocchetti I. Induction of nerve growth factor and basic fibroblast growth factor mRNA following clenbuterol: contrasting anatomical and cellular localization. *Exp Neurol* 1995; 132(1):33–41.

21. Tymianski M, Wallace MC, Spigelman I, Uno M, Carlen PL, Tator CH, Charlton MP. Cell-permeant Ca2+ chelators reduce early excitotoxic and ischemic neuronal injury in vitro and in vivo. *Neuron* 1993; 11(2):221–235.

25 Spinal Cord Injury Rehabilitation

GARY M. YARKONY, MD
MICHELLE GITTLER, MD

IN 1945, SIR LUDWIG GUTTMAN stated that, "Rehabilitation after spinal injuries seeks the fullest possible physical and psychological readjustment of the injured person to his permanent disability with a view to restoring his will to live and working capacity" (1). This comment is still poignant today, even as improvements in acute care and long-term medical management have resulted in increasing life spans for individuals with spinal cord injury. Although research continues toward a cure for the conditions resulting from spinal cord injury, these individuals must not let this hope interfere with their reintegration into society.

Although estimates of the exact number of spinal cord injuries per year vary, there are approximately 10,000 persons annually who survive these injuries and are hospitalized (2,3). The prevalence of spinal cord injury is estimated to be 721 spinal injuries per million persons at risk (3). Because this population is young, with most injuries occurring in the 16- to 30-year age group (mean age = 30.7, median = 26.0), the importance of rehabilitation and reintegration into the community is crucial (4). Recent studies indicate that post-injury life span is increasing (5).

Vital to rehabilitation after spinal cord injury is an interdisciplinary team (6) functioning in an appropriate facility (7–8). Comprehensive units with skilled therapists capable of providing all aspects of care for spinal cord injured persons are essential. The concept of specialized spinal cord injury units was first developed in the United States by Munro (9) and in England by Guttman (10). Care of spinal cord injuries in these units should provide for a coordinated system of care with decreased secondary complications and lifelong follow-up. A comprehensive rehabilitation program, which provides a full range of services and maximum patient participation, enhances the likelihood of achieving favorable outcomes, promotes the resumption of meaningful life roles, and facilitates the opportunities for community reintegration (8).

ASPECTS OF REHABILITATION IN THE ACUTE CARE PHASE

The most important aspects during the acute care phase relate to saving the life of the traumatized patient. Efforts to prevent further damage to the spinal cord include immobilization of the spine, correction of the deformity, administration of steroids, and maintenance of the cardiovascular and other biological parameters. It is essential that while these complex problems are being managed efforts are made to prevent secondary complications that may interfere with rehabilitation (11). Two of the most essential complications to be prevented are pressure sores and joint contracture. Consideration must also be given to the presence of concomitant head injury (12) and its affect on further rehabilitation and urologic management.

Prevention of deep venous thrombosis had been a perplexing problem during the acute care and initial rehabilitation phase. Low molecular weight heparin has resulted in a significant drop in the incidence of deep venous thrombosis and pulmonary embolism (12).

Joint range of motion can be maintained by range of motion (ROM) exercises and splinting. As the patient is initially flaccid, ROM exercises performed daily may be all that is necessary. Joints affected by local trauma or edema may require more. The best guide is careful reassessment and upgrading of the program if loss of range of motion occurs. As spasticity develops, ROM exercises may be necessary two or three times daily. Splinting of the wrist in a functional position of extension with the web space of the thumb maintained in abduction is a useful adjunct. Splinting of the ankles at 90 degrees may be necessary if plantar flexion contractures develop. Studies on contracture development after spinal cord injury show a decreased incidence of contracture development in a specialized system of acute care (13).

Although ROM exercises are generally in the domain of the therapist, it is essential that the nursing staff be able to perform these exercises. Frequently, family members can assist in these activities if they will not interfere with life support equipment. This not only prevents deformity but gives family members the satisfaction of contributing to the care of their loved one. Particular care should be given to the shoulder, as a tetraplegic suffering from adhesive capsulitis of this joint may have a more difficult and prolonged rehabilitation. Contractures most commonly occur during the acute care phase in the hip, knee, and ankle.

Prevention of pressure sores is best accomplished by frequent turning and careful skin inspection. Initially, the patient should be turned every 2 hours. Skin should be kept clean and dry. Shearing forces, particularly during transfers, should be avoided. Particular care should be exercised, when using a rotating bed, that the bed is not stopped frequently, thus defeating its usefulness. Pressure sores in the sacral area (4) are most common during the acute care phase of rehabilitation, but one must also be careful to protect the heels and other bony prominences.

Optimal urologic management in the acute care phase is often limited by the need to closely monitor fluid and electrolyte balance. An indwelling catheter may be the most practical method in these situations. When the patient is stabilized, intermittent catheterization should be considered. Because catheterizations should be performed every 4 hours initially and volumes maintained at less than 450 cc, it is essential that there be sufficient staff to manage the program. It is better to leave an indwelling catheter in place than to have a poorly managed intermittent catheterization program. Recent studies have shown that early intermittent catheterization does not produce any long-term advantages to spinal cord injured patients in terms of urinary infection rates, upper tract pathological abnormalities, or ultimate bladder drainage method. Urethral complications may be increased with long-term indwelling catheterization (>3 months) and these patients may benefit from suprapubic cystostomy if rehabilitation will be delayed (14).

Head trauma is a common problem that coexists with spinal cord injury. Up to 60 percent of patients may have concurrent head injury. It is important to assess this during the acute care phase because further medical intervention may be needed, and the patient's initial ability to comprehend his disability and cooperate with therapy may be limited.

THE REHABILITATION TEAM

A physician trained in spinal cord injury care coordinates the rehabilitation team and manages medical complications that may result from the spinal injury. This physician must also be responsible for the lifelong care of the patient. In the United States this physician is generally a physiatrist.

Consultants in urology, orthopedic surgery, neurologic surgery, plastic surgery, psychiatry, and internal medicine may assist the physiatrist because of the complex nature of the problems the patient may develop. However, it remains the responsibility of the primary physician to coordinate this care and make all decisions with the patient's input and consent. Particular medical issues common or unique to spinal cord injury are addressed later in this chapter.

The rehabilitation nurse (15) in a spinal injury unit has numerous responsibilities beyond providing basic nursing care. Nurses work closely with the physician and collaborate with the management of skin lesions and the neurogenic bowel and bladder. The nurse also assumes a major role in patient and family teaching. This teaching includes performance of catheterization and bowel management techniques, skin inspection, and medication and its side effects. Prevention and management of complications such as autonomic dysreflexia, deep venous thrombosis, pulmonary embolism, and urinary tract infection are key areas of an educational program that enhances quality of life and prevents long-term medical costs. The rehabilitation nurse collaborates with the therapists in ensuring that skills learned in therapy are practiced on the nursing unit.

Occupational therapists (16) provide training in activities of daily living, including dressing, feeding, writing, and homemaking. They may provide splints to maintain range of motion or dynamic splints that assist in the performance of functional skills. Occupational therapists should be able to evaluate and train spinal cord injured individuals in the use of environmental controls if needed to enhance their interaction with the environment. This is particularly important for the high-level tetraplegic. Occupational therapists and nurses often collaborate in training and modification of equipment necessary for self-catheterization and bowel management.

The physical therapist's (17) primary role is enhancement of mobility skills. Teaching may begin with basic tasks such as balance, sitting, and turning in bed and then progress to more complicated skills. The physical therapist can teach wheelchair use and safe transfers, instructing family members to assist or perform these tasks if necessary. In turn, patients are taught to instruct care providers in the safe performance of these skills. Gait training with braces, canes, crutches, or other devices as needed is provided. Equipment such as wheelchairs and shower and bathroom equipment are recommended by the therapist and obtained through durable equipment firms in the patient's community.

Rehabilitation engineering is an important part of a comprehensive spinal cord injury rehabilitation center. The rehabilitation engineer may assist in the design and construction of special wheelchair modifications to improve seating posture and prevent pressure sores. The engineer may also construct and modify environmental controls or other electronic and mechanical aids such as computers and electric wheelchairs.

Vocational rehabilitation counselors assist in the patient's return to work or school. They may guide the patient into new careers or work with the former employer to return patients to their former jobs. The counselor works with job placement specialists and representatives of the state offices of rehabilitation services. Driver education is an important component of vocational outcomes in patients undergoing spinal cord injury rehabilitation that is still needed. Employment status of spinal cord injured persons has been described (18). These services are generally provided after discharge as length of stay has shortened.

Social workers or case managers assist the team and the patient throughout the rehabilitation stay and coordinate discharge planning. They work closely with the psychologist to manage any psychosocial problems that may arise. The social worker is the main link between the patient's family and the rehabilitation team.

The clinical psychologist provides counseling services to the patient and family members. These services must be available to all spinal cord injured patients, as adaptation to this degree of injury has many difficulties. The interaction of each patient with a psychologist, therefore, is crucial. In addition, the psychologist should be able to provide neuropsychologic assessment to assist in the rehabilitation of the patient with concurrent brain injury or, when necessary, for vocational evaluation and planning. The psychologist may assist team members in management techniques to deal with patients who are having problems adapting to the rehabilitation unit.

Therapeutic recreation adds a dimension to rehabilitation far beyond a diversion for the hospitalized patient. Recreation therapists may assist the patient to return to pre-injury areas of interest or to develop new interests such as wheelchair sports. Activities may occur on the nursing unit, in special recreation areas, or in the community as permitted by the patient's medical condition.

The assistance of speech pathologists and audiologists may also be required. This is most often the case when swallowing problems or concurrent brain trauma is present.

Although the rehabilitation team has been described as a group of individuals with distinct responsibilities, the key to a successful rehabilitation of the spinal cord injured person is collaboration among all team members. This is necessary for such activities as community re-entry programs and wheelchair seating clinics that must be interdisciplinary. Therapists must be aware of each others' skills and limitations to achieve solutions to problems that arise as a result of the unique needs of the individual. Collaboration yields the unique solutions necessary to foster maximum independence (6,19).

FUNCTIONAL LEVELS AND REHABILITATION OUTCOMES

The classification system of the American Spinal Injury Association (ASIA) is used to define levels of injury and enhance communication for patient care and research (20). The level of injury is defined as the last (most caudal) level with normal sensory function in all modalities. This can be defined as two separate motor and two separate sensory segments on each side of the body

and a motor strength of grade 3 on a scale of 5 (fair strength) or better. The zone of partial preservation is used with a complete lesion and defined as the dermatomes and myotomes that remain partially innervated. A *complete injury* is present when motor and sensory function is absent in the lowest sacral segment. An *incomplete injury* occurs when there is partial preservation of sensory and/or motor functions. This must include the lowest sacral segment. A lesion is incomplete if either sensory or motor function is present in the rectum. Sensation is considered to be present if found at the anal mucocutaneous junction or if deep anal sensation is present (rectal exam). Motor function is considered to be present if voluntary contraction at the anal sphincter occurs on digital examination.

Motor level is determined by testing the key muscles (Table 25-1). A muscle with grade 3 strength is considered the intact muscle of the last normal level if the next most rostral key muscle has grade 5 strength. Sensation of pin prick and light touch are tested in the key areas of each dermatome (Fig. 25-1).

Tetraplegia is defined as damage of neural elements within the cervical segments of the spinal canal. The term quadriplegia was commonly used in the past. Paraplegia is defined as damage to the thoracic, lumbar, or sacral segments within the spinal canal including conus medullaris and cauda equina. These definitions exclude root avulsion and peripheral nerve injury outside the spinal canal.

The ASIA Impairment Scale is a modification of the Frankel scale used to describe impairment after spinal cord injury. The letters A through E are used. A complete lesion ASIA A has no sensory or motor function in the sacral segments S4-S5. An ASIA B Incomplete has sensory function below the neurologic level and this must include the S4-S5 sacral segments. Motor function is not preserved. ASIA C Incomplete has preserved motor function below the neurological level and more than half of the key muscles have a motor grade at less than 3. ASIA D Incomplete also has preserved motor function below the last normal level but at least half of the

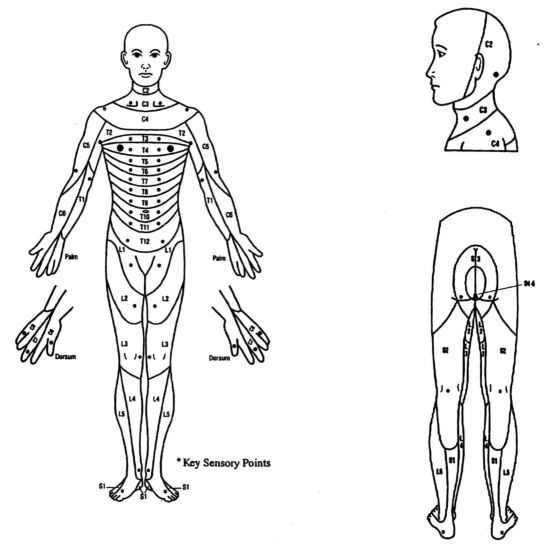

FIGURE 25-1 Sensory levels, with key points indicated by dots. Reproduced with permission of the American Spinal Injury Association 1996, Reference 20.

key muscles have a muscle grade greater than or equal to 3. When there is normal sensory and motor function, the classification ASIA E Normal is used.

Injuries may also be classified based on the anatomic area injured with the spinal cord. A *central cord syndrome* occurs within the cervical spinal cord. The upper limbs are weaker than the lower limbs, and there is sacral sparing. A *Brown–Sequard syndrome* produces greater sensory loss of pain and temperature on the side that is contralateral to the motor loss. In the *anterior*

cord syndrome, proprioception is preserved with sparing at the posterior column. There is a variable loss of motor function and sensitivity to pain and temperature, but proprioception is preserved.

Figure 25-2 describes injury to the conus medullaris and cauda equina. Conus lesions result in sacral cord and lumbar nerve root injury. At level A, bulbocavernous and micturition reflexes are preserved with areflexic lower limb. At level B, the legs, bowel, and bladder are areflexic. Cauda equina injuries at level C result

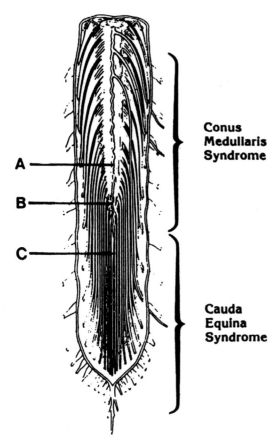

Conus Medullaris Syndrome

Cauda Equina Syndrome

FIGURE 25-2 Conus/cauda equina syndromes. Reproduced with permission of the American Spinal Injury Association 1996, Reference 20.

TABLE 25-1 Classification of Motor Level

Level	Muscle
C5	Elbow flexors (biceps, brachialis)
C6	Wrist extensors (extensor carpi radialis longus and brevis)
C7	Elbow extensors (triceps)
C8	Finger flexors (flexor digitorum profundus) to the middle finger
T1	Small finger abductors (abductor digiti minimi)
L2	Hip flexors (iliopsoas)
L3	Knee extensors (quadriceps)
L4	Ankle dorsiflexors (tibialis anterior)
L5	Long toe extensors (extensor hallucis longus)
S1	Ankle plantarflexors (gastrocnemius, soleus)

in injury to the lumbosacral nerve roots in the neural canal with areflexic bowel, bladder, and leg muscles.

The Functional Independence Measure (FIM) is recommended for descriptions of functional outcome. It does not describe the entire rehabilitation process but focuses on key areas using a seven-point scale. (See reference 20 for more detail on neurologic and functional classification.)

FUNCTIONAL OUTCOMES AFTER SPINAL CORD INJURY REHABILITATION

Prediction of functional abilities that can be achieved following rehabilitation can generally be guided by the degree of residual muscle function (21–24). These outcomes must be individualized because each person is unique and is affected by numerous factors including age, weight, endurance, and coexisting medical conditions. Patients at all levels of injury benefit from rehabilitation. Skills that the patient cannot perform must be taught through rehabilitation so that the patient can guide others in the performance of these skills. An educational program for these patients, their families, and their care givers is an essential component of the rehabilitation program. All concerned must be trained to recognize and prevent the medical and physical complications that may occur after spinal cord injury.

Skills learned in the rehabilitation setting must be generalized to the home environment and community before discharge to enhance reintegration into society after discharge. This can be accomplished through therapeutic weekend passes and community activities conducted during the rehabilitation stay. It is important to individualize the rehabilitation program for each patient. Patients who are motivated, if given the opportunity, may achieve goals expected for patients with greater motor skills. Allowing patients to attempt a complex skill and determine on their own if it is feasible is more valuable than an explanation by a staff member, which is often interpreted by the patient as a denial of any opportunity to achieve greater independence. Patients benefit from spinal cord injury rehabilitation at all ages (25). Older paraplegic patients may have difficulty performing more complex mobility and skills required for activities of daily living. Initially after discharge, patients can be expected to maintain the ability to perform functional tasks learned during the initial rehabilitation period (26). The aging process, however, has a tremendous impact on functional abilities as does degenerative changes at the extremities; this causes an increased need for assistance and power, as well as additional equipment. A description of functional outcomes, rehabilitation, equipment considerations at different levels of injuries is provided. This is intended to serve as a guide for the various levels and is not to be interpreted as a complete description of all equipment available and skills performed.

C1–C4 TETRAPLEGIA

Rehabilitation of high tetraplegics requires sophisticated electronic equipment and a staff trained in dealing with the respiratory problems that may develop. Patient with lesions at C1 and C2 may have sparing of the phrenic nerve and be managed with implanted phrenic nerve pacemakers. (Pacing of the diaphragm may be simultaneous or intermittent.) These patients have a lesser need for equipment than ventilator-dependent patients and are often easier to manage and discharge from the rehabilitation environment. They may also have their tracheostomies plugged or discontinued if secretions are not a problem. Patients with lesions above C4 who are ventilator-dependent participate in rehabilitation programs similar to those of the phrenic nerve pacemaker patients, although the equipment, respiratory circuitry, and tracheostomy interfere with communication and lead to greater discharge problems. Patients with lesions at the C4 level are often free of respiratory equipment beyond the initial acute care stage but require functional aids similar to those of patients with respiratory dependent injuries.

A major component of rehabilitation in these individuals is the use of technical aids such as environmental controls (16,27). Cooperation between an occupational therapist and rehabilitation engineer is often necessary to modify commercially available equipment for the individual patient. Equipment that may be necessary includes call systems, telephones, page turners, door openers, environmental control units, and computers. Environmental control units may access these devices or they may be prescribed individually. They may also be simple devices that access a few appliances or complex systems activated from a remote wheelchair unit. Control options include breath control (sip and puff), mouth sticks, or mechanically activated systems. Simple systems are available commercially as well but often require significant hand function. Computer modifications and programs are numerous and allow greater ease of use because of technological advances.

Power wheelchairs are essential at these levels of injury. They may be controlled by breath control, chin control, or voice activation or by hand control in patients with spared function. These chairs may be reclined by head-activated switches to perform pressure reliefs. A manual wheelchair is necessary, because the electric wheelchair may not be accessible to all environments, is not easily transportable, and may be in need of charging and repair. Lifts may be necessary for transfers because patients are dependent at this level.

C5 TETRAPLEGIA

Patients with lesions at the C5 level have functional deltoids and/or biceps. The presence of functional biceps and appropriate splinting allows for significant improvements in functional abilities (28). These patients may initially require use of a balanced forearm orthosis for arm placement during activities of daily living, such as feeding and typing (Fig. 25-3). This device is particularly useful for patients with partial C4 lesions with inadequate elbow flexors. A long opponens orthosis provides wrist stability

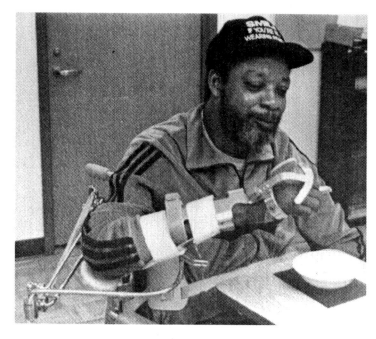

FIGURE 25-3 The balanced forearm orthosis.

and utensil slots and pen holders to allow these patients to perform activities such as feeding, writing, and typing. Other less commonly used devices include cable driven orthoses, electrically powered orthoses, or ratchet orthoses that provide tenodesis similar to that used by a C6 tetraplegic. With these assistive devices, C5 tetraplegics are able to feed with food cut up, perform oral facial hygiene with equipment set up, and assist with dressing.

Electric wheelchair propulsion may be performed with a hand control. Patients may propel a manual wheelchair with oblique projections indoors and occasionally on unlevel surfaces for short distances.

C6 TETRAPLEGIA

Active wrist extension and the presence of the C6 component in the proximal musculature enhances functional independence. Wrist extensor recovery is common, although its return can be delayed (29). Tenodesis, opposition of the thumb to the index finger with wrist extension, is used for functional activities. The RIC tenodesis orthosis (Fig. 25-4) is easily fabricated for tenodesis training during the early phases of

training. Infrequently, patients are provided with wrist-driven flexor hinge orthosis (Fig. 25-5) to perform tasks requiring increased pinch strength such as catheterization and feeding. Patients at this level often use short opponens orthoses with utensil slots and writing splints and simple D ring velcro handles to assist in feeding, writing, and oral facial hygiene. C6 tetraplegics usually feed with food provided, perform their oral facial hygiene, execute upper extremity dressing, and assist or are independent with lower extremity dressing. They may catheterize themselves and perform their bowel program with assistive devices (30).

Manual wheelchair propulsion is independent on level surfaces and is enhanced on rough terrain. Vertical wheelchair projections may be required in conjunction with wheelchair gloves. Some patients may require electric wheelchairs for work and school. Transfers may be independent or assisted from bed to wheelchair with a sliding board (17).

C7–C8 TETRAPLEGIA

The addition of functional triceps at C7 greatly enhances transfer and mobility skills. C7

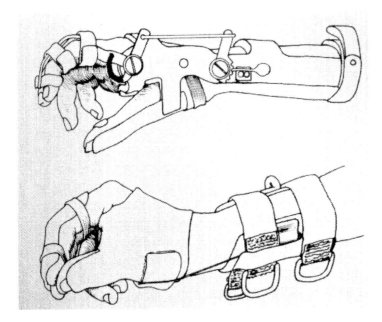

FIGURE 25-4 Top, wrist-driven flexor hinge splint; bottom, RIC tenodesis splint.

tetraplegics may also benefit from enhanced finger extension. Tenodesis splints may be used to assist in activities of daily living, most of which are independent at this level. Wheelchair and transfer skills are markedly enhanced, and wheelchair propulsion is improved on rough terrain and slopes (23). A case of a C7 tetraplegic who was able to walk a short distance with a specially modified walker has been reported (19). Although this is far from the norm, it is an exam-

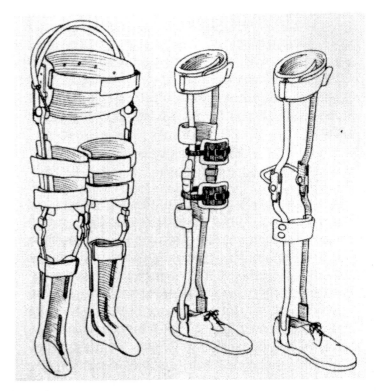

FIGURE 25-5 Three designs of orthosis for ambulation (right) Scott-Craig orthosis (center) standard knee ankle foot orthosis; (left) reciprocating gait orthosis (LSU-RGO)

ple of the importance of allowing a patient to attempt functional skills far beyond that predicated at a given level of musculature functioning.

THORACIC PARAPLEGIA

The T1 level is the first level with normal hand function. Because thoracic levels proceed caudally, intercostal and abdominal musculature is present, leading to enhanced respiratory function and trunk balance. Patients at all thoracic levels may be independent from a wheelchair level and able to manage their bowel and bladder function. Variable outcomes at the thoracic level are often described based on various levels of injury within the thoracic spinal cord. Our studies in a large series of thoracic patients show that this is not generally true. Patients at all levels should attempt complex transfers, standing, and ambulation because most descriptions based on thoracic levels are artificial (31). Also, this prevents the person from believing that he or she could have obtained skills if only he or she had been given a chance.

LUMBAR PARAPLEGIA

Hip flexion is present at the L2 level, knee extension at L3, and dorsiflexion at L4. The L5 level adds the extensor hallucis longus, and the S1 level adds the gastrocnemius and soleus muscles. Lumbar patients may all be independent from the wheelchair level, and ambulation is common. Community ambulators generally have proprioception at the hips and ankles, good pelvic control, hip flexors, and a quadriceps muscle on one side. Lack of hip extension and abduction may be compensated for by canes or crutches, and loss of ankle control by ankle-foot orthoses.

ORTHOTIC DEVICES

There are numerous orthotic devices that have been developed for paraplegic ambulation (32); Fig. 25-5 depicts three such devices. The standard metal upright knee-ankle-foot orthoses (KAFO) generally has upper and lower thigh bands, drop locks, a calf band, and a single-action (Klenzak) or double-action ankle joint. A pelvic band and a hip joint are rarely added, except in children, because they add increased weight and energy requirements and are not necessary because patients can extend at the hips using the ligaments of the hip to stabilize (33). The Scott-Craig (34) design, with a bale lock at the knee, a patellar tendon strap, and a rigid ankle support provides a lighter weight orthosis. The knee is eccentrically placed, and lower thigh and calf band closures are eliminated. Improved donning and doffing, standing, and more efficient ambulation results. There are two recent designs of orthoses that attempt to restore a reciprocating gait pattern: the reciprocating gait orthosis (RGO) or Louisiana State University orthosis (LSU) (35), and the adult hip guidance orthosis (Parawalker, HGO) (36). The RGO uses a Bowden cable system, commonly used in prosthetic devices, that allows alternate hip flexion as the hip is lifted and forces are transferred from the weight-bearing side via extension. Although this system yields a more aesthetic gait pattern, it is less efficient than the Scott-Craig orthosis and more cumbersome and expensive (37). The Parawalker combines a pair of rigid leg braces and a rigid pelvic brace articulating with ball bearing hinges. Hybrid systems using this brace, or the RGO, and functional neuromuscular stimulation have demonstrated the possibility of ambulation combining these two techniques of custom orthosis and electrical stimulation (38).

In spite of the development of numerous orthotic systems, it is uncommon for paraplegics to ambulate at the community level (39–42). Numerous studies have shown that with the six determinants of gait loss, the energy requirement per unit distance is at least six times that of normal levels (29,43,44). As in other disabilities, gait slows to a more tolerable level. The rejection of KAFOs for functional ambulation is therefore common (39,40,45,46). Patients may, however, use their braces for other purposes. Standing for short periods to reach objects at home or work or for short exercise periods during the day is found to be of value by many patients. Many paraplegics exercise with their KAFOs in home with parallel bars or with a walker or crutches. Brief periods of ambulation may be necessary in environments that are not wheelchair accessible. Many patients report enhanced bowel function from these periodic standing or walking times.

There are numerous approaches recommended in dealing with the paraplegic person who would like to ambulate (32). Although we advise our patients of the difficulties associated with ambulation—the high energy requirements and the dangers of falling—the decision to attempt ambulation lies with the patient. Temporary KAFOs are available; therefore, custom fitting is not necessary. Patients can discover on their own if ambulation is feasible, without feeling that they were denied their chance to walk. The patient must first learn the necessary prerequisite skills from the wheelchair level before the trial of gait training. This often enhances cooperation in these areas in individuals whose only stated goal is to "walk out of here." The trial of gait training often prevents patients from seeking out other rehabilitation facilities to obtain this goal and allows them to focus on more appropriate goals without feeling imposed upon.

AUTOMATIC DYSREFLEXIA AND AUTOMATIC DYSFUNCTION

Autonomic dysreflexia (AD) (47–50) has been reported to occur in 48 percent of patients with complete lesions above T6 and in 85 percent of tetraplegics. It is often referred to as autonomic hyperreflexia (AHR) and generally occurs in patients with lesions at or above T6. The syndrome develops secondary to a noxious stimulus below the level of injury. The afferent signals from this stimulus are transmitted via the spinothalamic tracts and dorsal columns to the sympathetic fibers in the lateral horns. An exaggerated sympathetic response results in increased levels of norepinephrine, resulting in hypertension, piloerection, nasal congestion, and sweating.

The most common symptoms are pounding headache caused by the reflex dilatation of cranial vessels, sweating, and cutaneous vasodilation. The common signs are hypertension, bladder and bowel distension, and tachycardia. Although reflex bradycardia is not commonly observed in this syndrome, it may occur. The diagnosis should not be excluded in the absence of bradycardia. Morbidity and mortality result from the effects of the hypertension. Mental status changes, seizures, and death caused by intracranial hemorrhage have been reported (47,51).

The first step in management of AD is prevention and patient and family education. Patients with adequate bladder and bowel management who follow their prescribed programs are less likely to develop these complications. They should be instructed to monitor their fluid intake, especially if they are on intermittent catheterization, to avoid overdistension or to catheterize more frequently if fluid intake is increased. Prescribed bowel regiments should be followed with proper diet and use of stool softeners as needed. Patients should be aware of the danger of AD and be knowledgeable of inciting factors such as tight clothing or urinary drainage leg bags, plugged or kinked catheters, pressure sores, urinary tract infections, or ingrown toenails.

Management of the acute episode rarely requires pharmacologic intervention. The patient should be sat up, tight clothing loosened, and a cause sought. Most often bladder distension is the causative factor and can be relieved by straight catheterization, unkinking or changing a blocked catheter, or draining a full urine collection bag. If a distended bladder is ruled out, fecal impaction should also be ruled out. An anesthetic ointment should be used to decrease the risk of aggravating the dysreflexia. Removal of the impaction often results in resolution of the symptoms.

If hypertension persists, pharmacologic intervention may be indicated. Nitrates and nifedipine are easy to use and may be effective. Nitrates may be given as amyl nitrate, sublingual nitroglycerin, or nitropaste. The cutaneous preparation is useful because it can be easily removed when the inciting stimulus resolves or the episode spontaneously ceases. Antihypertensives may be necessary when the aforementioned measures fail. Hydralazine, which may be given IM or IV, is probably the most practical drug, particularly if venous access is difficult. Diazoxide and nitroprusside are effective intravenous medications, but diazoxide is given via IV push, and nitroprusside is usually given in intensive care units.

Patients with recurrent AD may require prophylaxis with a-blocker, which is effective, and often only 10 mg to 30 mg is required daily (52). Many patients use a single daily dose; some are reluctant to use this medication because phenoxybenzamine has been associated with malignancy in laboratory animals. Other effective a-blocking agents include mecamylamine, guanethidine, prazosin, and clonidine. Clonidine has recently been reported to decrease spasticity and may be particularly advantageous (53,54).

Regular medical follow-up may identify and eliminate problems such as renal and bladder stones or ingrown toenails that may eventually cause AD. These problems should also be investigated in patients with recurrent episodes.

Sweating may be a manifestation of a noxious stimulus similar to that of AD. A cause should be sought before initiating treatment. Bladder stones are a common cryptic cause of sweating. Posttraumatic syringomyelia may cause sweating in the absence of other signs or symptoms. Recommended medications for sweating are mecamylamine or atropine (52). There have been anecdotal case reports of propoxyphene decreasing idiopathic sweating (55).

Orthostatic hypotension often interferes with remobilization after spinal cord injury. Because acute care stays have been shortened, it is less of a problem. Patients should be sat up slowly in bed before transferring. Support hose and an abdominal binder are worn. If a 90-degree sitting position in the wheelchair is not tolerated, a recliner chair is used. The tilt table may help restore postural reflexes. If physical measures are not successful, sodium chloride may be used alone or in combination with ephedrine. In rare cases use of mineral-corticoids is necessary. Long-term use of these medications is rarely needed.

Abnormalities of thermoregulation may interfere with community and other activities. Patients with lesions above T8 may be poikilothermic (10). Precautions must be taken during temperature extremes to prevent hypo- or hyperthermia. Patients often report febrile episodes after being in a warm environment. This should be assessed before initiating a medical workup for a source of infection.

HETEROTOPIC OSSIFICATION

Heterotopic ossification is also known as *ectopic bone* or *para-articular osteoarthropathy* (56,57). It is bone that forms in abnormal locations, most often around the hips and knees after spinal cord injury. The bone is true bone, as opposed to dystropic calcification. The incidence has been estimated to be from 16 percent to 53 percent (58).

There are numerous clinical presentations of heterotopic bone. It is often found on routine radiographs when it has not been clinically suspected. It may present as swelling around a joint or may first present as loss of range of motion. Heterotopic ossification may present with findings similar to a deep venous thrombosis with proximal hip swelling and distal edema resulting from vascular compression. It is crucial to rule out a deep venous thrombosis that may be life-threatening and not to assume that when heterotopic bone formation is present that a deep venous thrombosis is excluded (57,59).

Diagnosis is made most often by plain radiograph or bone scan. Suspected heterotopic ossification with positive clinical findings may initially present with negative radiographs. A radionuclide triple-phase bone scan is often positive in these situations (60). Bone is also identified on the initial angiographic phase in these instances. Alkaline phosphatase may be elevated as well, but by itself this is of little diagnostic value because most spinal cord injured patients have healing fractures or have undergone recent orthopaedic surgery.

Etidronate disodium (didronel) may be used prophylactically to decrease the amount but not the incidence of heterotopic ossification (58). Recommended dosages are 20 mg/kg daily for 2 weeks, followed by 10 mg/kg for 10 weeks in a single dosage. The most common side effects are gastrointestinal; when they occur the dosage may be split. In the presence of heterotopic ossification, Stover recommends continuing etidronate disodium for 6 months to one year (57).

Range of motion exercises are of the utmost importance for joints affected by heterotopic ossification (61). A joint not receiving ROM exercise ultimately leads to ankylosis. The best guideline to frequency of ROM exercises is the clinical response.

Surgical resection should be considered only for a clinical benefit to the patient. The mere presence of the bone is not sufficient reason to operate. The bone should be removed if a clinical problem exists, such as joint ankylosis with decreased functional abilities or pressure sores resulting from poor positioning. Surgical complications include infection, hemorrhage, and recurrence of the ossification. Bone should generally be present from 1 to 2 years, have a mature appearance on radiograph, and decreased uptake on serial bone scans. Etidronate disodium is given prophylactically before surgery and continued for 1 year (57).

PAIN

The incidence of pain after spinal cord injury has been reported to be as high as 100 percent. A useful classification system has been described (62):

1. Cauda equina (radicular)
2. Visceral
3. Mechanical (myofascial)
4. Psychioc
5. Spinal cord (dyesthetic)

Dyesthetic pain syndrome—pain distal to the injury and often described as *central pain* or *phantom pain*—may be extremely disabling. Patients often describe this pain as "cutting, burning, piercing, radiating, or tight" (63).

As with any medical problem that develops, a history and physical should be taken and any local or medical cause ruled out. Patients may have abdominal visceral complications; posttraumatic syringomyelia; or suffer from tendinitis, bursitis, or a similar condition that may occur in the general population.

Management of dyesthetic pain syndrome is difficult (64). When the condition exists it must be explained adequately to the patient. Pharmacologic intervention should be avoided unless pain interferes with activities, sleep, or mood state. The patient should be reassured as to the nature of the pain problem and the fact that it is not a sign of a medical problem. Therapy should be initiated with the most benign medications possible. Acetaminophen or nonsteroidal anti-inflammatory drugs (NSAIDs) may be attempted initially, although success is limited. Transcutaneous nerve stimulation benefits a small number of patients in our clinical experience. Of the centrally acting drugs used such as phenytoin, carbamazepine, clonazepam, gabapentin, and amitriptyline, amitriptyline appears to be the most effective. It acts centrally to decrease reuptake of serotonin and norepinephrine. A once-daily dosage at bedtime also enhances sleep. Gabapentin is frequently used with good results, although studies in SCI are not yet available.

SPASTICITY

Spasticity is a common complication of spinal cord injuries. It is defined as "a motor disorder characterized by a velocity-dependent increase in tonic stretch reflexes (muscle tone) with exaggerated tendon jerks, resulting from hyperexcitability of the stretch reflex, as one component of the upper motor neuron syndrome" (65). Spasticity is variable, but in general, initially follows a flexor pattern after the termination of spinal shock, followed by extensor spasticity in patients with lesions above the conus medullaris (66,67).

Spasticity may interfere with positioning functional activities and can cause discomfort or safety concerns. Therapeutic intervention should be initiated with a specific goal in mind. The mere presence of spasticity is not an indication for treatment. The patient should be made aware of the beneficial effects of spasticity, such as maintenance of muscle bulk and decreased lower extremity edema before initiating treatment.

The basic of control of spasticity is appropriate medical and nursing management. A patient's complaints of increased spasticity may indicate a urinary tract infection, a pressure sore, or insufficient ROM exercises. Spasticity often improves when these problems are treated. Frequently, patients awakening with increased spasms may require ROM exercises in the morning before beginning their daily routine. If this fails and bladder stones, bowel impactions, and other noxious stimuli are not found, pharmacologic intervention may be necessary.

Baclofen, diazepam, dantrolene, clonidine and most recently, tizanidine, are most commonly used to treat spasticity. Use of these agents for long-term management is considered "justifiable if the drug produces a notable reduction in painful or disabling symptoms and permits increased function by the patient, perhaps with a need for less intensive nursing care" (64). Care must be taken not to decrease useful spasticity that may serve as an aid for transfers. The minimal effective dosage should be used and tapered gradually if the medication(s) are discontinued.

Baclofen is considered by many to be the treatment of choice for spasticity after spinal cord injury. Its major site of action is the spinal cord, and it is equally effective in complete and incomplete lesions. Baclofen is given in dosages from 10 mg to a maximum of 80 mg daily, although there are reports of dosages beyond the maximum recommended by the manufacturer. The most common side effect is transient drowsiness, and sudden discontinuance may cause hallucinations (67,68).

Diazepam (66–68) is a centrally acting benzodiazepine useful in management of spasticity resulting from spinal cord injury. It may be used alone or in combination with baclofen and dantrium. Use of diazepam is limited primarily by its tranquilizing properties. Recommended dosage is 2 mg b.i.d., slowly increasing, if necessary, to 15 mg to 20 mg daily. Dosages greater than this may be tolerated by some patients but most find them oversedating.

Dantrolene (66,67,69) differs from the previously described medications in that it is peripherally acting. It suppresses the release of calcium from the sarcoplasmic reticulum, thus decreasing the activity of the contractile apparatus. Dantrium's usefulness is limited by its side effects. It may produce drowsiness, lightheadedness, or confusion. The potential for hepatic toxicity, particularly in females and patients older than 35 or in those on estrogen, limits its usefulness. Liver functions tests should be repeated regularly, making its usage difficult in outpatients in whom follow-up is often inconsistent because of transportation and other difficulties. Dosage begins with 25 mg twice a day and may be slowly increased to 100 mg four times a day. Dosages as high as 200 mg four times a day are rarely necessary (66,69).

Clonidine (53,67) is an antihypertensive agent that has recently been shown to be useful in spasticity management. Clonidine's primary action is as a central a-adrenergic blocker. It may be given orally or through a transdermal delivery system. Dosage is in the range of 0.1 mg to 0.5 mg daily. Major side effects are dry mouth, drowsiness, and sedation. Hypotension may occur, and the drug should be withdrawn slowly.

Tizanidine (67) is similar to clonidine. It binds to α-2 adrenergic, and imidazole receptors in the central nervous system. Dosage ranges from an initial dose of 4 mg titrated by 2 to 4 mg up to 36 mg daily. Major side effects are dry mouth, somnolence, fatigue, and dizziness. Liver functions should be monitored.

Botulinum toxin (72) is one of the newest agents for spasticity management. It is a purified neurotoxin that is injected directly into muscle, blocking the release of acetylcholine from the nerve terminal. A local denervation with partial paralysis occurs. It can be used to target muscles to decrease spasticity and associated pain or to improve function. The duration of benefit is variable and repeat injections may be required. It has significantly reduced the usage of phenol because it is reversible.

Surgical procedures most commonly performed are tendon lengthening procedures (71,72). The tendons most commonly lengthened are the heel cords and adductors. The need for destructive rhizotomies and myelotomies has been replaced by continuous intrathecal baclofen (71–74). A baclofen pump is placed in the abdominal wall and attached to a lumbar subarachnoid catheter. Dosages as high as 900 micrograms are programmed externally by a computer and radiofrequency transmitter. This technique initially described by Penn, may allow for lower doses of baclofen to be used because they are delivered to the site needed with markedly enhanced control of spasticity (73,74).

NEUROGENIC BLADDER MANAGEMENT

There are numerous classification schemes for abnormalities of bladder and sphincter control after spinal cord injury or other nervous system trauma. The simplest classification for management in spinal cord injured persons is upper and lower motor neuron lesions (75,76). An upper motor neuron (UMN) bladder may be described as a spastic or reflexic bladder. The isolated bladder maintains its contractile function and may contract and attempt to empty spontaneously. This action may be coordinated with sphincter relaxation (a synergic pattern) or uncoordinated sphincter contraction (a dysynergic pattern). Patients with UMN bladders have an intact bulbocavernosus reflex on physical examination. Lower motor neuron (LMN) bladders are flaccid because of the distal cord involvement. They are generally found with more distal cord lesions but may be seen with high cervical and thoracic lesions with associated lumbar fractures.

Management options for bladder dysfunction are numerous. Of major consideration in selection of a management technique is the patient's lifestyle and preferences in cooperation with the optimal medical situation to decrease renal and bladder complications. Although a technique may be optimal medically, it should not be chosen if it will require significant assistance or require the patient to become homebound for proper and consistent performance. The performance of surgical procedures such as suprapubic catheterization on a routine basis as the preferred method of management is not justified. Several management techniques are described below. Although intermittent catheterization may be the preferred method, its practicality for each patient must be considered.

Intermittent catheterization decreases the risks of infection and stones caused by the presence of an indwelling catheter (45,77–81). Although some C6 tetraplegics can perform self-catheterization, it generally requires good hand function and the ability to manage lower extremity clothing in an efficient manner. The patient must be well motivated to perform the procedure on a regular basis and have adequate facilities available when away from the home environment. For patients with UMN bladder with a synergic pattern, this technique is often used until satisfactory voiding with low residuals (generally less than 100 cc) is obtained. Patients may use this technique in conjunction with medications that inhibit voiding such as oxybutynin (Ditropan) or propantheline bromide (Pro-Banthine), or with external (condom) catheters. Intermittent catheterization techniques may take advantage of the safe emptying interval as described by Wu (82) to prevent and treat urinary tract infections.

External catheters are generally used in spinal cord injured males who void between catheterizations or who have developed a balanced bladder. Patients who have contractile bladders but void with a dysynergic pattern may undergo external sphincterotomy and become free of an indwelling catheter or intermittent catheterization (73,83–86). Patients should be aware of the difficulties associated with the usage of external catheters, such as local irritation or breakdown of the penis; leakage and improper tight fitting can lead to infection and upper tract abnormalities (87).

Suprapubic catheters (88) offer many advantages over indwelling catheters. Complications such as penile-scrotal fistulas and urethral injury are diminished. The catheter is easy to change and long-term studies in a small series of patients have not shown any major adverse long-term effects (78).

Indwelling catheters, although not ideal from the medical standpoint (76), are preferred by many patients. Ease of management and the absence of need for a surgical procedure are two advantages. Disadvantages are risks of infection, bladder stones, urethral damage, fistulas, and a reported increased incidence of bladder carcinoma. On the other hand, many patients have found that this secure, leak-free method allows for easier reintegration into society and return to work. The ileal conduit should be reserved for patients with progressive hydronephrosis not manageable by other means (89).

Long-term follow-up of patients with neurogenic bladders is essential. There are three methods commonly used. Intravenous pyelograms (IVP) were traditionally performed on an annual basis. This technique is invasive and may be unsafe in patients with impaired renal function or dye allergy. Poor compliance often results from the discomfort associated with the procedure. Renal ultrasonography is a viable replacement for IVP (90,91). It is noninvasive and offers diagnostic capabilities similar to those of the IVP. Renal scintography has been proposed as a more accurate diagnostic technique (78).

Pharmacologic intervention may assist in management of the neurogenic bladder. Bethanechol (Urecholine) may stimulate bladder contraction, although its usefulness in UMN lesions has been questioned (92). It may enhance dyssynergia in high level patients by stimulating the sympathetic ganglions as well. Pro-banthine and Ditropan, discussed earlier, may be useful to decrease bladder contractibility in patients with a spastic bladder or in patients who prefer not to void between intermittent catheterizations. α-adrenergic agents such as phenylpropanolamine or ephedrine may be both helpful and harmful after spinal cord injury. In patients with high

level lesions who void spontaneously, these agents may stimulate the internal sphincter, inhibit voiding, and enhance autonomic dysreflexia. In patients with lower level lesions, these sympathomimetic agents may be used to prevent voiding. Phenylpropanolamine (Ornade Spansule Capsules) may be conveniently administered for this purpose.

GASTROINTESTINAL FUNCTION

Abnormalities resulting in impaired defecation follow neurologic patterns similar to that of the neurogenic bladder. The goal of a bowel program is to develop a predictable time of elimination that is most effective, most convenient, and least expensive for the patient (15).

A proper diet is essential in management of the neurogenic bowel. Sufficient fluid and fiber intake is essential. Dietary instruction and awareness of foods with high fiber content, such as bran, should be instituted as soon as feasible. Patients may often be asked to make a major dietary change after their injury. Stool softeners such as docusate sodium (Colace) or bulk softeners such as psyllium (Metamucil) are the most commonly used supplements. A mild laxative such as casanthranol may be used in combination with docusate sodium (Peri-Colace) when motility is a problem.

There are two general patterns of bowel regulation (93). Patients with upper motor neuron neurogenic bowel are generally regulated with suppositories and/or digital stimulation on a daily or every-other-day basis. Recent evidence suggests that polyethylene glycol-based suppositories are more effective than vegetable oil-based suppositories. A schedule that can easily be incorporated into a person's lifestyle should be determined. Lower motor neuron lesions are more difficult to regulate and may require manual removal. Patients often tend to decrease the frequency of their bowel program performance, which may lead to fecal impaction and diarrhea. This is often misinterpreted as a primary problem; antidiarrheal agents, which compound the problem, are sometimes erroneously used.

Bowel management has been extensively reviewed by Stiens and associates (92).

WHEELCHAIR CONSIDERATIONS

Proper seating in a wheelchair is of utmost importance (16,94). The seating system must allow the individual to propel the chair properly and should not contribute to spinal deformity or pressure sore development. A high back and head support may be needed for patients who cannot propel their wheelchair manually. Patients who propel their chair require freedom of movement and the back of the wheelchair should be below the scapula. A lumbar support that maintains the lumbar lordosis or a firm back support may be necessary. The seat should be inclined to prevent forward sliding; a firm seat prevents the sling effect and decrease abnormal positioning and pressure sore development. Trunk and arm supports may be necessary in higher levels. Difficult positioning problems may require custom molded seating systems.

Cushions help to decrease pressure and the incidence of pressure sores. A common misconception regarding wheelchair cushions is the erroneous conclusion that they eliminate the need for pressure reliefs. Pressure reliefs every 10 to 15 minutes must be continued on all seating surfaces. Considerations in choosing cushions include effect on posture, transfer skills, heat, and moisture.

SEXUAL FUNCTION

Sexual function in spinal cord injured males varies with the location and extent of the lesion (95,96). Erections are more common in injured patients with upper motor neuron lesions as compared to those with lower motor neuron lesions, particularly if the lesion is more cranial in location. Reflex erections occur with an intact sacral cord and psychogenic erections that are cerebrally mediated in lower motor neuron lesions. Ejaculation increases in frequency if the lesion is caudal and is more common in partial lower motor neuron lesions. Males with incom-

plete lesions have better erectile and ejaculatory function.

Sexual dysfunction must be approached from two aspects. Psychological counseling, training, and education is the first component (96,97). The second component is provision to the person of technologic advances that may enhance erectile or ejaculatory function.

Restoration of erections may be mechanical, pharmacologic, or surgical. There are many commonly used external aids for the restoration of erections. They use a vacuum system to cause tumescence of the penis. The systems (98,99) consist of a plastic cylinder and a vacuum pump after which a constrictive band is placed at the base of the penis. This is left in place for 30 minutes and decreases blood flow to the penis. Nonerectile tissue becomes engorged and the penis pivots over the constriction band.

Numerous medications have been used for restoration of erection (100–103). The most common are papaverine and phentolamine, each used alone or in combination, and prostaglandins. In clinical practice, most patients respond to papaverine alone in dosages of 3 mg to 30 mg (102). Use of one agent as opposed to a combination may produce fewer side effects. An injection is given in the proximal third of the penis in the midline of the lateral aspect (101). Pressure and massage is then applied for several minutes. A tourniquet may be applied during this period. The major side effect is priapism and, as a result, a low test dosage should be used on the first visit. This is particularly important in patients with UMN lesions and reflex erections that are present but transient and are too brief for sexual intercourse. Urethral delivery of prostaglandin is limited in effectiveness and may result in hypotension, which can be limited by the use of a constriction band.

The latest drug now available for erection is sildenafil (Viagra). This drug has received much notoriety in the lay press. It acts by inhibiting cyclic guanosine monophosphate (cGMP)-specific phosphodiesterase resulting in increased cGMP levels, which is a mediator of nitric oxide, a smooth muscle relaxant and vasodilator, the key neurotransmitter for erections. It is taken orally and is effective in up to 78 percent of spinal cord injured men. The response is better if there is some residual erectile function.

Surgical management for restoration of erections involves the use of semirigid or inflatable penile prosthesis. Semirigid protheses (42,104,105) may be used for sexual intercourse and for maintenance of external urinary appliances. Spinal cord injured patients are at greater risk due to sensory loss, vasomotor abnormalities, and the associated pressure from the implant. Complications include extrusion and infection. An inflatable penile prosthesis decreases the risk of erosion; mechanical breakdown is the major problem (106). The choice of the technique to enhance erectile function depends on patient preference and experiences with the various techniques. Patients will often choose the method they find to be most natural or simple to use. Nonsurgical treatment should be explored before using surgical means.

Male fertility after spinal cord injury has been estimated at 5 percent (95,96). Techniques under development may increase this severalfold (107). More caudal incomplete lesions generally have the best prognosis. The earliest technique to stimulate ejaculation was intrathecal neostigmine, which was described by Guttman (108). This technique is not in common usage, and deaths have been reported. Recently, injection of subcutaneous physostigmine has been proposed as the alternative of choice (19). The most commonly used techniques at this time are vibratory ejaculation and electroejaculation.

Vibratory ejaculation is noninvasive with few side effects (74,109). It requires intact thoracolumbar sympathetics from T11 to L2 and an intact conus medullaris cauda equina reflex. The technique has been well studied by Brindley and by Sarkarati and others (109,110). The Ling 201 vibrator, at approximately 80 Hz and 2.5 mm peak-to-peak amplitude, appears to be the most effective. Other vibrators may be used, but response is variable. If success is obtained with the Ling vibrator, we attempt use of other commercially available vibrators that can be used at home. Vibration is applied to the lower ventral surface of the glans penis for 3-$\frac{1}{2}$ minutes, followed by a 1-$\frac{1}{2}$ minute pause for four cycles, totalling 20 minutes. Vibratory stimulation usually fails within the first 6 months. It is usually successful if the hip flexion response is present; the hip flexes when the sole of the foot is scratched. There are contradictory reports as to whether semen quality improves with repeated attempts.

Rectal probe electroejaculation may be attempted when vibratory ejaculation is not successful. There are several devices used for this technique (65,110–113). Seminal emission results when the right or left obturator point is found. Patients must be monitored for autonomic dysreflexia. Pain may limit this procedure's utility in patients with incomplete lesions, and rectal mucosal damage is a possible complication. This technique causes emission by stimulating sympathetic efferent fibers. Fertility may be enhanced by decreasing scrotal temperature. A simple technique of sitting with the legs abducted in the wheelchair may be satisfactory (22).

In females, normal menstruation lost after a spinal cord injury usually returns within several months to a year, if affected. Fertility is usually unimpaired. Potential problems during labor include autonomic dysreflexia. Studies on sexual functioning in females after spinal cord injury are limited by small series with varying levels of injury. Sexual relationships for females with spinal cord injury may be enhanced by appropriate training and counseling (96).

RESPIRATORY DYSFUNCTION

Respiratory problems are a significant cause of morbidity and mortality after spinal cord injury. With the intercostals and abdominal muscles paralyzed, the diaphragm is often the only functional muscle. Vital capacity is generally diminished by one-third, and expiratory reserve volume is markedly diminished. Rehabilitation efforts should be directed toward improving vital capacity, chest mobility, and cough (15,59,114).

There are numerous methods to enhance vital capacity. Incentive spirometry encourages chest expansion. Inspiratory training devices that have variable resistance to inspiratory force are available and may enhance maximum inspiratory pressure and endurance. Exercise programs should be instituted to strengthen the remaining muscles of respiration. Diaphragmatic strengthening is an important component of this, as well as strengthening of the remaining accessory muscles in the neck. Glossopharyngeal breathing (17) uses the muscles of the mouth, pharynx, and larynx to swallow air into the lungs. This technique enhances vital capacity, promotes chest expansion, and assists in weaning from the ventilator. An abdominal corset supports the abdominal contents when erect and allows for a more normal positioning of the diaphragm. This enhances diaphragmatic excursion from the erect position. Chest mobility is maintained by methods described previously, such as incentive spirometry and glossopharyngeal breathing. The chest may be stretched manually as well once or twice a day to maintain or increase range of motion.

Enhancement of active expiration and cough is crucial to maintain bronchial hygiene. The clavicular portion of the pectoralis major is a muscle of active expiration in tetraplegic patients. Potentially strengthening this muscle may improve cough effectiveness and long-term respiratory outlook. Assistive cough is performed by applying pressure inwardly and upwardly to the upper abdomen. This technique enhances peak flow during cough and assists in clearing of secretions.

PSYCHOLOGICAL COUNSELING AND LIFELONG FOLLOW-UP

The clinical psychologist is a vital member of the rehabilitation team (97,115,116). Psychological services should be routinely available to all patients. Additional support should be available from peer visitors who can share their experiences with the newly injured person. Group sessions help patients to better adjust to their dis-

abilities and gain insight into their situation. The psychologist may be active in sexual and family counseling and in helping the team develop strategies to foster a more successful rehabilitation outcome.

Comprehensive follow-up services of the rehabilitation team should be available to all patients. An annual history, physical, and urologic workup is mandatory. Services that may not have been appropriate initially, such as vocational rehabilitation, may benefit outpatients who are ready to reach their maximum rehabilitation potential. Spinal cord injured individuals also benefit from services provided by independent living centers and collaboration with societies that provide information, promote research, and advocate on their behalf.

REFERENCES

1. Guttmann L. New hope for spinal cord injury sufferers. *Paraplegia* 1979; 17:6.
2. Anderson DW, McLaurin RL. The national head and spinal cord injury survey. *J Neurosurg* 1980; 53:S1.
3. Berkowitz M, O'Leary PK, Kruse DL, Harvey L. *Spinal Cord Injury: An Analysis of Medical and Social Costs.* New York: Demos Medical Publishing, 1998.
4. Stover SL, Delisa JA, Whiteneck GG. *Spinal Cord Injury, Clinical Outcomes from the Model Systems.* Gaithersburg, Maryland: Aspen, 1995.
5. Geisler WO, Jousse AT, Waynne-Jones M, et al. Survival in traumatic spinal cord injury. *Paraplegia* 1983; 21:364.
6. Fordyce WE. On interdisciplinary peers. *Arch Phys Med Rehabil* 1981; 62:51.
7. Bedbrook GM. Spinal injuries with tetraplegia and paraplegia. *J Bone Joint Surg* 1979; 61B:267.
8. Yarkony GM, Roth EJ, Heinemann AW, et al. Benefits of rehabilitation for traumatic spinal cord injury: multivariate analysis in 711 patients. *Arch Neurol* 1987; 44:93.
9. Freed ML. Traumatic and congenital lesions of the spinal cord. In Kottke FJ, Stillwell GK, Lehmann JF, eds., *Krusen's Handbook of Physical Medicine and Rehabilitation* 3rd ed. Philadelphia: W.B. Saunders, 1982. Pp. 643.
10. Guttmann L. *Spinal Cord Injuries Comprehensive Management and Research* 2nd ed. Boston: Blackwell Scientific Publications 1976.
11. Davidoff G, Morris J, Roth E, et al. Closed head

injury in spinal cord injured patients: retrospective study of the loss of consciousness and post traumatic amnesia. *Arch Phys Med Rehabil* 1985; 66:41.

12. Green D, Lee M, Lim A, et al. Prevention of thromboembolism after spinal cord injury using low-molecular weight heparin. *Ann Int Med* 1990; 113:571–574.

13. Yarkony GM, Bass LM, Keenan V III, Meyer PR Jr. Contractures complicating spinal cord injury: incidence and comparison between spinal cord centre and general hospital acute care. *Paraplegia* 1985; 23:265.

14. Lloyd LK, Kuhlemeier KV, Fine PR, Stover SL. Initial bladder management in spinal cord injury: does it make a difference? J Urol 1986; 135:523.

15. Matthews PJ, Carlson CE. *Spinal Cord Injury: A Guide to Rehabilitation Nursing.* Rockville, Maryland: Aspen, 1987.

16. Hill JP. *Spinal Cord Injury: A Guide to Functional Outcomes in Occupational Therapy.* Rockville, Maryland: Aspen, 1986.

17. Nixon V. Spinal Cord Injury: A Guide to *Functional Outcomes in Physical Therapy Management.* Rockville, Maryland: Aspen, 1985.

18. DeVivo MJ, Fine PR. Employment status of spinal cord injured patients three years after injury. *Arch Phys Med Rehabil* 1982; 63:200.

19. Yarkony GM, Jones R, Hdman G, O'Donnell A. Jones-Hedman walker modification for C7 quadriplegic patient: case study in team cooperation. *Arch Phys Med Rehabil* 1986; 67:54.

20. *American Spinal Injury Association: International Standards for Neurological and Functional Classification of Spinal Injury Patients.* Chicago: American Spinal Injury Association, 1996.

21. Bergstrom EMK, Frankel HR, Galer IAR, et al. Physical ability in relation to anthropometric measurements in persons with complete spinal cord lesion below the sixth cervical segment. *Int Rehabil Med* 1985; 7:51.

22. Whiteneck G, et al. *Outcomes Following Traumatic Spinal Cord Injury: Clinical Practice Guidelines for Health Care Professionals.* Washington, D.C.: Paralyzed Veterans of America, 1999.

23. Bromley I. *Tetraplegia and Paraplegia: A Guide for Physiotherapist* 2nd ed. New York: Churchill Livingstone, 1981. P. 37.

24. Woolsey RM: Rehabilitation outcome following spinal cord injury. *Arch Neurol* 1985; 42:116.

25. Yarkony GM , Roth EJ, Heinemann AW, Lovell L. Spinal cord injury rehabilitation outcome: The impact of age.

26. Yarkony GM, Roth EJ, Heinemann AW, et al. Functional skills after spinal cord injury: three-year longitudinal followup. *Arch Phys Med Rehabil* 1988; 69:111.

27. Voda JA, Gordon RE. Environmental control and augmentative communication program for nonverbal physically disabled persons. *Arch Phys Med Rehabil* 1982; 63:511.

28. Yarkony GM, Roth E, Lovell L, et al. Rehabilitation outcomes in complete C5 quadriplegia. *Am J Phys Med Rehabil* 1988; 67:73.

29. Ditunno JF, Sipski ML, Posuniak EA, et al. Wrist extensor recovery in traumatic quadriplegia. *Arch Phys Med Rehabil* 1987; 68:287.

30. Yarkony GM, Roth EJ, Heinemann AW, Lovell L. Rehabilitation outcomes in C6 tetraplegia. *Paraplegia* 1988; 26:177.

31. Yarkony GM, Roth EJ, Meyer PR, et al. Rehabilitation outcomes in complete thoracic spinal cord injury. *Am J Phys Med Rehabil* 1990; 69:23.

32. Merritt JL. Knee-ankle-foot orthotics: Long leg braces and their practical applications. In Redford JB, ed. *Physical Medicine and Rehabilitation: State of the Art Reviews*, Vol. 1. Philadelphia: Hanley and Belfus, 1987. P. 67.

33. Warren CG, Lehmann JF, deLateur BJ. Pelvic band use in orthotics for adult paraplegic patients. *Arch Phys Med Rehabil* 1978; 56:221.

34. Lehmann JF, Warren CG, Hertling D, et al. Craig-Scott orthosis: a biomechanical and functional evaluation. *Arch Phys Med Rehabil* 1976; 57:438.

35. Douglas R, Larson PF, D'Ambrosia R, McCall RE. The LSO reciprocation-gait orthosis. *Orthopaedics* 1983; 6:834.

36. Patrick TH, McClelland MR. Low energy cost reciprocal walking for the adult paraplegic. *Paraplegia* 1985; 23:113.

37. Merrit JL, Miller NE, Houston TJ. Preliminary studies of energy expenditure in paraplegics using swing-through and reciprocating gait pattern. (Abstract). *ArchPhys Med Rehabil* 1987; 64:510.

38. McClelland M, Andrews BT, Patrick JH, et al. Augmentation of the Oswestry Parawalker Orthosis by means of surface electrical stimulation: gait analysis of three patients. *Paraplegia* 1987; 25:32.

39. Coughlan JK, Robinson CE, Newmarch B, Jackson G. Lower extremity bracing in paraplegia: a follow-up study. *Paraplegia* 1980; 18:25.

40. Heinemann A, Magiera-Planey R, Schiro-Geist C, Gimenes G. Mobility for persons with SCI: an evaluation of two systems. *Arch Phys Med Rehabil* 1987; 68:60.

41. Mikelberg R, Reid S. Spinal cord lesions and lower extremity bracing: an overview and follow-up study. *Paraplegia* 1981; 19:379.

42. Rossier AB, Fam BA. Indication and results of semirigid penile prosthesis in spinal cord injury patients: long-term followup. *J Urol* 1984; 131:59.

43. Fisher SV, Gullickson G. Energy cost of ambulation in health and disability: a literature review. *Arch Phys Med Rehabil* 1978; 59:124.

44. Merkel KD, Miller NE, Merrit JL. Energy expenditure in patients with low-, mid-, or high-thoracic paraplegia using Scott-Craig knee-ankle-foot orthoses. *Mayo Clinic Proc* 1985; 60:165.

45. Nanninga JB, Wu Y, Hamilton B. Long-term intermittent catheterization in the spinal cord injury patient. *J Urol* 1982; 128:760.

46. O'Daniel WE, Hahn HR. Follow-up usage of the Scott-Craig orthosis in paraplegia. *Paraplegia* 1981; 19:373.

47. Erikson RP: Autonomic hyperreflexia: pathophysiology and medical management. *Arch Phy Med Rehabil* 1980; 61:431.

48. Kurnick NB. Autonomic hyperreflexia and its control in patients with spinal cord lesions. *Ann Intern Med* 1956; 44:678.

49. Kursh ED, Freehafer A, Pursky L. Complications of autonomic dysreflexia. *J Urol* 1978; 118:70.

50. Lindan R, Joiner E, Frehafer AA, Hazel C. Incidence and clinical features of autonomic dysreflexia in patients with spinal cord injury. *Paraplegia* 1980; 18:285.

51. Yarkony, GM, Katz RT, Wu Y. Seizures secondary to autonomic dysreflexia. *Arch Phys Med Rehabil* 1986; 67:834.

52. Halstead LS, Claus-Weker J. *Neuroactive Drugs of Choice in Spinal Cord Injury.* Houston: The Institute for Rehabilitation and Research, 1980.

53. Donovan WH, Carter E, Ross CD, Wilkerson MA. Clonidine-effect on spasticity: a clinical trial. *Arch Phys Med Rehabil* 1988; 69:193.

54. Maynard FM. Early clinical experience with clonidine in spinal spasticity. *Paraplegia* 1986; 24:175.

55. Tashjian EA, Richfor KJ. The value of propoxyphene hydrochloride (Darvon)® for the treatment of hyperhidrosis in the spinal cord injured patient: an anecdotal experience and case reports. *Paraplegia* 1995; 23:349.

56. Kewalramani LS, Ortho MS. Ectopic ossification. *Am J Phys Med Rehabil* 1977; 56:99.

57. Stover SL. Heterotropic ossification. In Bloch RF, Basbaum M ,eds., *Management of Spinal Cord Injuries.* Baltimore: Williams and Wilkins, 1986. P. 284.

58. Finerman G, Stover SL. Heterotopic ossification following hip replacement or spinal cord injury: two clinical studies with EHDP. *Metabol Bone Dis Relat Res* 1981; 4, 5:337.

59. Venier LH, Ditunno JF. Heterotopic ossification in paraplegic patient. *Arch Phys Med Rehabil* 1971; 54:475.

60. Freed JH, Hahn H, Menter R, Dillon T. The use of the three-phase bone scan in the early diagnosis of heterotopic ossification and in the evaluation of Didronel therapy. *Paraplegia* 1982; 20:208.

61. Stover SL, Hataway CT, Zeiger HE. Heterotopic ossification in spinal cord injured patients. *Arch Phys Med Rehabil* 1975; 56:199.

62. Donovan WH, Dimitrijevic MR, Dahm L, Dimitrijevic M. Neurophysiological approaches to chronic pain following spinal cord injury. *Paraplegia* 1982; 20:135.

63. Davidoff G, Roth E, Guarracini M, et al. Function-limiting dyesthetic pain syndrome among traumatic spinal cord injury patients: a cross-sectional study. *Pain* 1987; 29:39.

64. Davidoff G, Guarracini M, Roth E, et al. Trazadone hydrochloride in the treatment of dyesthetic pain in traumatic myelopathy: a randomized double-blind placebo-controlled study. *Pain* 1987; 29:151.

65. Brindley GS. Electroejaculation and the fertility of paraplegic men. *Sexuality and Disability* 1980; 3:223.

66. Davidoff RA. Antispasticity drugs: mechanisms of action. *Ann Neurol* 1985; 17:107.

67. Merritt JL. Management of spasticity in spinal cord injury. *Mayo Clin Proc* 1981; 56:614.

68. Young RR, Delwaide PT. Drug therapy: spasticity. *N Eng J Med* 1981; 304:28.

69. Young RR, Delwaide PT. Drug therapy: spasticity. *N Eng J Med* 1981; 304:96.

70. Nance PW, Bugorest J, Shellenger K. Efficacy and safety of Tizanidine in the treatment of spasticity in patients with spinal cord injury. *Neurology* 1994; 44S:S44–52.

71. Hertz DA, Parsons KC, Pearl L. Percutaneous radio-frequency foramenal rhizotomies. *Spine* 1983; 6:729.

72. Pierson SH, Katz DI, Tarsy D. Botulinum toxin A in the treatment of spasticity: functional implications and patient selection. *Arch Phys Med Rehabil* 1996: 77:717–21.

73. Penn RD, Krois JS. Continuous intrathecal baclofen for severe spasticity. *Lancet* 1985; 2:125.

74. Penn RD, Krois JS. Long-term intrathecal baclofen infusion for treatment of spasticity. *J Neurosurg* 1987; 66:181.

75. Bedbrook GM, Sedgley GY. The management of spinal injuries, past and present. *Int Rehabil Med* 1980; 2:45.

76. Borkin M, Dolfin D, Herschorn S, et al. The urologic care of the spinal cord injury patient. *J Urol* 1983; 129:335.

77. Guttman L, Frankel H. The value of intermittent catheterization in the early management of traumatic paraplegia and tetraplegia. *Paraplegia* 1966; 4:63.

78. Kuhlmeir KV, Lloyd LK, Stover DL. Long-term follow-up of renal function after spinal cord injury. *J Urol* 1985; 134:510.

79. Maynard FM, Diokno AC. Urinary infection and complications during clean intermittent catheterization following spinal cord injury. *J Urol* 1984; 132:943.

80. Maynard FM, Glass T. Management of the neuropathic bladder by clean intermittent catheterization: 5-year outcomes. *Paraplegia* 1987; 25:106.

81. McGuire E, Savastano JA. Long-term follow-up spinal cord injury patients managed by intermittent catheterization. *J Urol* 1983; 129:775.

82. Wu YC. Total bladder care for the spinal cord injured patient. *Ann Acad Med Singapore* 1983; 12:387.

83. Golji H: Urethral sphincterotomy for chronic spinal cord injury. *J Urol* 1986; 123:204.

84. Jameson RM. The long-term results of transurethral division of the external urethral sphincter in the neuropathic urethra with reference to potency. *Paraplegia* 1982; 20:299.

85. Morrow JW, Bogaard TP. Bladder rehabilitation in patients with old spinal cord injuries with bladder neck incision and external sphincterotomy. *J Urol* 1977; 117:164.

86. Schellhamer PF, Hackler RH, Bunts RC. External sphinctorotomy: rationale for the procedure and experiences with 150 patients. *Paraplegia* 1979; 1A: 5.

87. Newman E, Price M. External catheters: hazards and benefits of their use by men with spinal cord lesions. *Arch Phys Med Rehabil* 1985; 66:310.

88. Grundy DJ, Fellows GJ, Gillett AP, et al. A comparison of fine-bore suprapubic and intermittent urethral catheterization regime after spinal cord injury. *Paraplegia* 1987; 21:227.

89. Hackler RH. When is an ileal conduit indicated in the spinal cord injured patient? *Paraplegia* 1987; 16:257.

90. Calenoff L, Neiman HL, Kaplan PE, et al. Ultrasonography in spinal cord injury patients. *J Urol* 1982; 128:1234.

91. Rao KG, Hackler RH, Woodlief RM, et al. Real-time renal sonography in spinal cord injury patients: prospective comparison with excretory urography. *J Urol* 1986; 135:72.

92. Awad SA. Clinical use of Bethanecol. *J Urol* 1981; 133:523.

93. Stiens SA, Biener Bergman S, Goetz LL. Neurogenic bowel dysfunction after spinal cord injury: clinical evaluation and rehabilitative management (Focused review). *Arch Phys Med Rehabil* 1997; 78:S86–102.

94. Zacharkow D. *Wheelchair Posture and Pressure Sores.* Springfield, Illinois: Charles C. Thomas, 1984.

95. Bors E, Commorr AE. Neurological disturbances of sexual function with special reference to 529 patients with spinal cord injury. *Urol Survey* 1960; 10:191.

96. Sha'ked A. *Human Sexuality and Rehabilitation Medicine: Sexual Functioning Following Spinal Cord Injury.* Baltimore: Williams and Wilkins, 1981.

97. Trieschmann RB. *Spinal Cord Injuries, Psychological, Social and Vocational Adjustment.* New York: Pergamon Press, 1980.

98. Nadig PW, Ware JC, Blomoft R. Noninvasive device to produce and maintain an erection-like state. *Urology* 1985; 27:126.

99. Witherington R. External aids for treatment for impotence. *J Urol Nurs* 1987; 6:1.

100. Am Sidi A, Cameron JS, Duffy LM, Lange PH. Intracavernous drug-induced erections in the management of male erectile dysfunction: experience with 100 patients. *J Urol* 1986; 135:704.

101. Brindley GSL. Pilot experiments on the actions of drugs injected into the human corpus cavernosum penis. *Br J Phamacol* 1986; 87:495.

102. Monga M, Bernie J, Rajasekaran M. Male infertility and erectile dysfunction in spinal cord Injury: a review. *Arch Phys Med Rehabil* 1999; 80:1331–1339.

103. Wyndaele JT. DeMeyur JM, deSy WA, Closens H. Intracavernous injections of vasoactive drugs for treating impotence in spinal cord injury patients. *Paraplegia* 1986; 24:271.

104. Golji H. Experience with penile prosthesis in spinal cord injury patients. *J Urol* 1979; 121:288.

105. Iwatsubo L, Tanaka M, Takahoshi K, Akasto T. Non-inflatable penile prosthesis for the management of urinary incontinence and sexual disability of patients with spinal cord injury. *Paraplegia* 1986; 24:307.

106. Light JK, Scott FB. Management of neurogenic impotence with inflatable penile prosthesis. *Urology* 1981; 26:341.

107. Brindley GS. The fertility of men with spinal injuries. *Paraplegia* 1984; 22:337.

108. Otani T, Kondo A, Takita T. A paraplegic fathering a child after an intrathecal injection of neostigmine: case report. *Paraplegia* 1985; 23:32.

109. Brindley GS. Reflex ejaculation under vibratory stimulation in paraplegic men. *Paraplegia* 1981; 10:299.

110. Sakarati M, Rossier AB, Fam BA. Experience in vibratory and electroejaculation techniques in spinal cord injury patients: a preliminary report. *J Urol* 1987; 138:59.

111. Brindley GS. Electroejaculation: its technique, neurological implications and uses. *J Neurol Neurosurg Psychiatry* 1981; 44:9.

112. Halsted LS, VerVoort S, Seager SWJ. Rectal probe electrostimulation in the treatment of nonejaculatory spinal cord injured man. *Paraplegia* 1987; 25:120.

113. Martin DE, Warner H. Crenshaw T, et al. Initiation of erection and semen release by rectal probe electrostimulation (RPE). *J Urol* 1983; 129:637.

114. Haas A, Pineda H, Haas F, Axen K. *Pulmonary Therapy and Rehabilitation Principles and Practice.* Baltimore: Williams and Wilkins, 1979. Pp. 92, 133.

115. Bracket TO, Condon N, Kindelan KM, et al. The emotional care of a person with a spinal cord injury. J 116. Tucker SJ: The psychological of spinal cord injury: patient-staff interaction. *Rehabil Lit* 1980; 41:114, 160.

26 Omental Transposition to the Spinal Cord

HARRY S. GOLDSMITH, MD

THE SERIOUSNESS OF A SPINAL CORD INJURY has been known since the time of Hippocrates. He reported that a spinal cord injury (SCI) was a disaster with no medical treatment being available and, as now, little possibility of a favorable result following such an injury.

In spite of some improvement in the post-traumatic care of spinal cord injured patients, there have been no major therapeutic break-throughs in the field. However, placement of a pedicled omental graft on an injured spinal cord has been shown experimentally and clinically to offer some hope that the procedure can benefit patients who have injured their spinal cord (1).

PATHOPHYSIOLOGY OF SPINAL CORD INJURY (SCI)

Following a SCI, two major factors come into play regarding the potential return of function of the spinal cord: the force of the impact delivered to the cord and the pathologic cascade that subsequently occurs in the cord at the area of impact. Obviously, there is no way to have an effect on the amount of force presented to the cord at the time of injury, but the pathologic activities that occur within the cord following trauma may, in the future, be altered to allow the therapeutic window of opportunity that has been sought for so many years.

One of the most important factors responsible for the irreversible damage that can occur after SCI results from the formation of vasogenic edema that develops at the site of injury. The production of this edema fluid is very rapid, with the cord trying to compensate for this localized fluid collection by dynamic movement of the fluid up and down the cord (2). However, this action is inadequate to decrease the high tissue pressure that develops at the point of a severe SCI. The swelling of the cord from the edema fluid occurs within the confines of the non-yielding dura mater covering and the rigid vertebral canal (Fig. 26-1). This situation in which there is a rising tissue pressure in the spinal cord, which is surrounded by the firm dural covering, leads to a progressive loss of capillary perfusion pressure within the small blood vessels located in and adjacent to the site of SCI. The inverse ratio of a high tissue pressure and a low capillary perfusion pressure that can fall to zero results in ischemia and eventual destruction in the area of cord impaction.

Because a lowering of the elevated tissue pressure following SCI was considered important, various surgical attempts were carried out in the past to try to accomplish this. Myelotomy and decompressive laminectomy were operations performed for this purpose, but the unpredictability of the results of these procedures

381

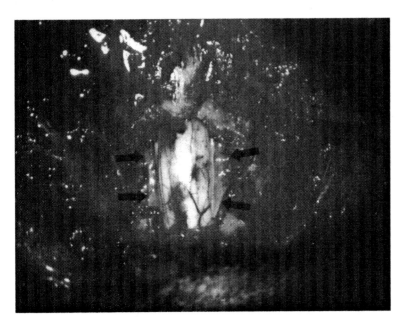

FIGURE 26-1 Photograph of injured spinal cord in a cat 5 hours following standard (450 gm/cm) injury. Black arrows show edges of incised dura lying at sides of edematous cord. The restrictive nature of the intact dura on spinal cord capillaries is readily apparent.

failed to justify their continued performance. A likely cause of these failures was that neither operation addressed the problem of the absorption of vasogenic edema that follows SCI.

The spinal cord lacks the ability to absorb edema fluid because it has no lymphatic system. Experimental work from our laboratory demonstrated that if the edema fluid at the site of cord injury is not absorbed, the fluid itself leads to fibrosis, which has a subsequent constricting effect on underlying spinal cord capillaries (3). This con-

stricting effect caused by the fibrosis results in a progressive ischemic state that hinders the possible healing process of still-viable nervous tissue present at the site of the SCI. With this physiologic scenario, it is important to absorb edema fluid after SCI because fibrinogen, which is a component of the edema fluid, can be converted to fibrin and scar formation. Since a major function of the omentum is its ability to absorb fluid (4), such absorption should theoretically prove critical if there is to be a beneficial effect following a SCI.

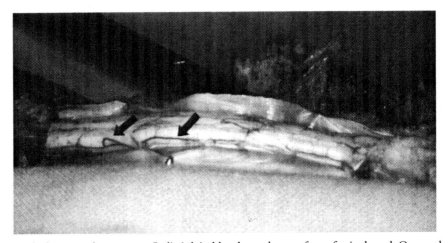

FIGURE 26-2 Black arrows demonstrate India ink in blood vessel on surface of spinal cord. Omental-spinal cord specimen was removed intact and the dye marker injected invitro into an omental artery.

OMENTAL TRANSPOSITION TO SPINAL CORD—EXPERIMENTAL

Placing the omentum directly on the spinal cord results in the development of vascular connections that penetrate through the omental–spinal cord interface (5). These blood vessels were confirmed by injecting a dye marker (India ink) into an omental artery supplying the intact omental pedicle to the spinal cord with the subsequent appearance of the dye in blood vessels present on the surface (Fig. 26-2) and in those deeply positioned within the spinal cord (Fig. 26-3A, B).

It was also shown that when the omentum was placed on the site of a complete spinal cord transection, blood vessels grew through the cut ends of the spinal cord stumps in a longitudinal fashion (Fig. 26-4). This is believed to be important, because if axons were eventually found to connect between the divided proximal and distal spinal cord segments, they would be expected to grow longitudinally.

Of major importance was the finding in early experiments in our laboratory that blood vessels developed from the omentum into the spinal cord by 72 hours; there was presumptive evidence that this event occurred even more rapidly (5). The speed in which omental blood vessels grew into the spinal cord was subsequently confirmed (6). These observations showing the rapidity of blood vessel growth from the omentum into the spinal cord were made on normal spinal cords, but the revascularization process was even more rapid when the omentum was placed on a traumatized cord (7) (Fig. 26-5).

OMENTAL ABSORPTION

As mentioned, a major function of the omentum is its ability to absorb edema fluid (8). A simple experiment to demonstrate this effectiveness is to place an intact pedicled omentum in a beaker filled with saline and India ink. Within minutes the dye can be seen in omental lymphatics (Fig. 26-6). It has been shown that the omentum can absorb one third of the entire cerebrospinal fluid reservoir, a function that in the future might be effective in treating hydrocephalus (6).

The importance of fluid absorption can be seen in a traumatized spinal cord where swelling begins to develop almost immediately after injury. If one studies spinal cords weeks later in the SCI animal, fibrosis is seen at the site of cord trauma (9) (Fig. 26-7). However, when the pedicled omentum is laid on the cord immediately after trauma, little or no fibrosis develops (3) (Fig. 26-8). It was theorized that the lack of

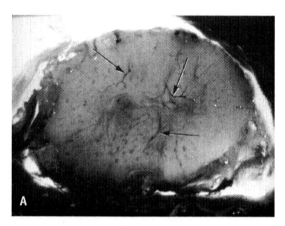

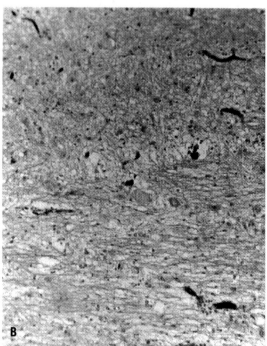

FIGURE 26-3 **A.** Macroscopic evidence of India ink within spinal cord. **B.** Microscopic evidence of India ink in deep-seated capillaries within the spinal cord.

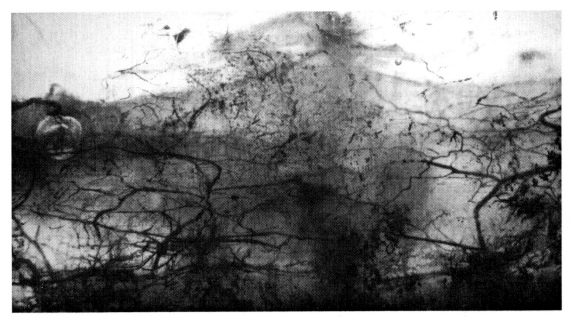

FIGURE 26-4 Corrosion cast model using methyl salicylate shows blood vessels growing longitudinally through a spinal cord transection site.

fibrosis resulted from the omentum's ability to absorb vasogenic edema following SCI. This lack of scarring at the site of injury is believed to be the result of a dynamic equilibrium that develops between the production of vasogenic edema from within the injured spinal cord and the absorption of this fluid by the omentum. Decreasing the volume of vasogenic edema in the area is theorized to decrease fibrinogen levels in this plasma-derived fluid; fibrinogen being the agent that leads to fibrin formation by the activation of blood in the area of injury (10).

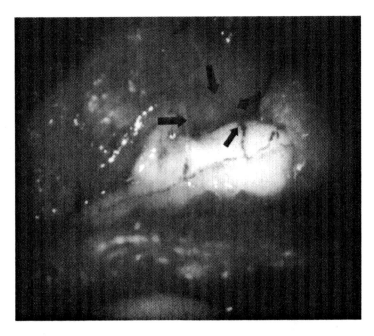

FIGURE 26-5 Autopsy of a cat, 52 hours after standard SCI that was treated by omental transposition. Arrows show rapid revascularization by blood vessels from omentum to markedly edematous spinal cord.

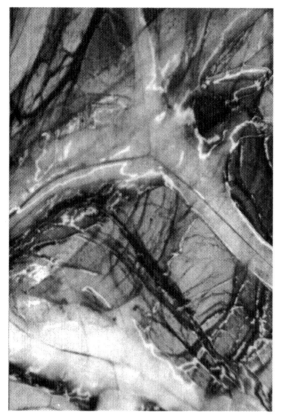

FIGURE 26-6 India ink seen in 30 seconds within omental lymphatics.

Another possible explanation of impeded scar development that occurs when the omentum is placed on the spinal cord at an injury site is that there might be an antifibrotic agent originating in the omentum. This possibility is raised given the large variety of biologic substances that are present in omental tissue (11–13).

Although the absorption of vasogenic edema fluid by the omentum is believed important in decreasing the formation of subsequent scar tissue following SCI, of equal importance might be the simple placement of the omentum on an acutely injured spinal cord. The reason for this is that the necessary laminectomy and opening of the dura, allows the cord to expand, which decreases the high tissue pressure caused by the edema fluid within the cord, thus increasing capillary perfusion pressure at the site of injury. This hypothesis strongly suggests that the earlier the omentum can be placed on a SCI site, the greater the potential for posttraumatic recovery as measured by improved motor and neuroelectrical activity.

EXPERIMENTAL STUDIES

To test the above hypothesis, a series of experiments (3) were performed in cats who were subjected to a standard 450 gm/cm injury to their spinal cord using the weight dropping technique described by Allen (14). Motor and neuroelectrical

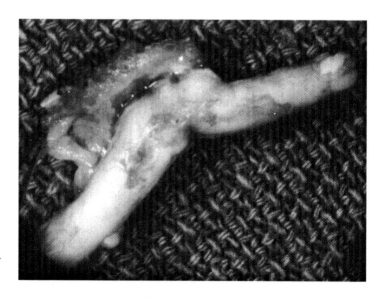

FIGURE 26-7 Severe surface and circumferential fibrosis 1 month after injury. Note the persistence of fluid accumulation.

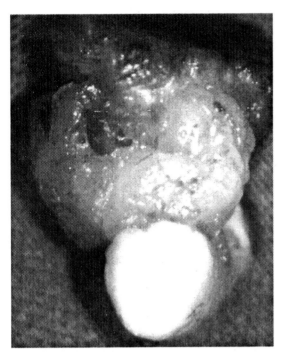

FIGURE 26-8 Note the absence of fibrosis or edema at the omental-spinal cord interface 3 weeks after injury in cat.

studies were done on all control and experimental cats 30 days after injury, at which time they were euthanized to evaluate by histologic examination the status of their spinal cords.

Control Cats

There were 11 cats who had their spinal cord injured in a standard fashion. Three hours after injury, the dura overlying the site of injury was excised. Nine of these animals had persistent paralysis of their hind limbs. Of the two remaining cats in this group, one regained the ability to walk, and the other animal could push up on its hind legs. Positive somatosensory evoked potentials (SEP) returned in five of the 20 hind limbs in this group (25 percent). One animal died during the study.

Early Omental Application

There were 11 cats in this group. Five of these animals had their omentum placed on the site of

their SCI exactly 3 hours after injury. These animals all showed varying degrees of walking ability at the time of their death (30 days posttrauma). Two additional cats never were able to walk, but they could push up into a standing position. The remaining four cats in this group remained permanently paralyzed. SEPs were taken in the hind limbs of these animals; 18 of the 22 limbs demonstrated positive SEPs.

Late Omental Application (14 Cats)

The animals in this experiment had their omentum placed on the site of their standard SCI 6 to 8 hours after injury. The hind limbs of all animals in this group remained paralyzed at the time of their deaths. A positive SEP was recorded in only one hind limb of one cat in this group (1 of 28, or 4 percent).

The above experiments strongly suggests that placing the omentum on a recently injured spinal cord as early as possible after injury could lead to improved motor and neuroelectrical activity. This was evident by the statistically significant differences noted between the control and experimental groups; using the Mann-Whitney test, P values ranged from 0.005 to 0.05.

Although the early placement of the omentum on a SCI can be easily accomplished in the laboratory, a limited time restriction imposes great difficulty in trying to carry out a comparable clinical experiment in humans. To learn if it might be possible to extend the window of opportunity for the successful placement of omentum on an injured spinal cord, a series of experiments were performed on cats using a variety of pharmaceutical agents. Following a standard injury, the omentum was laid on the spinal cord 6 to 8 hours later. The agents given intravenously included methyl prednisolone, dexamethasone, and banamine. None of these agents showed any beneficial effects. However, when dimethyl sulfuxide (DMSO) was used in conjunction with omental placement on the cord 6 to 8 hours after injury, a statistically significant improvement was noted in comparison with control animals in preventing paralysis (P < 0.02) and in the differences between the return of positive SEPs (P < 0.04) (3).

In studying the beneficial effects of DMSO, it should be noted that the drug was administered intravenously in a 40 percent solution as a single bolus 1 hour after injury with the omentum being applied to the spinal cord 6 to 8 hours following trauma. One might wonder: If DMSO was administered at varying time periods over several days following injury or given continuously for an extended period, would this allow for a longer time period prior to omental placement on an injured spinal cord with an expectation of improved neurologic function? The answer to this question awaits future research evaluation of DMSO in conjunction with omental transposition for SCI.

Axonal Regeneration

Over a period of many years, work in our laboratory has attempted to prove that a totally transected spinal cord in animals has the capacity to have axons regenerate through a spinal cord transection site with the subsequent development of coordinated walking (15). This has been accomplished, but it did not occur before several experimental techniques were attempted.

The first experiment aimed at axonal regeneration following total spinal cord transection required three separate operative steps (16). The first step involved the excision of a 5-mm piece of ice-hardened spinal cord using an ultra-sharp stainless steel blade. To prevent the possibility that neurologic improvement could occur as a result of axonal growth from dorsal root ganglia into the healing spinal cord, spinal nerves were divided outside the dorsal sheath but flush with the cord so that ganglia were widely separated from the spinal cord.

So that the stumps of the divided spinal cord be placed in apposition without tension, a lumbar vertebrectomy was performed. The vertebrae above and below the previously performed vertebrectomy were then solidly fixed by placement of stainless steel plates and screws.

At this point the abdominal cavity was entered, and a long intact pedicle graft of the omentum was made. The pedicle was then placed in a subcutaneous tunnel developed around the flank of the animal and brought to the level of the divided ends of the transected spinal cord. The divided spinal cord stumps were then apposed without tension because of the previous vertebrectomy.

The proximal and distal spinal cord ends were then fused together by laser-welding the outer edges of spinal cord transected stumps using a carbon dioxide laser at 1 to 2 watts of energy. The laser beam was carefully directed under microscopic control at the transection site.

The last step in this particular experiment was to totally envelop the spinal cord transection site by omentum, which was used to absorb postoperative edema accumulation at the transection site and to revascularize the location (Fig. 26-9).

Of interest in this experiment was the return of positive SEPs, which occurred within 2 months in seven of the 15 animals who were long-term survivors of the operation. Their spinal cords were carefully studied at autopsy and clearly demonstrated the presence of axons at the spinal cord transection site (Fig. 26-10). No positive SEPs occurred in control animals, and there were no axons noted at their transection sites.

Even though this experiment showed that it was possible for a transected spinal cord to regain SEP activity and have axons regenerate through a spinal cord transection site, none of the animals demonstrated any return of motor function by the time of their sacrifice (45 days). Without any return of function in the animals described above, a new and simpler surgical technique was developed in a further attempt to show not only axonal regeneration, but also motor function—the ability to achieve coordinated walking. The new surgical technique involved placement of collagen between proximal and distal spinal cord stumps that would act as a biological bridge through which axons could grow (17,18).

A series of cats had their spinal cord and surrounding dura mater completely transected,

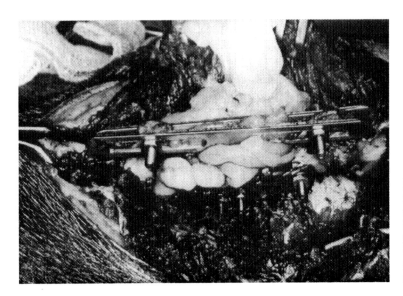

FIGURE 26-9 Completed operation. Short metal struts have been secured by screws through vertebral bodies. Large metal struts are placed through spinous processes. Omentum completely envelops the area of the laser-fused spinal cord.

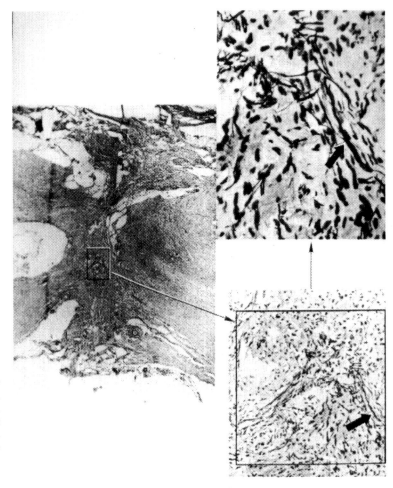

FIGURE 26-10 Left. Macrophoto showing spinal cord transection site and its reapproximation. Solid bridging of transection site is observed. Right. Black arrows in successive photo enlargements point to axons at transection site. Bodian silver stain X 250.

which resulted in a cord separation of approximately 5 to 6 mm because of the cord's elasticity. The spinal cord stumps were irrigated with a polyvinyl alcohol and chlorpromazine solution to reduce axoplasmic extrusion, which routinely follows spinal cord transection.

Animals were randomly placed in one of three groups (A, B, or C) to determine which surgical preparation increased spinal cord blood flow (SCBF) at the cord transection site. Group A had the transected spinal cord gap filled with collagen. Group B had the transected spinal cord gap filled with gelfoam. In Group C the transected spinal cord gap was filled with collagen, but in addition, the pedicled omentum was placed on top of the collagen bridge and on the proximal and distal spinal cord stumps. All animals in these three groups were killed 90 days after surgery.

Results of the above experiment were as follows: Group C (collagen and omentum) showed an increase of 65 and 83 percent, respectively, in blood flow to the spinal cord transection site when compared to Group A (collagen alone) and Group B (gelfoam) (Fig. 26-11). In addition, blood vessel density counts in Group C showed a 3-to-1 increase as compared with the number of blood vessels in Groups A and B. Of particular interest was the presence in Group C of immunoreactive catecholaminergic axons that grew through the collagen bridge and continued into the distal cord stump. These axons were found in abundance in Group C. It is believed that the blood supply from the omentum was the primary factor in the development of these axons. But there is also the possibility that the omentum supplied circulating proteins and neurotrophic factors that had a favorable effect on sprouting nerve fibers.

The experiments involving the use of the collagen-omentum preparation further showed that placing the pedicled omentum on the spinal cord transection site allowed the development of dopaminergic and noradrenergic fibers through the collagen bridge and into distal spinal cord tissue (19). These fibers grew distally through a smaller (3 mm) transection gap for a maximum distance of 90 mm during a 12-week recovery period (Fig. 26-12). In addition, it was also shown in these animals that the blood flow in the spinal cord tissue distal to the cord transection site was 58 percent greater when compared to control cats. Also noted was the return of SEPs when neuroelectrical stimulus was applied below the lesion site (17).

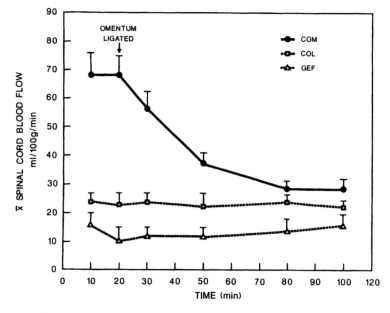

FIGURE 26-11 Group A (COL), Group B (CEF), Group C (COM). Mean averages of six serial blood flow measurements using a hydrogen clearance technique. Microelectrodes placed 6 mm distal to spinal cord 90 days after surgery. Analysis of variance comparing blood flow increases of Group C to Group A and Group B were P<0.0001 and P<0.001, respectively.

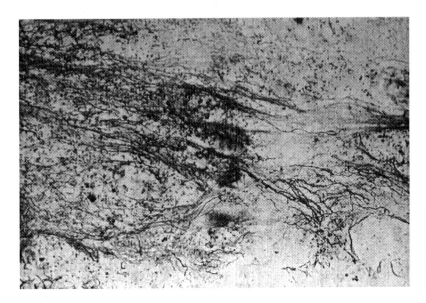

FIGURE 26-12 Axons exiting the distal end of the biodegrading collagen–omental bridge. These axons are growing into the distal spinal cord for an extended distance.

What was believed to be convincing evidence that the collagen–omentum preparation allowed for axonal transport across a spinal cord transection gap was shown using the retrograde axonal marker Fluoro-Gold. When this marker is injected into the distal spinal cord of a normal cat, it follows a retrograde axonal pathway to the brain and is seen mainly in the cytoplasm and processes of neurons located in the locus coeruleus, Kolliker-Fuse nucleus, and regions in the medulla. When Fluoro-Gold was injected below a spinal cord transection site, no marker was subsequently seen in the cat's brain. In contrast, when Fluoro-Gold was injected distal to a spinal cord transection site bridged by collagen and the omentum, an accumulation of this marker was found in the brain (Fig. 26-13) in locations where the Fluoro-Gold marker is normally located following its injection into an intact spinal cord.

A summary of the changes that were seen in animals who had their transected spinal cord bridged by collagen and omentum, but were not seen in control cats whose cord was not reconstructed, were as follows:

- An increase of spinal cord blood flow (SCBF) at the cord transection site. This SCBF increase was caused by supplemented blood flow coming from the omentum, which increased the SCBF by a mean of 58 percent compared to the SCBF of control cats.

- Placement of the omentum on a collagen bridge connecting transected spinal cord stumps prevented hind-limb muscle atrophy. Such atrophy was always apparent and extensive in control animals.

- Well-coordinated hind-forelimb locomotion occurred in collagen–omental treated cats when the lower body was supported (Fig. 26-14). This had occurred by the time the animals were sacrificed 3 months after surgery.

- Supraspinal fibers grew through the collagen–omental bridge and continued to grow into the distal spinal cord. The growth rate of the regenerating fibers was approximately 1 mm per day, roughly the same growth rate that occurs in peripheral axonal regeneration.

- The injection of the marker (synaptophysin), which is an indicator that synaptogenesis has occurred, showed the marker above and below a spinal cord transection site and was found adjacent to preganglionic sympathetic neurons, suggestive of synaptic connection to these targets.

- Fluoro-Gold particles were located in the brain following retrograde labeling. This confirmed that this labeled marker, when

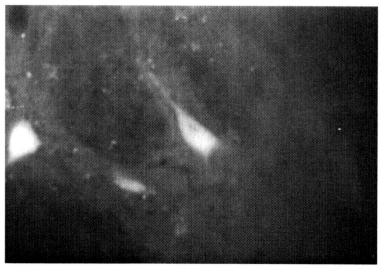

FIGURE 26-13 Typical Fluoro-Gold accumulation in Kollicker–Fuse nucleus. The marker was injected distal to the spinal cord transection site, which was bridged by omental–collagen reconstruction.

injected distal to the spinal cord transection, moved in a retrograde fashion through the collagen–omental bridge up to the brain.

CLINICAL FINDINGS

Over the past years, the omentum has been placed on the spinal cord of patients with a chronic SCI of long duration. There have been many reports that this procedure has resulted in postoperative improvement in some patients

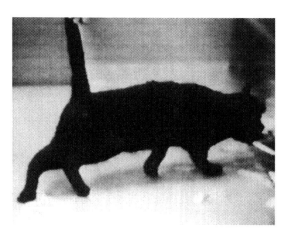

FIGURE 26-14 Picture taken from a video showing front and hind limb coordinated walking with tail support at 3 months after cord transection.

regarding various aspects of their motor, sensory, bladder, rectal, and thermoregulatory systems (20–24).

The technical steps in transposing the omentum to the spinal cord have been reported in detail in an earlier publication and are not repeated here (25). It should be stressed, however, that if one is to carry out omental transposition to a chronically injured spinal cord, the scar tissue over the cord and adjacent spinal nerves must be carefully excised under an operating microscope. I say this because I am aware of patients who have failed omental transposition onto their injured spinal cord because they did not have the scar tissue over the cord removed prior to omental placement. This is an extremely important part of the operation.

A logical question to ask is, why should placement of the omentum on a chronically injured cord result in neurologic improvement? If the operation were done on a patient with an acute spinal cord injury, improvement could be theorized to be caused mainly by the absorption of vasogenic edema by the omentum. But with chronic SCI, vasogenic edema is not a factor. The most likely cause for improvement in chronic spinal cord injuries is probably two-fold. The first of these is the removal of scar tissue on the spinal cord and spinal nerves in the area of injury. The scar tissue has a constricting effect on the underlying spinal cord that is readily seen as the cord becomes mobile after scar excision. Releasing the scar tissue decreases the compression it has exerted on capillaries, both on the surface and within the depths of the spinal cord. Removing this compressive effect on the capillaries would be expected to allow some increase in blood flow to the area of chronic injury.

The second reason why the omentum has been shown to be clinically effective in some patients with a chronically injured spinal cord could be caused by the large amount of blood flow that the omentum adds to the cord, along with neurobiologic agents that the omentum presents to any viable but poorly functioning neural elements in the area of SCI. Angiogenic (11,26) neurotransmitter (13,27) and nerve growth factors (12) are known to be present in omental tissue, and it is these substances that could be responsible for the favorable neurologic changes that have occurred in some patients following omental transposition to their spinal cord. It must be stressed, however, that intensive postoperative physiotherapy is very important if there is to be the possibility of a favorable outcome following the operation.

A clinical area that should be evaluated in the future is to learn whether very early placement of the omentum on an acutely injured spinal cord can lead to improved clinical results, results that have not improved over the years. Experimental data in animals have shown that the pedicled omentum can improve neuroelectrical and functional results after SCI and that the best time to apply the omentum surgically is as early after injury as practical. A patient with multiple trauma would not be a candidate for this, but a healthy patient with an isolated spinal cord injury might be suitable for the operation. This is a possibility that has been described in a recent article (28).

The experimental studies mentioned above have shown it is possible to bridge a major defect in the spinal cord using an omental–collagen bridge. This technique has now been applied clinically. The patient was a 24-year-old woman who had what was initially reported by MRI as a "total anatomical spinal cord transection" at the T6 level as a result of a high-speed skiing accident.

Three and a half years after her injury, surgery was performed. A massive formation of scar tissue was found at the injury site. After this had been removed, a large defect in the spinal cord was present, extending from T5 to T7 and measuring 1.6 inches in length. In this large defect remained 5 to 10 percent of still-intact cord. Into the extensive spinal cord defect was placed 4 to 5 cc of collagen (Fig. 26-15); the area was then cov-

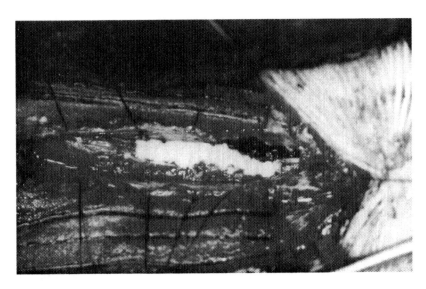

FIGURE 26-15 Operative photo showing collagen forming a bridge between extensive defect between proximal and distal spinal cord segments.

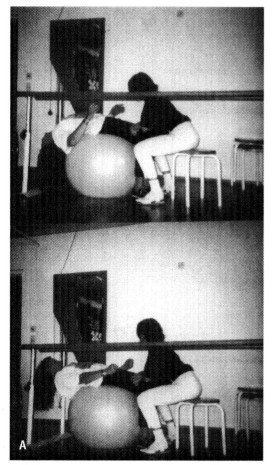 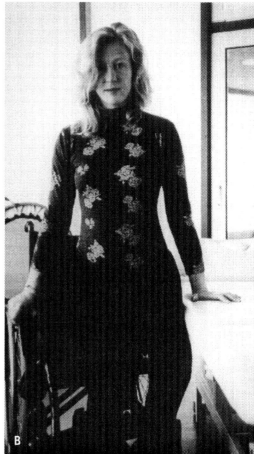

FIGURE 26-16   Photos (A and B) showing increased motor power below T6 level after reconstruction of near total spinal cord transection.

ered with omentum. The patient has achieved continuing and progressive improvement in motor function over the past several years (29) (Fig. 26-16A, B). The future role of the omentum in spinal cord regeneration and clinical application following SCI appears optimistic.

REFERENCES

1. Goldsmith HS. The 0mentum: present status and future applications. In Goldsmith HS, ed., *The Omentum: Research and Clinical Applications.* New York: Springer-Verlag, 1990. Pp. 131–145.
2. Nemecek ST, Peter R, Suba P, Rozsival V, Melka O. Longitudinal extension of edema in experimental spinal cord injury. *Acta Neurochir* 1977; 37:7–16.
3. Goldsmith HS, Steward E, Duckett S. Early application of pedicled omentum to the acutely traumatized spinal cord. *Paraplegia* 1985; 23:100–112.
4. Goldsmith HS, de los Santos R, Beattie EJ. The relief of chronic lymphedema by omental transposition. *Ann Surg* 1967; 166:573–585.
5. Goldsmith HS, Duckett S, Chen W. Spinal cord vascularization by intact omentum. *Am J Surg* 1975; 129:262–265.
6. Levander B, Zwetnow NW. Bulk flow of CSF through a lumbo-omental pedicled graft in the dog. *Acta Neurochir* 1978; 41:147–155.
7. Goldsmith HS, Steward E, Chen WF, Duckett S. Application of intact omentum to the normal and traumatized spinal cord. In Kao C, Bunge RP, Reier PJ, eds., *Spinal Cord Reconstruction.* New York: Raven Press, 1983. Pp. 235–244.
8. Goldsmith HS. Revascularization and edema absorption of the brain and spinal cord. In Liebermann-Meffert D, White H, eds., *The*

Greater Omentum. Berlin: Springer-Verlag, 1983. Pp. 189–197.

9. Goodkin R, Campbell JB. Sequential pathologic changes in spinal cord injury. *Surg Forum* 1969; 20:430–432.

10. Ryan GB, Grobety J, Majno G. Postoperative peritoneal adhesions. *Am J Path* 1971; 65:117–148.

11. Goldsmith HS, Griffith AL, Kupferman A, Catsimpoolas N. Lipid angiogenic factor from omentum. *JAMA* 1984; 252:2034–2036.

12. Seik GC, Marquis JK, Goldsmith HS. Experimental studies of omentum derived neurotrophic factors. In Goldsmith HS, ed., *The Omentum—Research and Clinical Applications*. Berlin: Springer-Verlag, 1990. Pp. 83–95.

13. Goldsmith HS, McIntosh T, Vezena RM, Colton T. Vasoactive neurochemicals identified in omentum. *Br J Neurosurg* 1987; 1:359–364.

14. Allen AR. Surgery of experimental lesions of spinal cord Equivalent to Crush Injury of Fracture—Dislocation of Spinal Cord. *JAMA* 1911; 57:878.

15. de la Torre JC, Goldsmith HS. Supraspinal outgrowth and apparent synaptic remodeling across transected-reconstructed feline spinal cord. *Acta Neurochir (Wein)* 1992 114:118–127.

16. Goldsmith HS. The omentum in spinal cord injury. In Lee, Ostrander, Cochran, Shaw, eds., *The Spinal Cord Injured Patient: Comprehensive Management*. Philadelphia: W.B. Saunders, 1991. Pp. 313–329.

17. Goldsmith HS, de la Torre JC. Axonal regeneration after spinal cord transection and reconstruction. Brain Research 1992; 589:217–224.

18. de la Torre JC, Goldsmith HS. Experimental reconstruction of transected spinal cord using a collagen–pedicle omentum graft. *Acta Neurochir* 1990; 102:152–163.

19. de la Torre JC, Goldsmith HS. Coerulospinal fiber regeneration in transected feline spinal cord. *Brain Res Bull* 1994; 35:413–417.

20. Goldsmith HS. Brain and spinal cord revascularization by omental transposition. *Neurological Research* 1994; 16:159–162.

21. Abraham J, Paterson A, Bothra M, et al. Omentomyelo-synangiosis in the management of chronic traumatic paraplegia. *Paraplegia* 1987; 25:44–49.

22. Nagashima C, Masumori Y, Hod E, et al. Omental transposition to the cervical cord with macroangio anastomosis. *No Shinkei Geka* 1991; 19:309–318.

23. Rafael H. Omental transposition in the management of chronic traumatic paraplegia. *Acta Neurochir* 1992; 114:145–146.

24. Goldsmith HS. The first international of omentum in CNS. *Surg Neurol* 1996; 45:87–90.

25. Goldsmith HS. Omental transposition to the brain and spinal cord. *Surg Rounds* 1986; 9:22–23.

26. Cartier R, Brunette I, Hashimoto K, et al. Angiogenic factor: a possible mechanism for neurovascularization produced by omental pedicles. *J Thorac Cardiovascular Surgery* 1990; 99:264–268.

27. Goldsmith HS, Marquis JK, Siek G. Choline acetyltransferase activity in omental tissue. *Br J Neurosurgery* 1987; 1:463–466.

28. Goldsmith HS. Acute spinal cord injuries: a search for functional improvement. *Surg Neurol* 1995; 51:231–233.

29. Goldsmith HS, Brandt M, Walz T. Near total transection of human spinal cord: functional return following omentum–collagen reconstruction. In Goldsmith, HS, ed., *The Omentum-Application to Brain and Spinal Cord*. Wilton, Connecticut: Forefront Publishing, 2000. Pp. 61–75.

Index

Note: Boldface numbers indicate illustrtions; italic *t* indicates a table.